P9-CAB-096

Elaine

Quick Check
FOOD
FACTS

Third Edition

Compiled by the Editorial Staff
of Barron's Educational Series, Inc.

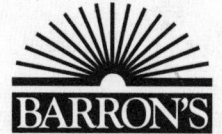

BARRON'S

Acknowledgments
The publisher gratefully acknowledges the participating national restaurant chains for allowing inclusion of nutritional data of selected menu items in this edition.

Nutritional data for Dunkin' Donuts® and Applebee's® current as of 2011.

McDonald's® trademarks and nutritional information used with permission from McDonald's Corporation.

Red Mango® trademarks and nutritional information are used with permission from Red Mango, Inc. Nutritional data current as of May 2011 and is subject to change.

Subway® trademarks and nutritional information used with permission from Subway.

TCBY® nutritional information is subject to change without notice. For the most up-to-date nutritional information, please visit TCBY.com.

Wendy's® nutrition information is based on standard product formulations. Variations may occur due to differences in suppliers, ingredient substitutions, recipe revisions, product assembly at the restaurant level, and/or season of the year. Nutrition calculations follow federal regulations regarding the rounding of nutritional data. This information is effective as of June 2011. For the most comprehensive and up-to-date information, or to calculate nutrition facts, visit *www.wendys.com.*

All inquiries should be addressed to:
Barron's Educational Series, Inc.
250 Wireless Boulevard
Hauppauge, New York, 11788
www.barronseduc.com

ISBN: 978-1-4380-0010-7

Library of Congress Control Number: 2011034299

Library of Congress Cataloging-in-Publication Data

Quick check food facts / compiled by the Editorial Staff. -- 3rd ed.
  p. cm.
 ISBN 978-1-4380-0010-7
 1. Food--Composition--Tables. 2. Nutrition--Tables. I. Barron's Educational Series, Inc.
  TX551.Q53 2012
  613.2'8--dc23

2011034299

Printed in the United States of America

9 8 7 6 5 4 3 2

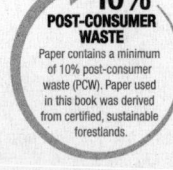

10%
POST-CONSUMER WASTE
Paper contains a minimum of 10% post-consumer waste (PCW). Paper used in this book was derived from certified, sustainable forestlands.

Contents

Preface

The information in this book (excluding the nutritional counts of selected menu items from national restaurant chains) is based on the *USDA National Nutrient Database for Standard Reference, Release 23*, published in computer-readable form by the U.S. Department of Agriculture. The original database is very large and unwieldy, and we have extracted just the most useful information for publication here.

For each food we list serving size, and then, per serving:

> **Total calories** *(kcal)*
> **Total fat** *(grams)*
> **Saturated fat** *(grams)*
> **Cholesterol** *(milligrams)*
> **Carbohydrates** *(grams)*
> **Fiber** *(grams)*
> **Sugar** *(grams)*
> **Protein** *(grams)*
> **Sodium** *(milligrams)*

In a very few cases, numbers were missing from the USDA database. They are left blank here.

About the Author

Linda McDonald, MS, RD, LD, owns SUPERMARKET SAVVY, an information and resource service focused on making healthy shopping easy. Her national newsletter, teaching tools, and website (*www.supermarketsavvy.com*) assist health professionals and consumers to shop healthy.

Mrs. McDonald is a graduate of the University of Houston with a Master of Science from the University of Texas Graduate School of Biomedical Sciences. She works with Dietetic Interns from the University of Houston, Texas Women's University, and University of Texas School of Public Health.

Introduction

Food is a fact of life! In fact, you can't live long without food. And the food decisions you make affect the health of you and your family. So, you want to make the best food choices. This book will help you with those decisions.

Healthy Eating Tips

1. Think Variety

There are over 40 essential nutrients that you can only get from the foods you eat. Since each food contains only a few of these nutrients in limited amounts, you can see why eating a variety of foods is important. Not only do you need to eat foods from each of the food categories—grains, vegetables, fruits, dairy, proteins—but within each food category, you should eat a variety of foods. For instance, eating a rainbow of colors of fruits and vegetables will provide a variety of different nutrients—vitamins A, C, and other antioxidants.

2. Slash Sodium

The U.S. Dietary Guidelines for Americans and the American Heart Association recommend limiting sodium to less than 2,300 mg a day (the amount in 1 teaspoon of salt) for healthy adults and 1,500 mg per day for those who are salt sensitive—individuals who have high blood pressure, are 40 years of age or older, or who are African-Americans. More than two-thirds of the adult population falls into one or more of these categories.

3. Choose Healthy Fats

Research has shown that it is the type of fat, not the amount, that has the biggest effect on your health. Fats are essential because they deliver essential fatty acids that your body can't manufacture, such as omega-3 fats. Also, certain vitamins are fat-soluble (vitamins A, D, E, and K), meaning they need fat to be digested and metabolized. However, fats are high in calories and should be enjoyed in moderation. The good fats are those that are poly- or monounsaturated. The unhealthy fats include saturated and trans fats.

4. Practice Portion Control

It is not just what you eat but how much you eat that determines a healthy diet. Most people eat more than they need. Start by paying attention to the serving sizes recommended by the Choose MyPlate program and those given in the Nutrition Facts Boxes on food labels. You may also want to measure foods and beverages with a scale, measuring cups, or spoon. Use the MyPlate recommendation to make half your plate fruits and vegetables, a quarter of your plate grains, and the final quarter protein. Use the suggested portion sizes given in this book to help you with portion control.

5. Go for Whole Grains

The U.S. Dietary Guidelines recommend that you make half your grains whole. Research has shown that eating 2½ servings of grains per day is enough to lower your risk of heart disease. And it appears that a greater whole grain intake is associated with reduced obesity, diabetes, high blood pressure, and high cholesterol. All grains contains three components—the germ, endosperm and bran but during processing one or more of these components are lost. The bran is full of fiber, while the germ and endosperm contain valuable phytonutrients. Eat the whole grain for the best nutrition.

6. Cut Added Sugar

We are drowning in sugar! The U.S.D.A. recommends we get no more than 10 teaspoons a day, while the average American downs about 34 teaspoons. In fact, the amount of sugar we eat and drink every year has soared nearly 30 percent since 1983 and is a major contributor to the soaring rates of overweight and obesity. Sugar often hides under several names and turns up in the most innocuous foods like bread, crackers, salad dressing, ketchup, and mustard. Check the ingredients list for added sugars.

7. Go Fish

Seafood contains a variety of nutrients, notably the omega-3 fatty acids, EPA, and DHA. The U.S. Dietary Guidelines recommend eating about 8 ounces per week. Eating seafood contributes to the prevention of heart disease. Seafood varieties that are commonly consumed that are higher in EPA and DHA and lower in mercury include salmon, anchovies, herring, sardines, Pacific oysters, trout, and Atlantic and Pacific mackerel.

8. Use MyPlate

The U.S. Dietary Guidelines form the basis for the federal government's nutrition education program, Choose-MyPlate. This program uses a portioned plate logo to divide food choices into five food groups. This logo shows that half your plate should be fruits and vegetables, one quarter grain, and the last quarter protein with a glass of milk. The ChooseMyPlate program provides recommended food plans, food lists, serving sizes, health benefits, nutrients, and tips for making wise choices. Find MyPlate diet recommendations, serving sizes, and tips throughout this book.

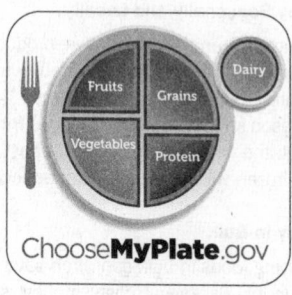

Healthy Shopping Tips

1. Shop with a List

Planning ahead is important for saving money and eating healthy. Plan meals for a week at a time and keep a running grocery list in a central location where family members can add items as they are needed. Organize your list in categories based on the way you travel through the supermarket.

2. Comparison Shop

Compare the prices of similar items. Most shelf tags have a total price and a price per unit that provides an easy way to compare apples to apples. Should you buy apples in a 3-pound bag for $4.99 or individual apples that are $0.99 each? Scan supermarket ads, circulars, and the Internet for specials and coupons. Use coupons only for foods that are on your list.

3. Start on the Perimeter

Most fresh foods are on the perimeter of the supermarket—fresh fruits and vegetables; meats, poultry, and fish; dairy products; and the bakery. This is where you can be assured of natural nutrients without many preservatives or artificial ingredients. Some fresh items are in the interior—grains, rice, flours, and nuts. Make the majority of your purchases from the perimeter before shopping the aisles.

4. Buy Seasonally and Locally

Seasonal and locally grown products are usually cheaper and healthier. They maintain more nutrients because they have not travelled as far from picking to store. They are cheaper because there are more available. Stay attuned to the season so that you can purchase fruits and vegetables that are the most economical, the freshest, and the cheapest. When produce is not in season, buy canned or frozen without sauces and added salt.

5. Buy in Bulk

Buying foods in bulk can often save you money, but only if you can use the larger amount. Packaging costs money, so the less package the more you save. For instance, steel-cut oats in bulk are $0.89 a pound, while a tin runs $3.35 a pound. Other items you can save on by buying in bulk are grains, lentils, dried beans, and rice. Check out the unit price to see how much you save by buying the larger size.

6. Read Nutrition Facts Labels and Ingredients Lists

The front of a package may make claims like "Healthy," "Natural," and "Contains" but the back or side of the package will give you the real scoop. Check out the Nutrition Facts Box that gives you the amount of individual nutrients. Compare these nutrients between products to see which is better. Read the ingredients list to check for partially hydrogenated fats, which mean "trans fats" and added sugars.

7. Understand Health and Nutrition Claims

You'll find a variety of health and nutrition claims on labels. These can be a help to those who need to find foods that are heart healthy or low in sodium, but be sure to check the Nutrition Facts numbers to make sure the food fits into your food plan.

8. Store Brands vs. National Brands

It used to be that store brands were cheaper and lower quality versions of national brands. Now store brands are quality lines of products that can save you money. Statistics say that store brands can save 30% over nationally branded products. In some supermarkets, store brands account for as much as 35% of total sales. Check out the store brands and compare them to their national counterparts.

What Does "Healthy" Mean?

Food labeling allows manufacturers to make a "healthy" claim on a food or beverage label if it meets specific nutrient criteria. The basic requirements are:

- Low in fat: 3 g or less or 30% or less fat calories
- Low in sodium: 140 mg or less except for meal-type products (6 oz or more) that require 360 mg for individual foods and 480 mg for meal-type foods
- 10% or more of at least one of the following:
  - Vitamin A
  - Vitamin C
  - Iron
  - Calcium
  - Protein
  - Fiber

How to Use This Book

This book can help you plan your menus and make a shopping list.

- Read the MyPlate recommendations for each food category for number of servings and serving sizes. The servings given are for an adult consuming 2000 calories per day. For a personalized food plan based on your age, sex, weight, and activity level, go to www.choosemyplate.gov.
- Make your shopping list by multiplying the number of people in your family by the recommended number of servings.
- Check the list of foods in each category provided in this book and choose a variety of items.
- Compare nutrients within categories for the best food choices for positive nutrients such as protein, fiber, calcium, vitamins, and minerals. Also check nutrients for foods with negative nutrients such as total fat, saturated fat, cholesterol, and sodium.
- Read the Shopping Tips and Shopping List Essentials for each category and include these suggestions into your meal planning and shopping list.
- Highlight the foods that are presently in your food plan and use a different color highlighter for the foods you want to try. Make a goal to try a new food each week. Remember that variety is important for healthy eating.
- Take this book to the supermarket for a quick check on the nutrients in foods that may not have nutrition facts—fruits, vegetables, bulk items, meat, poultry, and fish.

Using Nutrition Facts

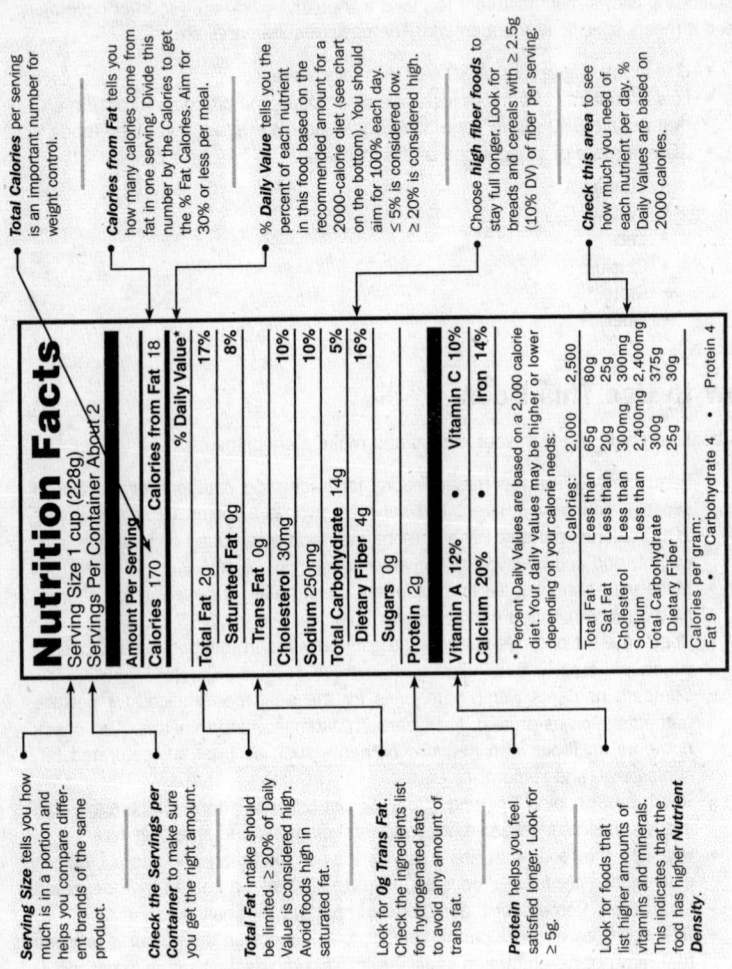

Serving Size tells you how much is in a portion and helps you compare different brands of the same product.

Check the Servings per Container to make sure you get the right amount.

Total Fat intake should be limited. ≥ 20% of Daily Value is considered high. Avoid foods high in saturated fat.

Look for **0g Trans Fat**. Check the ingredients list for hydrogenated fats to avoid any amount of trans fat.

Protein helps you feel satisfied longer. Look for ≥ 5g.

Look for foods that list higher amounts of vitamins and minerals. This indicates that the food has higher **Nutrient Density**.

Total Calories per serving is an important number for weight control.

Calories from Fat tells you how many calories come from fat in one serving. Divide this number by the Calories to get the % Fat Calories. Aim for 30% or less per meal.

% **Daily Value** tells you the percent of each nutrient in this food based on the recommended amount for a 2000-calorie diet (see chart on the bottom). You should aim for 100% each day. ≤ 5% is considered low. ≥ 20% is considered high.

Choose **high fiber foods** to stay full longer. Look for breads and cereals with ≥ 2.5g (10% DV) of fiber per serving.

Check this area to see how much you need of each nutrient per day. % Daily Values are based on 2000 calories.

Nutrition Facts

Serving Size 1 cup (228g)
Servings Per Container About 2

Amount Per Serving

Calories 170	Calories from Fat 18
	% Daily Value*
Total Fat 2g	17%
Saturated Fat 0g	8%
Trans Fat 0g	
Cholesterol 30mg	10%
Sodium 250mg	10%
Total Carbohydrate 14g	5%
Dietary Fiber 4g	16%
Sugars 0g	
Protein 2g	

Vitamin A 12%	•	Vitamin C	10%
Calcium 20%	•	Iron	14%

*Percent Daily Values are based on a 2,000 calorie diet. Your daily values may be higher or lower depending on your calorie needs:

	Calories:	2,000	2,500
Total Fat	Less than	65g	80g
Sat Fat	Less than	20g	25g
Cholesterol	Less than	300mg	300mg
Sodium	Less than	2,400mg	2,400mg
Total Carbohydrate		300g	375g
Dietary Fiber		25g	30g

Calories per gram:
Fat 9 • Carbohydrate 4 • Protein 4

MyPlate Key Messages

Take action on the Dietary Guidelines by making changes in these three areas. Choose steps that work for you and start today.

Balancing Calories

- Enjoy your food, but eat less.
- Avoid oversized portions.

Foods to Increase

- Make half your plate fruits and vegetables.
- Switch to fat-free or low-fat (1%) milk.
- Make at least half your grains whole grains.

Foods to Reduce

- Compare sodium in foods like soup, bread, and frozen meals—and choose foods with lower numbers.
- Drink water instead of sugary drinks.

Go to ChooseMyPlate.gov for a personalized food plan based on your age, sex, weight, and activity level. Find food lists and specific serving size photos.

Ideal Weight Chart

Height	Ideal Male Weight	Ideal Female Weight
4'6"	63–77 lbs.	63–77 lbs.
4'7"	68–84 lbs.	68–83 lbs.
4'8"	74–90 lbs.	72–88 lbs.
4'9"	79–97 lbs.	77–94 lbs.
4'10"	85–103 lbs.	81–99 lbs.
4'11"	90–110 lbs.	86–105 lbs.
5'0"	95–117 lbs.	90–110 lbs.
5'1"	101-123 lbs.	95–116 lbs.
5'2"	106–130 lbs.	99–121 lbs.
5'3"	112–136 lbs.	104–127 lbs.
5'4"	117–143 lbs.	108–132 lbs.
5'5"	122–150 lbs.	113–138 lbs.
5'6"	128–156 lbs.	117–143 lbs.
5'7"	133–163 lbs.	122–149 lbs.
5' 8"	139–169 lbs.	126–154 lbs.
5' 9"	144–176 lbs.	131–160 lbs.
5'10"	149–183 lbs.	135–165 lbs.
5'11"	155–189 lbs.	140-171 lbs.
6'0"	160–196 lbs.	144–176 lbs.
6'1"	166–202 lbs.	149–182 lbs.
6'2"	171–209 lbs.	153–187 lbs.
6'3"	176–216 lbs.	158–193 lbs.
6'4"	182–222 lbs.	162–198 lbs.
6'5"	187–229 lbs.	167–204 lbs.
6'6"	193–235 lbs.	171–209 lbs.
6'7"	198–242 lbs.	176–215 lbs.
6'8"	203–249 lbs.	180–220 lbs.
6'9"	209–255 lbs.	185–226 lbs.
6'10"	214–262 lbs.	189–231 lbs.
6'11"	220–268 lbs.	194–237 lbs.
7'0"	225–275 lbs.	198–242 lbs.

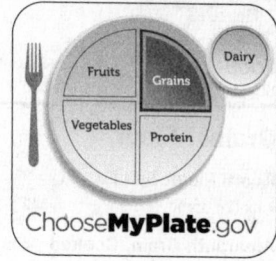

Grains

Why Eat Grains?

Grains are important sources of many nutrients, including dietary fiber, several B vitamins (thiamin, riboflavin, niacin, and folate), and minerals (iron, magnesium, and selenium). Eating whole grains as part of a healthy diet may reduce the risk of heart disease and help with weight management. Additionally, consuming foods containing fiber, such as whole grains, may reduce constipation and diverticulitis. B vitamins play a role in metabolism and are essential for a healthy nervous system. Folate (folic acid), a B vitamin, is important before and during pregnancy because it helps prevent birth defects.

Daily Goal

6 one-ounce servings for an adult on a 2000-calorie diet
48 grams of whole grains
One-ounce equivalents:
    1 slice bread
    1 cup dry cereal
    ½ cup cooked rice or pasta
    1 six-inch tortilla

Shopping Tips

- Make at least half your grains whole grains.
- Look for a whole grain as the first ingredient—whole wheat, brown rice, oatmeal, bulgur, or whole corn meal are examples of whole grains.
- Substitute whole wheat flour for up to half of regular flour in baking.

Shopping List Essentials

Whole wheat bread	Whole wheat pasta	Popcorn
Brown rice	Whole grain cereal	
Whole wheat flour	Oatmeal	

Red Flags

"Wheat flour" or "corn starch" are not whole grains. If a product claims "whole grain" or sounds like it is made with whole grains, look for the amount of whole grains on the label or the Whole Grain Stamp found on many but not all whole grain foods.

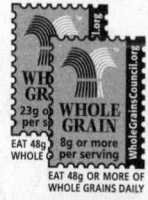

THE BASIC STAMP

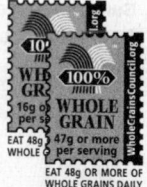

THE 100% STAMP

Food Serving size	Cal.	(g) Total Fat	(g) Sat. Fat	(mg) Chol.	(g) Carb.	(g) Fiber	(g) Sug.	(g) Prot.	(mg) Sod.
Grains, Flour									
Acorn Flour, Full Fat 1 oz (28.35g)	142	9	1	0	15	--	--	2	0
Amaranth Grain, Cooked 1 cup (246g)	251	4	--	--	46	5.2	--	9	15
Amaranth, Uncooked 1 cup (193g)	716	14	3	0	126	12.9	3	26	8
Arrowroot Flour 1 cup (128g)	457	0	0	0	113	4.4	--	0	3
Barley Flour or Meal 1 cup (148g)	511	2	0	0	110	14.9	1	16	6
Barley Malt Flour 1 cup (162g)	585	3	1	0	127	11.5	1	17	18
Barley, Hulled 1 cup (184g)	651	4	1	0	135	31.8	1	23	22
Barley, Pearled, Cooked 1 cup (157g)	193	1	0	0	44	6.0	0	4	5
Barley, Pearled, Raw 1 cup (200g)	704	2	0	0	155	31.2	2	20	18
Buckwheat 1 cup (170g)	583	6	1	0	122	17.0	--	23	2
Buckwheat Flour, Whole Groat 1 cup (120g)	402	4	1	0	85	12.0	3	15	13
Buckwheat Groats, Roasted, Cooked 1 cup (168g)	155	1	0	0	33	4.5	2	6	7
Buckwheat Groats, Roasted, Dry 1 cup (164g)	567	4	1	0	123	16.9	--	19	18
Bulgur, Cooked 1 tbsp (8.4g)	7	0	0	0	2	0.4	0	0	0
Bulgur, Dry 1 cup (140g)	479	2	0	0	106	25.6	1	17	24
Carob Flour 1 tbsp (6g)	13	0	0	0	5	2.4	3	0	2
Chickpea Flour (Besan) 1 cup (92g)	356	6	1	0	53	9.9	10	21	59

Food Serving size	Cal.	(g) Total Fat	(g) Sat. Fat	(mg) Chol.	(g) Carb.	(g) Fiber	(g) Sug.	(g) Prot.	(mg) Sod.
Corn Bran, Crude									
1 cup (76g)	170	1	0	0	65	60.0	0	6	5
Corn Flour, Whole-grain, Blue (Harina de Maiz Morado)									
1 tbsp (6.9g)	25	0	--	--	5	0.6	--	1	0
Corn Flour, Degermed, Unenriched, Yellow									
1 cup (126g)	473	2	0	0	104	2.4	1	7	1
Corn Flour, Masa, Enriched, White									
1 cup (114g)	416	4	1	0	87	7.3	2	11	6
Corn Flour, Masa, Enriched, Yellow									
1 cup (114g)	416	4	1	0	87	7.3	--	11	6
Corn Flour, Masa, Unenriched, White									
1 cup (114g)	416	4	1	0	87	7.3	2	11	6
Corn Flour, Whole-grain, White									
1 cup (117g)	422	5	1	0	90	8.5	1	8	6
Corn Flour, Whole-grain, Yellow									
1 cup (117g)	422	5	1	0	90	8.5	1	8	6
Cornmeal, Degermed, Enriched, White									
1 cup (157g)	581	3	0	0	125	6.1	3	11	11
Cornmeal, Degermed, Enriched, Yellow									
1 cup (157g)	581	3	0	0	125	6.1	3	11	11
Cornmeal, Degermed, Unenriched, White									
1 cup (157g)	581	3	0	0	125	6.1	3	11	11
Cornmeal, Degermed, Unenriched, Yellow									
1 cup (157g)	581	3	0	0	125	6.1	3	11	11
Cornmeal, Self-rising, Bolted, Plain, Enriched, White									
1 cup (122g)	407	4	1	0	86	8.2	--	10	1521
Cornmeal, Self-rising, Bolted, Plain, Enriched, Yellow									
1 cup (122g)	407	4	1	0	86	8.2	--	10	1521
Cornmeal, Self-rising, Bolted, with Wheat Flour, Enriched, White									
1 cup (170g)	592	5	1	0	125	10.7	--	14	2242
Cornmeal, Self-rising, Bolted, with Wheat Flour, Enriched, Yellow									
1 cup (170g)	592	5	1	0	125	10.7	--	14	2242
Cornmeal, Self-rising, Degermed, Enriched, White									
1 cup (138g)	490	2	0	0	103	9.8	--	12	1860
Cornmeal, Self-rising, Degermed, Enriched, Yellow									
1 cup (138g)	490	2	0	0	103	9.8	--	12	1860

Food Serving size	Cal.	(g) Total Fat	(g) Sat. Fat	(mg) Chol.	(g) Carb.	(g) Fiber	(g) Sug.	(g) Prot.	(mg) Sod.
Cornmeal, Whole-grain, White 1 cup (122g)	442	4	1	0	94	8.9	1	10	43
Cornmeal, Whole-grain, Yellow 1 cup (122g)	442	4	1	0	94	8.9	1	10	43
Cottonseed Flour, Low Fat (Glandless) 1 oz (28.35g)	94	0	0	0	10	--	--	14	10
Cottonseed Flour, Part Defatted (Glandless) 1 tbsp (5g)	18	0	0	0	2	0.2	--	2	2
Cottonseed Kernels, Roasted (Glandless) 1 tbsp (10g)	51	4	1	0	2	0.6	--	3	3
Cottonseed Meal, Part Defatted (Glandless) 1 oz (28.35g)	104	1	0	0	11	--	--	14	10
Couscous, Cooked 1 cup, dry, yields (528g)	591	1	0	0	123	7.4	1	20	26
Couscous, Dry 1 cup (173g)	650	1	0	0	134	8.7	--	22	17
Hominy, Canned, White 1 cup (165g)	119	1	0	0	24	4.1	3	2	347
Hominy, Canned, Yellow 1 cup (160g)	115	1	0	0	23	4.0	--	2	336
Leavening Agents, Baking Powder, Double-acting, Sodium Aluminum Sulfate .5 tsp (2.3g)	1	0	0	0	1	0.0	0	0	244
Leavening Agents, Baking Powder, Double-acting, Straight Phosphate .5 tsp (2.3g)	1	0	0	0	1	0.0	0	0	182
Leavening Agents, Baking Powder, Low Sodium .5 tsp (2.5g)	2	0	0	0	1	0.1	0	0	2
Leavening Agents, Baking Soda .5 tsp (2.3g)	0	0	0	0	0	0.0	0	0	629
Leavening Agents, Yeast, Baker's, Active Dry 1 tbsp (12g)	39	1	0	0	5	3.2	0	5	6
Millet Flour 1 cup (119g)	444	5	1	--	87	4.2	2	13	5
Millet, Raw 1 cup (200g)	756	8	1	0	146	17.0	--	22	10
Miso 1 cup (275g)	547	17	3	0	73	14.9	17	32	10252

Food Serving size	Cal.	(g) Total Fat	(g) Sat. Fat	(mg) Chol.	(g) Carb.	(g) Fiber	(g) Sug.	(g) Prot.	(mg) Sod.
Oat Bran, Cooked 1 cup (219g)	88	2	0	0	25	5.7	--	7	2
Oat Bran, Raw 1 cup (94g)	231	7	1	0	62	14.5	1	16	4
Oats 1 cup (156g)	607	11	2	0	103	16.5	--	26	3
Pancakes, Blueberry, Prepared from Recipe 1 pancake (4" dia) (38g)	84	3	1	21	11	--	--	2	157
Pancakes, Buttermilk, Prepared from Recipe 1 pancake (4" dia) (38g)	86	4	1	22	11	--	--	3	198
Pancakes, Plain, Dry Mix, Complete (Includes Buttermilk) 1 cup, poured from box (130g)	489	6	1	27	93	3.5	--	13	1580
Pancakes, Plain, Dry Mix, Complete, Prepared 1 pancake (4" dia) (38g)	74	1	0	5	14	0.5	--	2	239
Pancakes, Plain, Dry Mix, Incomplete (Includes Buttermilk) 1 cup, poured from box (112g)	398	2	0	0	82	6.0	2	11	1220
Pancakes, Plain, Dry Mix, Incomplete, Prepared 1 pancake (4" dia) (38g)	83	3	1	27	11	0.7	--	3	192
Pancakes, Plain, Frozen, Ready-to-heat (Includes Buttermilk) 1 pancake (41g)	92	2	0	7	16	1.0	4	2	207
Pancakes, Plain, Frozen, Ready-to-heat, Microwave (Including Buttermilk) 1 pancake (38g)	91	2	0	--	16	1.0	3	2	215
Pancakes, Plain, Prepared from Recipe 1 pancake (4" dia) (38g)	86	4	1	22	11	--	--	2	167
Pancakes, Whole Wheat, Dry Mix, Incomplete, Prepared 1 pancake (4" dia) (44g)	92	3	1	27	13	1.2	--	4	252
Rice Flour, Brown 1 cup (158g)	574	4	1	0	121	7.3	1	11	13
Rice Flour, White 1 cup (158g)	578	2	1	0	127	3.8	0	9	0
Rye 1 cup (169g)	571	3	0	0	128	25.5	2	17	3
Rye Flour, Dark 1 cup (128g)	416	3	0	0	88	30.5	3	20	3
Rye Flour, Light 1 cup (102g)	364	1	0	0	78	8.2	1	10	2

Food Serving size	Cal.	(g) Total Fat	(g) Sat. Fat	(mg) Chol.	(g) Carb.	(g) Fiber	(g) Sug.	(g) Prot.	(mg) Sod.
Rye Flour, Medium 1 cup (102g)	356	2	0	0	77	12.0	1	11	2
Semolina, Enriched 1 cup (167g)	601	2	0	0	122	6.5	--	21	2
Semolina, Unenriched 1 cup (167g)	601	2	0	0	122	6.5	--	21	2
Sesame Flour, High Fat 1 oz (28.35g)	149	11	1	0	8	--	--	9	12
Sesame Flour, Low Fat 1 oz (28.35g)	94	0	0	0	10	--	--	14	11
Sesame Flour, Part Defatted 1 oz (28.35g)	108	3	0	0	10	--	--	11	12
Sesame Meal, Part Defatted 1 oz (28.35g)	161	14	2	0	7	--	--	5	11
Sesame Sticks, Wheat-based, Salted 2 oz (57g)	308	21	4	0	27	1.6	0	6	848
Sesame Sticks, Wheat-based, Unsalted 2 oz (57g)	308	21	4	0	27	--	--	6	17
Sorghum 1 cup (192g)	651	6	1	0	143	12.1	--	22	12
Sorghum Flour 1 cup (121g)	437	4	1	--	94	8.0	2	10	5
Soy Flour, Defatted 1 tbsp (6.6g)	22	0	0	0	3	1.2	1	3	1
Soy Flour, Defatted, Crude Protein Basis (N x 6.25) 1 cup, stirred (100g)	372	9	1	0	31	16.0	15	50	9
Soy Flour, full-fat, raw 1 tbsp (5.2g)	23	1	0	0	2	0.5	0	2	1
Soy Flour, Full-fat, Raw, Crude Protein Basis (N x 6.25) 1 cup, stirred (85g)	369	18	3	0	27	8.2	--	32	11
Soy Flour, Full-fat, Roasted 1 cup, stirred (85g)	375	19	3	0	29	8.2	6	30	10
Soy Flour, Full-fat, Roasted, Crude Protein Basis (N x 6.25) 1 cup, stirred (85g)	373	19	3	0	26	--	--	32	10
Soy Flour, Low Fat 1 tbsp (5.5g)	21	0	0	0	2	0.9	1	3	0

Food Serving size	Cal.	(g) Total Fat	(g) Sat. Fat	(mg) Chol.	(g) Carb.	(g) Fiber	(g) Sug.	(g) Prot.	(mg) Sod.
Soy Flour, Low Fat, Crude Protein Basis (N x 6.25)									
1 cup, stirred (88g)	325	6	1	0	30	9.0	17	45	16
Soy Meal, Defatted, Raw									
1 cup (122g)	414	3	0	0	49	--	--	55	4
Soy Meal, Defatted, Raw, Crude Protein Basis (N x 6.25)									
1 cup (122g)	411	3	0	0	44	--	--	60	4
Spelt, Cooked									
1 cup (194g)	246	2	--	0	51	7.6	--	11	10
Spelt, Uncooked									
1 cup (174g)	588	4	1	0	122	18.6	12	25	14
Teff, Cooked									
1 cup (252g)	255	2	--	0	50	7.1	--	10	20
Teff, Uncooked									
1 cup (193g)	708	5	1	--	141	15.4	4	26	23
Tortillas, Ready-to-bake or Fry, Flour									
1 tortilla, medium (approx 6" dia) (30g)	94	2	1	0	15	0.9	1	2	191
Tortillas, Ready-to-bake or Fry, Flour, Without Calcium									
1 tortilla, medium (approx 6" dia) (32g)	104	2	1	0	18	1.1	--	3	153
Triticale									
1 cup (192g)	645	4	1	0	138	--	--	25	10
Triticale Flour, Whole Grain									
1 cup (130g)	439	2	0	0	95	19.0	--	17	3
Wheat Bran, Crude									
1 cup (58g)	125	2	0	0	37	24.8	0	9	1
Wheat Flour, Bread, Unenriched									
1 cup, unsifted, dipped (137g)	495	2	0	0	99	3.3	0	16	3
Wheat Flour, White, All Purpose, Enriched, Bleached									
1 cup (125g)	455	1	0	0	95	3.4	0	13	3
Wheat Flour, White, All Purpose, Enriched, Calcium-fortified									
1 cup (125g)	455	1	0	0	95	3.4	--	13	3
Wheat Flour, White, All Purpose, Enriched, Unbleached									
1 cup (125g)	455	1	0	0	95	3.4	0	13	3
Wheat Flour, White, All Purpose, Self-rising, Enriched									
1 cup (125g)	443	1	0	0	93	3.4	0	12	1588

Food Serving size	Cal.	(g) Total Fat	(g) Sat. Fat	(mg) Chol.	(g) Carb.	(g) Fiber	(g) Sug.	(g) Prot.	(mg) Sod.
Wheat Flour, White, All Purpose, Unenriched 1 cup (125g)	455	1	0	0	95	3.4	0	13	3
Wheat Flour, White, Bread, Enriched 1 cup (137g)	495	2	0	0	99	3.3	0	16	3
Wheat Flour, White, Cake, Enriched 1 cup, unsifted, dipped (137g)	496	1	0	0	107	2.3	0	11	3
Wheat Flour, White, Tortilla, Mix, Enriched 1 cup (111g)	450	12	5	0	75	--	--	11	751
Wheat Flour, Whole Grain 1 cup (120g)	408	3	1	0	86	12.8	0	16	2
Wheat Germ, Crude 1 cup (115g)	414	11	2	0	60	15.2	--	27	14
Wheat, Durum 1 cup (192g)	651	5	1	0	137	--	--	26	4
Wheat, Hard Red Spring 1 cup (192g)	632	4	1	0	131	23.4	1	30	4
Wheat, Hard Red Winter 1 cup (192g)	628	3	1	0	137	23.4	1	24	4
Wheat, Hard White 1 cup (192g)	657	3	1	0	146	23.4	1	22	4
Wheat, Soft Red Winter 1 cup (168g)	556	3	0	0	125	21.0	1	17	3
Wheat, Soft White 1 cup (168g)	571	3	1	0	127	21.3	1	18	3
Wheat, Sprouted 1 cup (108g)	214	1	0	0	46	1.2	--	8	17
Whelk, Unspecified, Cooked, Moist Heat 3 oz (85g)	234	1	0	111	13	0.0	--	41	350
Whey, Acid, Dried 1 tbsp (2.9g)	10	0	0	0	2	0.0	2	0	28
Whey, Acid, Fluid 1 quart (984g)	236	1	1	10	50	0.0	50	7	472
Whey, Sweet, Dried 1 tbsp (7.5g)	26	0	0	0	6	0.0	6	1	81
Whey, Sweet, Fluid 1 quart (984g)	266	4	2	20	51	0.0	51	8	531

Food Serving size	Cal.	(g) Total Fat	(g) Sat. Fat	(mg) Chol.	(g) Carb.	(g) Fiber	(g) Sug.	(g) Prot.	(mg) Sod.
Yeast Extract Spread 1 tsp (6g)	9	0	0	0	1	0.2	0	2	216

Pastas and Pasta Products

Food Serving size	Cal.	(g) Total Fat	(g) Sat. Fat	(mg) Chol.	(g) Carb.	(g) Fiber	(g) Sug.	(g) Prot.	(mg) Sod.
Kamut, Cooked 1 cup (172g)	251	2	--	0	52	6.7	--	11	10
Kamut, Uncooked 1 cup (186g)	627	4	0	--	131	16.9	15	27	11
Macaroni and Cheese, Canned Entrée 1 serving (244g)	200	6	2	15	28	1.2	12	8	737
Macaroni, Cooked, Enriched 1 cup, spiral shaped (134g)	212	1	0	0	41	2.4	1	8	1
Macaroni, Cooked, Unenriched 1 cup, elbow shaped (140g)	221	1	0	0	43	2.5	1	8	1
Macaroni, Dry, Enriched 1 cup, spiral shaped (84g)	312	1	0	0	63	2.7	2	11	5
Macaroni, Dry, Unenriched 2 oz (57g)	211	1	0	0	43	1.8	2	7	3
Macaroni, Protein-fortified, Cooked, Enriched (N x 5.70) 1 cup, small shells (115g)	189	0	0	0	36	--	--	9	6
Macaroni, Protein-fortified, Cooked, Enriched (N x 6.25) 1 cup, small shells (115g)	189	0	0	0	36	1.7	--	10	6
Macaroni, Protein-fortified, Dry, Enriched (N x 5.70) 2 oz (57g)	214	1	0	0	39	1.4	--	11	5
Macaroni, Protein-fortified, Dry, Enriched (N x 6.25) 2 oz (57g)	213	1	0	0	37	1.4	--	12	5
Macaroni, Vegetable, Cooked, Enriched 1 cup, spiral shaped (134g)	172	0	0	0	36	5.8	2	6	8
Macaroni, Vegetable, Dry, Enriched 2 oz (57g)	209	1	0	0	43	2.5	--	7	25
Macaroni, Whole Wheat, Cooked 1 cup, elbow shaped (140g)	174	1	0	0	37	3.9	1	7	4
Macaroni, Whole Wheat, Dry 2 oz (57g)	198	1	0	0	43	4.7	--	8	5

Food Serving size	Cal.	(g) Total Fat	(g) Sat. Fat	(mg) Chol.	(g) Carb.	(g) Fiber	(g) Sug.	(g) Prot.	(mg) Sod.
Noodles, Chinese, Cellophane or Long Rice (Mung Beans), Dehydrated									
1 cup (140g)	491	0	0	0	121	0.7	0	0	14
Noodles, Chinese, Chow Mein									
1.5 oz (43g)	227	13	2	0	25	1.7	0	4	189
Noodles, Egg, Cooked, Enriched									
1 cup (160g)	221	3	1	46	40	1.9	1	7	8
Noodles, Egg, Cooked, Enriched, with Salt									
1 cup (160g)	221	3	1	46	40	1.9	1	7	264
Noodles, Egg, Cooked, Unenriched, with Salt									
1 cup (160g)	221	3	1	46	40	1.9	1	7	264
Noodles, Egg, Cooked, Unenriched, Without Salt									
1 cup (160g)	221	3	1	46	40	1.9	1	7	8
Noodles, Egg, Dry, Enriched									
2 oz (57g)	219	3	1	48	41	1.9	1	8	12
Noodles, Egg, Dry, Unenriched									
1 cup (38g)	146	2	0	32	27	1.3	1	5	8
Noodles, Egg, Spinach, Cooked, Enriched									
1 cup (160g)	211	3	1	53	39	3.7	1	8	19
Noodles, Egg, Spinach, Dry, Enriched									
2 oz (57g)	218	3	1	54	40	3.9	--	8	41
Noodles, Japanese, Soba, Cooked									
1 cup (114g)	113	0	0	0	24	--	--	6	68
Noodles, Japanese, Soba, Dry									
2 oz (57g)	192	0	0	0	43	--	--	8	451
Noodles, Japanese, Somen, Cooked									
1 cup (176g)	231	0	0	0	48	--	--	7	283
Noodles, Japanese, Somen, Dry									
2 oz (57g)	203	0	0	0	42	2.5	--	6	1049
Pasta with Meatballs in Tomato Sauce, Canned Entrée									
1 cup (255g)	273	13	5	23	28	6.9	6	11	742
Pasta with Sliced Franks in Tomato Sauce, Canned Entrée									
1 serving, (1 cup) (252g)	227	6	2	23	32	4.0	10	11	600
Pasta with Tomato Sauce, No Meat, Canned									
1 serving, 1 cup (252g)	189	2	1	3	37	3.3	10	6	630

Food Serving size	Cal.	(g) Total Fat	(g) Sat. Fat	(mg) Chol.	(g) Carb.	(g) Fiber	(g) Sug.	(g) Prot.	(mg) Sod.
Pasta, Corn, Cooked 1 cup (140g)	176	1	0	0	39	6.7	--	4	0
Pasta, Corn, Dry 2 oz (57g)	203	1	0	0	45	6.3	--	4	2
Pasta, Fresh-refrigerated, Plain, as Purchased 4.5 oz (128g)	369	3	0	93	70	--	--	14	33
Pasta, Fresh-refrigerated, Plain, Cooked 2 oz (57g)	75	1	0	19	14	--	--	3	3
Pasta, Fresh-refrigerated, Spinach, as Purchased 4.5 oz (128g)	370	3	1	93	71	--	--	14	35
Pasta, Fresh-refrigerated, Spinach, Cooked 2 oz (57g)	74	1	0	19	14	--	--	3	3
Pasta, Homemade, Made with Egg, Cooked 2 oz (57g)	74	1	0	23	13	--	--	3	47
Pasta, Homemade, Made Without Egg, Cooked 2 oz (57g)	71	1	0	0	14	--	--	2	42
Spaghetti with Meat Sauce, Frozen Entrée 1 oz (28.35g)	26	0	0	2	4	0.5	1	1	60
Spaghetti with Meatballs, Canned 1 cup (255g)	273	13	5	23	28	--	8	11	1035
Spaghetti, Cooked, Enriched, with Salt 1 cup (140g)	220	1	0	0	43	2.5	1	8	183
Spaghetti, Cooked, Enriched, Without Salt 1 cup (140g)	221	1	0	0	43	2.5	1	8	1
Spaghetti, Cooked, Unenriched, with Salt 1 cup (140g)	220	1	0	0	43	2.5	1	8	183
Spaghetti, Cooked, Unenriched, Without Salt 1 cup (140g)	221	1	0	0	43	2.5	1	8	1
Spaghetti, Dry, Enriched 2 oz (57g)	211	1	0	0	43	1.8	2	7	3
Spaghetti, Dry, Unenriched 2 oz (57g)	211	1	0	0	43	1.8	2	7	3
Spaghetti, Protein-fortified, Cooked, Enriched (N x 5.70) 1 cup (140g)	230	0	0	0	44	2.4	--	11	7
Spaghetti, Protein-fortified, Cooked, Enriched (N X 6.25) 1 cup (140g)	230	0	0	0	43	2.8	--	12	7

Food Serving size	Cal.	(g) Total Fat	(g) Sat. Fat	(mg) Chol.	(g) Carb.	(g) Fiber	(g) Sug.	(g) Prot.	(mg) Sod.
Spaghetti, Protein-fortified, Dry, Enriched (N x 5.70) 2 oz (57g)	214	1	0	0	39	--	--	11	5
Spaghetti, Protein-fortified, Dry, Enriched (N X 6.25) 2 oz (57g)	213	1	0	0	37	1.4	--	12	5
Spaghetti, Spinach, Cooked 1 cup (140g)	182	1	0	0	37	--	--	6	20
Spaghetti, Spinach, Dry 2 oz (57g)	212	1	0	0	43	6.0	2	8	21
Spaghetti, Whole Wheat, Cooked 1 cup (140g)	174	1	0	0	37	6.3	1	7	4
Spaghetti, Whole Wheat, Dry 2 oz (57g)	198	1	0	0	43	--	--	8	5
Tortellini, Pasta with Cheese Filling, Fresh-refrigerated .75 cup (81g)	249	6	3	34	38	1.5	2	11	499
Vermicelli, Made from Soy 1 cup (140g)	463	0	0	0	115	5.5	0	0	6
Wonton Wrappers (Including Egg Roll Wrappers) 1 wrapper, eggroll (7" square) (32g)	93	0	0	3	19	0.6	--	3	183

Rice

Food Serving size	Cal.	(g) Total Fat	(g) Sat. Fat	(mg) Chol.	(g) Carb.	(g) Fiber	(g) Sug.	(g) Prot.	(mg) Sod.
Rice Bowl with Chicken, Frozen Entrée, Prepared 1 bowl (340g)	428	5	1	54	76	2.4	80	19	1132
Rice Bran, Crude 1 cup (118g)	373	25	5	0	59	24.8	1	16	6
Rice Cake, Cracker (Including Hain Mini Rice Cakes) 1 cubic inch (4.2g)	16	0	0	0	3	0.2	--	0	3
Rice Cakes, Brown Rice, Buckwheat 2 cakes (18g)	68	1	0	0	14	0.7	--	2	21
Rice Cakes, Brown Rice, Buckwheat, Unsalted 2 cakes (18g)	68	1	0	0	14	--	--	2	1
Rice Cakes, Brown Rice, Multi-grain 2 cakes (18g)	70	1	0	0	14	0.5	--	2	45

Food Serving size	Cal.	(g) Total Fat	(g) Sat. Fat	(mg) Chol.	(g) Carb.	(g) Fiber	(g) Sug.	(g) Prot.	(mg) Sod.
Rice Cakes, Brown Rice, Multi-grain, Unsalted 2 cakes (18g)	70	1	0	0	14	--	--	2	1
Rice Cakes, Brown Rice, Plain 2 cakes (18g)	70	1	0	0	15	0.8	0	1	59
Rice Cakes, Brown Rice, Plain, Unsalted 2 cakes (18g)	70	1	0	0	15	0.8	0	1	5
Rice Cakes, Brown Rice, Rye 2 cakes (18g)	69	1	0	0	14	0.7	--	1	20
Rice Cakes, Brown Rice, Sesame Seed 2 cakes (18g)	71	1	0	0	15	1.0	--	1	41
Rice Cakes, Brown Rice, Sesame Seed, Unsalted 2 cakes (18g)	71	1	0	0	15	--	--	1	1
Rice Noodles, Cooked 1 cup (176g)	192	0	0	0	44	1.8	--	2	33
Rice Noodles, Dry 2 oz (57g)	207	0	0	0	47	0.9	--	2	104
Rice, Brown, Long-grain, Cooked 1 cup (195g)	216	2	0	0	45	3.5	1	5	10
Rice, Brown, Long-grain, Raw 1 cup (185g)	685	5	1	0	143	6.5	2	15	13
Rice, Brown, Medium-grain, Cooked 1 cup (195g)	218	2	0	0	46	3.5	--	5	2
Rice, Brown, Medium-grain, Raw 1 cup (190g)	688	5	1	0	145	6.5	--	14	8
Rice, White, Glutinous, Cooked 1 cup (174g)	169	0	0	0	37	1.7	0	4	9
Rice, White, Glutinous, Raw 1 cup (185g)	685	1	0	0	151	5.2	--	13	13
Rice, White, Long-grain, Parboiled, Enriched, Cooked 1 cup (158g)	194	1	0	0	41	1.4	0	5	3
Rice, White, Long-grain, Parboiled, Enriched, Dry 1 cup (185g)	692	2	1	0	150	3.3	1	14	4
Rice, White, Long-grain, Parboiled, Unenriched, Cooked 1 cup (158g)	194	1	0	0	41	1.4	0	5	3

Food Serving size	Cal.	(g) Total Fat	(g) Sat. Fat	(mg) Chol.	(g) Carb.	(g) Fiber	(g) Sug.	(g) Prot.	(mg) Sod.
Rice, White, Long-grain, Parboiled, Unenriched, Dry									
1 cup (185g)	692	2	1	0	150	3.3	1	14	4
Rice, White, Long-grain, Precooked or Instant, Enriched, Dry									
1 cup (95g)	361	1	0	0	78	1.8	0	7	10
Rice, White, Long-grain, Precooked or Instant, Enriched, Prepared									
1 cup (165g)	193	1	0	0	41	1.0	0	4	7
Rice, White, Long-grain, Regular, Cooked									
1 cup (158g)	205	0	0	0	45	0.6	0	4	2
Rice, White, Long-grain, Regular, Cooked, Enriched, with Salt									
1 cup (158g)	205	0	0	0	45	0.6	0	4	604
Rice, White, Long-grain, Regular, Cooked, Unenriched, with Salt									
1 cup (158g)	205	0	0	0	45	0.6	0	4	604
Rice, White, Long-grain, Regular, Cooked, Unenriched, Without Salt									
1 cup (158g)	205	0	0	0	45	0.6	0	4	2
Rice, White, Long-grain, Regular, Raw, Enriched									
1 cup (185g)	675	1	0	0	148	2.4	0	13	9
Rice, White, Long-grain, Regular, Raw, Unenriched									
1 cup (185g)	675	1	0	0	148	2.4	0	13	9
Rice, White, Medium-grain, Cooked									
1 cup (186g)	242	0	0	0	53	0.6	--	4	0
Rice, White, Medium-grain, Cooked, Unenriched									
1 cup (186g)	242	0	0	0	53	--	--	4	0
Rice, White, Medium-grain, Raw, Enriched									
1 cup (195g)	702	1	0	0	155	2.7	--	13	2
Rice, White, Medium-grain, Raw, Unenriched									
1 cup (195g)	702	1	0	0	155	--	--	13	2
Rice, White, Short-grain, Cooked									
1 cup (186g)	242	0	0	0	53	--	--	4	0
Rice, White, Short-grain, Cooked, Unenriched									
1 cup (205g)	267	0	0	0	59	--	--	5	0
Rice, White, Short-grain, Raw									
1 cup (200g)	716	1	0	0	158	5.6	--	13	2
Rice, White, Short-grain, Raw, Unenriched									
1 cup (200g)	716	1	0	0	158	--	--	13	2
Rice, White, with Pasta, Cooked									
1 cup (202g)	246	6	1	2	43	5.1	--	5	1147

Food Serving size	Cal.	(g) Total Fat	(g) Sat. Fat	(mg) Chol.	(g) Carb.	(g) Fiber	(g) Sug.	(g) Prot.	(mg) Sod.
Rice, White, with Pasta, Dry 1 cup (163g)	600	4	1	3	123	--	--	15	3042
Wild Rice, Cooked 1 cup (164g)	166	1	0	0	35	3.0	1	7	5
Wild Rice, Raw 1 cup (160g)	571	2	0	0	120	9.9	4	24	11

Cereals and Cereal Bars

Food Serving size	Cal.	(g) Total Fat	(g) Sat. Fat	(mg) Chol.	(g) Carb.	(g) Fiber	(g) Sug.	(g) Prot.	(mg) Sod.
Amaranth Flakes 1 cup (38g)	134	3	1	0	27	3.6	5	6	13
Breakfast Bar, Corn Flake Crust with Fruit 1 oz (28.35g)	107	2	0	0	21	0.6	0	1	47
Cereal Ready-to-eat, Crispy Brown Rice 1 cup (32g)	124	1	0	0	28	2.3	--	2	4
Cereals Ready-to-eat, Familia 1 cup (122g)	473	8	1	0	90	10.4	--	12	61
Cereals Ready-to-eat, Frosted Oat Cereal, with Marshmallows .75 cup (30g)	116	1	0	0	25	1.3	--	2	150
Cereals Ready-to-eat, Marshmallow Alpha-Bits 1 cup (1 NLEA serving) (29g)	115	1	0	0	25	0.5	0	2	206
Cereals Ready-to-eat, Muesli, Dried Fruits and Nuts 1 cup (85g)	289	4	1	0	66	6.2	--	8	196
Cereals Ready-to-eat, Oat Bran Flakes, Health Valley 1 cup (47g)	166	1	0	0	37	6.1	--	5	17
Cereals Ready-to-eat, Post Banana Nut Crunch 1 cup (1 NLEA serving) (59g)	249	6	1	0	44	4.0	2	5	230
Cereals Ready-to-eat, Post Great Grains, Raisin, Date and Pecan .667 cup (1 NLEA serving) (54g)	204	5	1	0	40	4.0	--	4	160
Cereals Ready-to-eat, Post Honey Bunches of Oats, Honey Roasted .75 cup (1 NLEA serving) (30g)	118	1	0	0	25	1.4	2	2	150
Cereals Ready-to-eat, Post Honey Bunches of Oats, with Almonds .75 cup (1 NLEA serving) (31g)	126	3	0	0	24	1.4	--	2	136
Cereals Ready-to-eat, Weetabix, Whole Wheat Cereal 1 biscuit (18g)	67	1	0	0	14	2.1	--	2	70
Cereals Ready-to-eat, Wheat and Bran, Presweetened with Nuts and Fruits 1 cup (1 NLEA serving) (55g)	212	3	0	0	42	5.3	1	4	280

Food Serving size	Cal.	(g) Total Fat	(g) Sat. Fat	(mg) Chol.	(g) Carb.	(g) Fiber	(g) Sug.	(g) Prot.	(mg) Sod.
Cereals Ready-to-eat, Whole Wheat, Rolled Oats, Presweetened with Pecans .667 cup (1 NLEA serving) (53g)									
	216	6	1	0	38	3.7	--	5	214
Cereals, Corn Grits, White, Regular and Quick, Enriched, Cooked with Water, with Salt 1 tbsp (16g)	11	0	0	0	2	0.1	0	0	36
Cereals, Corn Grits, White, Regular and Quick, Enriched, Cooked with Water, Without Salt 1 tbsp (16g)	11	0	0	0	2	0.1	0	0	0
Cereals, Corn Grits, White, Regular and Quick, Enriched, Dry 1 tbsp (9.7g)	36	0	0	0	8	0.4	0	1	0
Cereals, Corn Grits, White, Regular and Quick, Unenriched, Cooked with Water, with Salt .75 cup (182g)	109	0	0	0	24	0.4	--	3	406
Cereals, Corn Grits, White, Regular and Quick, Unenriched, Cooked with Water, Without Salt .75 cup (182g)	107	0	0	0	23	0.5	0	3	4
Cereals, Corn Grits, White, Regular and Quick, Unenriched, Dry 1 tbsp (9.7g)	36	0	0	0	8	0.2	0	1	0
Cereals, Corn Grits, Yellow, Regular and Quick, Enriched, Cooked with Water, with Salt 1 cup (233g)	151	1	0	0	32	1.6	0	3	520
Cereals, Corn Grits, Yellow, Regular and Quick, Enriched, Cooked with Water, Without Salt 1 cup (233g)	151	1	0	0	32	1.6	0	3	5
Cereals, Corn Grits, Yellow, Regular and Quick, Enriched, Dry 1 cup (170g)	626	3	0	0	136	6.6	1	11	3
Cereals, Corn Grits, Yellow, Regular and Quick, Unenriched, Cooked with Water, with Salt .75 cup (182g)	107	0	0	0	23	0.5	0	3	406
Cereals, Corn Grits, Yellow, Regular and Quick, Unenriched, Cooked with Water, Without Salt .75 cup (182g)	107	0	0	0	23	0.5	0	3	4
Cereals, Corn Grits, Yellow, Regular and Quick, Unenriched, Dry 1 tbsp (9.7g)	36	0	0	0	8	0.2	0	1	0

Food Serving size	Cal.	(g) Total Fat	(g) Sat. Fat	(mg) Chol.	(g) Carb.	(g) Fiber	(g) Sug.	(g) Prot.	(mg) Sod.
Cereals, Cream of Rice, Cooked with Water, with Salt									
.75 cup (183g)	95	0	0	0	21	0.2	0	2	317
Cereals, Cream of Rice, Cooked with Water, Without Salt									
1 tbsp (15g)	8	0	0	0	2	0.0	0	0	0
Cereals, Cream of Rice, Dry									
.25 cup (1 NLEA serving) (46g)	170	0	0	0	38	0.3	0	3	3
Cereals, Cream of Wheat, 1 Minute Cook Time, Dry									
1 tbsp (13.7g)	49	0	0	--	10	0.6	0	2	1
Cereals, Cream of Wheat, 1 Minute, Cooked with Water, Microwaved, Without Salt									
1 cup (237g)	130	1	0	--	25	3.6	7	5	9
Cereals, Cream of Wheat, 1 Minute, Cooked with Water, Stove-top, Without Salt									
1 cup (245g)	137	1	0	--	27	1.0	0	4	10
Cereals, Cream of Wheat, 2 1/2 Minutes, Cooked with Water, Microwaved									
1 cup (231g)	120	1	0	--	23	1.6	1	4	104
Cereals, Cream of Wheat, 2 1/2 Minutes, Cooked, Dry									
1 tbsp (13.8g)	49	0	0	--	10	0.6	0	2	45
Cereals, Cream of Wheat, 2 1/2 Minutes, Cooked, Stove-top, Without Salt									
1 cup (244g)	137	0	0	--	29	1.7	0	4	83
Cereals, Cream of Wheat, Instant, Dry									
1 tbsp (11.5g)	42	0	0	0	9	0.4	0	1	2
Cereals, Cream of Wheat, Instant, Prepared with Water, with Salt (Wheat)									
.75 cup (181g)	112	0	0	0	24	1.1	0	3	273
Cereals, Cream of Wheat, Instant, Prepared with Water, Without Salt									
1 tbsp (15g)	9	0	0	0	2	0.1	0	0	1
Cereals, Cream of Wheat, Mix 'n Eat, Apple, Banana and Maple Flavors, Dry									
1 packet (35g)	131	0	--	0	29	0.9	--	2	238
Cereals, Cream of Wheat, Mix 'n Eat, Apple, Banana and Maple Flavors, Prepared									
1 packet, prepared (150g)	132	0	0	0	29	0.5	--	2	242
Cereals, Cream of Wheat, Mix 'n Eat, Plain, Dry									
1 packet (28g)	101	0	0	0	21	0.6	--	3	238
Cereals, Cream of Wheat, Mix 'n Eat, Plain, Prepared with Water									
1 packet, prepared (142g)	102	0	0	0	21	0.4	--	3	241
Cereals, Cream of Wheat, Regular (10 Minutes), Cooked with Water, with Salt									
1 cup (1 serving) (251g)	126	1	0	0	27	1.3	0	4	324

Food Serving size	Cal.	(g) Total Fat	(g) Sat. Fat	(mg) Chol.	(g) Carb.	(g) Fiber	(g) Sug.	(g) Prot.	(mg) Sod.
Cereals, Cream of Wheat, Regular (10 Minutes), Cooked with Water, Without Salt									
1 tbsp (16g)	8	0	0	0	2	0.1	0	0	1
Cereals, Cream of Wheat, Regular, 10 Minutes Cooking, Dry									
1 serving (3 tbsp) (33g)	122	0	0	0	25	1.3	0	3	2
Cereals, Farina, Enriched, Assorted Brands, Dry									
1 tbsp (11g)	40	0	0	0	8	0.5	0	1	14
Cereals, Farina, Enriched, Assorted Brands, Quick, Cooked with Water, Without Salt									
1 tbsp (14.9g)	8	0	0	0	2	0.1	0	0	3
Cereals, Farina, Enriched, Cooked with Water, with Salt									
1 cup (233g)	123	1	0	0	25	1.9	2	4	294
Cereals, Farina, Enriched, Cooked with Water, Without Salt									
1 tbsp (15g)	8	0	0	0	2	0.1	0	0	3
Cereals, Farina, Unenriched, Dry									
1 tbsp (10.9g)	40	0	0	0	9	0.2	--	1	0
Cereals, Kashi GoLean Hot Cereal, Hearty Honey and Cinnamon, Dry									
1 packet (1 NLEA serving) (40g)	145	2	0	0	25	7.8	6	9	100
Cereals, Kashi, Heart to Heart, Instant Oatmeal, Apple Cinnamon, Dry									
1 packet (1 NLEA serving) (43g)	161	2	0	0	34	4.9	12	5	108
Cereals, Kashi, Heart to Heart, Instant Oatmeal, Maple, Dry									
1 packet (1 NLEA serving) (43g)	162	2	0	0	33	5.0	12	5	99
Cereals, Kashi, Kashi GoLean Hot Cereal, Truly Vanilla, Dry									
1 packet (1 NLEA serving) (40g)	145	2	0	0	26	5.1	7	8	99
Cereals, Maltex, Cooked with Water, with Salt									
.75 cup (187g)	142	1	0	0	30	1.7	0	4	142
Cereals, Maltex, Cooked with Water, Without Salt									
1 tbsp (16g)	12	0	0	0	3	0.1	0	0	1
Cereals, Maltex, Dry									
.25 cup (38g)	134	1	0	0	29	1.6	0	4	6
Cereals, Malt-O-Meal, Chocolate, Dry									
1 tbsp (10.3g)	39	0	0	0	8	0.4	3	1	1

Food Serving size	Cal.	(g) Total Fat	(g) Sat. Fat	(mg) Chol.	(g) Carb.	(g) Fiber	(g) Sug.	(g) Prot.	(mg) Sod.
Cereals, Malt-O-Meal, Chocolate, Prepared with Water, Without Salt									
1 serving (3 T dry cereal plus 1 cup water) (268g)									
	118	0	0	0	25	1.3	8	3	8
Cereals, Malt-O-Meal, Farina Hot Wheat Cereal, Dry									
3 tbsp (35g)	127	0	0	0	26	1.4	0	5	4
Cereals, Malt-O-Meal, Plain, Dry									
1 tbsp (10.3g)	37	0	0	0	8	0.4	0	1	1
Cereals, Malt-O-Meal, Plain, Prepared with Water, Without Salt									
1 serving (3 T dry cereal plus 1 cup water) (268g)									
	113	0	0	0	23	1.3	0	4	8
Cereals, Maypo, Cooked with Water, with Salt									
.75 cup (180g)	128	2	0	0	24	3.6	11	4	194
Cereals, Maypo, Cooked with Water, Without Salt									
1 tbsp (15g)	11	0	0	0	2	0.4	1	0	1
Cereals, Maypo, Dry									
.5 cup (47g)	181	2	0	0	34	5.1	16	6	9
Cereals, Oats, Instant, Fortified, Plain, Dry									
1 packet (28g)	105	2	0	0	19	2.8	0	4	78
Cereals, Oats, Instant, Fortified, Plain, Prepared with Water									
1 cup, dry, yields (501g)	341	7	1	0	58	8.5	2	12	245
Cereals, Oats, Instant, Fortified, with Cinnamon and Spice, Dry									
1 packet (46g)	170	2	0	0	35	3.0	16	4	222
Cereals, Oats, Instant, Fortified, with Cinnamon and Spice, Prepared with Water									
1 tbsp (15g)	16	0	0	0	3	0.3	1	0	20
Cereals, Oats, Instant, Fortified, with Raisins and Spice, Dry									
1 packet (43g)	155	2	0	0	33	2.7	16	3	209
Cereals, Oats, Instant, Fortified, with Raisins and Spice, Prepared with Water									
1 tbsp (15g)	15	0	0	0	3	0.2	1	0	23
Cereals, Oats, Regular and Quick and Instant, Not Fortified, Dry									
.333 cup (27g)	102	2	0	0	18	2.7	0	4	2
Cereals, Oats, Regular and Quick and Instant, Unenriched, Cooked with Water, with Salt									
.75 cup (175g)	124	3	1	0	21	3.0	0	4	124
Cereals, Oats, Regular and Quick and Instant, Unenriched, Cooked with Water, Without Salt									
1 tbsp (14.6g)	10	0	0	0	2	0.2	0	0	1

Food Serving size	Cal.	(g) Total Fat	(g) Sat. Fat	(mg) Chol.	(g) Carb.	(g) Fiber	(g) Sug.	(g) Prot.	(mg) Sod.
Cereals, Quaker, Corn Grits, Instant, Butter Flavor, Dry 1 packet (28g)	102	2	1	0	21	1.3	0	2	367
Cereals, Quaker, Corn Grits, Instant, Cheddar Cheese Flavor, Dry 1 packet (28g)	102	2	0	1	20	1.2	1	2	522
Cereals, Quaker, Corn Grits, Instant, Cheddar Cheese Flavor, Prepared with Water 1 packet, prepared (142g)	102	2	0	0	20	1.1	1	2	508
Cereals, Quaker, Corn Grits, Instant, Country Bacon (Imitation Bacon Bits) Prepared with Water 1 packet, prepared (141g)	97	0	0	0	21	1.4	0	3	413
Cereals, Quaker, Corn Grits, Instant, Plain, Dry 1 tbsp (7g)	25	0	0	0	5	0.3	0	1	74
Cereals, Quaker, Corn Grits, Instant, Plain, Prepared Without Salt 1 cup (219g)	166	1	0	--	35	2.4	0	3	412
Cereals, Quaker, Corn Grits, Instant, with Imitation Bacon Bits, Dry 1 packet (28g)	98	0	0	0	22	1.5	0	3	341
Cereals, Quaker, Farina, Creamy Wheat, Enriched, Dry .25 cup, (1 NLEA serving) (44g)	154	0	0	0	33	1.3	0	5	1
Cereals, Quaker, Hominy Grits, White, Quick, Dry .25 cup (37g)	128	1	0	0	29	1.8	0	3	1
Cereals, Quaker, Hominy Grits, White, Regular, Dry .25 cup (41g)	142	1	0	0	32	2.0	0	3	1
Cereals, Quaker, Hominy Grits, Yellow, Quick, Dry .25 cup (37g)	125	1	0	0	29	2.1	0	3	1
Cereals, Quaker, Instant Grits Product with American Cheese Flavor, Dry 1 packet (28g)	102	1	0	0	21	1.2	1	2	425
Cereals, Quaker, Instant Grits Product with Ham-n-Cheese 1 packet (28g)	101	1	0	0	20	1.2	--	3	540
Cereals, Quaker, Instant Grits Product with Imitation Bacon Bits and Cheddar Flavor, Dry 1 packet (28g)	102	1	0	0	20	1.3	1	3	436
Cereals, Quaker, Instant Grits, with Redeye Gravy and Imitation Ham Bits, Dry 1 packet (28g)	97	0	0	0	21	1.3	--	3	494
Cereals, Quaker, Instant Oat, Maple and Brown Sugar, Prepared with Boiling Water 1 packet, prepared (155g)	157	2	0	0	31	2.8	13	4	253

Food Serving size	Cal.	(g) Total Fat	(g) Sat. Fat	(mg) Chol.	(g) Carb.	(g) Fiber	(g) Sug.	(g) Prot.	(mg) Sod.
Cereals, Quaker, Instant Oatmeal Express Cinnamon Roll, Dry									
1 cup (54g)	200	3	0	0	41	3.6	17	5	246
Cereals, Quaker, Instant Oatmeal Express, Baked Apple, Dry									
1 cup (54g)	198	2	0	0	42	3.9	19	4	319
Cereals, Quaker, Instant Oatmeal, Apples and Cinnamon, Dry									
1 packet (35g)	128	2	0	0	27	2.8	12	3	177
Cereals, Quaker, Instant Oatmeal, Apples and Cinnamon, Prepared with Boiling Water									
1 packet, prepared (149g)	130	1	0	0	26	2.7	12	3	165
Cereals, Quaker, Instant Oatmeal, Baked Apple, Prepared with Boiling Water									
1 packet, prepared (159g)	153	2	0	0	31	2.9	14	3	229
Cereals, Quaker, Instant Oatmeal, Banana Bread, Dry									
1 packet (41g)	151	2	0	0	31	2.6	12	4	287
Cereals, Quaker, Instant Oatmeal, Cinnamon Roll, Prepared with Boiling Water									
1 packet, prepared (173g)	209	3	0	0	41	3.6	17	5	249
Cereals, Quaker, Instant Oatmeal, Cinnamon Spice, Dry									
1 packet (46g)	170	2	0	0	35	3.0	16	4	222
Cereals, Quaker, Instant Oatmeal, Cinnamon Spice, Prepared with Boiling Water									
1 packet, prepared (165g)	177	2	0	0	36	3.0	16	4	223
Cereals, Quaker, Instant Oatmeal, Dinosaur Eggs with Dinosaur Bones, Brown Sugar Cinnamon, Dry									
1 packet (50g)	195	4	2	0	38	2.8	20	4	262
Cereals, Quaker, Instant Oatmeal, Dinosaur Eggs with Dinosaur Bones, Brown Sugar Cinnamon, Prepared with Boiling Water									
1 packet, prepared (167g)	199	4	2	0	38	2.8	19	4	261
Cereals, Quaker, Instant Oatmeal, Express Baked Apple, Prepared with Boiling Water									
1 packet, prepared (173g)	208	3	0	0	42	4.0	19	4	322
Cereals, Quaker, Instant Oatmeal, Express, Golden Brown Sugar, Prepared with Boiling Water									
1 packet, prepared (173g)	209	3	0	0	42	3.5	18	5	294
Cereals, Quaker, Instant Oatmeal, Express, Golden Brown Sugar, Dry									
1 cup (54g)	201	3	0	0	42	3.3	18	5	291
Cereals, Quaker, Instant Oatmeal, French Vanilla, Prepared with Boiling Water									
1 packet, prepared (162g)	165	2	0	0	33	2.9	13	4	249
Cereals, Quaker, Instant Oatmeal, Fruit and Cream Variety, Dry									
1 packet (35g)	135	3	1	0	26	2.0	11	3	176

Food Serving size	Cal.	(g) Total Fat	(g) Sat. Fat	(mg) Chol.	(g) Carb.	(g) Fiber	(g) Sug.	(g) Prot.	(mg) Sod.
Cereals, Quaker, Instant Oatmeal, Fruit and Cream, Prepared with Boiling Water									
1 packet, prepared (193g)	139	3	1	0	26	2.1	11	3	178
Cereals, Quaker, Instant Oatmeal, Honey Nut, Prepared with Boiling Water									
1 packet, prepared (162g)	173	4	0	0	31	2.8	13	4	238
Cereals, Quaker, Instant Oatmeal, Low Sodium, Dry									
1 packet (28g)	102	2	0	0	19	2.7	0	4	78
Cereals, Quaker, Instant Oatmeal, Maple and Brown Sugar, Dry									
1 packet (43g)	157	2	0	0	32	2.8	13	4	261
Cereals, Quaker, Instant Oatmeal, Nutrition for Women, Apple Spice, Prepared with Boiling Water									
1 packet, prepared (166g)	178	2	0	0	35	3.2	16	5	319
Cereals, Quaker, Instant Oatmeal, Nutrition for Women, Brown Sugar, Prepared with Boiling Water									
1 packet, prepared (165g)	173	2	0	0	33	2.8	13	5	328
Cereals, Quaker, Instant Oatmeal, Raisin and Spice, Dry									
1 packet (43g)	155	2	0	0	33	2.7	16	3	209
Cereals, Quaker, Instant Oatmeal, Raisin and Spice, Prepared with Boiling Water									
1 packet, prepared (162g)	162	2	0	0	33	2.6	16	3	211
Cereals, Quaker, Instant Oatmeal, Raisins, Dates and Walnuts, Dry									
1 packet (37g)	135	2	0	0	27	2.4	--	3	191
Cereals, Quaker, Instant Oatmeal, Treasure Hunt, Prepared with Boiling Water									
1 packet, prepared (166g)	179	2	1	0	36	2.7	17	4	257
Cereals, Quaker, Mother's Instant Oatmeal (Non-fortified), Dry									
.25 cup (1 NLEA serving) (40g)	144	3	1	0	26	3.8	1	5	1
Cereals, Quaker, Multigrain Oatmeal, Dry									
.5 cup (1 NLEA serving) (40g)	133	1	0	0	29	4.8	0	5	1
Cereals, Quaker, Oat Bran, Quaker/Mother's Oat Bran, Dry									
.5 cup (1 NLEA serving) (40g)	146	3	1	0	25	5.7	1	7	2
Cereals, Quaker, Quick Oat, Dry									
.5 cup (40g)	148	3	0	0	27	3.8	1	5	1
Cereals, Ralston, cooked with Water, with Salt									
.75 cup (190g)	101	1	0	0	21	4.6	--	4	357
Cereals, Ralston, cooked with Water, Without Salt									
1 tbsp (16g)	8	0	0	0	2	0.4	--	0	0
Cereals, Ralston, Dry									
.25 cup (30g)	102	1	--	0	22	4.0	--	4	3

Food Serving size	Cal.	(g) Total Fat	(g) Sat. Fat	(mg) Chol.	(g) Carb.	(g) Fiber	(g) Sug.	(g) Prot.	(mg) Sod.
Cereals, Ready-to-eat, Alpen 1 cup (113g)	398	4	1	0	86	10.3	--	13	241
Cereals, Ready-to-eat, Apple Cinnamon Squares Mini-Wheats .75 cup (1 NLEA serving) (55g)	182	1	0	0	44	4.7	12	4	20
Cereals, Ready-to-eat, Bran Flakes, Single Brand .75 cup (1 NLEA serving) (30g)	96	1	0	0	24	5.3	6	3	220
Cereals, Ready-to-eat, Chocolate-flavored Frosted Puffed Corn 1 cup (30g)	122	1	0	0	26	1.1	14	1	201
Cereals, Ready-to-eat, Corn Flakes 1 oz (28.35g)	113	0	0	0	25	0.3	2	2	3
Cereals, Ready-to-eat, Cranberry Macadamia Nut Cereal 1 cup (60g)	245	6	1	--	46	3.6	17	4	251
Cereals, Ready-to-eat, General Mills Cinnamon Chex .75 cup (1 NLEA serving) (30g)	121	2	0	0	25	0.7	8	1	184
Cereals, Ready-to-eat, General Mills Peanut Butter Toast Crunch .75 cup (30g)	130	4	1	0	23	1.0	13	2	135
Cereals, Ready-to-eat, General Mills, Apple Cinnamon Cheerios .75 cup (1 NLEA serving) (30g)	120	2	0	0	25	1.2	13	2	133
Cereals, Ready-to-eat, General Mills, Basic 4 1 cup (1 NLEA serving) (55g)	197	2	1	0	43	3.5	14	4	322
Cereals, Ready-to-eat, General Mills, Berry Berry Kix .75 cup (1 NLEA serving) (26g)	99	1	0	0	23	0.9	8	1	179
Cereals, Ready-to-eat, General Mills, Berry Burst Cheerios, All Flavors .75 cup (1 NLEA serving) (27g)	99	1	0	0	22	2.0	8	3	173
Cereals, Ready-to-eat, General Mills, Boo Berry 1 cup (1 NLEA serving) (33g)	127	1	0	0	29	1.1	12	2	195
Cereals, Ready-to-eat, General Mills, Cheerios 1 cup (1 NLEA serving) (28g)	103	2	0	0	21	2.8	1	3	160
Cereals, Ready-to-eat, General Mills, Cheerios, Banana Nut .75 cup (1 NLEA serving) (28g)	105	1	0	0	24	1.7	9	2	160
Cereals, Ready-to-eat, General Mills, Cheerios, Chocolate .75 cup (1 NLEA serving) (27g)	103	1	0	0	23	1.7	9	2	170
Cereals, Ready-to-eat, General Mills, Cheerios, Yogurt Burst .75 cup (1 NLEA serving) (30g)	120	2	1	0	25	2.0	10	2	175
Cereals, Ready-to-eat, General Mills, Chocolate Chex .75 cup (1 NLEA serving) (32g)	132	3	0	0	26	0.6	8	2	238

Food Serving size	Cal.	(g) Total Fat	(g) Sat. Fat	(mg) Chol.	(g) Carb.	(g) Fiber	(g) Sug.	(g) Prot.	(mg) Sod.
Cereals, Ready-to-eat, General Mills, Chocolate Lucky Charms									
.75 cup (1 NLEA serving) (28g)	106	1	0	0	24	1.5	12	1	159
Cereals, Ready-to-eat, General Mills, Cinnamon Grahams									
.75 cup (30g)	113	1	0	0	26	1.0	11	2	237
Cereals, Ready-to-eat, General Mills, Cinnamon Toast Crunch									
.75 cup (1 NLEA serving) (31g)	128	3	0	0	25	1.2	10	2	217
Cereals, Ready-to-eat, General Mills, Cocoa Puffs									
.75 cup (1 NLEA serving) (27g)	104	1	0	0	23	1.8	11	1	147
Cereals, Ready-to-eat, General Mills, Cookie Crisp									
1 oz (28.35g)	107	1	0	0	24	1.3	11	1	157
Cereals, Ready-to-eat, General Mills, Corn Chex									
1 cup (1 NLEA serving) (31g)	114	1	0	0	26	1.2	3	2	236
Cereals, Ready-to-eat, General Mills, Count Chocula									
.75 cup (1 NLEA serving) (27g)	103	1	0	0	23	1.0	12	1	158
Cereals, Ready-to-eat, General Mills, Dora the Explorer									
.75 cup (1 NLEA serving) (27g)	100	2	0	0	23	3.0	6	1	174
Cereals, Ready-to-eat, General Mills, Fiber One									
.5 cup (1 NLEA serving) (30g)	60	1	0	0	25	14.2	0	2	106
Cereals, Ready-to-eat, General Mills, Fiber One, Caramel Delight									
1 cup (1 NLEA serving) (50g)	176	3	1	0	41	8.4	11	3	226
Cereals, Ready-to-eat, General Mills, Fiber One, Honey Clusters									
1 cup (1 NLEA serving) (52g)	157	1	0	0	44	12.7	6	3	240
Cereals, Ready-to-eat, General Mills, Fiber One, Raisin Bran Clusters									
1 cup (1 NLEA serving) (55g)	171	1	0	0	47	11.6	14	3	211
Cereals, Ready-to-eat, General Mills, Fiber One, Shredded Wheat									
1 cup (1 NLEA serving) (60g)	193	1	0	0	49	8.2	12	5	1
Cereals, Ready-to-eat, General Mills, Franken Berry									
1 cup (1 NLEA serving) (33g)	127	1	0	0	29	1.1	12	2	195
Cereals, Ready-to-eat, General Mills, French Toast Crunch									
.75 cup (1 NLEA serving) (31g)	136	3	0	0	24	1.0	11	2	223
Cereals, Ready-to-eat, General Mills, Frosted Cheerios									
.75 cup (1 NLEA serving) (28g)	106	1	0	0	23	1.7	10	2	173
Cereals, Ready-to-eat, General Mills, Frosted Chex									
.75 cup (1 NLEA serving) (30g)	110	1	0	0	27	0.0	10	1	180

Food Serving size	Cal.	(g) Total Fat	(g) Sat. Fat	(mg) Chol.	(g) Carb.	(g) Fiber	(g) Sug.	(g) Prot.	(mg) Sod.
Cereals, Ready-to-eat, General Mills, Fruity Cheerios									
.75 cup (1 NLEA serving) (27g)	100	1	0	0	23	1.6	9	2	133
Cereals, Ready-to-eat, General Mills, Golden Grahams									
.75 cup (1 NLEA serving) (30g)	113	1	0	0	25	1.3	10	2	256
Cereals, Ready-to-eat, General Mills, Harmony									
1.25 cup (55g)	201	1	0	0	43	2.2	13	6	355
Cereals, Ready-to-eat, General Mills, Honey Nut Cheerios									
.75 cup (1 NLEA serving) (28g)	110	2	0	0	22	2.0	9	3	159
Cereals, Ready-to-eat, General Mills, Honey Nut Chex									
.75 cup (1 NLEA serving) (32g)	128	1	0	0	28	0.3	10	2	198
Cereals, Ready-to-eat, General Mills, Honey Nut Clusters									
1 cup (1 NLEA serving) (57g)	218	3	0	0	48	3.1	18	4	294
Cereals, Ready-to-eat, General Mills, Kaboom									
1.25 cup (1 NLEA serving) (30g)	120	1	0	0	26	1.0	6	1	190
Cereals, Ready-to-eat, General Mills, Kix									
1 cup (24g)	88	1	0	0	20	2.1	2	2	151
Cereals, Ready-to-eat, General Mills, Lucky Charms									
1 cup (35g)	142	1	0	0	29	1.6	14	2	252
Cereals, Ready-to-eat, General Mills, Multi-Bran Chex									
.75 cup (1 NLEA serving) (47g)	154	1	0	0	40	5.7	10	3	265
Cereals, Ready-to-eat, General Mills, Multi-Grain Cheerios									
1 cup (1 NLEA serving) (29g)	110	1	0	0	24	2.7	6	2	161
Cereals, Ready-to-eat, General Mills, Nature Valley Low Fat Fruit Granola									
.667 cup (1 NLEA serving) (55g)	212	3	0	0	44	2.8	18	4	207
Cereals, Ready-to-eat, General Mills, Oatmeal Crisp with Almonds									
1 cup (1 NLEA serving) (60g)	240	5	1	0	46	4.5	17	5	124
Cereals, Ready-to-eat, General Mills, Oatmeal Crisp, Apple Cinnamon									
1 cup (1 NLEA serving) (55g)	210	2	1	0	46	4.0	19	4	270
Cereals, Ready-to-eat, General Mills, Oatmeal Crisp, Raisin									
1 cup (1 NLEA serving) (62g)	237	2	0	0	52	4.7	20	5	122
Cereals, Ready-to-eat, General Mills, Raisin Nut Bran									
.75 cup (1 NLEA serving) (49g)	178	3	0	0	37	4.8	13	4	226
Cereals, Ready-to-eat, General Mills, Reese's Puffs									
.75 cup (1 NLEA serving) (29g)	126	3	0	0	22	1.2	12	2	192

Food Serving size	Cal.	(g) Total Fat	(g) Sat. Fat	(mg) Chol.	(g) Carb.	(g) Fiber	(g) Sug.	(g) Prot.	(mg) Sod.
Cereals, Ready-to-eat, General Mills, Rice Chex									
1 cup (1 NLEA serving) (27g)	103	0	0	0	23	0.3	2	2	246
Cereals, Ready-to-eat, General Mills, Total Blueberry Pomegranate									
1 cup (1 NLEA serving) (49g)	173	2	0	0	38	3.9	11	5	96
Cereals, Ready-to-eat, General Mills, Total Corn Flakes									
1.333 cup (1 NLEA serving) (30g)	112	0	0	0	26	0.8	3	2	209
Cereals, Ready-to-eat, General Mills, Total Cranberry Crunch									
1.25 cup (1 NLEA serving) (58g)	194	1	0	0	46	4.2	16	4	194
Cereals, Ready-to-eat, General Mills, Total Raisin Bran									
1 cup (1 NLEA serving) (53g)	164	1	0	0	40	4.8	18	3	232
Cereals, Ready-to-eat, General Mills, Trix									
1 cup (1 NLEA serving) (32g)	123	1	0	0	27	1.4	11	2	188
Cereals, Ready-to-eat, General Mills, Trix, Reduced Sugar, Bowlpak									
1 bowlpak (21g)	84	1	0	0	18	1.0	6	1	120
Cereals, Ready-to-eat, General Mills, Wheat Chex									
.75 cup (1 NLEA serving) (47g)	169	1	0	0	38	5.1	5	5	298
Cereals, Ready-to-eat, General Mills, Wheaties									
.75 cup (1 NLEA serving) (27g)	94	0	0	0	22	3.2	4	3	199
Cereals, Ready-to-eat, General Mills, Wheaties Raisin Bran									
1 cup (1 NLEA serving) (55g)	183	1	0	0	45	5.0	18	4	251
Cereals, Ready-to-eat, General Mills, Wheaties FUEL									
.75 cup (1 NLEA serving) (55g)	206	3	0	0	46	5.3	14	3	152
Cereals, Ready-to-eat, General Mills, Whole Grain Total									
.75 cup (1 NLEA serving) (30g)	96	1	0	0	22	2.7	5	3	197
Cereals, Ready-to-eat, Granola, Homemade									
1 oz (28.35g)	139	7	1	0	15	2.6	6	4	7
Cereals, Ready-to-eat, Health Valley, Fiber 7 Flakes									
.75 cup (1 NLEA serving) (31g)	109	0	0	0	24	4.4	1	4	16
Cereals, Ready-to-eat, Just Right with Crunchy Nuggets									
1 cup (1 NLEA serving) (55g)	204	1	0	0	46	2.8	12	4	338
Cereals, Ready-to-eat, Kashi 7 Whole Grain Flakes									
1 cup (1 NLEA serving) (50g)	175	1	0	0	41	5.7	4	6	152
Cereals, Ready-to-eat, Kashi 7 Whole Grain Honey Puffs									
1 cup (1 NLEA serving) (30g)	114	1	0	0	25	2.0	7	3	3

Food Serving size	Cal.	(g) Total Fat	(g) Sat. Fat	(mg) Chol.	(g) Carb.	(g) Fiber	(g) Sug.	(g) Prot.	(mg) Sod.
Cereals, Ready-to-eat, Kashi 7 Whole Grain Nuggets									
.5 cup (1 NLEA serving) (58g)	206	2	0	0	47	6.8	3	7	260
Cereals, Ready-to-eat, Kashi GoLean									
1 cup (1 NLEA serving) (52g)	148	1	0	0	30	10.2	6	14	86
Cereals, Ready-to-eat, Kashi GoLean Crunch!									
1 cup (1 NLEA serving) (53g)	200	3	0	0	36	8.1	13	9	101
Cereals, Ready-to-eat, Kashi GoLean Crunch!, Honey Almond Flax									
1 cup (1 NLEA serving) (53g)	202	4	0	0	36	8.6	12	9	138
Cereals, Ready-to-eat, Kashi Good Friends									
1 cup (1 NLEA serving) (53g)	167	2	0	0	43	11.8	9	5	106
Cereals, Ready-to-eat, Kashi Granola, Cocoa Beach Cereal									
.5 cup (1 NLEA serving) (55g)	226	9	2	0	34	7.0	11	6	138
Cereals, Ready-to-eat, Kashi Granola, Mountain Medley Cereal									
.5 cup (1 NLEA serving) (55g)	218	7	1	0	37	6.3	12	6	121
Cereals, Ready-to-eat, Kashi Granola, Orchard Spice Cereal									
.5 cup (1 NLEA serving) (55g)	222	7	1	0	37	6.3	11	6	132
Cereals, Ready-to-eat, Kashi Granola, Summer Berry Cereal									
.5 cup (1 NLEA serving) (55g)	215	6	1	0	37	6.8	9	7	132
Cereals, Ready-to-eat, Kashi Heart to Heart Warm Cinnamon									
.75 cup (1 NLEA serving) (33g)	117	2	0	0	25	4.7	5	4	80
Cereals, Ready-to-eat, Kashi Heart to Heart, Honey Toasted Oat									
.75 cup (1 NLEA serving) (33g)	118	2	0	0	25	4.4	6	4	83
Cereals, Ready-to-eat, Kashi Mighty Bites, Honey Crunch Cereal									
1 cup (1 NLEA serving) (33g)	116	1	0	0	23	3.0	6	6	159
Cereals, Ready-to-eat, Kashi Organic Promise Cinnamon Harvest									
1 cup (1 NLEA serving) (54g)	184	1	0	0	44	5.6	9	4	5
Cereals, Ready-to-eat, Kashi Organic Promise Island Vanilla Biscuit									
27 biscuits (1 NLEA serving) (55g)	193	1	0	0	44	5.9	9	6	6
Cereals, Ready-to-eat, Kashi Organic Promise Strawberry Fields									
1 cup (1 NLEA serving) (32g)	118	0	0	0	28	1.1	9	2	200
Cereals, Ready-to-eat, Kashi, Cinna-Raisin Crunch									
1 cup (50g)	165	1	0	0	41	7.6	13	4	104
Cereals, Ready-to-eat, Kashi, Heart to Heart, Wild Blueberry									
1 cup (1 NLEA serving) (55g)	204	3	0	0	42	3.9	12	6	133

Food Serving size	Cal.	(g) Total Fat	(g) Sat. Fat	(mg) Chol.	(g) Carb.	(g) Fiber	(g) Sug.	(g) Prot.	(mg) Sod.
Cereals, Ready-to-eat, Kashi, Kashi U 1 cup (1 NLEA serving) (55g)	202	4	0	0	42	6.6	10	6	127
Cereals, Ready-to-eat, Kashi, Organic Promise Autumn Wheat 1 cup (1 NLEA serving) (54g)	191	1	0	0	45	6.0	7	5	0
Cereals, Ready-to-eat, Kellogg's Corn Flakes 1 cup (1 NLEA serving) (28g)	101	0	0	0	24	0.7	3	2	202
Cereals, Ready-to-eat, Kellogg's Frosted Mini-Wheats, Original 5 biscuits (1 NLEA serving) (51g)	175	1	0	0	42	5.1	11	5	5
Cereals, Ready-to-eat, Kellogg's Fruit Harvest Strawberry/Blueberry .75 cup (1 NLEA serving) (29g)	107	0	0	0	25	1.3	10	2	137
Cereals, Ready-to-eat, Kellogg's Honey Crunch Corn Flakes .75 cup (1 NLEA serving) (30g)	116	1	0	0	26	1.0	10	2	210
Cereals, Ready-to-eat, Kellogg's Mini-Wheats, Frosted Strawberry Delight 24 biscuit (1 NLEA serving) (52g)	180	1	0	0	43	5.0	12	4	0
Cereals, Ready-to-eat, Kellogg's Special K, Vanilla Almond .75 cup (1 NLEA serving) (30g)	115	1	0	0	25	1.7	8	2	170
Cereals, Ready-to-eat, Kellogg's Special K, Low Carb Lifestyle Protein Plus .75 cup (1 NLEA serving) (29g)	101	3	1	0	14	4.9	2	10	110
Cereals, Ready-to-eat, Kellogg's, All-Bran Buds .333 cup (1 NLEA serving) (30g)	75	1	0	0	24	12.9	8	2	204
Cereals, Ready-to-eat, Kellogg's, All-Bran Strawberry Medley 1 cup (1 NLEA serving) (55g)	175	2	0	0	44	9.9	10	6	231
Cereals, Ready-to-eat, Kellogg's, All-Bran with Extra Fiber .5 cup (1 NLEA serving) (26g)	50	1	0	0	20	13.0	0	3	124
Cereals, Ready-to-eat, Kellogg's, All-Bran Yogurt Bites 1.25 cup (1 NLEA serving) (56g)	192	3	2	0	44	10.1	7	6	235
Cereals, Ready-to-eat, Kellogg's, All-Bran, Original .5 cup (1 NLEA serving) (31g)	81	2	0	0	23	9.1	5	4	81
Cereals, Ready-to-eat, Kellogg's, Apple Jacks 1 cup (1 NLEA serving) (28g)	102	1	0	0	25	2.6	12	1	124
Cereals, Ready-to-eat, Kellogg's, Berry Rice Krispies 1 cup (1 NLEA serving) (30g)	115	0	0	0	26	0.1	9	2	218
Cereals, Ready-to-eat, Kellogg's, Cinnabon Cereal 1 cup (1 NLEA serving) (30g)	123	2	0	0	25	1.2	12	2	116

Food Serving size	Cal.	(g) Total Fat	(g) Sat. Fat	(mg) Chol.	(g) Carb.	(g) Fiber	(g) Sug.	(g) Prot.	(mg) Sod.
Cereals, Ready-to-eat, Kellogg's, Cinnamon Mini Swirlz									
1 cup (1 NLEA serving) (30g)	122	2	0	0	25	1.0	3	2	116
Cereals, Ready-to-eat, Kellogg's, Cocoa Krispies									
.75 cup (1 NLEA serving) (31g)	118	1	1	0	27	0.6	11	2	131
Cereals, Ready-to-eat, Kellogg's, Complete Oat Bran Flakes									
.75 cup (1 NLEA serving) (30g)	105	1	0	0	23	3.9	6	3	210
Cereals, Ready-to-eat, Kellogg's, Complete Wheat Flakes									
.75 cup (1 NLEA serving) (29g)	92	1	0	0	23	5.1	5	3	209
Cereals, Ready-to-eat, Kellogg's, Corn Pops									
1 cup (1 NLEA serving) (32g)	124	0	0	0	29	2.9	10	1	124
Cereals, Ready-to-eat, Kellogg's, Cracklin' Oat Bran									
.75 cup (1 NLEA serving) (49g)	197	7	3	0	35	6.2	16	4	151
Cereals, Ready-to-eat, Kellogg's, Crispix									
1 cup (laboratory weight) (30g)	113	0	0	0	26	0.3	4	2	225
Cereals, Ready-to-eat, Kellogg's, Eggo Crunch Cereal, Maple Flavor									
1 cup (1 NLEA serving) (31g)	117	1	0	0	26	1.8	12	2	146
Cereals, Ready-to-eat, Kellogg's, Froot Loops									
1 cup (1 NLEA serving) (29g)	108	1	1	0	25	2.8	12	1	132
Cereals, Ready-to-eat, Kellogg's, Frosted Flakes									
1 cup (39g)	143	0	0	0	35	0.7	15	2	180
Cereals, Ready-to-eat, Kellogg's, Frosted Mini-Wheats, Bite-size									
24 biscuit (1 NLEA serving) (59g)	203	1	0	0	48	5.9	12	6	6
Cereals, Ready-to-eat, Kellogg's, Frosted Mini-Wheats, Bite-size Strawberry									
24 biscuits (1 NLEA serving) (52g)	180	1	0	0	43	5.0	12	4	0
Cereals, Ready-to-eat, Kellogg's, Frosted Mini-Wheats, Maple and Brown Sugar, Bite-size									
24 biscuit (1 NLEA serving) (52g)	185	1	0	0	43	5.0	12	4	1
Cereals, Ready-to-eat, Kellogg's, Frosted Rice Krispies									
.75 cup (1 NLEA serving) (30g)	115	0	0	0	27	0.1	12	2	111
Cereals, Ready-to-eat, Kellogg's, Honey Smacks									
.75 cup (1 NLEA serving) (27g)	105	1	0	0	24	1.0	15	2	51
Cereals, Ready-to-eat, Kellogg's, Just Right Fruit and Nut									
.75 cup (1 NLEA serving) (53g)	194	2	0	0	43	2.8	13	4	243

Food Serving size	Cal.	(g) Total Fat	(g) Sat. Fat	(mg) Chol.	(g) Carb.	(g) Fiber	(g) Sug.	(g) Prot.	(mg) Sod.
Cereals, Ready-to-eat, Kellogg's, Low Fat Granola with Raisins .667 cup (1 NLEA serving) (60g)									
	226	3	1	0	47	4.2	17	5	144
Cereals, Ready-to-eat, Kellogg's, Low Fat Granola Without Raisins .5 cup (1 NLEA serving) (49g)	190	3	1	0	40	3.0	14	4	107
Cereals, Ready-to-eat, Kellogg's, Marshmallow Froot Loops 1 cup (1 NLEA serving) (30g)	112	1	0	0	26	2.0	15	1	115
Cereals, Ready-to-eat, Kellogg's, Mueslix .667 cup (1 NLEA serving) (55g)	196	3	0	0	40	4.0	17	5	170
Cereals, Ready-to-eat, Kellogg's, Product 19 1 cup (1 NLEA serving) (30g)	100	0	0	0	25	1.0	4	2	207
Cereals, Ready-to-eat, Kellogg's, Puffed Wheat .75 cup (1 NLEA serving) (9g)	29	0	0	0	7	1.4	0	1	0
Cereals, Ready-to-eat, Kellogg's, Raisin Bran 1 cup (1 NLEA serving) (59g)	190	1	0	0	46	6.5	18	5	251
Cereals, Ready-to-eat, Kellogg's, Raisin Bran Crunch 1 cup (1 NLEA serving) (53g)	188	1	0	0	45	4.0	20	3	207
Cereals, Ready-to-eat, Kellogg's, Reduced Sugar Froot Loops 1.25 cup (1 NLEA serving) (32g)									
	126	1	0	0	27	3.3	10	2	179
Cereals, Ready-to-eat, Kellogg's, Reduced Sugar Frosted Flakes Cereal 1 cup (1 NLEA serving) (31g)	117	0	0	0	28	0.3	8	2	177
Cereals, Ready-to-eat, Kellogg's, Rice Krispies 1 cup (28g)	108	0	0	0	24	0.2	3	2	157
Cereals, Ready-to-eat, Kellogg's, Rice Krispies Treats Cereal .75 cup (1 NLEA serving) (30g)	120	1	0	0	25	0.1	9	1	165
Cereals, Ready-to-eat, Kellogg's, Shredded Wheat Miniatures 30 biscuits (1 NLEA serving) (30g)									
	102	1	0	0	24	3.9	1	3	0
Cereals, Ready-to-eat, Kellogg's, Smart Start Antioxidants Cereal 1 cup (1 NLEA serving) (50g)	183	1	0	0	43	2.7	14	4	275
Cereals, Ready-to-eat, Kellogg's, Smart Start Strong Heart, Original 1.25 cup (1 NLEA serving) (60g)									
	220	2	0	0	47	5.3	17	6	140

Food Serving size	Cal.	(g) Total Fat	(g) Sat. Fat	(mg) Chol.	(g) Carb.	(g) Fiber	(g) Sug.	(g) Prot.	(mg) Sod.
Cereals, Ready-to-eat, Kellogg's, Smart Start, Maple Brown Sugar 1.25 cup (1 NLEA serving) (60g)	220	2	0	0	47	5.1	17	6	138
Cereals, Ready-to-eat, Kellogg's, Smorz 1 cup (1 NLEA serving) (30g)	122	2	1	0	25	0.8	13	1	138
Cereals, Ready-to-eat, Kellogg's, Special K 1 cup (1 NLEA serving) (31g)	117	1	0	0	23	2.6	4	6	204
Cereals, Ready-to-eat, Kellogg's, Special K Low Fat Granola .75 cup (1 NLEA serving) (52g)	198	3	1	0	39	6.1	9	7	125
Cereals, Ready-to-eat, Kellogg's, Special K Red Berries 1 cup (1 NLEA serving) (31g)	111	0	0	0	27	2.5	9	2	190
Cereals, Ready-to-eat, Kellogg's, Special K, Blueberry .75 cup (1 NLEA serving) (30g)	109	0	0	0	26	3.0	8	2	141
Cereals, Ready-to-eat, Kellogg's, Special K, Chocolatey Delight .75 cup (1 NLEA serving) (31g)	122	2	2	1	25	2.2	9	2	179
Cereals, Ready-to-eat, Kellogg's, Special K, Cinnamon Pecan .75 cup (1 NLEA serving) (30g)	115	2	0	0	24	2.4	7	2	195
Cereals, Ready-to-eat, Kellogg's, Special K, Fruit and Yogurt .75 cup (1 NLEA serving) (32g)	119	1	0	0	27	1.5	11	2	146
Cereals, Ready-to-eat, Malt-O-Meal, Apple Zings 1 cup (33g)	130	1	0	0	29	0.9	14	2	150
Cereals, Ready-to-eat, Malt-O-Meal, Berry Colossal Crunch .75 cup (1 NLEA serving) (30g)	124	2	0	0	26	1.0	12	1	220
Cereals, Ready-to-eat, Malt-O-Meal, Blueberry Muffin Tops Cereal .75 cup (30g)	133	3	1	0	24	1.4	11	1	140
Cereals, Ready-to-eat, Malt-O-Meal, Cinnamon Toasters .75 cup (30g)	129	3	1	0	24	1.4	10	2	138
Cereals, Ready-to-eat, Malt-O-Meal, Cocoa Dyno-Bites .75 cup (29g)	117	1	1	0	26	0.3	13	1	150
Cereals, Ready-to-eat, Malt-O-Meal, Coco-Roos .75 cup (1 NLEA serving) (30g)	119	1	0	0	27	0.5	14	1	135
Cereals, Ready-to-eat, Malt-O-Meal, Colossal Crunch .75 cup (30g)	125	2	0	0	26	0.2	12	1	230
Cereals, Ready-to-eat, Malt-O-Meal, Corn Bursts 1 cup (31g)	122	0	0	0	29	0.6	14	1	270

Food Serving size	Cal.	(g) Total Fat	(g) Sat. Fat	(mg) Chol.	(g) Carb.	(g) Fiber	(g) Sug.	(g) Prot.	(mg) Sod.
Cereals, Ready-to-eat, Malt-O-Meal, Crispy Rice									
1 cup (1 NLEA serving) (33g)	126	0	0	0	29	0.3	3	2	300
Cereals, Ready-to-eat, Malt-O-Meal, Frosted Flakes									
1 cup (40g)	155	0	0	0	36	0.8	15	2	229
Cereals, Ready-to-eat, Malt-O-Meal, Frosted Mini Spooners									
1 cup (55g)	213	1	0	1	46	5.8	10	5	10
Cereals, Ready-to-eat, Malt-O-Meal, Fruity Dyno-Bites									
.75 cup (27g)	109	1	0	0	24	0.3	12	1	170
Cereals, Ready-to-eat, Malt-O-Meal, Golden Puffs									
1 cup (37g)	147	0	0	0	33	1.0	19	2	89
Cereals, Ready-to-eat, Malt-O-Meal, Honey Buzzers									
1.333 cup (29g)	115	1	0	0	25	0.8	11	2	220
Cereals, Ready-to-eat, Malt-O-Meal, Honey Graham Squares									
.75 cup (1 NLEA serving) (30g)	130	3	1	0	24	1.0	10	1	270
Cereals, Ready-to-eat, Malt-O-Meal, Honey Nut Toasty O's Cereal									
1 cup (30g)	117	1	0	0	24	1.7	12	3	210
Cereals, Ready-to-eat, Malt-O-Meal, Maple & Brown Sugar Hot Wheat Cereal, Dry									
.25 cup (45g)	170	0	0	0	38	1.4	16	4	5
Cereals, Ready-to-eat, Malt-O-Meal, Marshmallows Mateys									
1 cup (30g)	118	1	0	0	25	1.4	13	2	200
Cereals, Ready-to-eat, Malt-O-Meal, Puffed Rice Cereal									
1 cup (15g)	60	0	0	0	14	0.2	0	1	1
Cereals, Ready-to-eat, Malt-O-Meal, Puffed Wheat Cereal									
1 cup (15g)	59	0	0	0	12	1.1	0	2	2
Cereals, Ready-to-eat, Malt-O-Meal, Raisin Bran Cereal									
1 cup (59g)	213	1	0	1	45	8.0	18	5	340
Cereals, Ready-to-eat, Malt-O-Meal, Toasty O's									
1 cup (1 NLEA serving) (30g)	121	2	0	0	22	3.2	1	4	269
Cereals, Ready-to-eat, Malt-O-Meal, Tootie Fruities									
1 cup (1 NLEA serving) (32g)	128	1	0	0	28	0.8	15	2	148
Cereals, Ready-to-eat, Nature's Path, Optimum									
1 cup (55g)	190	3	0	0	40	10.0	16	8	230
Cereals, Ready-to-eat, Nature's Path, Optimum Slim									
1 cup (55g)	180	3	0	0	38	11.0	10	9	290

Food Serving size	Cal.	(g) Total Fat	(g) Sat. Fat	(mg) Chol.	(g) Carb.	(g) Fiber	(g) Sug.	(g) Prot.	(mg) Sod.
Cereals, Ready-to-eat, Oat, Corn & Wheat Squares, Presweetened, Maple Flavor									
1 cup (1 NLEA serving) (30g)	129	3	0	0	24	0.5	11	2	130
Cereals, Ready-to-eat, Post Blueberry Morning									
1.25 cup (1 NLEA serving) (55g)	211	2	0	0	44	2.1	11	4	260
Cereals, Ready-to-eat, Post Raisin Bran Cereal									
1 cup (1 NLEA serving) (59g)	187	1	0	0	45	7.1	17	6	250
Cereals, Ready-to-eat, Post Selects, Cranberry Almond Crunch									
.75 cup (1 NLEA serving) (51g)	197	3	0	0	40	3.1	13	4	115
Cereals, Ready-to-eat, Post Shredded Wheat n' Bran, Spoon-size									
1.25 cup (1 NLEA serving) (59g)	197	1	0	0	47	7.9	9	7	3
Cereals, Ready-to-eat, Post Toasties Corn Flakes									
1 box, single serving (.75 oz) (21g)	76	0	0	0	18	0.9	1	1	150
Cereals, Ready-to-eat, Post, 100% Bran Cereal									
.333 cup (1 NLEA serving) (29g)	83	1	0	0	23	8.3	7	4	121
Cereals, Ready-to-eat, Post, Alpha-Bits									
1 box, single serving (.75 oz) (21g)	85	1	0	0	18	0.9	8	2	120
Cereals, Ready-to-eat, Post, Cocoa Pebbles									
.75 cup (1 NLEA serving) (30g)	119	1	1	0	26	0.5	13	1	190
Cereals, Ready-to-eat, Post, Fruity Pebbles									
.75 cup (1 NLEA serving) (30g)	120	1	0	0	26	0.2	13	1	190
Cereals, Ready-to-eat, Post, Golden Crisp									
.75 cup (1 NLEA serving) (27g)	107	0	0	0	25	0.0	15	1	25
Cereals, Ready-to-eat, Post, Grape-Nuts Cereal									
1 cup (115g)	413	2	0	0	92	10.1	15	14	575
Cereals, Ready-to-eat, Post, Grape-Nuts Flakes									
.75 cup (1 NLEA serving) (29g)	106	1	0	0	24	2.6	5	3	125
Cereals, Ready-to-eat, Post, Great Grains Crunchy Pecan Cereal									
.667 cup (1 NLEA serving) (53g)	216	6	1	0	38	3.7	8	5	214
Cereals, Ready-to-eat, Post, Honey Nut Shredded Wheat									
1 cup (1 NLEA serving) (52g)	200	2	0	0	42	4.0	12	5	70

Food Serving size	Cal.	(g) Total Fat	(g) Sat. Fat	(mg) Chol.	(g) Carb.	(g) Fiber	(g) Sug.	(g) Prot.	(mg) Sod.
Cereals, Ready-to-eat, Post, Honeycomb Cereal 1.5 cup (1 NLEA serving) (32g)	126	1	0	0	28	0.8	12	2	180
Cereals, Ready-to-eat, Post, Oreo O's Cereal .75 cup (27g)	112	2	0	0	22	1.5	13	1	128
Cereals, Ready-to-eat, Post, Shredded Wheat, Bite-size 1 cup (1 NLEA serving) (52g)	183	1	0	0	44	5.0	12	4	10
Cereals, Ready-to-eat, Post, Shredded Wheat, Spoon-size 1 box, single serving (.875 oz) (25g)	85	0	0	0	21	2.9	0	3	2
Cereals, Ready-to-eat, Puffed Kashi 1 cup (1 NLEA serving) (19g)	64	0	0	0	15	1.5	1	2	2
Cereals, Ready-to-eat, Quaker Apple Zaps .75 cup (1 NLEA serving) (30g)	118	1	0	0	27	0.7	14	1	135
Cereals, Ready-to-eat, Quaker Cocoa Blasts 1 cup (1 NLEA serving) (33g)	130	1	0	0	29	0.8	16	1	135
Cereals, Ready-to-eat, Quaker Fruitangy Oh!s 1 cup (1 NLEA serving) (31g)	122	1	0	0	27	0.8	13	2	152
Cereals, Ready-to-eat, Quaker Oat Cinnamon Life .75 cup (1 NLEA serving) (32g)	119	1	0	0	25	2.0	8	3	153
Cereals, Ready-to-eat, Quaker, 100% Natural Cereal with Oats, Honey and Raisins .5 cup (1 NLEA serving) (51g)	213	6	4	1	38	3.3	15	5	127
Cereals, Ready-to-eat, Quaker, 100% Natural Granola Oats and Honey .5 cup (1 NLEA serving) (48g)	206	6	4	0	35	3.3	12	5	24
Cereals, Ready-to-eat, Quaker, Cap'n Crunch .75 cup (1 NLEA serving) (27g)	109	2	1	0	23	0.7	12	1	211
Cereals, Ready-to-eat, Quaker, Cap'n Crunch with Crunchberries .75 cup (1 NLEA serving) (26g)	105	1	1	0	22	0.7	12	1	186
Cereals, Ready-to-eat, Quaker, Cap'n Crunch's Peanut Butter Crunch .75 cup (1 NLEA serving) (27g)	112	2	1	0	21	0.7	9	2	200
Cereals, Ready-to-eat, Quaker, Cinnamon Oatmeal Squares 1 cup (1 NLEA serving) (60g)	227	3	0	0	48	4.9	13	6	263
Cereals, Ready-to-eat, Quaker, Honey Graham Life Cereal .75 cup (1 NLEA serving) (32g)	119	1	0	0	25	2.0	7	3	156
Cereals, Ready-to-eat, Quaker, Honey Graham Oh!s .75 cup (1 NLEA serving) (27g)	111	2	2	0	23	0.5	12	1	165

Food Serving size	Cal.	(g) Total Fat	(g) Sat. Fat	(mg) Chol.	(g) Carb.	(g) Fiber	(g) Sug.	(g) Prot.	(mg) Sod.
Cereals, Ready-to-eat, Quaker, King Vitaman									
1.5 cup (1 NLEA serving) (31g)	120	1	0	0	26	1.1	6	2	259
Cereals, Ready-to-eat, Quaker, Kretschmer Honey Crunch Wheat Germ									
1.667 tbsp (1 NLEA serving) (14g)	52	1	0	0	8	1.4	3	4	2
Cereals, Ready-to-eat, Quaker, Kretschmer Toasted Wheat Bran									
.25 cup (1 NLEA serving) (16g)	32	1	0	0	10	6.6	--	3	1
Cereals, Ready-to-eat, Quaker, Kretschmer Wheat Germ, Regular									
1.67 tbsp (14g)	51	1	0	0	7	1.7	--	4	1
Cereals, Ready-to-eat, Quaker, Low Fat 100% Natural Granola with Raisins									
.67 cup (1 NLEA serving) (55g)	215	3	1	0	45	3.1	18	4	139
Cereals, Ready-to-eat, Quaker, Marshmallow Safari									
.75 cup (1 NLEA serving) (30g)	119	2	0	0	25	1.3	14	2	192
Cereals, Ready-to-eat, Quaker, Mother's Cinnamon Oat Crunch									
1 cup (1 NLEA serving) (60g)	228	3	0	0	48	5.0	15	6	251
Cereals, Ready-to-eat, Quaker, Mother's Cocoa Bumpers									
1 cup (1 NLEA serving) (33g)	124	1	0	0	29	1.0	14	2	156
Cereals, Ready-to-eat, Quaker, Mother's Toasted Oat Bran Cereal, Brown Sugar									
.75 cup (1 NLEA serving) (32g)	119	2	0	--	24	2.8	5	4	202
Cereals, Ready-to-eat, Quaker, Oat Bran Cereal									
1.25 cup (57g)	212	3	1	0	43	5.6	9	7	207
Cereals, Ready-to-eat, Quaker, Oatmeal Cereal, Brown Sugar Bliss									
1 cup (49g)	188	3	1	0	39	3.6	--	4	249
Cereals, Ready-to-eat, Quaker, Oatmeal Squares									
1 cup (1 NLEA serving) (56g)	212	2	1	0	44	4.0	9	6	250
Cereals, Ready-to-eat, Quaker, Puffed Rice									
1 cup (1 NLEA serving) (14g)	54	0	0	0	12	0.2	0	1	1
Cereals, Ready-to-eat, Quaker, Puffed Wheat									
1.25 cup (1 NLEA serving) (15g)	55	0	0	0	11	1.4	0	2	1
Cereals, Ready-to-eat, Quaker, Quaker Crunchy Bran									
.75 cup (1 NLEA serving) (27g)	90	1	1	0	23	4.7	6	2	234
Cereals, Ready-to-eat, Quaker, Quaker Oat Life, Plain									
.75 cup (1 NLEA serving) (32g)	119	1	0	0	25	2.1	6	3	176
Cereals, Ready-to-eat, Quaker, Sun Country Granola with Almonds									
.5 cup (1 NLEA serving) (57g)	266	10	1	0	38	3.0	12	7	19

Food Serving size	Cal.	(g) Total Fat	(g) Sat. Fat	(mg) Chol.	(g) Carb.	(g) Fiber	(g) Sug.	(g) Prot.	(mg) Sod.
Cereals, Ready-to-eat, Quaker, Sweet Crunch/Quisp									
1 cup (1 NLEA serving) (27g)	109	2	1	0	23	0.6	12	1	200
Cereals, Ready-to-eat, Quaker, Sweet Puffs									
1 cup (34g)	133	1	0	0	30	1.2	16	2	80
Cereals, Ready-to-eat, Quaker, Toasted Oatmeal Cereal									
1 cup (1 NLEA serving) (49g)	188	2	1	--	39	2.7	12	5	274
Cereals, Ready-to-eat, Quaker, Toasted Oatmeal Cereal, Honey Nut									
1 cup (1 NLEA serving) (49g)	188	2	1	0	40	2.7	12	4	228
Cereals, Ready-to-eat, Ralston Corn Biscuits									
1 cup (31g)	114	0	0	--	27	0.8	3	2	332
Cereals, Ready-to-eat, Ralston Corn Flakes									
1 cup (31g)	111	0	0	--	27	0.8	2	2	220
Cereals, Ready-to-eat, Ralston Crispy Hexagons									
1 cup (28g)	106	0	0	--	24	0.4	3	2	228
Cereals, Ready-to-eat, Ralston Crispy Rice									
1 cup (28g)	102	0	0	0	24	0.2	2	2	214
Cereals, Ready-to-eat, Ralston Tasteeos									
1 cup (28g)	111	2	0	0	21	3.0	1	3	239
Cereals, Ready-to-eat, Ralston, Enriched Bran Flakes									
1 cup (42g)	130	1	0	--	34	7.1	7	4	341
Cereals, Ready-to-eat, Rice, Puffed, Fortified									
.5 oz (14.2g)	57	0	0	0	13	0.2	--	1	0
Cereals, Ready-to-eat, Rolled Oats, Whole Wheat, Rice, Maple flavor, with Pecans									
1 serving (1 NLEA serving) (52g)	219	5	2	0	40	3.1	13	4	145
Cereals, Ready-to-eat, Uncle Sam Cereal									
1 cup (1 serving) (55g)	237	6	1	0	36	11.2	1	9	113
Cereals, Ready-to-eat, Waffelos									
1 oz (28.35g)	115	1	--	0	24	--	--	2	118
Cereals, Ready-to-eat, Wheat and Malt Barley Flakes									
1 box, single serving (.75 oz) (21g)	77	1	0	0	17	1.8	4	2	101
Cereals, Ready-to-eat, Wheat Germ, Toasted, Plain									
1 oz (28.35g)	108	3	1	0	14	4.3	2	8	1
Cereals, Ready-to-eat, Wheat, Puffed, Fortified									
.5 oz (14.2g)	52	0	0	0	11	0.6	--	2	1

Food Serving size	Cal.	(g) Total Fat	(g) Sat. Fat	(mg) Chol.	(g) Carb.	(g) Fiber	(g) Sug.	(g) Prot.	(mg) Sod.
Cereals, Ready-to-eat, Wheat, Shredded, Plain, Sugar and Salt-free									
1 serving (46g)	155	1	0	0	36	5.5	0	5	3
Cereals, Roman Meal with Oats, Cooked with Water, with Salt									
.75 cup (180g)	128	1	0	0	26	6.1	--	5	405
Cereals, Roman Meal with Oats, Cooked with Water, Without Salt									
.75 cup (180g)	128	1	0	0	26	5.2	--	5	7
Cereals, Roman Meal, Plain, Cooked with Water, with Salt									
.75 cup (181g)	110	1	0	0	25	6.2	--	5	148
Cereals, Roman Meal, Plain, Cooked with Water, Without Salt									
.75 cup (181g)	110	1	0	0	25	6.2	--	5	2
Cereals, Roman Meal, Plain, Dry									
1 tbsp (5.8g)	19	0	0	0	4	1.0	--	1	0
Cereals, Wafer Straws, Kellogg's, Apple Jacks Cereal Straws									
3 straws (1 NLEA serving) (31g)	136	4	2	3	24	0.0	12	2	16
Cereals, Wafer Straws, Kellogg's, Cocoa Krispies Cereal Straws									
3 straws (1 NLEA serving) (31g)	136	4	2	0	24	0.5	12	2	16
Cereals, Wafer Straws, Kellogg's, Froot Loops Cereal Straws									
3 straws (1 NLEA serving) (31g)	136	4	2	5	24	1.0	12	2	15
Cereals, Wheatena, Cooked with Water									
.75 cup (182g)	102	1	0	0	21	4.9	--	4	4
Cereals, Wheatena, Cooked with Water, with Salt									
.75 cup (182g)	107	1	0	0	21	3.6	0	4	433
Cereals, Wheatena, Dry									
.25 cup (35g)	125	1	0	0	26	4.5	1	5	5
Cereals, Whole Wheat Hot Natural Cereal, Cooked with Water, with Salt									
.75 cup (182g)	113	1	0	0	25	2.9	0	4	424
Cereals, Whole Wheat Hot Natural Cereal, Cooked with Water, Without Salt									
.75 cup (182g)	113	1	0	0	25	2.9	0	4	0
Cereals, Whole Wheat Hot Natural Cereal, Dry									
.333 cup (31g)	106	1	0	0	23	2.9	0	3	1
Crisped Rice Bar, Chocolate Chip									
1 bar (1 oz) (28g)	113	4	1	0	20	0.6	--	1	78
Granola Bars, Hard, Almond									
1 bar (24g)	119	6	3	0	15	1.2	--	2	61

Food Serving size	Cal.	(g) Total Fat	(g) Sat. Fat	(mg) Chol.	(g) Carb.	(g) Fiber	(g) Sug.	(g) Prot.	(mg) Sod.
Granola Bars, Hard, Chocolate Chip 1 bar (24g)	105	4	3	0	17	1.1	--	2	83
Granola Bars, Hard, Peanut 1 oz (28.35g)	136	6	1	0	18	1.2	10	3	79
Granola Bars, Hard, Peanut Butter 1 bar (24g)	116	6	1	0	15	0.7	--	2	68
Granola Bars, Hard, Plain 1 bar (1 oz) (28g)	132	6	1	0	18	1.5	--	3	82
Granola Bars, Oats, Fruits and Nuts 1 oz (28.35g)	113	2	0	0	22	1.5	12	2	71
Granola Bars, Soft, Coated, Milk Chocolate Coating, Chocolate Chip 1 bar (1 oz) (28g)	130	7	4	1	18	1.0	--	2	56
Granola Bars, Soft, Coated, Milk Chocolate Coating, Peanut Butter 1 bar (37g)	188	12	6	4	20	1.0	--	4	71
Granola Bars, Soft, Milk Chocolate Coated, Peanut Butter 1 oz (28.35g)	152	9	5	3	15	1.1	--	3	55
Granola Bars, Soft, Uncoated, Chocolate Chip 1 bar (1 oz) (28g)	117	5	2	0	20	1.1	8	2	50
Granola Bars, Soft, Uncoated, Chocolate Chip, Graham and Marshmallow 1 bar (1 oz) (28g)	120	4	3	0	20	1.1	--	2	88
Granola Bars, Soft, Uncoated, Nut and Raisin 1 bar (1 oz) (28g)	127	6	3	0	18	1.6	--	2	71
Granola Bars, Soft, Uncoated, Peanut Butter 1 bar (1 oz) (28g)	119	4	1	0	18	1.2	--	3	115
Granola Bars, Soft, Uncoated, Peanut Butter and Chocolate Chip 1 bar (1 oz) (28g)	121	6	2	0	17	1.2	--	3	92
Granola Bars, Soft, Uncoated, Plain 1 bar (1 oz) (28g)	124	5	2	0	19	1.3	--	2	78
Granola Bars, Soft, Uncoated, Raisin 1 bar (1 oz) (28g)	125	5	3	0	19	1.2	--	2	79
Granola Bars, with Coconut, Chocolate Coated 1 oz (28.35g)	151	9	6	0	16	1.8	--	1	43
Kashi, GoLean Crisp, Toasted Berry Crumble .75 cup (1 NLEA serving) (51g)	188	4	1	0	35	7.6	11	9	124

Food Serving size	Cal.	(g) Total Fat	(g) Sat. Fat	(mg) Chol.	(g) Carb.	(g) Fiber	(g) Sug.	(g) Prot.	(mg) Sod.
Rice and Wheat Cereal Bar 1 bar (22g)	90	2	0	0	16	0.4	7	2	110
Snacks, Granola Bars, Fruit-filled, Nonfat 1 oz (28.35g)	97	0	0	0	22	2.1	16	2	5
Snacks, Granola Bars, Soft Almond, Confectioners Coating 1 bar (35g)	159	7	2	1	21	1.5	0	3	170
Snacks, Granola Bites, Mixed Flavors 1 pkg (20g)	90	4	2	0	13	1.1	0	1	7
Snacks, Kellogg, Kellogg's Rice Krispies Treats Square 1 bar (37g)	153	3	1	0	30	0.2	--	1	130
Snacks, Kellogg's Low Fat Granola Bar, Crunchy Almond/Brown Sugar 1 bar (37g)	144	3	0	0	29	2.3	--	3	108
Snacks, Rice Cakes, Brown Rice, Corn 2 cakes (18g)	69	1	0	0	15	0.5	--	2	30

Breads

Food Serving size	Cal.	(g) Total Fat	(g) Sat. Fat	(mg) Chol.	(g) Carb.	(g) Fiber	(g) Sug.	(g) Prot.	(mg) Sod.
Bread, Banana, Prepared from Recipe, Made with Margarine 1 individual, loaf (include Keebler Elfin Loaves) (57g)	186	6	1	25	31	0.6	--	2	172
Bread, Boston Brown, Canned 1 slice (45g)	88	1	0	0	19	2.1	1	2	284
Bread, Cornbread, Dry Mix, Enriched (Including Corn Muffin Mix) 1 pkg (8.5 oz) (241g)	1007	29	7	5	167	15.7	49	17	1969
Bread, Cornbread, Dry Mix, Prepared 1 piece (60g)	188	6	2	37	29	1.4	--	4	467
Bread, Cornbread, Dry Mix, Unenriched (Including Corn Muffin Mix) 1 pkg (8.5 oz) (241g)	1007	29	7	5	167	15.7	--	17	2678
Bread, Cornbread, Prepared from Recipe, Made with Low Fat (2%) Milk 1 piece (65g)	173	5	1	26	28	--	--	4	428
Bread, Cracked Wheat 1 cubic inch (3.2g)	8	0	0	0	2	0.2	--	0	17
Bread, Egg 1 slice (5" x 3" x 1/2") (40g)	113	2	1	20	19	0.9	1	4	165

Food Serving size	Cal.	(g) Total Fat	(g) Sat. Fat	(mg) Chol.	(g) Carb.	(g) Fiber	(g) Sug.	(g) Prot.	(mg) Sod.
Bread, Egg, Toasted 1 slice (5" x 3" x 1/2") (37g)	117	2	1	21	19	0.9	1	4	200
Bread, French or Vienna (Includes Sourdough) 1 slice, small (2" x 2-1/2" x 1-3/4") (32g)	92	1	0	0	18	0.8	1	4	164
Bread, French or Vienna, Toasted (Includes Sourdough) 1 slice, small (29g)	93	1	0	0	18	0.9	1	4	209
Bread, Irish Soda, Prepared from Recipe 1 oz (28.35g)	82	1	0	5	16	0.7	--	2	113
Bread, Italian 1 slice, large (4-1/2" x 3-1/4" x 3/4") (30g)	81	1	0	0	15	0.8	0	3	175
Bread, Multi-grain (Includes Whole Grain) 1 slice, regular (26g)	69	1	0	0	11	1.9	2	3	109
Bread, Multi-grain, Toasted (Includes Whole Grain) 1 slice, regular (24g)	69	1	0	0	11	1.9	2	3	110
Bread, Oat Bran 1 slice (30g)	71	1	0	0	12	1.4	2	3	122
Bread, Oat Bran, Toasted 1 slice (27g)	70	1	0	0	12	1.3	2	3	121
Bread, Oatmeal 1 slice (27g)	73	1	0	0	13	1.1	2	2	127
Bread, Oatmeal, Toasted 1 slice (25g)	73	1	0	0	13	1.1	2	2	163
Bread, Pan Dulce, Sweet Yeast Bread 1 slice, (average weight of 1 slice) (63g)	231	7	1	--	36	1.4	8	6	144
Bread, Pita, White, Enriched 1 pita, small (4" dia) (28g)	77	0	0	0	16	0.6	0	3	150
Bread, Pita, White, Unenriched 1 pita, large (6-1/2" dia) (60g)	165	1	0	0	33	1.3	--	5	322
Bread, Pita, Whole Wheat 1 pita, small (4" dia) (28g)	74	1	0	0	15	2.1	0	3	149
Bread, Pound Cake Type, Pan de Torta Salvadoran 1 cake, square (622g)	2426	109	19	--	319	10.6	113	44	2426

Food Serving size	Cal.	(g) Total Fat	(g) Sat. Fat	(mg) Chol.	(g) Carb.	(g) Fiber	(g) Sug.	(g) Prot.	(mg) Sod.
Bread, Protein (Including Gluten) 1 slice (19g)	47	0	0	0	8	0.6	0	2	91
Bread, Protein, Toasted (Including Gluten) 1 slice (17g)	46	0	0	0	8	0.6	0	2	102
Bread, Pumpernickel 1 slice, regular (26g)	65	1	0	0	12	1.7	0	2	174
Bread, Pumpernickel, Toasted 1 slice (5" x 4" x 3/8") (29g)	80	1	0	0	15	2.1	0	3	214
Bread, Raisin, Enriched 1 slice, large (32g)	88	1	0	0	17	1.4	2	3	100
Bread, Raisin, Toasted, Enriched 1 slice, large (29g)	86	1	0	0	17	1.4	2	2	123
Bread, Raisin, Unenriched 1 slice, large (32g)	88	1	0	0	17	1.4	--	3	125
Bread, Reduced-calorie, Oat Bran 1 slice (23g)	46	1	0	0	9	2.8	1	2	132
Bread, Reduced-calorie, Oat Bran, Toasted 1 slice (19g)	45	1	0	0	9	2.7	1	2	79
Bread, Reduced-calorie, Oatmeal 1 slice (23g)	48	1	0	0	10	--	--	2	89
Bread, Reduced-calorie, Rye 1 slice (23g)	47	1	0	0	9	2.8	1	2	118
Bread, Reduced-calorie, Wheat 1 slice (23g)	46	1	0	0	10	2.8	1	2	118
Bread, Reduced-calorie, White 1 slice (23g)	48	1	0	0	10	2.2	1	2	104
Bread, Rice Bran 1 slice (27g)	66	1	0	0	12	1.3	1	2	82
Bread, Rice Bran, Toasted 1 slice (25g)	66	1	0	0	12	1.3	1	2	120
Bread, Rye 1 slice, regular (32g)	83	1	0	0	15	1.9	1	3	211
Bread, Rye, Toasted 1 slice, large (29g)	82	1	0	0	15	1.9	1	3	210

Food Serving size	Cal.	(g) Total Fat	(g) Sat. Fat	(mg) Chol.	(g) Carb.	(g) Fiber	(g) Sug.	(g) Prot.	(mg) Sod.
Bread, Salvadoran Sweet Cheese (Quesadilla Salvadorena)									
1 cake, square (average weight of whole item) (399g)	1492	68	18	235	191	2.8	99	28	2035
Bread, Wheat 1 slice (25g)	67	1	0	0	12	0.9	1	3	130
Bread, Wheat Bran 1 slice (36g)	89	1	0	0	17	1.4	3	3	175
Bread, Wheat Germ 1 slice (28g)	73	1	0	0	14	0.6	1	3	155
Bread, Wheat Germ, Toasted 1 slice (25g)	73	1	0	0	14	0.6	1	3	155
Bread, Wheat, Toasted 1 slice (24g)	75	1	0	0	13	1.1	2	3	147
Bread, White, Commercially Prepared (Including Soft Bread Crumbs) 1 cup, crumbs (45g)	120	1	0	0	23	1.1	2	3	230
Bread, White, Commercially Prepared, Low Sodium, No Salt 1 cup, crumbs (45g)	120	2	0	0	22	1.0	2	4	12
Bread, White, Commercially Prepared, Toasted 1 cup, crumbs (45g)	132	2	0	0	24	1.1	2	4	266
Bread, White, Commercially Prepared, Toasted, Low Sodium, No Salt 1 slice (23g)	67	1	0	0	13	--	--	2	7
Bread, White, Prepared from Recipe, Made with Low Fat (2%) Milk 1 slice (42g)	120	2	0	1	21	0.8	--	3	151
Bread, White, Prepared from Recipe, Made with Nonfat Dry Milk 1 slice (44g)	121	1	0	0	24	0.9	--	3	148
Bread, Whole Wheat, Commercially Prepared 1 slice (28g)	69	1	0	0	12	1.9	2	4	132
Bread, Whole Wheat, Commercially Prepared, Toasted 1 slice (25g)	77	1	0	0	13	2.3	1	4	146
Bread, Whole Wheat, Prepared from Recipe 1 slice, regular (4" x 5" x 3/4") (46g)	128	2	0	0	24	2.8	2	4	159
Bread, Whole Wheat, Prepared from Recipe, Toasted 1 slice (42g)	128	2	0	0	24	2.8	2	4	160

Food Serving size	Cal.	(g) Total Fat	(g) Sat. Fat	(mg) Chol.	(g) Carb.	(g) Fiber	(g) Sug.	(g) Prot.	(mg) Sod.
George Weston Bakeries, Thomas' English Muffins									
1 serving (57g)	132	1	0	--	26	--	--	5	197
Rolls, Dinner, Egg									
1 roll (2-1/2" dia) (35g)	107	2	1	18	18	1.3	2	3	161
Rolls, Dinner, Oat Bran									
1 roll (33g)	78	2	0	0	13	1.4	2	3	136
Rolls, Dinner, Plain, Commercially Prepared (Including brown-n-serve)									
1 each (pan, dinner, or small roll) (2" square, 2" high) (25g)	78	2	0	1	13	0.5	1	3	134
Rolls, Dinner, Plain, Prepared from Recipe, Made with Low Fat (2%) Milk									
1 large, roll or bun (3-1/2" dia) (43g)	136	3	1	15	23	0.8	--	4	178
Rolls, Dinner, Rye									
1 medium (36g)	103	1	0	0	19	1.8	0	4	234
Rolls, Dinner, Wheat									
1 roll (1 oz) (28g)	76	2	0	0	13	1.1	0	2	136
Rolls, Dinner, Whole Wheat									
1 roll (hamburger, frankfurter roll) (43g)	114	2	0	0	22	3.2	4	4	172
Rolls, French									
1 roll (38g)	105	2	0	0	19	1.2	0	3	193
Rolls, Hamburger or Hot Dog, Mixed-grain									
1 roll (43g)	113	3	1	0	19	1.6	3	4	197
Rolls, Hamburger or Hot Dog, Plain									
1 roll (43g)	120	2	0	0	21	0.9	3	4	206
Rolls, Hamburger or Hot Dog, Reduced-calorie									
1 roll (43g)	84	1	0	0	18	2.7	2	4	190
Rolls, Hard (Including Kaiser)									
1 roll (3-1/2" dia) (57g)	167	2	0	0	30	1.3	1	6	310
Rolls, Pumpernickel									
1 roll (pan, dinner, or small roll) (2" square, 2" high) (28g)	78	1	0	0	15	1.5	0	3	198
Shortening Bread, Soybean (Hydrogenated) and Cottonseed									
1 cup (205g)	1812	205	45	0	0	0.0	0	0	0

Food Serving size	Cal.	(g) Total Fat	(g) Sat. Fat	(mg) Chol.	(g) Carb.	(g) Fiber	(g) Sug.	(g) Prot.	(mg) Sod.
Baked Products (Including Mixes and Refrigerated Doughs)									
Archway Home Style Cookies, Apple Filled Oatmeal									
1 serving (25g)	98	3	1	2	17	0.4	8	1	83
Archway Home Style Cookies, Apricot Filled									
1 serving (25g)	100	3	1	2	16	0.6	8	1	80
Archway Home Style Cookies, Cherry Filled									
1 serving (25g)	101	4	1	5	16	0.5	8	1	87
Archway Home Style Cookies, Chocolate Chip Drop									
1 serving (25g)	102	4	1	3	16	0.4	7	1	98
Archway Home Style Cookies, Chocolate Chip Ice Box									
1 serving (24g)	119	6	2	3	16	0.5	8	1	65
Archway Home Style Cookies, Coconut Macaroon									
1 serving (22g)	101	5	4	0	13	1.1	10	1	44
Archway Home Style Cookies, Cookies Jar Hermits									
1 serving (25g)	98	2	1	3	18	0.5	9	1	164
Archway Home Style Cookies, Dark Molasses									
1 serving (28g)	114	4	1	0	19	0.3	10	1	155
Archway Home Style Cookies, Date Filled Oatmeal									
1 serving (25g)	100	3	1	2	17	0.5	9	1	83
Archway Home Style Cookies, Dutch Cocoa									
1 serving (24g)	103	4	1	2	17	0.6	8	1	92
Archway Home Style Cookies, Fat-free Devil's Food Cookie									
1 serving (20g)	68	0	0	0	16	0.6	8	1	79
Archway Home Style Cookies, Fat-free Oatmeal Raisin									
1 serving (31g)	108	0	0	14	25	0.7	15	1	179
Archway Home Style Cookies, Frosty Lemon									
1 serving (26g)	112	4	2	0	17	0.2	9	1	117
Archway Home Style Cookies, Fruit & Honey Bar									
1 serving (26g)	106	3	1	4	18	0.5	10	1	107
Archway Home Style Cookies, Gourmet Apple 'n Raisin									
1 serving (26g)	113	4	1	2	17	0.7	9	1	137
Archway Home Style Cookies, Gourmet Oatmeal Pecan									
1 serving (28g)	132	6	2	2	17	0.9	8	2	97
Archway Home Style Cookies, Gourmet Rocky Road									
1 serving (28g)	129	6	1	3	18	0.7	10	1	79

Food Serving size	Cal.	(g) Total Fat	(g) Sat. Fat	(mg) Chol.	(g) Carb.	(g) Fiber	(g) Sug.	(g) Prot.	(mg) Sod.
Archway Home Style Cookies, Gourmet Ruth's Golden Oatmeal									
1 serving (28g)	121	5	1	2	18	0.8	9	2	109
Archway Home Style Cookies, Iced Molasses									
1 serving (28g)	118	4	1	3	19	0.3	11	1	169
Archway Home Style Cookies, Iced Oatmeal									
1 serving (28g)	122	5	1	2	19	0.6	10	1	106
Archway Home Style Cookies, Molasses									
1 serving (26g)	105	3	1	7	18	0.3	9	1	150
Archway Home Style Cookies, Oatmeal									
1 serving (25g)	105	4	1	3	17	0.7	9	1	99
Archway Home Style Cookies, Oatmeal Raisin									
1 serving (26g)	106	3	1	2	18	0.7	10	1	88
Archway Home Style Cookies, Old Fashioned Molasses									
1 serving (26g)	106	3	1	7	18	0.3	9	1	146
Archway Home Style Cookies, Old Fashioned Windmill Cookies									
1 serving (20g)	94	4	1	0	14	0.4	7	1	94
Archway Home Style Cookies, Peanut Butter									
1 serving (21g)	101	5	1	8	12	0.6	7	2	85
Archway Home Style Cookies, Pecan Ice Box									
1 serving (24g)	120	6	1	7	15	0.3	7	1	76
Archway Home Style Cookies, Raspberry Filled									
1 serving (25g)	100	3	1	2	16	0.6	8	1	84
Archway Home Style Cookies, Reduced-fat Ginger Snaps									
1 serving (32g)	136	4	1	0	24	0.4	12	1	130
Archway Home Style Cookies, Ruth's Oatmeal									
1 serving (26g)	111	4	1	4	17	0.7	9	2	114
Archway Home Style Cookies, Strawberry Filled									
1 serving (25g)	100	3	1	2	16	0.6	8	1	94
Archway Home Style Cookies, Sugar									
1 serving (24g)	99	3	1	4	17	0.4	--	1	154
Archway Home Style Cookies, Sugar Free Chocolate Chip									
1 serving (24g)	117	5	2	0	16	0.3	0	1	64
Archway Home Style Cookies, Sugar Free Oatmeal									
1 serving (24g)	106	5	1	0	16	0.5	0	1	74

Food Serving size	Cal.	(g) Total Fat	(g) Sat. Fat	(mg) Chol.	(g) Carb.	(g) Fiber	(g) Sug.	(g) Prot.	(mg) Sod.
Archway Home Style Cookies, Sugar Free Rocky Road									
1 serving (24g)	112	5	1	0	15	0.7	0	1	68
Artificial Blueberry Muffin, Mix, Dry									
1 muffin (31g)	126	3	1	--	24	--	--	1	236
Bagel, Plain, Toasted, Enriched with Calcium Propionate (Includes Onion, Poppy, Sesame)									
1 small bagel (3" dia) (69g)	177	1	0	0	35	1.5	3	7	357
Bagels, Cinnamon-raisin									
1 small bagel (3" dia) (69g)	188	1	0	0	38	1.6	4	7	299
Bagels, Cinnamon-raisin, Toasted									
1 small bagel (3-1/2" to 4" dia) (65g)	191	1	0	0	39	1.6	4	7	225
Bagels, Egg									
1 mini bagel (2-1/2" dia) (26g)	72	1	0	6	14	0.6	--	3	131
Bagels, Oat Bran									
1 small bagel (3" dia) (69g)	176	1	0	0	37	2.5	1	7	407
Bagels, Plain, Enriched, Without Calcium Propionate (Including Onion, Poppy, Sesame)									
1 mini bagel (2-1/2" dia) (26g)	72	0	0	0	14	0.6	--	3	139
Bagels, Plain, Toasted, Enriched with Calcium Propionate (Includes Onion, Poppy, Sesame)									
1 small bagel (3" dia) (65g)	187	1	0	0	37	1.7	4	7	312
Bagels, Plain, Unenriched, with Calcium Propionate (Including Onion, Poppy, Sesame)									
1 mini bagel (2-1/2" dia) (26g)	72	0	0	0	14	0.6	--	3	139
Bagels, Plain, Unenriched, Without Calcium Propionate (Including Onion, Poppy, Sesame)									
1 mini bagel (2-1/2" dia) (26g)	72	0	0	0	14	0.6	--	3	139
Baking Chocolate, Mars Snackfood US, M&M's Milk Chocolate Mini Baking Bits									
1 serving, 0.5 oz, about 1 tbsp (14g)	70	3	2	2	10	0.4	9	1	10
Baking Chocolate, Mars Snackfood US, M&M's Semisweet Chocolate Mini Baking Bits									
1 pkg (net weight, 12 oz) (340g)	1758	89	53	10	224	22.8	180	15	7
Baking Chocolate, Mexican, Squares									
1 tablet (20g)	85	3	2	0	15	0.8	14	1	1

Food Serving size	Cal.	(g) Total Fat	(g) Sat. Fat	(mg) Chol.	(g) Carb.	(g) Fiber	(g) Sug.	(g) Prot.	(mg) Sod.
Baking Chocolate, Unsweetened, Liquid 1 oz (28.35g)	134	14	7	0	10	5.1	0	3	3
Baking Chocolate, Unsweetened, Squares 1 cup, grated (132g)	661	69	43	0	39	21.9	1	17	32
Biscuit, Plain or Buttermilk, Refrigerated Dough, Higher Fat 1 biscuit (43g)	138	6	2	0	19	0.3	3	3	430
Biscuits, Mixed Grain, Refrigerated Dough 1 biscuit (2-1/2" dia) (44g)	116	2	1	0	21	--	--	3	295
Biscuits, Plain or Buttermilk, Commercially Baked 1 large (77g)	281	13	2	1	37	1.0	3	5	607
Biscuits, Plain or Buttermilk, Dry Mix 1 cup, poured from box (128g)	548	20	5	3	81	2.7	15	10	1295
Biscuits, Plain or Buttermilk, Dry Mix, Prepared 1 oz (28.35g)	95	3	1	1	14	0.5	--	2	271
Biscuits, Plain or Buttermilk, Prepared from Recipe 1 biscuit (4" dia) (101g)	357	16	4	3	45	1.5	2	7	586
Biscuits, Plain or Buttermilk, Refrigerated Dough, Higher Fat, Baked 1 biscuit (2-1/2" dia) (27g)	95	4	1	0	13	0.2	2	2	292
Biscuits, Plain or Buttermilk, Refrigerated Dough, Lower Fat 1 biscuit (2" dia) (23g)	59	1	0	0	11	0.4	2	2	227
Biscuits, Plain or Buttermilk, Refrigerated Dough, Lower Fat, Baked 1 biscuit (2-1/4" dia) (21g)	63	1	0	0	12	0.4	2	2	305
Bread Sticks, Plain 1 stick, small (approx 4-1/4" long) (5g)	21	0	0	0	3	0.2	0	1	33
Bread Stuffing, Bread, Dry Mix 1 pkg (6 oz) (170g)	656	6	1	2	130	5.4	14	19	2389
Bread Stuffing, Bread, Dry Mix, Prepared .5 cup (100g)	177	9	2	0	22	2.9	2	3	524
Bread Stuffing, Cornbread, Dry Mix 1 pkg (6 oz) (170g)	661	7	2	0	130	24.3	8	17	2181
Bread Stuffing, Cornbread, Dry Mix, Prepared .5 cup (100g)	179	9	2	0	22	2.9	4	3	455
Cake, Angel Food, Commercially Prepared 1 cake (9" dia x 4") (340g)	877	3	0	0	197	5.1	--	20	2547

Food Serving size	Cal.	(g) Total Fat	(g) Sat. Fat	(mg) Chol.	(g) Carb.	(g) Fiber	(g) Sug.	(g) Prot.	(mg) Sod.
Cake, Angel Food, Dry Mix 1 pkg (14.5 oz) (411g)	1533	2	0	0	350	1.2	182	37	2006
Cake, Angel Food, Dry Mix, Prepared 1 tube, cake (10" dia, 4-3/8" high) (596g)	1532	2	0	0	350	1.2	182	36	3046
Cake, Boston Cream Pie, Commercially Prepared 1 piece (1/6 of pie) (92g)	232	8	2	34	39	1.3	33	2	234
Cake, Carrot, Dry Mix, Pudding Type 1 pkg (18 oz) (510g)	2117	50	8	0	404	--	--	26	2892
Cake, Cherry Fudge with Chocolate Frosting 1 piece (1/8 cake) (71g)	187	9	4	30	27	0.9	23	2	185
Cake, Chocolate, Commercially Prepared with Chocolate Frosting 1 piece (1/8 of 18 oz cake) (64g)	235	10	3	27	35	1.8	--	3	214
Cake, Chocolate, Dry Mix, Pudding Type 1 pkg (18.25 oz) (517g)	2047	48	10	0	407	18.1	238	24	4617
Cake, Chocolate, Dry Mix, Regular 1 pkg (18.50 oz) (524g)	2243	82	17	0	383	12.6	201	31	4323
Cake, Chocolate, Prepared from Recipe Without Frosting 1 piece (1/12 of 9" dia) (95g)	352	14	5	55	51	1.5	--	5	299
Cake, Fruit Cake, Commercially Prepared 1 piece (43g)	139	4	0	2	26	1.6	13	1	138
Cake, German Chocolate, Dry Mix, Pudding Type 1 pkg (18.25 oz) (517g)	2073	49	17	0	414	18.1	256	21	4203
Cake, Gingerbread, Dry Mix 1 pkg (14.5 oz) (411g)	1796	57	14	0	307	7.0	192	18	2700
Cake, Gingerbread, Prepared from Recipe 1 piece (1/9 of 8" square) (74g)	263	12	3	24	36	--	--	3	242
Cake, Marble, Dry Mix, Pudding Type 1 pkg (18.25 oz) (517g)	2151	60	13	0	410	15.0	298	18	3392
Cake, Pineapple Upside-down, Prepared from Recipe 1 piece (1/9 of 8" square) (115g)	367	14	3	25	58	0.9	--	4	367
Cake, Pound, Bimbo Bakeries USA, Panque Casero, Home Baked Style 1 loaf (311g)	1300	67	--	--	152	3.1	89	21	1110

Food Serving size	Cal.	(g) Total Fat	(g) Sat. Fat	(mg) Chol.	(g) Carb.	(g) Fiber	(g) Sug.	(g) Prot.	(mg) Sod.
Cake, Pound, Commercially Prepared, Butter 1 piece (1/12 of 12 oz cake) (28g)									
	109	6	3	62	14	0.1	--	2	111
Cake, Pound, Commercially Prepared, Fat Free 1 cake (340g)	962	4	1	0	207	3.7	117	18	1159
Cake, Pound, Commercially Prepared, Other than All Butter, Enriched 1 piece (1/12 of 12 oz cake) (28g)									
	109	5	1	16	15	0.3	--	1	112
Cake, Pound, Commercially Prepared, Other than All Butter, Unenriched 1 piece (1/12 of 12 oz cake) (28g)	109	5	1	16	15	0.3	--	1	112
Cake, Shortcake, Biscuit-type, Prepared from Recipe 1 oz (28.35g)	98	4	1	1	14	--	--	2	143
Cake, Snack Cakes, Créme-filled, Chocolate with Frosting 1 cupcake (50g)	200	8	2	0	30	1.6	19	2	166
Cake, Snack Cakes, Créme-filled, Sponge 1 cake (42g)	157	5	2	17	27	0.4	16	1	215
Cake, Snack Cakes, Cupcakes, Chocolate with Frosting, Low Fat 1 cupcake (43g)	131	2	0	0	29	1.8	--	2	178
Cake, Sponge, Commercially Prepared 1 piece (1/12 of 16 oz cake) (38g)									
	110	1	0	39	23	0.2	14	2	54
Cake, Sponge, Prepared from Recipe 1 piece (1/12 of 10 inch cake) (63g)									
	187	3	1	107	36	--	--	5	144
Cake, White, Dry Mix, Pudding Type, Enriched 1 pkg (18.50 oz) (524g)	2217	50	12	0	424	3.7	256	20	3485
Cake, White, Dry Mix, Pudding Type, Unenriched 1 pkg (18.50 oz) (524g)	2217	50	12	0	424	3.7	--	20	3485
Cake, White, Dry Mix, Regular 1 pkg (18.50 oz) (524g)	2232	57	9	0	409	4.7	286	24	3479
Cake, White, Dry Mix, Special Dietary (Including Lemon-flavored) 1 pkg (8 oz) (227g)	901	19	3	0	181	--	--	7	590
Cake, White, Prepared from Recipe with Coconut Frosting 1 piece (1/12 of 9" dia) (112g)	399	12	4	1	71	1.1	64	5	318
Cake, White, Prepared from Recipe, Without Frosting 1 piece (1/12 of 9" dia) (74g)	264	9	2	1	42	0.6	26	4	242

Food Serving size	Cal.	(g) Total Fat	(g) Sat. Fat	(mg) Chol.	(g) Carb.	(g) Fiber	(g) Sug.	(g) Prot.	(mg) Sod.
Cake, Yellow, Commercially Prepared, with Chocolate Frosting									
1 piece (1/8 of 18 oz cake) (64g)	243	11	3	35	35	1.2	--	2	216
Cake, Yellow, Commercially Prepared, with Vanilla Frosting									
1 piece (1/8 of 18 oz cake) (64g)	239	9	2	35	38	0.2	--	2	220
Cake, Yellow, Dry Mix, Light									
1 pkg (18.50 oz) (524g)	2117	29	7	0	441	6.8	--	25	3165
Cake, Yellow, Dry Mix, Pudding Type									
1 pkg (18.50 oz) (524g)	2217	51	13	0	419	3.7	232	21	3600
Cake, Yellow, Dry Mix, Regular, Enriched									
1 pkg (18.50 oz) (524g)	2264	61	9	10	409	5.8	227	23	3443
Cake, Yellow, Dry Mix, Regular, Unenriched									
1 pkg (18.50 oz) (524g)	2264	61	9	10	409	5.8	--	23	3443
Cake, Yellow, Prepared from Recipe, Without Frosting									
1 piece (1/12 of 8" dia) (68g)	245	10	3	37	36	0.5	--	4	233
Cheesecake, Commercially Prepared									
1 piece (1/6 of 17 oz cake) (80g)	257	18	8	44	20	0.3	17	4	166
Cheesecake, Prepared from Mix, No-bake-type									
1 piece (1/12 of 9" dia) (99g)	271	13	7	29	35	1.9	--	5	376
Coffee Cake, Cheese									
1 piece (1/6 of 16 oz cake) (76g)	258	12	4	65	34	0.8	--	5	258
Coffee Cake, Cinnamon with Crumb Topping, Commercially Prepared, Enriched									
1 individual, cake (57g)	238	13	3	18	27	1.1	--	4	200
Coffee Cake, Cinnamon with Crumb Topping, Commercially Prepared, Unenriched									
1 individual, cake (57g)	238	13	3	18	27	1.1	--	4	200
Coffee Cake, Cinnamon with Crumb Topping, Dry Mix									
1 pkg (10.5 oz) (298g)	1299	36	9	0	232	5.4	127	14	1776
Coffee Cake, Cinnamon with Crumb Topping, Dry Mix, Prepared									
1 piece (1/8 of 8" x 5-3/4" cake) (56g)	178	5	1	27	30	0.7	17	3	236
Coffee Cake, Créme-filled, with Chocolate Frosting									
1 piece (1/6 of 19 oz cake) (90g)	298	10	3	62	48	1.8	--	5	291

Food Serving size	Cal.	(g) Total Fat	(g) Sat. Fat	(mg) Chol.	(g) Carb.	(g) Fiber	(g) Sug.	(g) Prot.	(mg) Sod.
Coffee Cake, Fruit									
1 piece (1/8 cake) (50g)	156	5	1	4	26	1.3	--	3	193
Cookies, Animal Crackers (Including Arrowroot, Tea Biscuits)									
1 Arrowroot biscuit (include Arrowroot cookie) (4.9g)									
	22	1	0	0	4	0.1	1	0	24
Cookies, Brownies, Commercially Prepared									
1 square, large (2-3/4" sq x 7/8") (56g)									
	227	9	2	10	36	1.2	21	3	144
Cookies, Brownies, Dry Mix, Regular									
1 pkg (21.5 oz) (610g)	2647	91	15	0	467	--	--	24	1848
Cookies, Brownies, Dry Mix, Special Dietary									
1 pkg (8.5 oz) (241g)	1027	30	5	0	194	10.1	--	7	200
Cookies, Brownies, Dry Mix, Special Dietary, Prepared									
1 brownie (2" square) (22g)	84	2	1	0	16	0.8	0	1	21
Cookies, Brownies, Prepared from Recipe									
1 brownie (2" square) (24g)	112	7	2	18	12	--	--	1	82
Cookies, Butter, Commercially Prepared, Enriched									
1 cookie (5g)	23	1	1	6	3	0.0	1	0	12
Cookies, Butter, Commercially Prepared, Unenriched									
1 cookie (5g)	23	1	1	6	3	0.0	--	0	18
Cookies, Chocolate Chip, Commercially Prepared, Regular, Higher Fat, Enriched									
1 cookie, bite size (2.2g)	10	1	0	0	1	0.1	1	0	8
Cookies, Chocolate Chip, Commercially Prepared, Regular, Higher Fat, Unenriched									
1 cookie, medium (2-1/4" dia) (10g)									
	48	2	1	0	7	0.3	--	1	32
Cookies, Chocolate Chip, Commercially Prepared, Regular, Lower Fat									
1 cookie (10g)	45	2	0	0	7	0.4	--	1	38
Cookies, Chocolate Chip, Commercially Prepared, Soft-type									
1 cookie (average weight of 1 cookie) (12.2g)									
	55	3	1	--	8	0.3	5	1	33
Cookies, Chocolate Chip, Commercially Prepared, Special Dietary									
1 cookie, medium (1-5/8" dia) (7g)									
	32	1	0	0	5	0.1	3	0	1
Cookies, Chocolate Chip, Dry Mix									
1 pkg (17.5 oz) (496g)	2465	125	41	0	328	--	--	23	1438

Food Serving size	Cal.	(g) Total Fat	(g) Sat. Fat	(mg) Chol.	(g) Carb.	(g) Fiber	(g) Sug.	(g) Prot.	(mg) Sod.
Cookies, Chocolate Chip, Prepared from Recipe, Made with Butter 1 cookie, medium (2-1/4" dia) (16g)	78	5	2	11	9	--	--	1	55
Cookies, Chocolate Chip, Prepared from Recipe, Made with Margarine 1 bar (2" square) (32g)	156	9	3	10	19	0.9	--	2	116
Cookies, Chocolate Chip, Refrigerated Dough 1 portion, dough spoon from roll (29g)	128	6	2	7	18	0.4	--	1	61
Cookies, Chocolate Chip, Refrigerated Dough, Baked 1 cookie, medium (2-1/4" dia) (12g)	59	3	1	3	8	0.2	--	1	28
Cookies, Chocolate Sandwich, with Créme Filling, Regular 3 cookies (1 NLEA serving) (34g)	159	7	2	0	24	1.0	14	2	171
Cookies, Chocolate Sandwich, with Créme Filling, Regular, Chocolate-coated 1 cookie (17g)	82	4	1	0	11	0.9	11	1	55
Cookies, Chocolate Sandwich, with Créme Filling, Special Dietary 1 cookie (10g)	46	2	0	0	7	0.4	2	0	24
Cookies, Chocolate Sandwich, with Extra Créme Filling 1 cookie (13g)	65	3	1	0	9	0.4	6	1	46
Cookies, Chocolate Wafers 1 cup, crumbs (112g)	485	16	5	2	81	3.8	33	7	773
Cookies, Coconut Macaroons, Prepared from Recipe 1 cookie, medium (2" dia) (24g)	97	3	3	0	17	0.4	17	1	59
Cookies, Fig Bars 1 Figaroo (2 square halves) (43g)	150	3	0	0	30	2.0	20	2	151
Cookies, Fortune 1 cookie (8g)	30	0	0	0	7	0.1	4	0	22
Cookies, Fudge, Cake-type (Including Trolley Cakes) 1 cookie (21g)	73	1	0	0	16	0.6	--	1	40
Cookies, Ginger Snaps 1 cookie (7g)	29	1	0	0	5	0.2	1	0	39
Cookies, Graham Crackers, Chocolate-coated 1 cracker (2-1/2" square) (14g)	68	3	2	0	9	0.4	6	1	36

Food Serving size	Cal.	(g) Total Fat	(g) Sat. Fat	(mg) Chol.	(g) Carb.	(g) Fiber	(g) Sug.	(g) Prot.	(mg) Sod.
Cookies, Graham Crackers, Plain or Honey (Including Cinnamon)									
1 cup, crushed (84g)	355	8	1	0	65	2.4	26	6	401
Cookies, Ladyfingers, with Lemon Juice and Rind									
1 anisette sponge (4" x 1-1/8" x 7/8") (13g)	47	1	0	29	8	0.1	3	1	19
Cookies, Ladyfingers, Without Lemon Juice and Rind									
1 anisette sponge (4" x 1-1/8" x 7/8") (13g)	47	1	0	29	8	0.1	--	1	19
Cookies, Marshmallow, Chocolate-coated (Including Marshmallow Pies)									
1 Fudge Marshmallow (28g)	118	5	1	0	19	0.6	13	1	47
Cookies, Molasses									
1 large (3-1/2" to 4" dia) (include Archway brand) (32g)	138	4	1	0	24	0.3	6	2	147
Cookies, Oatmeal, Commercially Prepared, Fat Free									
1 oz (28.35g)	92	0	0	0	22	2.1	12	2	62
Cookies, Oatmeal, Commercially Prepared, Regular									
1 cookie, big (3-1/2" - 4" dia) (include Archway brand, Grandma brand) (25g)	113	5	1	0	17	0.7	6	2	96
Cookies, Oatmeal, Commercially Prepared, Soft-type									
1 cookie (15g)	61	2	1	1	10	0.4	--	1	52
Cookies, Oatmeal, Commercially Prepared, Special Dietary									
1 cookie, medium (1-5/8" dia) (7g)	31	1	0	0	5	0.2	2	0	1
Cookies, Oatmeal, Dry Mix									
1 pkg (17.5 oz) (496g)	2292	95	24	0	334	--	--	32	2346
Cookies, Oatmeal, Prepared from Recipe, with Raisins									
1 cookie (2-5/8" dia) (15g)	65	2	0	5	10	--	--	1	81
Cookies, Oatmeal, Prepared from Recipe, Without Raisins									
1 cookie (2-5/8" dia) (15g)	67	3	1	5	10	--	--	1	90
Cookies, Oatmeal, Refrigerated Dough									
1 portion, dough for 1 cookie (16g)	68	3	1	4	9	0.4	--	1	47
Cookies, Oatmeal, Refrigerated Dough, Baked									
1 cookie (12g)	57	3	1	3	8	0.3	--	1	39
Cookies, Peanut Butter Sandwich, Regular									
1 cookie (14g)	67	3	1	0	9	0.3	5	1	52

Food Serving size	Cal.	(g) Total Fat	(g) Sat. Fat	(mg) Chol.	(g) Carb.	(g) Fiber	(g) Sug.	(g) Prot.	(mg) Sod.
Cookies, Peanut Butter Sandwich, Special Dietary 1 cookie (10g)	54	3	0	0	5	--	--	1	41
Cookies, Peanut Butter, Commercially Prepared, Regular 1 cookie (15g)	72	4	1	0	9	0.3	5	1	62
Cookies, Peanut Butter, Commercially Prepared, Soft-type 1 cookie (15g)	69	4	1	0	9	0.3	--	1	50
Cookies, Peanut Butter, Prepared from Recipe 1 cookie (3" dia) (20g)	95	5	1	6	12	--	--	2	104
Cookies, Peanut Butter, Refrigerated Dough 1 portion, dough for 1 cookie (16g)	73	4	1	4	8	0.2	--	1	64
Cookies, Peanut Butter, Refrigerated Dough, Baked 1 cookie (12g)	60	3	1	4	7	0.1	--	1	52
Cookies, Raisin, Soft-type 1 cookie (15g)	60	2	1	0	10	0.2	7	1	51
Cookies, Shortbread, Commercially Prepared, Pecan 1 cookie (2" dia) (14g)	76	5	1	5	8	0.3	--	1	39
Cookies, Shortbread, Commercially Prepared, Plain 1 cookie (1-5/8" square) (8g)	40	2	0	2	5	0.1	1	0	36
Cookies, Sugar Wafers with Créme Filling, Regular 1 cookie (10.1g)	51	2	1	0	7	0.2	4	0	10
Cookies, Sugar Wafers with Créme Filling, Special Dietary 1 wafer (4g)	20	1	0	0	3	--	--	0	0
Cookies, Sugar, Commercially Prepared, Regular (Including Vanilla) 1 cookie (15g)	72	3	1	8	10	0.1	6	1	54
Cookies, Sugar, Commercially Prepared, Special Dietary 1 cookie, medium (1-5/8" dia) (7g)	30	1	0	0	5	0.1	2	0	0
Cookies, Sugar, Prepared from Recipe, Made with Margarine 1 cookie (3" dia) (14g)	66	3	1	4	8	0.2	3	1	69
Cookies, Sugar, Refrigerated Dough 1 cookie, dough for 1 rolled cookie (17g)	74	4	1	5	10	0.1	4	1	72
Cookies, Sugar, Refrigerated Dough, Baked 1 cookie, 1 rolled cookie dough (15g)	73	3	1	5	10	0.1	4	1	70

Food Serving size	Cal.	(g) Total Fat	(g) Sat. Fat	(mg) Chol.	(g) Carb.	(g) Fiber	(g) Sug.	(g) Prot.	(mg) Sod.
Cookies, Vanilla Sandwich with Créme Filling 1 cookie, oval (3-1/8" x 1-1/4" x 3/8") (15g)	72	3	0	0	11	0.2	6	1	52
Cookies, Vanilla Wafers, Higher Fat 1 wafer (6g)	28	1	0	0	4	0.1	--	0	18
Cookies, Vanilla Wafers, Lower Fat 1 cup, crumbs (80g)	353	12	3	41	59	1.5	30	4	310
Corn Cakes 2 cakes (18g)	70	0	0	0	15	0.3	4	1	88
Corn Cakes, Very Low Sodium 2 cakes (18g)	70	0	0	0	15	--	--	1	5
Corn-based, Extruded, Cones, Plain 1 oz (28.35g)	145	8	6	0	18	0.3	--	2	290
Cornstarch 1 cup (128g)	488	0	0	0	117	1.2	0	0	12
Cracker Meal 1 cup (115g)	440	2	0	0	93	3.0	0	11	18
Crackers, Cheese, Low Sodium 1 cup, Cheez-its (62g)	312	16	6	8	36	1.5	0	6	284
Crackers, Cheese, Regular 1 cup, bite size (62g)	312	16	6	8	36	1.5	0	6	617
Crackers, Cheese, Sandwich-type with Cheese Filling 1 sandwich (6.5g)	32	2	--	0	4	0.1	1	1	57
Crackers, Cheese, Sandwich-type, with Peanut Butter Filling 1 cup, crushed (83g)	412	21	4	0	47	2.8	6	10	758
Crackers, Cream, Gamesa Sabrosas 1 cracker (3.1g)	15	1	0	--	2	0.1	0	0	36
Crackers, Cream, La Moderna Rikis Cream Crackers 1 cracker (3.1g)	13	1	0	--	2	0.1	0	0	23
Crackers, Crispbread, Rye 1 cup, crushed (55g)	201	1	0	0	45	9.1	1	4	249
Crackers, Matzo, Egg 1 matzo (28g)	109	1	0	23	22	0.8	--	3	6
Crackers, Matzo, Egg and Onion 1 matzo (28g)	109	1	0	13	22	1.4	--	3	80

Food Serving size	Cal.	(g) Total Fat	(g) Sat. Fat	(mg) Chol.	(g) Carb.	(g) Fiber	(g) Sug.	(g) Prot.	(mg) Sod.
Crackers, Matzo, Plain 1 matzo (28g)	111	0	0	0	23	0.8	0	3	0
Crackers, Matzo, Whole Wheat 1 matzo (28g)	98	0	0	0	22	3.3	--	4	1
Crackers, Melba Toast, Plain 1 cup, pieces (30g)	117	1	0	0	23	1.9	0	4	179
Crackers, Melba Toast, Plain, Without Salt 1 cup, crushed (70g)	273	2	0	0	54	4.4	--	8	13
Crackers, Melba Toast, Rye (Including Pumpernickel) 1 toast (5g)	19	0	0	0	4	0.4	--	1	45
Crackers, Melba Toast, Wheat 1 toast (5g)	19	0	0	0	4	0.4	--	1	42
Crackers, Milk 1 cracker (11g)	50	2	0	1	8	0.2	2	1	65
Crackers, Rusk Toast 1 rusk (10g)	41	1	0	8	7	--	--	1	25
Crackers, Rye, Sandwich-type, with Cheese Filling 1 cracker, sandwich (7g)	34	2	0	1	4	0.3	--	1	73
Crackers, Rye, Wafers, Plain 1 cup, crushed (61g)	204	1	0	0	49	14.0	1	6	340
Crackers, Rye, Wafers, Seasoned 1 cracker, triple (22g)	84	2	0	0	16	4.6	--	2	195
Crackers, Saltines (Including Oyster, Soda, Soup) 1 cup, crushed (70g)	295	6	1	0	52	2.0	2	7	781
Crackers, Saltines, Fat Free, Low-sodium 6 saltines (30g)	118	0	0	0	25	0.8	0	3	215
Crackers, Saltines, Low Salt (Including Oyster, Soda, Soup) 1 cup, oyster crackers (45g)	189	4	1	0	33	1.3	1	4	89
Crackers, Saltines, Unsalted Tops (Including Oyster, Soda, Soup) 1 cracker (3g)	13	0	0	0	2	0.1	--	0	23
Crackers, Snack, Goya Crackers 1 cracker (12.7g)	55	2	1	--	8	0.5	0	2	84
Crackers, Standard Snack-type, Regular 1 cracker, round (3.2g)	16	1	0	0	2	0.1	0	0	28

Food Serving size	Cal.	(g) Total Fat	(g) Sat. Fat	(mg) Chol.	(g) Carb.	(g) Fiber	(g) Sug.	(g) Prot.	(mg) Sod.
Crackers, Standard Snack-type, Regular, Low Salt									
1 cup, bite size (62g)	311	16	2	0	38	1.0	1	5	134
Crackers, Standard Snack-type, Sandwich, with Cheese Filling									
1 cracker, sandwich (7g)	33	1	0	0	4	0.1	0	1	62
Crackers, Standard Snack-type, Sandwich, with Peanut Butter Filling									
1 cracker, sandwich (7g)	35	2	0	0	4	0.2	1	1	63
Crackers, Wheat, Low Salt									
1 cup, crushed (83g)	393	17	4	0	54	3.7	11	7	158
Crackers, Wheat, Reduced Fat									
1 cracker (1.8g)	8	0	0	0	1	0.1	0	0	16
Crackers, Wheat, Regular									
1 cracker, thin square (2g)	9	0	0	0	1	0.1	0	0	18
Crackers, Wheat, Sandwich, with Cheese Filling									
1 cracker, sandwich (7g)	35	2	0	0	4	0.2	--	1	64
Crackers, Wheat, Sandwich, with Peanut Butter Filling									
1 cracker, sandwich (7g)	35	2	0	0	4	0.3	--	1	56
Crackers, Whole Wheat									
6 crackers, Triscuits, regular size (28g)	120	4	1	0	19	2.9	0	3	197
Crackers, Whole Wheat, Low Salt									
1 cup, crushed (94g)	416	16	3	0	64	9.9	0	8	175
Crackers, Whole Wheat, Reduced Fat									
1 cracker (4.2g)	17	0	0	0	3	0.5	0	0	31
Cream Puffs, Prepared from Recipe, Shell (Including Éclair)									
1 eclair (5" x 2" x 1-3/4") (48g)	174	12	3	94	11	0.4	0	4	267
Cream Puffs, Prepared from Recipe, Shell, with Custard Filling									
1 cream puff (130g)	335	20	5	174	30	0.5	12	9	443
Croissants, Apple									
1 croissant, medium (57g)	145	5	3	18	21	1.4	--	4	156
Croissants, Butter									
1 croissant, mini (28g)	114	6	3	19	13	0.7	3	2	97
Croissants, Cheese									
1 croissant, small (42g)	174	9	4	24	20	1.1	5	4	152

Food Serving size	Cal.	Total Fat (g)	Sat. Fat (g)	Chol. (mg)	Carb. (g)	Fiber (g)	Sug. (g)	Prot. (g)	Sod. (mg)
Croutons, Plain 1 cup (30g)	122	2	0	0	22	1.5	--	4	209
Croutons, Seasoned 1 cup (40g)	186	7	2	3	25	2.0	2	4	436
Danish Pastry, Cheese 1 pastry (71g)	266	16	5	16	26	0.7	5	6	229
Danish Pastry, Cinnamon, Enriched 1 large (approx 7" dia) (142g)	572	32	8	30	63	1.8	28	10	527
Danish Pastry, Cinnamon, Unenriched 1 large (approx 7" dia) (142g)	572	32	8	30	63	1.7	--	10	527
Danish Pastry, Fruit, Enriched 1 large (approx 7" dia) (142g)	527	26	7	162	68	2.7	39	8	503
Danish Pastry, Fruit, Unenriched (Including Apple, Cinnamon, Raisin, Strawberry) 1 container (3 oz) (142g)	527	26	4	57	68	2.7	--	8	503
Danish Pastry, Lemon, Unenriched 1 pastry (71g)	263	13	2	28	34	1.3	--	4	251
Danish Pastry, Nut (Including Almond, Raisin Nut, Cinnamon Nut) 1 pastry (4-1/4" dia) (65g)	280	16	4	30	30	1.3	17	5	194
Danish Pastry, Raspberry, Unenriched 1 pastry (4-1/4" dia) (71g)	263	13	2	28	34	1.3	--	4	251
Desserts, Apple Crisp, Prepared from Recipe 1 recipe, yield (844g)	1359	29	6	0	260	11.8	166	15	2962
Desserts, Egg Custard, Baked, Prepared from Recipe 1 recipe, yield (563g)	586	26	12	473	62	0.0	62	28	343
Doughnuts, Cake-type, Chocolate, Sugared or Glazed 1 doughnut (3-3/4" dia) (60g)	250	12	3	34	34	1.3	19	3	238
Doughnuts, Cake-type, Plain (Includes Unsugared, Old-fashioned) 1 doughnut, stick (52g)	217	12	4	5	24	0.8	8	3	290
Doughnuts, Cake-type, Plain, Chocolate-coated or Frosted 1 donettes (2" dia) (18g)	81	5	2	3	9	0.3	5	1	59
Doughnuts, Cake-type, Plain, Sugared or Glazed 1 doughnut, medium (approx 3" dia) (45g)	192	10	3	14	23	0.7	--	2	181
Doughnuts, Cake-type, Wheat, Sugared or Glazed 1 doughnut (2" dia) (28g)	101	5	1	6	12	0.6	6	2	120

Food Serving size	Cal.	(g) Total Fat	(g) Sat. Fat	(mg) Chol.	(g) Carb.	(g) Fiber	(g) Sug.	(g) Prot.	(mg) Sod.
Doughnuts, French Crullers, Glazed									
1 cruller (3" dia) (41g)	169	8	2	5	24	0.5	14	1	141
Doughnuts, Yeast-leavened, Glazed, Enriched (Including Honey Buns)									
1 doughnut, hole (13g)	52	2	1	4	7	0.3	3	1	41
Doughnuts, Yeast-leavened, Glazed, Unenriched (Including Honey Buns)									
1 doughnut, medium (3-1/4" dia) (60g)	242	14	3	4	27	0.7	--	4	205
Doughnuts, Yeast-leavened, with Créme Filling									
1 doughnut, oval (3-1/2" x 2-1/2") (85g)	307	21	5	20	26	0.7	12	5	263
Doughnuts, Yeast-leavened, with Jelly Filling									
1 doughnut, oval (3-1/2" x 2-1/2") (85g)	289	16	4	22	33	0.8	18	5	204
Éclairs, Custard-filled, with Chocolate Glaze, Prepared from Recipe									
1 cream puff (3-1/2" x 2") (112g)	293	18	5	142	27	0.7	7	7	377
English Muffin, Plain, Enriched, with Calcium Propionate (Including Sourdough)									
1 muffin (57g)	129	1	0	0	25	2.0	2	5	206
English Muffin, Plain, Toasted, Enriched, with Calcium Propionate (Including Sourdough)									
1 muffin (52g)	140	1	0	0	27	1.5	2	5	248
English Muffins, Mixed-grain (Including Granola)									
1 muffin (66g)	155	1	0	0	31	1.8	1	6	220
English Muffins, Mixed-grain, Toasted (Including Granola)									
1 muffin (61g)	156	1	0	0	31	1.8	1	6	276
English Muffins, Plain, Enriched, Without Calcium Propionate (Including Sourdough)									
1 muffin (57g)	134	1	0	0	26	1.5	--	4	264
English Muffins, Plain, Unenriched, with Calcium Propionate (Including Sourdough)									
1 muffin (57g)	134	1	0	0	26	1.5	--	4	264
English Muffins, Plain, Unenriched, without Calcium Propionate (Including Sourdough)									
1 muffin (57g)	134	1	0	0	26	1.5	--	4	264
English Muffins, Raisin-cinnamon (Includes Apple-cinnamon)									
1 muffin (57g)	137	1	0	0	27	1.5	8	5	158

Food Serving size	Cal.	(g) Total Fat	(g) Sat. Fat	(mg) Chol.	(g) Carb.	(g) Fiber	(g) Sug.	(g) Prot.	(mg) Sod.
English Muffins, Raisin-cinnamon, Toasted (Including Apple-cinnamon)									
1 muffin (52g)	144	1	0	0	29	1.6	7	5	192
English Muffins, Wheat									
1 muffin (57g)	127	1	0	0	26	2.6	1	5	218
English Muffins, Wheat, Toasted									
1 muffin (52g)	126	1	0	0	25	2.6	1	5	216
English Muffins, Whole Wheat									
1 muffin (66g)	134	1	0	0	27	4.4	5	6	240
English Muffins, Whole Wheat, Toasted									
1 muffin (61g)	135	1	0	0	27	4.5	5	6	422
French Toast, Prepared from Recipe, Made with Low Fat (2%) Milk									
1 slice (65g)	149	7	2	75	16	--	--	5	311
General Mills, Betty Crocker Supermoist Yellow Cake Mix, Dry									
1 serving (43g)	178	3	1	--	35	--	19	2	289
Hush Puppies, Prepared from Recipe									
1 cup (152g)	512	21	3	68	70	4.3	3	12	1015
Interstate Brands Corp., Wonder Hamburger Rolls									
1 serving (43g)	117	2	0	--	22	1.1	5	3	210
Keebler, Keebler Chocolate Graham Selects									
1 serving (31g)	144	5	1	--	22	--	8	2	111
Keebler, Keebler Golden Vanilla Wafers, Artificially Flavored									
1 serving (31g)	147	6	1	--	22	--	8	2	120
Keikitos (Muffins), Latino Bakery Item									
1 piece (42g)	196	11	--	--	22	0.5	11	3	216
Kellogg's Eggo Lowfat Nutri-Grain Waffles									
1 serving (70g)	142	2	0	0	28	2.6	4	4	391
Kellogg's Low Fat Pop Tarts, Frosted Brown Sugar Cinnamon									
1 pastry (50g)	188	3	1	0	39	0.6	18	2	210
Kellogg's Low Fat Pop Tarts, Frosted Chocolate Fudge									
1 pastry (52g)	190	3	1	0	40	0.6	19	3	249
Kellogg's Low Fat Pop Tarts, Frosted Strawberry									
1 pastry (52g)	191	3	1	0	40	0.6	21	2	201
Kellogg's Low Fat Pop Tarts, Strawberry									
1 pastry (52g)	192	3	1	0	40	0.6	19	2	182

Food Serving size	Cal.	(g) Total Fat	(g) Sat. Fat	(mg) Chol.	(g) Carb.	(g) Fiber	(g) Sug.	(g) Prot.	(mg) Sod.
Kellogg's Nutri-Grain Cereal Bars, Mixed Berry									
1 bar (NLEA serving) (116g)	429	9	2	0	84	2.2	39	5	329
Kellogg's Pop-Tarts Pastry Swirls, Apple Cinnamon Danish									
1 pastry (62g)	256	11	3	0	37	0.9	11	3	190
Kellogg's Pop-Tarts Pastry Swirls, Cheese Danish									
1 pastry (62g)	252	11	3	1	37	0.3	12	3	180
Kellogg's Pop-Tarts Pastry Swirls, Strawberry Danish									
1 pastry (62g)	254	11	3	0	37	1.1	16	3	170
Kraft Foods, Shake 'N' Bake Original Recipe, Coating for Pork, Dry									
1 serving (28g)	106	1	--	--	22	--	--	2	611
Krusteaz Almond Poppyseed Muffin Mix, Artificially Flavored, Dry									
1 serving (40g)	167	4	1	--	30	0.7	16	2	236
Leavening Agents, Cream of Tartar									
.5 tsp (1.5g)	4	0	0	0	1	0.0	0	0	1
Leavening Agents, Yeast, Baker's, Compressed									
1 cake (0.6 oz) (17g)	18	0	0	0	3	1.4	0	1	5
Martha White Foods, Martha White's Buttermilk Biscuit Mix, Dry									
1 serving (41g)	159	5	2	1	24	0.6	2	3	531
Martha White Foods, Martha White's Chewy Fudge Brownie Mix									
1 serving (28g)	114	2	0	0	23	0.8	15	1	128
Millet, Cooked									
1 cup (174g)	207	2	0	0	41	2.3	0	6	3
Millet, Puffed									
1 cup (21g)	74	1	0	0	17	0.6	--	3	1
Mission Foods, Mission Flour Tortillas, Soft Taco, 8 Inch									
1 serving (51g)	146	3	0	--	25	--	--	4	458
Muffins, Blueberry, Commercially Prepared (Includes Mini-muffins)									
1 mini (1-1/4" dia) (17g)	67	3	1	7	8	0.3	5	1	59
Muffins, Blueberry, Commercially Prepared, Low Fat									
1 oz (28.35g)	72	1	0	8	14	1.2	8	1	117
Muffins, Blueberry, Dry Mix									
1 pkg, mix + drained berries (356g)	1303	36	9	0	225	--	--	17	1951
Muffins, Blueberry, Prepared from Recipe, Made with Low Fat (2%) Milk									
1 muffin (57g)	162	6	1	21	23	--	--	4	251

Food Serving size	Cal.	(g) Total Fat	(g) Sat. Fat	(mg) Chol.	(g) Carb.	(g) Fiber	(g) Sug.	(g) Prot.	(mg) Sod.
Muffins, Blueberry, Toaster-type									
1 muffin, toaster (33g)	103	3	0	2	18	0.6	2	2	82
Muffins, Blueberry, Toaster-type, Toasted									
1 muffin, toaster (31g)	103	3	0	2	18	0.6	4	2	158
Muffins, Corn, Commercially Prepared									
1 mini (17g)	52	1	0	4	9	0.6	1	1	109
Muffins, Corn, Dry Mix, Prepared									
1 oz (28.35g)	91	3	1	18	14	0.7	--	2	225
Muffins, Corn, Prepared from Recipe, Made with Low Fat (2%) Milk									
1 muffin (2-3/4" dia x 2") (57g)	180	7	1	24	25	--	--	4	333
Muffins, Corn, Toaster-type									
1 muffin, toaster (33g)	114	4	1	4	19	0.5	--	2	142
Muffins, Oat Bran									
1 mini (17g)	46	1	0	0	8	0.8	1	1	67
Muffins, Plain, Prepared from Recipe, Made with Low Fat (2%) Milk									
1 muffin (57g)	169	6	1	22	24	1.5	--	4	266
Muffins, Wheat Bran, Dry Mix									
1 pkg (7 oz) (198g)	784	24	6	0	145	--	--	14	1386
Muffins, Wheat Bran, Toaster-type with Raisins, Toasted									
1 muffin, toaster (34g)	106	3	1	3	19	2.8	8	2	179
Muffins, Wheat Bran, Toaster-type, with Raisins									
1 muffin, toaster (36g)	106	3	0	6	19	2.8	5	2	178
Nabisco Graham Crackers									
1 serving (28g)	119	3	0	0	21	1.0	6	2	185
Nabisco Oreo Crunchies, Cookie Crumb Topping									
1 serving (11g)	52	2	0	--	8	0.4	4	1	58
Nabisco Ritz Crackers									
5 crackers (1 NLEA serving) (16g)	79	4	1	--	10	0.4	1	1	141
Nabisco Snackwell's Fat-free Devil's Food Cookie Cakes									
1 serving (16g)	49	0	0	0	12	0.3	7	1	28
Noodles, Flat, Crunchy, Chinese Restaurant									
1 cup (45g)	234	14	2	0	23	0.9	0	5	170
Pan Dulce, La Ricura, Salpora De Arroz, Cookie-like									
1 piece (1 serving) (42g)	187	7	--	--	28	0.5	9	4	187

Food Serving size	Cal.	(g) Total Fat	(g) Sat. Fat	(mg) Chol.	(g) Carb.	(g) Fiber	(g) Sug.	(g) Prot.	(mg) Sod.
Pastry, Pastelitos De Guava (Guava Pastries)									
1 piece (86g)	326	16	5	9	41	1.9	15	5	199
Phyllo Dough									
1 sheet, dough (19g)	57	1	0	0	10	0.4	0	1	92
Pie Crust, Cookie-type, Chocolate, Ready Crust									
1 crust (182g)	881	41	9	0	117	4.9	48	11	915
Pie Crust, Cookie-type, Graham Cracker, Ready Crust									
1 oz (28.35g)	142	7	1	0	18	0.5	5	1	94
Pie Crust, Cookie-type, Prepared from Recipe, Chocolate Wafer, Chilled									
1 piece (1/8 of 9" crust) (28g)	142	9	2	0	15	0.4	6	1	188
Pie Crust, Cookie-type, Prepared from Recipe, Graham Cracker, Baked									
1 tart shell (22g)	109	5	1	0	14	0.3	8	1	126
Pie Crust, Cookie-type, Prepared from Recipe, Graham Cracker, Chilled									
1 piece (1/8 of 9" crust) (30g)	145	7	2	0	19	0.5	11	1	168
Pie Crust, Cookie-type, Prepared from Recipe, Vanilla Wafer, Chilled									
1 crust, single 9" (176g)	935	64	13	69	88	0.2	13	7	906
Pie Crust, Deep Dish, Frozen, Baked, Made with Enriched Flour									
1 pie crust (average weight) (202g)	1052	64	18	--	106	4.6	--	12	794
Pie Crust, Deep Dish, Frozen, Unbaked, Made with Enriched Flour									
1 pie crust (average weight) (225g)	1053	65	18	--	105	3.2	--	12	794
Pie Crust, Refrigerated, Regular, Baked									
1 pie crust (198g)	1002	57	22	--	116	2.8	--	7	935
Pie Crust, Standard-type, Dry Mix, Prepared, Baked									
1 piece (1/8 of 9" crust) (20g)	100	6	2	0	10	0.4	--	1	146
Pie Crust, Standard-type, Frozen, Ready-to-bake, Enriched, Baked									
1 pie crust (average weight of 1 baked crust) (154g)	782	44	14	0	87	5.1	7	10	719
Pie Crust, Standard-type, Frozen, Ready-to-bake, Unenriched									
1 piece (1/8 of 9" crust) (16g)	73	5	1	0	7	0.1	--	1	92
Pie Crust, Standard-type, Prepared from Recipe, Baked									
1 piece (1/8 of 9" crust) (23g)	121	8	2	0	11	0.4	0	1	125
Pie Crust, Standard-type, Prepared from Recipe, Unbaked									
1 piece (1/8 of 9" crust) (24g)	113	7	2	0	10	0.8	0	1	116

Food Serving size	Cal.	(g) Total Fat	(g) Sat. Fat	(mg) Chol.	(g) Carb.	(g) Fiber	(g) Sug.	(g) Prot.	(mg) Sod.
Pie, Apple, Commercially Prepared, Enriched Flour									
1 piece (1/8 of 9" dia) (125g)	296	14	5	0	43	2.0	20	2	251
Pie, Apple, Commercially Prepared, Unenriched Flour									
1 piece (1/8 of 9" dia) (125g)	296	14	5	0	43	2.0	--	2	333
Pie, Apple, Prepared from Recipe									
1 piece (1/8 of 9" dia) (155g)	411	19	5	0	58	--	--	4	327
Pie, Banana Cream, Prepared from Mix, No-bake-type									
1 piece (1/8 of 9" dia) (92g)	231	12	6	27	29	0.6	--	3	267
Pie, Banana Cream, Prepared from Recipe									
1 pie (9" dia) (1186g)	3190	161	45	605	390	8.3	143	52	2846
Pie, Blueberry, Commercially Prepared									
1 piece (1/8 of 9" dia) (125g)	290	13	2	0	44	1.3	12	2	274
Pie, Blueberry, Prepared from Recipe									
1 piece (1/8 of 9" dia) (147g)	360	17	4	0	49	--	--	4	272
Pie, Cherry, Commercially Prepared									
1 piece (1/8 of 9" dia) (125g)	325	14	3	0	50	1.0	18	3	308
Pie, Cherry, Prepared from Recipe									
1 piece (1/8 of 9" dia) (180g)	486	22	5	0	69	--	--	5	344
Pie, Chocolate Créme, Commercially Prepared									
1 piece (1/4 of 6" pie) (99g)	301	19	5	5	33	2.0	--	3	135
Pie, Chocolate Mousse, Prepared from Mix, No-bake-type									
1 piece (1/8 of 9" dia) (95g)	247	15	8	33	28	--	--	3	437
Pie, Coconut Créme, Commercially Prepared									
1 piece (1/6 of 7" pie) (64g)	191	11	4	0	24	0.8	23	1	193
Pie, Coconut Créme, Prepared from Mix, No-bake-type									
1 piece (1/8 of 9" dia) (94g)	259	17	8	22	27	0.5	--	3	309
Pie, Coconut Custard, Commercially Prepared									
1 piece (1/6 of 8" pie) (104g)	270	14	6	36	31	1.9	--	6	348
Pie, Crust, Refrigerated, Regular, Unbaked									
1 pie crust (average weight) (229g)	1019	58	22	--	117	4.1	--	7	937
Pie, Dutch Apple, Commercially Prepared									
1 slice (137g)	397	16	3	0	61	2.2	30	3	274
Pie, Egg Custard, Commercially Prepared									
1 piece (1/6 of 8" pie) (105g)	221	12	2	35	22	1.7	12	6	158

Food Serving size	Cal.	(g) Total Fat	(g) Sat. Fat	(mg) Chol.	(g) Carb.	(g) Fiber	(g) Sug.	(g) Prot.	(mg) Sod.
Pie, Fried Pies, Cherry 1 pie (5" x 3-3/4") (128g)	404	21	3	0	55	3.3	--	4	479
Pie, Fried Pies, Fruit 1 pie (5" x 3-3/4") (128g)	404	21	3	0	55	3.3	27	4	479
Pie, Fried Pies, Lemon 1 pie (5" x 3-3/4") (128g)	404	21	3	0	55	3.3	--	4	479
Pie, Lemon Meringue, Commercially Prepared 1 piece (1/6 of 8" pie) (113g)	303	10	2	51	53	1.4	27	2	194
Pie, Lemon Meringue, Prepared from Recipe 1 piece (1/8 of 9" dia) (127g)	362	16	4	67	50	--	--	5	307
Pie, Mince, Prepared from Recipe 1 piece (1/8 of 9" dia) (165g)	477	18	4	0	79	4.3	47	4	419
Pie, Peach 1 piece (1/6 of 8" pie) (117g)	261	12	2	0	38	0.9	7	2	227
Pie, Pecan, Commercially Prepared 1 slice (133g)	541	22	4	56	79	2.8	33	6	210
Pie, Pecan, Prepared from Recipe 1 piece (1/8 of 9" dia) (122g)	503	27	5	106	64	--	--	6	320
Pie, Pumpkin, Commercially Prepared 1 slice (133g)	323	13	3	35	46	2.4	25	5	450
Pie, Pumpkin, Prepared from Recipe 1 piece (1/8 of 9" dia) (155g)	316	14	5	65	41	--	--	7	349
Pie, Vanilla Cream, Prepared from Recipe 1 piece (1/8 of 9" dia) (126g)	350	18	5	78	41	0.8	16	6	328
Pillsbury Golden Layer Buttermilk Biscuits, Artificially Flavored, Refrigerated Dough 1 serving (34g)	104	5	1	0	14	0.4	2	2	360
Pillsbury Grands, Buttermilk Biscuits, Refrigerated Dough 1 serving (61g)	193	8	3	0	25	0.7	4	4	631
Pillsbury, Buttermilk Biscuits, Artificially Flavored, Refrigerated Dough 1 serving (64g)	150	2	0	0	29	1.0	4	4	570
Pillsbury, Chocolate Chip Cookies, Refrigerated Dough 1 serving (28g)	135	7	2	5	17	0.6	10	1	85
Pillsbury, Cinnamon Rolls, with Icing, Refrigerated Dough 1 serving (44g)	145	5	1	0	23	0.5	10	2	340

Food Serving size	Cal.	(g) Total Fat	(g) Sat. Fat	(mg) Chol.	(g) Carb.	(g) Fiber	(g) Sug.	(g) Prot.	(mg) Sod.
Pillsbury, Crusty French Loaf, Refrigerated Dough 1 serving (62g)	149	2	1	0	29	1.1	2	5	358
Pillsbury, Traditional Fudge Brownie Mix, Dry 1 serving (30g)	132	4	1	--	23	--	15	1	88
Puff Pastry, Frozen, Ready-to-bake, Baked 1 sheet (245g)	1367	94	13	0	112	3.7	2	18	620
Shortening Cake Mix, Soybean (Hydrogenated) and Cottonseed (Hydrogenated) 1 cup (205g)	1812	205	56	0	0	0.0	0	0	0
Shortening Confectionery, Coconut (Hydrogenated) and/or Palm Kernel (Hydrogenated) 1 cup (205g)	1812	205	187	0	0	0.0	0	0	0
Shortening Frying (Heavy Duty) Beef Tallow and Cottonseed 1 cup (205g)	1845	205	92	205	0	0.0	--	0	0
Shortening Frying (Heavy Duty), Palm (Hydrogenated) 1 cup (205g)	1812	205	97	0	0	0.0	--	0	0
Shortening Frying Heavy Duty, Soybean Hydrogenated, Linoleic (Less than 1%) 1 cup (205g)	1812	205	43	0	0	0.0	0	0	0
Shortening Household Soybean (Hydrogenated) and Palm 1 cup (205g)	1812	205	51	0	0	0.0	--	0	0
Shortening Industrial, Lard and Vegetable Oil 1 cup (205g)	1845	205	73	115	0	0.0	--	0	0
Shortening Industrial, Soybean (Hydrogenated) and Cottonseed 1 cup (205g)	1812	205	52	0	0	0.0	0	0	0
Shortening, Confectionery, Fractionated Palm 1 cup (218g)	1927	218	143	0	0	0.0	--	0	0
Shortening, Household, Lard and Vegetable Oil 1 cup (205g)	1845	205	83	115	0	0.0	0	0	0
Shortening, Household, Partially Hydrogenated Soybean and Cottonseed 1 cup (205g)	1812	205	51	0	0	0.0	0	0	0
Shortening, Special Purpose for Baking, Soybean (Hydrogenated) Palm and Cottonseed 1 cup (205g)	1812	205	59	0	0	0.0	0	0	0
Shortening, Special Purpose for Cakes and Frostings, Soybean (Hydrogenated) 1 cup (205g)	1812	205	41	0	0	0.0	0	0	0
Strudel, Apple 1 piece (71g)	195	8	1	4	29	1.6	18	2	111

Food Serving size	Cal.	(g) Total Fat	(g) Sat. Fat	(mg) Chol.	(g) Carb.	(g) Fiber	(g) Sug.	(g) Prot.	(mg) Sod.
Sweet Rolls, Cheese 1 roll (66g)	238	12	4	50	29	0.8	--	5	236
Sweet Rolls, Cinnamon, Commercially Prepared with Raisins 1 large (83g)	309	14	3	55	42	2.0	26	5	252
Sweet Rolls, Cinnamon, Refrigerated Dough with Frosting 1 roll (30g)	100	4	1	0	15	--	--	2	230
Sweet Rolls, Cinnamon, Refrigerated Dough with Frosting, Baked 1 roll (30g)	109	4	1	0	17	--	--	2	250
Taco Shells, Baked 1 large (6-1/2" dia) (21g)	98	4	1	0	13	1.0	0	1	82
Taco Shells, Baked, Without Salt 1 medium (approx 5" dia) (13g)	61	3	0	0	8	1.0	--	1	2
Toaster Pastries, Brown Sugar Cinnamon 1 toaster pastry (50g)	206	7	2	0	34	0.5	--	3	212
Toaster Pastries, Fruit 1 toaster pastry (54g)	211	6	1	0	37	0.6	15	3	180
Toaster Pastries, Fruit, Frosted 1 oz (28.35g)	111	3	1	0	20	0.2	10	1	88
Toaster Pastries, Fruit, Toasted (Apple, Blueberry, Cherry, Strawberry) 1 pastry (51g)	209	6	1	--	37	0.5	15	2	181
Toaster Pastries, Kellogg's Pop Tarts, Apple Cinnamon 1 pastry (52g)	205	5	1	0	37	0.6	18	2	174
Toaster Pastries, Kellogg's Pop Tarts, Blueberry 1 pastry (52g)	212	7	1	0	36	0.6	16	2	182
Toaster Pastries, Kellogg's Pop Tarts, Brown Sugar Cinnamon 1 pastry (50g)	219	9	1	0	32	0.8	13	3	190
Toaster Pastries, Kellogg's Pop Tarts, Cherry 1 pastry (52g)	204	5	1	0	37	0.6	16	2	220
Toaster Pastries, Kellogg's Pop Tarts, Frosted Blueberry 1 pastry (52g)	203	5	1	0	37	0.6	16	2	166
Toaster Pastries, Kellogg's Pop Tarts, Frosted Brown Sugar Cinnamon 1 pastry (50g)	211	7	1	0	34	0.7	15	3	175
Toaster Pastries, Kellogg's Pop Tarts, Frosted Cherry 1 pastry (52g)	204	5	1	0	37	0.5	19	2	166

Food Serving size	Cal.	(g) Total Fat	(g) Sat. Fat	(mg) Chol.	(g) Carb.	(g) Fiber	(g) Sug.	(g) Prot.	(mg) Sod.
Toaster Pastries, Kellogg's Pop Tarts, Frosted Chocolate Fudge									
1 pastry (52g)	201	5	1	0	37	0.6	20	3	229
Toaster Pastries, Kellogg's Pop Tarts, Frosted Chocolate Vanilla Cream									
1 pastry (52g)	203	5	1	0	37	0.5	19	3	229
Toaster Pastries, Kellogg's Pop Tarts, Frosted Grape									
1 pastry (52g)	203	5	1	0	38	0.5	18	2	173
Toaster Pastries, Kellogg's Pop Tarts, Frosted Raspberry									
1 pastry (52g)	205	6	1	0	37	0.5	18	2	166
Toaster Pastries, Kellogg's Pop Tarts, Frosted Strawberry									
1 pastry (52g)	203	5	1	0	38	0.5	20	2	169
Toaster Pastries, Kellogg's Pop Tarts, Frosted Wild Berry									
1 pastry (54g)	210	5	1	0	39	0.5	21	2	168
Toaster Pastries, Kellogg's Pop Tarts, S'mores									
1 pastry (52g)	204	5	1	0	36	0.7	19	3	213
Toaster Pastries, Kellogg's Pop Tarts, Strawberry									
1 pastry (52g)	205	5	2	0	37	0.6	17	2	185

Vegetables

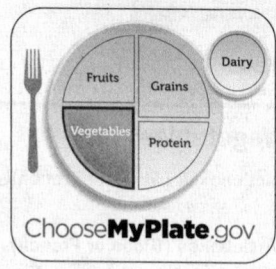

Choose**MyPlate**.gov

Why Eat Vegetables?

Eating a diet rich in vegetables and fruits as part of an overall healthy diet may reduce the risk of heart disease, including heart attack and stroke. Most vegetables are naturally low in fat and calories, and none have cholesterol, although added sauces or seasonings may add fat, calories, or cholesterol. Vegetables are important sources of many nutrients, including potassium, dietary fiber, folate (folic acid), vitamin A, and vitamin C. Diets rich in potassium may help to maintain healthy blood pressure. Vitamin A keeps eyes and skin healthy and helps to protect against infections. Vitamin C helps heal cuts and wounds, keeps teeth and gums healthy, and aids in iron absorption.

Daily Goal

2½ cups for an adult on a 2000-calorie diet
One-cup equivalents:

1 cup cooked vegetable	1 three-inch tomato
2 cups raw vegetables	1 cup cooked dry peas or beans
2 medium carrots	1 cup starchy vegetable

Shopping Tips

- Choose vegetables rich in color—red, orange, or dark green.
- Buy fresh vegetables in season.
- Purchase locally grown vegetables when possible.
- Stock up on frozen or canned vegetables for fast preparation.
- Remember that over a quarter of your plate should be vegetables.

Shopping List Essentials

Tomatoes	Broccoli	Spinach
Peppers	Cauliflower	Sweet potatoes/yams
Carrots	Green beans	Squash

Red Flags

Canned vegetables can be high in sodium. Look for salt-free canned vegetables or rinse canned vegetables before using. Frozen vegetables may have added sauces that add calories, fat, and salt. Choose frozen vegetables without sauces and seasonings.

Food Serving size	Cal.	(g) Total Fat	(g) Sat. Fat	(mg) Chol.	(g) Carb.	(g) Fiber	(g) Sug.	(g) Prot.	(mg) Sod.
Vegetables									
Artichokes (Globe or French), Cooked, Boiled, Drained, with Salt									
.5 cup, hearts (84g)	45	0	0	0	10	7.2	1	2	50
Artichokes (Globe or French), Cooked, Boiled, Drained, Without Salt									
.5 cup, hearts (84g)	45	0	0	0	10	7.2	1	2	50
Artichokes (Globe or French), Frozen, Cooked, Boiled, Drained, with Salt									
1 pkg (9 oz), yields (240g)	108	1	0	0	22	11.0	2	7	694
Artichokes (Globe or French), Frozen, Cooked, Boiled, Drained, Without Salt									
1 pkg (9 oz), yields (240g)	108	1	0	0	22	11.0	2	7	127
Artichokes (Globe or French), Frozen, Unprepared									
1 pkg (9 oz) (255g)	97	1	0	0	20	9.9	--	7	120
Artichokes (Globe or French), Raw									
1 artichoke, large (162g)	76	0	0	0	17	8.7	2	5	152
Arugula, Raw									
.5 cup (10g)	3	0	0	0	0	0.2	0	0	3
Asparagus, Canned, Drained, Solids									
1 spear (about 5" long) (18g)	3	0	0	0	0	0.3	0	0	52
Asparagus, Canned, No Salt, Solids and Liquids									
1 can (300 x 407) (411g)	62	1	0	0	10	4.1	4	7	107
Asparagus, Canned, Regular Pkg, Solids and Liquids									
1 can (300 x 407) (411g)	62	1	0	0	10	4.1	--	7	1167
Asparagus, Cooked, Boiled, Drained									
4 spears (1/2" base) (60g)	13	0	0	0	2	1.2	1	1	8
Asparagus, Cooked, Boiled, Drained, with Salt									
4 spears (1/2" base) (60g)	13	0	0	0	2	1.2	1	1	144
Asparagus, Frozen, Cooked, Boiled, Drained, with Salt									
1 pkg (10 oz), yields (293g)	53	1	0	0	6	4.7	1	9	703
Asparagus, Frozen, Cooked, Boiled, Drained, Without Salt									
1 pkg (10 oz), yields (293g)	53	1	0	0	6	4.7	1	9	9
Asparagus, Frozen, Unprepared									
4 spears (58g)	14	0	0	0	2	1.1	--	2	5

Food Serving size	Cal.	(g) Total Fat	(g) Sat. Fat	(mg) Chol.	(g) Carb.	(g) Fiber	(g) Sug.	(g) Prot.	(mg) Sod.
Asparagus, Raw 1 spear, small (5" long or less) (12g)	2	0	0	0	0	0.3	0	0	0
Avocados, Raw, All Commercial Varieties 1 cup, pureed (230g)	368	34	5	0	20	15.4	2	5	16
Avocados, Raw, California 1 fruit, without skin and seed (136g)	227	21	3	0	12	9.2	0	3	11
Avocados, Raw, Florida 1 fruit, without skin and seed (304g)	365	31	6	0	24	17.0	7	7	6
Basil, Fresh 5 leaves (2.5g)	1	0	0	0	0	0.0	0	0	0
Broccoli, Cooked, Boiled, Drained, with Salt 1 stalk, medium (7-1/2" - 8" long) (180g)	63	1	0	0	13	5.9	3	4	472
Broccoli, Cooked, Boiled, Drained, Without Salt 1 stalk, medium (7-1/2" - 8" long) (180g)	63	1	0	0	13	5.9	3	4	74
Broccoli, Flower Clusters, Raw 1 floweret (11g)	3	0	0	0	1	--	--	0	3
Garlic, Raw 1 tsp (2.8g)	4	0	0	0	1	0.1	0	0	0
Ginger Root, Raw .25 cup, slices (1" dia) (24g)	19	0	0	0	4	0.5	0	0	3
Lemon Grass (Citronella), Raw 1 tbsp (4.8g)	5	0	0	0	1	--	--	0	0
Lentils, Mature Seeds, Cooked, Boiled, Without Salt 1 tbsp (12.3g)	14	0	0	0	2	1.0	0	1	0
Lentils, Pink, Raw 1 cup (192g)	662	4	1	0	114	20.7	--	48	13
Lentils, Raw 1 tablespoon (12g)	42	0	0	0	7	3.7	0	3	1
Lentils, Sprouted, Raw 1 cup (77g)	82	0	0	0	17	--	--	7	8

Food Serving size	Cal.	(g) Total Fat	(g) Sat. Fat	(mg) Chol.	(g) Carb.	(g) Fiber	(g) Sug.	(g) Prot.	(mg) Sod.
Lettuce, Butterhead (Including Boston and Bibb Types), Raw									
1 head (5" dia) (163g)	21	0	0	0	4	1.8	2	2	8
Lettuce, Cos and Romaine, Raw									
1 leaf, inner (6g)	1	0	0	0	0	0.1	0	0	0
Lettuce, Green Leaf, Raw									
1 head (360g)	54	1	0	0	10	4.7	3	5	101
Lettuce, Iceberg (Including Crisphead Types), Raw									
1 cup, chopped (1/2" pieces, loosely packed) (57g)	8	0	0	0	2	0.7	1	1	6
Lettuce, Red Leaf, Raw									
1 leaf, inner (2.6g)	0	0	--	--	0	0.0	0	0	1
Lima Beans, Immature Seeds, Cooked, Boiled, Drained, with Salt									
1 cup (170g)	209	1	0	0	40	9.0	3	12	430
Lima Beans, Immature Seeds, Frozen, Baby, Cooked, Boiled, Drained, with Salt									
1 pkg (10 oz), yields (311g)	327	1	0	0	60	18.7	4	21	824
Lima Beans, Immature Seeds, Frozen, Fordhook, Cooked, Boiled, Drained, with Salt									
1 pkg (10 oz), yields (311g)	320	1	0	0	60	18.0	4	19	899
Lima Beans, Large, Mature Seeds, Canned									
1 cup (241g)	190	0	0	0	36	11.6	--	12	810
Lima Beans, Large, Mature Seeds, Cooked, Boiled, with Salt									
1 cup (188g)	216	1	0	0	39	13.2	5	15	447
Lima Beans, Large, Mature Seeds, Cooked, Boiled, Without Salt									
1 tbsp (11.7g)	13	0	0	0	2	0.8	0	1	0
Lima Beans, Large, Mature Seeds, Raw									
1 tbsp (11.1g)	38	0	0	0	7	2.1	1	2	2
Lima Beans, Thin Seeded (Baby), Mature Seeds, Cooked, Boiled, with Salt									
1 cup (182g)	229	1	0	0	42	14.0	--	15	435
Lima Beans, Thin Seeded (Baby), Mature Seeds, Cooked, Boiled, Without Salt									
1 cup (182g)	229	1	0	0	42	14.0	--	15	5
Lima Beans, Thin Seeded (Baby), Mature Seeds, Raw									
1 cup (202g)	677	2	0	0	127	41.6	17	42	26
Lotus Root, Cooked, Boiled, Drained, with Salt									
10 slices (2-1/2" dia) (89g)	59	0	0	0	14	2.8	--	1	250

Food Serving size	Cal.	(g) Total Fat	(g) Sat. Fat	(mg) Chol.	(g) Carb.	(g) Fiber	(g) Sug.	(g) Prot.	(mg) Sod.
Lotus Root, Cooked, Boiled, Drained, Without Salt 10 slices (2-1/2" dia) (89g)	59	0	0	0	14	2.8	0	1	40
Lotus Root, Raw 1 root (9-1/2" long) (115g)	85	0	0	0	20	5.6	--	3	46
Malabar Spinach, Cooked 1 bunch (17g)	4	0	--	0	0	0.4	--	1	9
Mountain Yam, Hawaii, Cooked, Steamed, with Salt 1 cup, cubes (145g)	119	0	0	0	29	--	--	3	360
Mountain Yam, Hawaii, Cooked, Steamed, Without Salt 1 cup, cubes (145g)	119	0	0	0	29	--	--	3	17
Mountain Yam, Hawaii, Raw 1 yam (420g)	281	0	0	0	69	--	--	6	55
Mushrooms, Brown, Italian or Crimini, Raw 1 cup, sliced (72g)	16	0	0	0	3	0.4	1	2	4
Mushrooms, Canned, Drained, Solid 1 can (132g)	33	0	0	0	7	3.2	3	2	561
Mushrooms, Chanterelle, Raw 1 piece (5.4g)	2	0	--	--	0	0.2	0	0	0
Mushrooms, Shiitake, Dried 4 mushrooms (15g)	44	0	0	0	11	1.7	0	1	2
Mushrooms, Enoki, Raw 1 medium (3g)	1	0	0	0	0	0.1	0	0	0
Mushrooms, Maitake, Raw 1 piece, whole (1.1g)	0	0	0	0	0	0.0	0	0	0
Mushrooms, Morel, Raw 1 piece (12.9g)	4	0	0	--	1	0.4	0	0	3
Mushrooms, Oyster, Raw 1 small (15g)	5	0	0	0	1	0.3	0	0	3
Mushrooms, Portobello, Exposed to Ultra-violet Light, Grilled 1 cup, sliced (121g)	35	1	0	--	5	2.7	3	4	13
Mushrooms, Portobello, Exposed to Ultra-violet Light, Raw 1 piece, whole (84g)	18	0	0	0	3	1.1	2	2	8
Mushrooms, Portobello, Grilled 1 cup, sliced (121g)	35	1	0	0	5	2.7	3	4	13

Food Serving size	Cal.	(g) Total Fat	(g) Sat. Fat	(mg) Chol.	(g) Carb.	(g) Fiber	(g) Sug.	(g) Prot.	(mg) Sod.
Mushrooms, Portobello, Raw 1 piece, whole (84g)	18	0	0	0	3	1.1	2	2	8
Mushrooms, Shiitake, Cooked, with Salt 4 mushrooms (72g)	40	0	0	0	10	1.5	3	1	173
Mushrooms, Shiitake, Cooked, Without Salt 4 mushrooms (72g)	40	0	0	0	10	1.5	3	1	3
Mushrooms, Shiitake, Raw 1 piece, whole (19g)	6	0	--	--	1	0.5	0	0	2
Mushrooms, Shiitake, Stir-fried 1 cup, sliced (97g)	38	0	0	0	7	3.5	0	3	5
Mushrooms, Straw, Canned, Drained, Solid 1 piece (5.5g)	2	0	0	0	0	0.1	--	0	21
Mushrooms, White, Cooked, Boiled, Drained, with Salt 1 tbsp (9.8g)	3	0	0	0	1	0.2	0	0	23
Mushrooms, White, Cooked, Boiled, Drained, Without Salt 1 tbsp (9.8g)	3	0	0	0	1	0.2	0	0	0
Mushrooms, White, Raw 1 cup, whole (96g)	21	0	0	0	3	1.0	2	3	5
Mushrooms, White, Stir-fried 1 cup, sliced (108g)	28	0	0	0	4	1.9	0	4	13
Mussel, Blue, Cooked, Moist Heat 3 oz (85g)	146	4	1	48	6	0.0	--	20	314
Mustard Greens, Cooked, Boiled, Drained, with Salt 1 cup, chopped (140g)	21	0	0	0	3	2.8	0	3	353
Mustard Greens, Cooked, Boiled, Drained, Without Salt 1 cup, chopped (140g)	21	0	0	0	3	2.8	0	3	22
Mustard Greens, Raw 1 cup, chopped (56g)	15	0	0	0	3	1.8	1	2	14
Mustard Spinach (Tendergreen), Raw 1 cup, chopped (150g)	33	0	0	0	6	4.2	--	3	32
New Zealand Spinach, Cooked, Boiled, Drained, with Salt 1 cup, chopped (180g)	22	0	0	0	4	--	--	2	617
New Zealand Spinach, Cooked, Boiled, Drained, Without Salt 1 cup, chopped (180g)	22	0	0	0	4	--	--	2	193

Food Serving size	Cal.	(g) Total Fat	(g) Sat. Fat	(mg) Chol.	(g) Carb.	(g) Fiber	(g) Sug.	(g) Prot.	(mg) Sod.
New Zealand Spinach, Raw 1 cup, chopped (56g)	8	0	0	0	1	--	--	1	73
Okra, Cooked, Boiled, Drained, with Salt 8 pods (3" long) (85g)	19	0	0	0	4	2.1	2	2	205
Okra, Cooked, Boiled, Drained, Without Salt 8 pods (3" long) (85g)	19	0	0	0	4	2.1	2	2	5
Okra, Frozen, Cooked, Boiled, Drained, with Salt .5 cup, slices (92g)	31	0	0	0	6	1.9	3	1	220
Okra, Frozen, Cooked, Boiled, Drained, Without Salt .5 cup, slices (92g)	27	0	0	0	6	1.9	3	1	3
Okra, Frozen, Unprepared 1 pkg (3 lb) (1361g)	408	3	1	0	90	29.9	40	23	41
Okra, Raw 8 pods (3" long) (95g)	29	0	0	0	7	3.0	1	2	8
Onions, Raw 1 cup, sliced (115g)	46	0	0	0	11	2.0	5	1	5
Onions, Spring or Scallions (Including Tops and Bulb), Raw 1 tbsp, chopped (6g)	2	0	0	0	0	0.2	0	0	1
Onions, Sweet, Raw 1 NLEA serving (148g)	47	0	--	0	11	1.3	7	1	12
Onions, Young Green, Tops Only 1 stalk (12g)	3	0	0	0	1	0.2	1	0	2
Parsley, Raw 1 tbsp (3.8g)	1	0	0	0	0	0.1	0	0	2
Parsnips, Cooked, Boiled, Drained, with Salt 1 parsnip (9" long) (160g)	114	0	0	0	27	6.4	8	2	394
Parsnips, Cooked, Boiled, Drained, Without Salt 1 parsnip (9" long) (160g)	114	0	0	0	27	5.8	8	2	16
Parsnips, Raw 1 cup, slices (133g)	100	0	0	0	24	6.5	6	2	13
Peas and Onions, Frozen, Cooked, Boiled, Drained, with Salt 1 cup (180g)	81	0	0	0	16	4.0	7	5	491
Peas, Edible-podded, Raw 1 cup, whole (63g)	26	0	0	0	5	1.6	3	2	3

Food Serving size	Cal.	(g) Total Fat	(g) Sat. Fat	(mg) Chol.	(g) Carb.	(g) Fiber	(g) Sug.	(g) Prot.	(mg) Sod.
Peas, Green, Frozen, Unprepared 1 pkg (284g)	219	1	0	0	39	12.8	14	15	307
Peas, Green, Raw 1 cup (145g)	117	1	0	0	21	7.4	8	8	7
Peas, Mature Seeds, Sprouted, Raw 1 cup (120g)	149	1	0	0	33	--	--	11	24
Peppers, Hot Chili, Red, Raw .5 cup, chopped or diced (75g)	30	0	0	0	7	1.1	4	1	7
Peppers, Hungarian, Raw 1 pepper (27g)	8	0	0	0	2	--	--	0	0
Peppers, Jalapeno, Raw 1 pepper (14g)	4	0	0	0	1	0.4	1	0	0
Peppers, Sweet, Green, Raw 1 cup, sliced (92g)	18	0	0	0	4	1.6	2	1	3
Peppers, Sweet, Yellow, Raw 10 strips (52g)	14	0	0	0	3	0.5	--	1	1
Poi 1 cup (240g)	269	0	0	0	65	1.0	1	1	29
Potato, Baked, Flesh and Skin, Without Salt 1 potato, medium (173g)	161	0	0	0	37	3.8	2	4	17
Potato, Flesh and Skin, Raw 1 Potato, medium (2-1/4" to 3-1/4" dia) (213g)	164	0	0	0	37	4.7	2	4	13
Potatoes, Baked, Flesh, Without Salt 1 potato (2-1/3" x 4-3/4") (156g)	145	0	0	0	34	2.3	3	3	8
Potatoes, Baked, Skin, with Salt 1 skin (58g)	115	0	0	0	27	4.6	1	2	149
Potatoes, Baked, Skin, Without Salt 1 skin (58g)	115	0	0	0	27	4.6	1	2	12
Potatoes, Boiled, Cooked in Skin, Flesh, with Salt 1 potato (2-1/2" dia, sphere) (136g)	118	0	0	0	27	2.7	1	3	326
Potatoes, Boiled, Cooked in Skin, Flesh, Without Salt 1 potato (2-1/2" dia, sphere) (136g)	118	0	0	0	27	2.4	1	3	5

Food Serving size	Cal.	(g) Total Fat	(g) Sat. Fat	(mg) Chol.	(g) Carb.	(g) Fiber	(g) Sug.	(g) Prot.	(mg) Sod.
Potatoes, Boiled, Cooked in Skin, with Salt									
1 skin (34g)	27	0	0	0	6	1.1	--	1	85
Potatoes, Boiled, Cooked in Skin, Without Salt									
1 skin (34g)	27	0	0	0	6	1.1	--	1	5
Potatoes, Boiled, Cooked Without Skin, Flesh, with Salt									
1 medium (2-1/4" to 2-1/4" dia.) (167g)	144	0	0	0	33	3.3	1	3	402
Potatoes, Boiled, Cooked Without Skin, Flesh, Without Salt									
1 medium (2-1/4" to 3-1/4" dia.) (167g)	144	0	0	0	33	3.0	1	3	8
Potatoes, Canned, Drained Solid									
1 potato (35g)	21	0	0	0	5	0.8	--	0	77
Potatoes, Canned, Drained Solid, No Salt									
1 cup (180g)	112	0	0	0	24	4.3	--	3	9
Potatoes, Canned, Solids and Liquids									
1 can (303 x 406) (454g)	200	0	0	0	45	6.4	--	5	985
Potatoes, Raw, Skin									
1 skin (38g)	22	0	0	0	5	1.0	--	1	4
Potatoes, Red, Flesh and Skin, Baked									
1 potato, medium (2-1/4" to 3-1/4" dia.) (173g)	154	0	0	0	34	3.1	2	4	21
Potatoes, Red, Flesh and Skin, Raw									
1 potato, medium (2-1/4" to 3-1/4" dia) (213g)	149	0	0	0	34	3.6	3	4	38
Potatoes, Russet, Flesh and Skin, Baked									
1 potato, medium (2-1/4" to 3-1/4" dia.) (173g)	168	0	0	0	37	4.0	2	5	24
Potatoes, Russet, Flesh and Skin, Raw									
1 potato, medium (2-1/4" to 3-1/4" dia) (213g)	168	0	0	0	38	2.8	1	5	11
Potatoes, White, Flesh and Skin, Baked									
1 potato, medium (2-1/4" to 3-1/4" dia) (138g)	130	0	0	0	29	2.9	2	3	10
Potatoes, White, Flesh and Skin, Raw									
1 potato, medium (2-1/4" to 3-1/4" dia) (213g)	147	0	0	0	33	5.1	2	4	34

Food Serving size	Cal.	(g) Total Fat	(g) Sat. Fat	(mg) Chol.	(g) Carb.	(g) Fiber	(g) Sug.	(g) Prot.	(mg) Sod.
Pumpkin, Raw 1 cup (1" cubes) (116g)	30	0	0	0	8	0.6	2	1	1
Purslane, Cooked, Boiled, Drained, Without Salt 1 squash (431g)	78	1	--	0	15	--	--	6	190
Purslane, Raw 1 plant (3g)	0	0	--	0	0	--	--	0	1
Quinoa, Cooked 1 cup (185g)	222	4	--	0	39	5.2	--	8	13
Quinoa, Uncooked 1 cup (170g)	626	10	1	0	109	11.9	--	24	9
Radicchio, Raw 1 leaf (8g)	2	0	0	0	0	0.1	0	0	2
Radish Seeds, Sprouted, Raw 1 cup (38g)	16	1	0	0	1	--	--	1	2
Radishes, Hawaiian Style, Pickled 1 cup (150g)	42	0	0	0	8	3.3	0	2	1184
Radishes, Oriental, Cooked, Boiled, Drained, with Salt 1 cup, slices (147g)	25	0	0	0	5	2.4	3	1	366
Radishes, Oriental, Cooked, Boiled, Drained, Without Salt 1 cup, sliced (147g)	25	0	0	0	5	2.4	3	1	19
Radishes, Oriental, Dried 1 cup (116g)	314	1	0	0	74	--	--	9	322
Radishes, Oriental, Raw 1 radish (7" long) (338g)	61	0	0	0	14	5.4	8	2	71
Radishes, Raw 1 large (1" to 1-1/4" dia) (9g)	1	0	0	0	0	0.1	0	0	4
Radishes, White Icicle, Raw 1 radish (7" long) (17g)	2	0	0	0	0	0.2	--	0	3
Refried Beans, Canned, Fat Free 1 can (445g)	352	2	0	0	60	20.9	3	24	1949
Refried Beans, Canned, Traditional Style 1 can (443g)	403	5	2	0	68	22.6	2	24	1989
Refried Beans, Canned, Vegetarian 1 can (444g)	369	4	1	--	60	20.9	3	23	1909

Food Serving size	Cal.	(g) Total Fat	(g) Sat. Fat	(mg) Chol.	(g) Carb.	(g) Fiber	(g) Sug.	(g) Prot.	(mg) Sod.
Rhubarb, Frozen, Cooked, with Sugar 1 cup (240g)	278	0	0	0	75	4.8	69	1	2
Rhubarb, Frozen, Uncooked 1 cup, diced (137g)	29	0	0	0	7	2.5	2	1	3
Rhubarb, Raw 1 stalk (51g)	11	0	0	0	2	0.9	1	0	2
Roselle, Raw 1 cup, without refuse (57g)	28	0	--	0	6	--	--	1	3
Roughy, Orange, Cooked, Dry Heat 3 oz (85g)	89	1	0	68	0	0.0	0	19	59
Rutabagas, Cooked, Boiled, Drained, with Salt .5 cup, mashed (120g)	47	0	0	0	10	--	7	2	305
Rutabagas, Cooked, Boiled, Drained, Without Salt 1 cup, mashed (240g)	94	1	0	0	21	4.3	14	3	48
Rutabagas, Raw 1 large (772g)	278	2	0	0	63	19.3	43	9	154
Salsify (Vegetable Oyster), Raw 1 cup, slices (133g)	109	0	--	0	25	4.4	--	4	27
Salsify, Cooked, Boiled, Drained, with Salt 1 cup, slices (135g)	92	0	--	0	21	4.2	4	4	340
Salsify, Cooked, Boiled, Drained, Without Salt 1 cup, sliced (135g)	92	0	0	0	21	4.2	4	4	22
Shallots, Freeze-dried .25 cup (3.6g)	13	0	0	0	3	--	--	0	2
Shallots, Raw 1 tbsp, chopped (10g)	7	0	0	0	2	--	--	0	1
Spinach, Canned, No Salt, Solids and Liquids 1 cup (234g)	44	1	0	0	7	5.1	--	5	176
Spinach, Canned, Regular Pack, Drained, Solid 1 cup (214g)	49	1	0	0	7	5.1	1	6	689
Spinach, Canned, Regular Pack, Solids and Liquids 1 cup (234g)	44	1	0	0	7	3.7	--	5	746
Spinach, Cooked, Boiled, Drained, with Salt 1 cup (180g)	41	0	0	0	7	4.3	1	5	551

Food Serving size	Cal.	(g) Total Fat	(g) Sat. Fat	(mg) Chol.	(g) Carb.	(g) Fiber	(g) Sug.	(g) Prot.	(mg) Sod.
Spinach, Cooked, Boiled, Drained, Without Salt 1 cup (180g)	41	0	0	0	7	4.3	1	5	126
Spinach, Frozen, Chopped or Leaf, Cooked, Boiled, Drained, with Salt .5 cup (95g)	32	1	0	0	5	3.5	0	4	306
Spinach, Frozen, Chopped or Leaf, Cooked, Boiled, Drained, Without Salt .5 cup (95g)	32	1	0	0	5	3.5	0	4	92
Spinach, Frozen, Chopped or Leaf, Unprepared 1 pkg (10 oz) (284g)	82	2	0	0	12	8.2	2	10	210
Spinach, Raw 1 bunch (340g)	78	1	0	0	12	7.5	1	10	269
Succotash (Corn and Limas), Canned, with Cream Style Corn 1 cup (266g)	205	1	0	0	47	8.0	--	7	652
Succotash (Corn and Limas), Canned, with Whole Kernel Corn, Solids and Liquids 1 cup (255g)	161	1	0	0	36	6.6	--	7	564
Succotash (Corn and Limas), Cooked, Boiled, Drained, with Salt 1 cup (192g)	213	2	0	0	47	--	--	10	486
Succotash (Corn and Limas), Cooked, Boiled, Drained, Without Salt 1 cup (192g)	221	2	0	0	47	8.6	--	10	33
Succotash (Corn and Limas), Frozen, Cooked, Boiled, Drained, with Salt 1 cup (170g)	158	2	0	0	34	7.0	4	7	478
Succotash (Corn and Limas), Frozen, Cooked, Boiled, Drained, Without Salt 1 cup (170g)	158	2	0	0	34	7.0	4	7	77
Succotash (Corn and Limas), Frozen, Unprepared 1 pkg (10 oz) (284g)	264	3	0	0	57	11.4	--	12	128
Tapioca, Pearl, Dry 1 cup (152g)	544	0	0	0	135	1.4	5	0	2
Taro Leaves, Cooked, Steamed, Without Salt 1 cup (145g)	35	1	0	0	6	2.9	--	4	3
Taro Leaves, Raw 1 leaf (11" x 6-1/2") (10g)	4	0	0	0	1	0.4	0	0	0
Taro Shoots, Cooked, Without Salt 1 cup, slices (140g)	20	0	0	0	4	--	--	1	3
Taro Shoots, Raw 1 shoot (83g)	9	0	0	0	2	--	--	1	1

Food Serving size	Cal.	(g) Total Fat	(g) Sat. Fat	(mg) Chol.	(g) Carb.	(g) Fiber	(g) Sug.	(g) Prot.	(mg) Sod.
Taro, Cooked, with Salt 1 cup, slices (132g)	187	0	0	0	46	6.7	1	1	331
Taro, Cooked, Without Salt 1 cup, sliced (132g)	187	0	0	0	46	6.7	1	1	20
Taro, Leaves, Cooked, Steamed, with Salt 1 cup (145g)	35	1	0	0	6	2.9	--	4	345
Taro, Raw 1 cup, sliced (104g)	116	0	0	0	28	4.3	0	2	11
Taro, Shoots, Cooked, with Salt 1 cup, slices (140g)	20	0	0	0	4	--	--	1	333
Taro, Tahitian, Cooked, with Salt 1 cup, slices (137g)	60	1	0	0	9	--	--	6	397
Taro, Tahitian, Cooked, Without Salt 1 cup, slices (137g)	60	1	0	0	9	--	--	6	74
Taro, Tahitian, Raw 1 cup, slices (125g)	55	1	0	0	9	--	--	3	63
Tomatoes, Green, Raw 1 large (182g)	42	0	0	0	9	2.0	7	2	24
Tomatoes, Orange, Raw 1 tomato (111g)	18	0	0	0	4	1.0	--	1	47
Tomatoes, Red, Ripe, Cooked 2 medium (246g)	44	0	0	0	10	1.7	6	2	27
Tomatoes, Red, Ripe, Cooked, Stewed 1 recipe, yield (604g)	477	16	3	0	79	10.3	--	12	2748
Tomatoes, Red, Ripe, Cooked, with Salt .5 cup (120g)	22	0	0	0	5	0.8	3	1	296
Tomatoes, Red, Ripe, Raw, Year Round Average 1 cup, chopped or sliced (180g)	32	0	0	0	7	2.2	5	2	9
Tomatoes, Sun-dried 1 piece (2g)	5	0	0	0	1	0.2	1	0	42
Tomatoes, Sun-dried, Packed in Oil, Drained 1 piece (3g)	6	0	0	0	1	0.2	--	0	8
Tomatoes, Yellow, Raw 1 tomato (212g)	32	1	0	0	6	1.5	--	2	49

Food Serving size	Cal.	(g) Total Fat	(g) Sat. Fat	(mg) Chol.	(g) Carb.	(g) Fiber	(g) Sug.	(g) Prot.	(mg) Sod.
Turnip Greens and Turnips, Frozen, Cooked, Boiled, Drained, with Salt .5 cup (86g)	29	0	0	0	4	2.7	1	3	219
Turnip Greens and Turnips, Frozen, Cooked, Boiled, Drained, Without Salt 1 cup (163g)	57	1	0	0	8	5.1	2	5	31
Turnip Greens and Turnips, Frozen, Unprepared 1 pkg (3 lb) (1361g)	286	3	0	0	46	32.7	--	33	245
Turnip Greens, Canned, No Salt 1 cup (144g)	27	0	0	0	4	1.9	1	2	42
Turnip Greens, Canned, Solids and Liquids 1 can, 15 oz (303 x 406) (425g)	60	1	0	0	10	7.2	--	6	1177
Turnip Greens, Cooked, Boiled, Drained, with Salt 1 cup, chopped (144g)	29	0	0	0	6	5.0	1	2	382
Turnip Greens, Cooked, Boiled, Drained, Without Salt 1 cup, chopped (144g)	29	0	0	0	6	5.0	1	2	42
Turnip Greens, Frozen, Cooked, Boiled, Drained, with Salt .5 cup (82g)	24	0	0	0	4	2.8	1	3	206
Turnip Greens, Frozen, Cooked, Boiled, Drained, Without Salt 1 pkg (10 oz), yields (220g)	64	1	0	0	11	7.5	2	7	33
Turnip Greens, Frozen, Unprepared 1 pkg (10 oz) (284g)	62	1	0	0	10	7.1	--	7	34
Turnip Greens, Raw 1 cup, chopped (55g)	18	0	0	0	4	1.8	0	1	22
Turnips, Cooked, Boiled, Drained, with Salt 1 cup, mashed (230g)	51	0	0	0	12	4.6	7	2	658
Turnips, Cooked, Boiled, Drained, Without Salt 1 cup, mashed (230g)	51	0	0	0	12	4.6	7	2	37
Turnips, Frozen, Cooked, Boiled, Drained, with Salt 1 cup (156g)	33	0	0	0	6	3.1	3	2	424
Turnips, Frozen, Unprepared .333 pkg, mashed (10 oz) (94g)	15	0	0	0	3	1.7	--	1	24
Turnips, Raw 1 large (183g)	51	0	0	0	12	3.3	7	2	123

Food Serving size	Cal.	(g) Total Fat	(g) Sat. Fat	(mg) Chol.	(g) Carb.	(g) Fiber	(g) Sug.	(g) Prot.	(mg) Sod.
Water Chestnuts, Chinese (Matai), Raw									
4 water chestnuts (36g)	35	0	0	0	9	1.1	2	1	5
Water Chestnuts, Chinese, Canned, Solids and Liquids									
4 water chestnuts (28g)	14	0	0	0	3	0.7	1	0	2
Watercress, Raw									
1 sprig (2.5g)	0	0	0	0	0	0.0	0	0	1
Waxgourd (Chinese Preserving Melon), Cooked, Boiled, Drained, with Salt									
1 cup, cubes (175g)	19	0	0	0	4	1.8	2	1	600
Waxgourd (Chinese Preserving Melon), Cooked, Boiled, Drained, Without Salt									
1 cup, cubes (175g)	25	0	0	0	5	1.8	2	1	187
Waxgourd (Chinese Preserving Melon), Raw									
1 waxgourd (5700g)	741	11	1	0	171	165.3	--	23	6327
Yam, Cooked, Boiled, Drained or Baked, Without Salt									
.5 cup, cubes (68g)	79	0	0	0	19	2.7	0	1	5
Yam, Cooked, Boiled, Drained, or Baked, with Salt									
.5 cup, cubes (68g)	78	0	0	0	18	2.7	0	1	166
Yam, Raw									
1 cup, cubes (150g)	177	0	0	0	42	6.2	1	2	14
Yambean (Jicama), Raw									
1 cup (130g)	49	0	0	0	11	6.4	2	1	5
Yardlong Bean, Cooked, Boiled, Drained, with Salt									
1 pod (14g)	7	0	0	0	1	--	--	0	34
Yardlong Bean, Cooked, Boiled, Drained, Without Salt									
1 pod (14g)	7	0	0	0	1	--	--	0	1
Yardlong Bean, Raw									
1 pod (12g)	6	0	0	0	1	--	--	0	0
Yardlong Beans, Mature Seeds, Cooked, Boiled, with Salt									
1 cup (171g)	202	1	0	0	36	6.5	--	14	412
Yardlong Beans, Mature Seeds, Cooked, Boiled, Without Salt									
1 cup (171g)	202	1	0	0	36	6.5	--	14	9
Yardlong Beans, Mature Seeds, Raw									
1 cup (167g)	579	2	1	0	103	18.4	--	41	28

Food Serving size	Cal.	(g) Total Fat	(g) Sat. Fat	(mg) Chol.	(g) Carb.	(g) Fiber	(g) Sug.	(g) Prot.	(mg) Sod.

Potatoes

Food Serving size	Cal.	Total Fat	Sat. Fat	Chol.	Carb.	Fiber	Sug.	Prot.	Sod.
Side Dishes, Potato Salad .333 cup (95g)	108	6	1	57	13	--	--	1	312
Sweet Potato Leaves, Cooked, Steamed, with Salt 1 cup (64g)	22	0	0	0	5	1.2	3	1	159
Sweet Potato Leaves, Cooked, Steamed, Without Salt 1 cup (64g)	22	0	0	0	5	1.2	3	1	8
Sweet Potato Leaves, Raw 1 leaf (12-1/4" long) (16g)	6	0	0	0	1	0.3	--	1	1
Sweet Potato, Canned, Mashed 1 can (404 x 307) (496g)	501	1	0	0	115	8.4	27	10	372
Sweet Potato, Canned, Syrup Packed, Drained, Solids 1 cup (196g)	212	1	0	0	50	5.9	11	3	76
Sweet Potato, Canned, Syrup Packed, Solids and Liquids 1 can (404 x 307) (638g)	568	1	0	0	134	16.0	98	6	281
Sweet Potato, Canned, Vacuum Pack 1 cup, pieces (200g)	182	0	0	0	42	3.6	10	3	106
Sweet Potato, Cooked, Baked in Skin, with Salt .5 cup, mashed (100g)	92	0	0	0	21	3.3	11	2	246
Sweet Potato, Cooked, Baked in Skin, Without Salt 1 large (180g)	162	0	0	0	37	5.9	12	4	65
Sweet Potato, Cooked, Boiled, Without Skin 1 medium (151g)	115	0	0	0	27	3.8	9	2	41
Sweet Potato, Cooked, Boiled, Without Skin, with Salt 1 medium (151g)	115	0	0	0	27	3.8	9	2	397
Sweet Potato, Cooked, Candied, Home-prepared 1 piece (2-1/2" x 2" dia) (105g)	151	3	1	8	29	2.5	--	1	74
Sweet Potato, Frozen, Cooked, Baked, with Salt 1 cup, cubes (176g)	176	0	0	0	41	3.2	--	3	429
Sweet Potato, Frozen, Cooked, Baked, Without Salt 1 cup, cubes (176g)	176	0	0	0	41	3.2	16	3	14
Sweet Potato, Frozen, Unprepared 1 cup, cubes (176g)	169	0	0	0	39	3.0	--	3	11
Sweet Potato, Raw, Unprepared 1 sweet potato, 5" long (130g)	112	0	0	0	26	3.9	5	2	72

Food Serving size	Cal.	(g) Total Fat	(g) Sat. Fat	(mg) Chol.	(g) Carb.	(g) Fiber	(g) Sug.	(g) Prot.	(mg) Sod.
Vegetable Products (Including Canned)									
Alfalfa Seeds, Sprouted, Raw									
1 tablespoon (3g)	1	0	0	0	0	0.1	0	0	0
Baked Beans, Canned, No Salt									
1 cup (253g)	266	1	0	0	52	13.9	--	12	3
Bamboo Shoots, Canned, Drained, Solids									
1 can (303 x 406) (262g)	50	1	0	0	8	3.7	5	5	18
Bamboo Shoots, Cooked, Boiled, Drained, with Salt									
1 shoot (144g)	16	0	0	0	2	1.4	--	2	346
Bamboo Shoots, Cooked, Boiled, Drained, Without Salt									
1 shoot (144g)	17	0	0	0	3	1.4	--	2	6
Bamboo Shoots, Raw									
.5 cup (1/2" pieces) (76g)	21	0	0	0	4	1.7	2	2	3
Beans, Adzuki, Mature Seeds, Canned, Sweetened									
1 cup (296g)	702	0	0	0	163	--	--	11	645
Beans, Adzuki, Mature Seeds, Cooked, Boiled, with Salt									
1 cup (230g)	294	0	0	0	57	16.8	--	17	561
Beans, Adzuki, Mature Seeds, Cooked, Boiled, Without Salt									
1 cup (230g)	294	0	0	0	57	16.8	--	17	18
Beans, Adzuki, Mature Seeds, Raw									
1 cup (197g)	648	1	0	0	124	25.0	--	39	10
Beans, Adzuki, Yokan, Mature Seeds									
1 slice (14g)	36	0	0	0	9	--	--	0	12
Beans, Baked, Canned, Plain or Vegetarian									
1 cup (254g)	239	1	0	0	54	10.4	20	12	871
Beans, Baked, Canned, with Beef									
1 cup (266g)	322	9	4	59	45	--	--	17	1264
Beans, Baked, Canned, with Franks									
1 cup (259g)	368	17	6	16	40	17.9	17	17	1114
Beans, Baked, Canned, with Pork									
1 cup (253g)	268	4	2	18	51	13.9	--	13	1047
Beans, Baked, Canned, with Pork and Sweet Sauce									
1 cup (253g)	283	4	1	18	53	10.6	22	13	845
Beans, Baked, Canned, with Pork and Tomato Sauce									
1 cup (246g)	231	2	1	17	46	9.8	14	13	1075

Food Serving size	Cal.	(g) Total Fat	(g) Sat. Fat	(mg) Chol.	(g) Carb.	(g) Fiber	(g) Sug.	(g) Prot.	(mg) Sod.
Beans, Baked, Home Prepared									
1 cup (253g)	392	13	5	13	55	13.9	--	14	1068
Beans, Black, Mature Seeds, Cooked, Boiled, with Salt									
1 cup (172g)	227	1	0	0	41	15.0	--	15	408
Beans, Black, Mature Seeds, Cooked, Boiled, Without Salt									
1 cup (172g)	227	1	0	0	41	15.0	--	15	2
Beans, Black, Mature Seeds, Raw									
1 tbsp (12.1g)	41	0	0	0	8	1.8	0	3	1
Beans, Black, Turtle Soup, Mature Seeds, Canned									
1 cup (240g)	218	1	0	0	40	16.6	--	14	922
Beans, Black, Turtle Soup, Mature Seeds, Cooked, Boiled, with Salt									
1 cup (185g)	241	1	0	0	45	9.8	1	15	442
Beans, Black, Turtle Soup, Mature Seeds, Cooked, Boiled, Without Salt									
1 cup (185g)	241	1	0	0	45	9.8	1	15	6
Beans, Black, Turtle Soup, Mature Seeds, Raw									
1 cup (184g)	624	2	0	0	116	45.8	4	39	17
Beans, Chili, Barbecue, Ranch Style, Cooked									
1 cup (253g)	245	3	0	0	43	10.6	0	13	1834
Beans, Cranberry (Roman), Mature Seeds, Canned									
1 cup (260g)	216	1	0	0	39	16.4	--	14	863
Beans, Cranberry (Roman), Mature Seeds, Cooked, Boiled, with Salt									
1 cup (177g)	241	1	0	0	43	17.7	--	17	419
Beans, Cranberry (Roman), Mature Seeds, Cooked, Boiled, Without Salt									
1 cup (177g)	241	1	0	0	43	17.7	--	17	2
Beans, Cranberry (Roman), Mature Seeds, Raw									
1 cup (195g)	653	2	1	0	117	48.2	--	45	12
Beans, Fava, in Pod, Raw									
1 pod (6.1g)	5	0	0	0	1	--	--	0	2
Beans, French, Mature Seeds, Cooked, Boiled, with Salt									
1 cup (177g)	228	1	0	0	43	16.6	--	12	428
Beans, French, Mature Seeds, Cooked, Boiled, Without Salt									
1 cup (177g)	228	1	0	0	43	16.6	--	12	11
Beans, French, Mature Seeds, Raw									
1 cup (184g)	631	4	0	0	118	46.4	--	35	33

Food Serving size	Cal.	(g) Total Fat	(g) Sat. Fat	(mg) Chol.	(g) Carb.	(g) Fiber	(g) Sug.	(g) Prot.	(mg) Sod.
Beans, Great Northern, Mature Seeds, Canned									
1 cup (262g)	299	1	0	0	55	12.8	--	19	10
Beans, Great Northern, Mature Seeds, Cooked, Boiled, with Salt									
1 cup (177g)	209	1	0	0	37	12.4	--	15	421
Beans, Great Northern, Mature Seeds, Cooked, Boiled, Without Salt									
1 cup (177g)	209	1	0	0	37	12.4	--	15	4
Beans, Great Northern, Mature Seeds, Raw									
1 cup (183g)	620	2	1	0	114	37.0	4	40	26
Beans, Kidney, All Types, Mature Seeds, Canned									
1 cup (256g)	215	2	0	0	37	13.6	5	13	758
Beans, Kidney, All Types, Mature Seeds, Cooked, Boiled, with Salt									
1 cup (177g)	225	1	0	0	40	11.3	1	15	421
Beans, Kidney, All Types, Mature Seeds, Cooked, Boiled, Without Salt									
1 tbsp (11g)	14	0	0	0	3	0.7	0	1	0
Beans, Kidney, All Types, Mature Seeds, Raw									
1 cup (184g)	613	2	0	0	110	45.8	4	43	44
Beans, Kidney, California Red, Mature Seeds, Cooked, Boiled, with Salt									
1 cup (177g)	219	0	0	0	40	16.5	--	16	425
Beans, Kidney, California Red, Mature Seeds, Cooked, Boiled, Without Salt									
1 cup (177g)	219	0	0	0	40	16.5	--	16	7
Beans, Kidney, California Red, Mature Seeds, Raw									
1 cup (184g)	607	0	0	0	110	45.8	--	45	20
Beans, Kidney, Mature Seeds, Sprouted, Raw									
1 cup (184g)	53	1	0	0	8	--	--	8	11
Beans, Kidney, Red, Mature Seeds, Canned									
1 tbsp (16g)	13	0	0	0	2	0.9	0	1	41
Beans, Kidney, Red, Mature Seeds, Cooked, Boiled, with Salt									
1 cup (177g)	225	1	0	0	40	13.1	1	15	421
Beans, Kidney, Red, Mature Seeds, Cooked, Boiled, Without Salt									
1 tbsp (11g)	14	0	0	0	3	0.8	0	1	0
Beans, Kidney, Red, Mature Seeds, Raw									
1 tbsp (12.2g)	41	0	0	0	7	1.9	0	3	1
Beans, Kidney, Royal Red, Mature Seeds, Cooked, Boiled with Salt									
1 cup (177g)	218	0	0	0	39	16.5	--	17	427

Food Serving size	Cal.	(g) Total Fat	(g) Sat. Fat	(mg) Chol.	(g) Carb.	(g) Fiber	(g) Sug.	(g) Prot.	(mg) Sod.
Beans, Kidney, Royal Red, Mature Seeds, Raw									
1 cup (184g)	605	1	0	0	107	45.8	--	47	24
Beans, Kidney, Royal Red, Mature sSeeds, Cooked, Boiled, Without Salt									
1 cup (177g)	218	0	0	0	39	16.5	--	17	9
Beans, Lima, Immature Seeds, Canned, Regular Packed, Solids and Liquid									
1 can (303 x 406) (454g)	322	1	0	0	61	16.3	--	18	1144
Beans, Lima, Immature Seeds, Cooked, Boiled, Drained, Without Salt									
1 cup (170g)	209	1	0	0	40	9.0	3	12	29
Beans, Lima, Immature Seeds, Fozen, Fordhook, Cooked, Boiled, Drained, Without Salt									
1 pkg (10 oz), yields (311g)	320	1	0	0	60	18.0	4	19	215
Beans, Lima, Immature Seeds, Frozen, Baby, Cooked, Boiled, Drained, Without Salt									
1 pkg (10 oz), yields (311g)	327	1	0	0	60	18.7	4	21	90
Beans, Lima, Immature Seeds, Frozen, Baby, Unprepared									
1 pkg (10 oz) (284g)	375	1	0	0	71	17.0	--	22	148
Beans, Lima, Immature Seeds, Frozen, Fordhook, Unprepared									
1 pkg (10 oz) (284g)	301	1	0	0	56	15.6	4	18	165
Beans, Lima, Immature Seeds, Raw									
1 cup (156g)	176	1	0	0	31	7.6	2	11	12
Beans, Liquid from Stewed Kidney Beans									
1 cup (240g)	113	8	3	10	7	0.2	0	4	5
Beans, Mung, Mature Seeds, Sprouted, Canned, Drained, Solids									
1 cup (125g)	15	0	0	0	3	1.0	2	2	175
Beans, Navy, Mature Seeds, Canned									
1 cup (262g)	296	1	0	0	54	13.4	1	20	1174
Beans, Navy, Mature Seeds, Cooked, Boiled, with Salt									
1 cup (182g)	255	1	0	--	47	19.1	1	15	431
Beans, Navy, Mature Seeds, Cooked, Boiled, Without Salt									
1 cup (182g)	255	1	0	--	47	19.1	1	15	0
Beans, Navy, Mature Seeds, Raw									
1 cup (208g)	701	3	0	--	126	50.8	8	46	10
Beans, Navy, Mature Seeds, Sprouted, Raw									
1 cup (104g)	70	1	0	0	14	--	--	6	14

Food Serving size	Cal.	(g) Total Fat	(g) Sat. Fat	(mg) Chol.	(g) Carb.	(g) Fiber	(g) Sug.	(g) Prot.	(mg) Sod.
Beans, Pink, Mature Seeds, Cooked, Boiled, with Salt 1 cup (169g)	252	1	0	0	47	9.0	1	15	402
Beans, Pink, Mature Seeds, Cooked, Boiled, Without Salt 1 cup (169g)	252	1	0	0	47	9.0	1	15	3
Beans, Pink, Mature Seeds, Raw 1 cup (210g)	720	2	1	0	135	26.7	4	44	17
Beans, Pinto, Immature Seeds, Frozen, Cooked, Boiled, Drained, with Salt .333 pkg (10 oz), yields (94g)	152	0	0	0	29	8.1	--	9	300
Beans, Pinto, Immature Seeds, Frozen, Cooked, Boiled, Drained, Without Salt .333 pkg (10 oz), yields (94g)	152	0	0	0	29	8.1	--	9	78
Beans, Pinto, Immature Seeds, Frozen, Unprepared .333 pkg (10 oz) (94g)	160	0	0	0	31	5.4	--	9	86
Beans, Pinto, Mature Seeds, Canned 1 cup (240g)	206	2	0	0	37	11.0	1	12	706
Beans, Pinto, Mature Seeds, Cooked, Boiled, with Salt 1 cup (171g)	245	1	0	0	45	15.4	1	15	407
Beans, Pinto, Mature Seeds, Cooked, Boiled, Without Salt 1 tbsp (10.6g)	15	0	0	0	3	1.0	0	1	0
Beans, Pinto, Mature Seeds, Raw 1 tbsp (12g)	42	0	0	0	8	1.9	0	3	1
Beans, Shellie, Canned, Solids and Liquids 1 cup (245g)	74	0	0	0	15	8.3	2	4	818
Beans, Small White, Mature Seeds, Cooked, Boiled, with Salt 1 cup (179g)	254	1	0	0	46	18.6	--	16	426
Beans, Small White, Mature Seeds, Cooked, Boiled, Without Salt 1 cup (179g)	254	1	0	0	46	18.6	--	16	4
Beans, Small White, Mature Seeds, Raw 1 cup (215g)	722	3	1	0	134	53.5	--	45	26
Beans, Snap, Canned, All Styles, Seasoned, Solids and Liquids 1 can (303 x 406) (439g)	70	1	0	0	15	6.6	--	4	1637
Beans, Snap, Green Variety, Canned, Regular Packed, Solids and Liquids 1 can (303 x 406) (439g)	66	0	0	0	15	6.6	--	4	1137

Food Serving size	Cal.	(g) Total Fat	(g) Sat. Fat	(mg) Chol.	(g) Carb.	(g) Fiber	(g) Sug.	(g) Prot.	(mg) Sod.
Beans, Snap, Green, Canned, No Salt, Drained, Solid 10 beans (62g)	12	0	0	0	3	1.2	0	1	1
Beans, Snap, Green, Canned, No Salt, Solids and Liquids 1 can (303 x 406) (439g)	66	0	0	0	15	6.6	--	4	61
Beans, Snap, Green, Canned, Regular Packed, Drained, Solids 10 beans (62g)	14	0	0	0	3	1.4	0	1	162
Beans, Snap, Green, Cooked, Boiled, Drained, with Salt 1 cup (125g)	44	0	0	0	10	4.0	2	2	299
Beans, Snap, Green, Cooked, Boiled, Drained, Without Salt 1 cup (125g)	44	0	0	0	10	4.0	2	2	1
Beans, Snap, Green, Frozen, All Styles, Microwaved 1 cup (111g)	44	0	0	--	8	3.8	3	2	3
Beans, Snap, Green, Frozen, All Styles, Unprepared 1 pkg (10 oz) (284g)	111	1	0	0	21	7.4	6	5	9
Beans, Snap, Green, Frozen, Cooked, Boiled, Drained, with Salt 1 cup (135g)	35	0	0	0	8	4.1	2	2	331
Beans, Snap, Green, Frozen, Cooked, Boiled, Drained, Without Salt 1 cup (135g)	38	0	0	0	9	4.1	2	2	1
Beans, Snap, Green, Microwaved 1 cup, 1/2" pieces (116g)	45	1	--	--	7	3.9	4	3	3
Beans, Snap, Green, Raw 10 beans (4" long) (55g)	17	0	0	0	4	1.5	2	1	3
Beans, Snap, Yellow Raw 10 beans (4" long) (55g)	17	0	0	0	4	1.9	--	1	3
Beans, Snap, Yellow, Canned, No Salt, Drained, Solids 10 beans (62g)	12	0	0	0	3	0.8	1	1	1
Beans, Snap, Yellow, Canned, No Salt, Solids and Liquids 1 can (303 x 406) (439g)	66	0	0	0	15	6.6	--	4	61
Beans, Snap, Yellow, Canned, Regular Pack, Drained, Solids 10 beans (62g)	12	0	0	0	3	0.8	1	1	156
Beans, Snap, Yellow, Canned, Regular Pack, Solids and Liquids 1 can (303 x 406) (439g)	66	0	0	0	15	6.6	--	4	1137
Beans, Snap, Yellow, Cooked, Boiled, Drained, with Salt 1 cup (125g)	44	0	0	0	10	4.1	2	2	299

Food Serving size	Cal.	(g) Total Fat	(g) Sat. Fat	(mg) Chol.	(g) Carb.	(g) Fiber	(g) Sug.	(g) Prot.	(mg) Sod.
Beans, Snap, Yellow, Cooked, Boiled, Drained, Without Salt									
1 cup (125g)	44	0	0	0	10	4.1	2	2	4
Beans, Snap, Yellow, Frozen, All Styles, Unprepared									
1 pkg (10 oz) (284g)	94	1	0	0	22	8.0	--	5	9
Beans, Snap, Yellow, Frozen, Cooked, Boiled, Drained, with Salt									
1 cup (135g)	35	0	0	0	8	4.1	2	2	331
Beans, Snap, Yellow, Frozen, Cooked, Boiled, Drained, Without Salt									
1 cup (135g)	38	0	0	0	9	4.1	2	2	12
Beans, White, Mature Seeds, Canned									
1 cup (262g)	299	1	0	0	56	12.6	1	19	13
Beans, White, Mature Seeds, Cooked, Boiled, with Salt									
1 cup (179g)	249	1	0	0	45	11.3	1	17	433
Beans, White, Mature Seeds, Cooked, Boiled, Without Salt									
1 tbsp (11.2g)	16	0	0	0	3	0.7	0	1	1
Beans, White, Mature Seeds, Raw									
1 tbsp (12.6g)	42	0	0	0	8	1.9	0	3	2
Beans, Yellow, Mature Seeds, Cooked, Boiled, with Salt									
1 cup (177g)	255	2	0	0	45	18.4	--	16	427
Beans, Yellow, Mature Seeds, Cooked, boiled, Without Salt									
1 cup (177g)	255	2	0	0	45	18.4	--	16	9
Beans, Yellow, Mature Seeds, Raw									
1 cup (196g)	676	5	1	0	119	49.2	--	43	24
Beef Broth and Tomato Juice, Canned									
1 can (5.5 oz) (168g)	62	0	0	0	14	0.2	--	1	220
Beet Greens, Cooked, Boiled, Drained, with Salt									
1 cup (1" pieces) (144g)	39	0	0	0	8	4.2	1	4	687
Beet Greens, Raw									
1 leaf (32g)	7	0	0	0	1	1.2	0	1	72
Beets Greens, Cooked, Boiled, Drained, Without Salt									
.5 cup (1" pieces) (72g)	19	0	0	0	4	2.1	0	2	174
Beets, Canned, Drained, Solids									
1 cup, shredded (195g)	60	0	0	0	14	3.5	11	2	378
Beets, Canned, No Salt, Solids and Liquids									
1 cup (246g)	69	0	0	0	16	3.0	13	2	52

Food Serving size	Cal.	(g) Total Fat	(g) Sat. Fat	(mg) Chol.	(g) Carb.	(g) Fiber	(g) Sug.	(g) Prot.	(mg) Sod.
Beets, Canned, Regular Pkg, Solids and Liquids 1 cup (246g)	74	0	0	0	18	3.0	16	2	352
Beets, Cooked, Boiled, Drained 2 beets (2" dia, sphere) (100g)	44	0	0	0	10	2.0	8	2	77
Beets, Cooked, Boiled, Drained, with Salt 2 beets (2" dia, sphere) (100g)	44	0	0	0	10	2.0	8	2	285
Beets, Harvard, Canned, Solids and Liquids 1 cup, slices (246g)	180	0	0	0	45	6.2	--	2	399
Beets, Pickled, Canned, Solids and Liquids 1 cup, slices (227g)	148	0	0	0	37	5.9	31	2	599
Beets, Raw 1 beet (2" dia) (82g)	35	0	0	0	8	2.3	6	1	64
Broccoli, Chinese, Cooked 1 cup (88g)	19	1	0	0	3	2.2	1	1	6
Broccoli, Frozen, Chopped, Cooked, Boiled, Drained, with Salt 1 cup (184g)	52	0	0	0	10	5.5	3	6	478
Broccoli, Frozen, Chopped, Cooked, Boiled, Drained, Without Salt 1 cup (184g)	52	0	0	0	10	5.5	3	6	20
Broccoli, Frozen, Chopped, Unprepared 1 pkg (10 oz) (284g)	74	1	0	0	14	8.5	4	8	68
Broccoli, Frozen, Spears, Cooked, Boiled, Drained, with Salt .5 cup (92g)	26	0	0	0	5	2.8	1	3	239
Broccoli, Frozen, Spears, Cooked, Boiled, Drained, Without Salt .5 cup (92g)	26	0	0	0	5	2.8	1	3	22
Broccoli, Frozen, Spears, Unprepared 1 pkg (2 lb) (907g)	263	3	0	0	49	27.2	13	28	154
Broccoli, Raab, Cooked 1 NLEA serving (85g)	28	0	0	--	3	2.4	1	3	48
Broccoli, Raab, Raw 1 stalk (19g)	4	0	0	--	1	0.5	0	1	6
Broccoli, Raw 1 bunch (608g)	207	2	0	0	40	15.8	10	17	201
Broccoli, Stalks, Raw 1 stalk (114g)	32	0	0	0	6	--	--	3	31

Food Serving size	Cal.	(g) Total Fat	(g) Sat. Fat	(mg) Chol.	(g) Carb.	(g) Fiber	(g) Sug.	(g) Prot.	(mg) Sod.
Brussels Sprouts, Cooked, Boiled, Drained, with Salt									
.5 cup (78g)	28	0	0	0	6	2.0	1	2	200
Brussels Sprouts, Cooked, Boiled, Drained, Without Salt									
.5 cup (78g)	28	0	0	0	6	2.0	1	2	16
Brussels Sprouts, Frozen, Cooked, Boiled, Drained, with Salt									
1 cup (155g)	65	1	0	0	13	6.4	3	6	401
Brussels Sprouts, Frozen, Cooked, Boiled, Drained, Without Salt									
1 cup (155g)	65	1	0	0	13	6.4	3	6	23
Brussels Sprouts, Frozen, Unprepared									
1 pkg (2 lb) (907g)	372	4	1	0	71	34.5	--	34	91
Brussels Sprouts, Raw									
1 sprout (19g)	8	0	0	0	2	0.7	0	1	5
Cabbage, Chinese (Pak-choi), Cooked, Boiled, Drained, with Salt									
1 cup, shredded (170g)	20	0	0	0	3	1.7	1	3	459
Cabbage, Chinese (Pak-choi), Cooked, Boiled, Drained, Without Salt									
1 cup, shredded (170g)	20	0	0	0	3	1.7	1	3	58
Cabbage, Chinese (Pak-choi), Raw									
1 head (840g)	109	2	0	0	18	8.4	10	13	546
Cabbage, Chinese (Pe-tsai), Cooked, Boiled, Drained, with Salt									
1 leaf (14g)	2	0	0	0	0	0.2	--	0	34
Cabbage, Chinese (Pe-tsai), Cooked, Boiled, Drained, Without Salt									
1 leaf (14g)	2	0	0	0	0	0.2	--	0	1
Cabbage, Chinese (Pe-tsai), Raw									
1 cup, shredded (76g)	12	0	0	0	2	0.9	1	1	7
Cabbage, Common (Danish, Domestic and Pointed Types), Stored, Raw									
.5 cup, shredded (35g)	8	0	0	0	2	0.8	--	0	6
Cabbage, Common, Cooked, Boiled, Drained, with Salt									
.5 cup, shredded (75g)	17	0	0	0	4	1.4	2	1	191
Cabbage, Common, Freshly Harvest, Raw									
.5 cup, shredded (35g)	8	0	0	0	2	0.8	--	0	6
Cabbage, Cooked, Boiled, Drained, Without Salt									
.5 cup, shredded (75g)	17	0	0	0	4	1.4	2	1	6
Cabbage, Japanese Style, Fresh, Pickled									
1 cup (150g)	45	0	0	0	9	4.7	1	2	416

Food Serving size	Cal.	(g) Total Fat	(g) Sat. Fat	(mg) Chol.	(g) Carb.	(g) Fiber	(g) Sug.	(g) Prot.	(mg) Sod.
Cabbage, Mustard, Salted 1 cup (128g)	36	0	0	0	7	4.0	27	1	918
Cabbage, Napa, Cooked 1 cup (109g)	13	0	--	0	2	--	--	1	12
Cabbage, Raw 1 cup, shredded (70g)	18	0	0	0	4	1.8	2	1	13
Cabbage, Red, Cooked, Boiled, Drained, with Salt .5 cup, shredded (75g)	22	0	0	0	5	2.0	2	1	183
Cabbage, Red, Cooked, Boiled, Drained, Without Salt .5 cup, shredded (75g)	22	0	0	0	5	2.0	2	1	21
Cabbage, Red, Raw 1 cup, shredded (70g)	22	0	0	0	5	1.5	3	1	19
Cabbage, Savoy, Cooked, Boiled, Drained, with Salt 1 cup, shredded (145g)	35	0	0	0	8	4.1	--	3	377
Cabbage, Savoy, Cooked, Boiled, Drained, Without Salt 1 cup, shredded (145g)	35	0	0	0	8	4.1	--	3	35
Cabbage, Savoy, Raw 1 cup, shredded (70g)	19	0	0	0	4	2.2	2	1	20
Campbell's V8 100% Vegetable Juice 1 serving (243g)	51	0	0	0	10	1.9	0	2	420
Carrot Juice, Canned 1 fl oz (29.5g)	12	0	0	0	3	0.2	1	0	9
Carrot, Dehydrated 1 cup (74g)	252	1	0	0	59	17.5	29	6	204
Carrots, Baby, Raw 1 medium (10g)	4	0	0	0	1	0.3	0	0	8
Carrots, Canned, No Salt, Drained Solid 1 cup, sliced (146g)	37	0	0	0	8	2.2	4	1	61
Carrots, Canned, No Salt, Solids and Liquids 1 can (303 x 406) (454g)	104	1	0	0	24	8.2	11	3	154
Carrots, Canned, Regular Packed, Drained Solids 1 cup, sliced (146g)	37	0	0	0	8	2.2	4	1	353
Carrots, Canned, Regular Packed, Solids and Liquids 1 can (303 x 406) (454g)	104	1	0	0	24	8.2	11	3	1090

Food Serving size	Cal.	(g) Total Fat	(g) Sat. Fat	(mg) Chol.	(g) Carb.	(g) Fiber	(g) Sug.	(g) Prot.	(mg) Sod.
Carrots, Cooked, Boiled, Drained, with Salt									
.5 cup, slices (78g)	27	0	0	0	6	2.3	3	1	236
Carrots, Cooked, Boiled, Drained, Without Salt									
.5 cup, slices (78g)	27	0	0	0	6	2.3	3	1	45
Carrots, Frozen, Cooked, Boiled, Drained, with Salt									
1 cup, slices (146g)	54	1	0	0	11	4.8	6	1	431
Carrots, Frozen, Cooked, Boiled, Drained, Without Salt									
1 cup, sliced (146g)	54	1	0	0	11	4.8	6	1	86
Carrots, Frozen, Unprepared									
.5 cup, slices (64g)	23	0	0	0	5	2.1	3	0	44
Carrots, Raw									
1 cup, grated (110g)	45	0	0	0	11	3.1	5	1	76
Cauliflower, Cooked, Boiled, Drained, with Salt									
3 flowerets (54g)	12	0	0	0	2	1.2	1	1	131
Cauliflower, Cooked, Boiled, Drained, Without Salt									
3 flowerets (54g)	12	0	0	0	2	1.2	1	1	8
Cauliflower, Frozen, Cooked, Boiled, Drained, with Salt									
1 cup (1" pieces) (180g)	31	0	0	0	6	4.9	1	3	457
Cauliflower, Frozen, Cooked, Boiled, Drained, Without Salt									
1 cup (1" pieces) (180g)	34	0	0	0	7	4.9	2	3	32
Cauliflower, Frozen, Unprepared									
.5 cup (1" pieces) (66g)	16	0	0	0	3	1.5	1	1	16
Cauliflower, Green, Cooked, No Salt Added									
.2 head (90g)	29	0	0	0	6	3.0	--	3	21
Cauliflower, Green, Cooked, with Salt									
.5 cup (1" pieces) (62g)	20	0	0	0	4	2.0	--	2	161
Cauliflower, Green, Raw									
1 floweret (25g)	8	0	0	0	2	0.8	1	1	6
Cauliflower, Raw									
1 floweret (13g)	3	0	0	0	1	0.3	0	0	4
Celery, Cooked, Boiled, Drained, with Salt									
2 stalks (75g)	14	0	0	0	3	1.2	2	1	245
Celery, Cooked, Boiled, Drained, Without Salt									
2 stalks (75g)	14	0	0	0	3	1.2	2	1	68

Food Serving size	Cal.	(g) Total Fat	(g) Sat. Fat	(mg) Chol.	(g) Carb.	(g) Fiber	(g) Sug.	(g) Prot.	(mg) Sod.
Celery, Raw 1 NLEA serving (110g)	18	0	0	0	3	1.8	2	1	88
Chard, Swiss, Cooked, Boiled, Drained, with Salt 1 cup, chopped (175g)	35	0	--	0	7	3.7	2	3	726
Chard, Swiss, Cooked, Boiled, Drained, Without Salt 1 cup, chopped (175g)	35	0	0	0	7	3.7	2	3	313
Chard, Swiss, Raw 1 leaf (48g)	9	0	0	0	2	0.8	1	1	102
Chicory Roots, Raw .5 cup (1" pieces) (45g)	32	0	0	0	8	0.7	4	1	23
Chicory, Greens, Raw 1 cup, chopped (29g)	7	0	0	0	1	1.2	0	0	13
Chicory, Witloof, Raw .5 cup (45g)	8	0	0	0	2	1.4	--	0	1
Chives, Freeze-dried .25 cup (0.8g)	2	0	0	0	1	0.2	--	0	1
Chives, Raw 1 tsp, chopped (1g)	0	0	0	0	0	0.0	0	0	0
Cole Slaw, Home Prepared .5 cup (60g)	47	2	0	5	7	0.9	--	1	14
Collards, Cooked, Boiled, Drained, with Salt 1 cup, chopped (190g)	49	1	0	0	9	5.3	1	4	479
Collards, Cooked, Boiled, Drained, Without Salt 1 cup, chopped (190g)	49	1	0	0	9	5.3	1	4	30
Collards, Frozen, Chopped, Cooked, Boiled, Drained, with Salt 1 cup, chopped (170g)	61	1	0	0	12	4.8	1	5	486
Collards, Frozen, Chopped, Cooked, Boiled, Drained, Without Salt 1 cup, chopped (170g)	61	1	0	0	12	4.8	1	5	85
Collards, Frozen, Chopped, Unprepared 1 pkg (3 lb) (1361g)	449	5	1	0	88	49.0	--	37	653
Collards, Raw 1 cup, chopped (36g)	11	0	0	0	2	1.3	0	1	7
Coriander (Cilantro) Leaves, Raw 9 sprigs (20g)	5	0	0	0	1	0.6	0	0	9

Food Serving size	Cal.	(g) Total Fat	(g) Sat. Fat	(mg) Chol.	(g) Carb.	(g) Fiber	(g) Sug.	(g) Prot.	(mg) Sod.
Coriander Leaf, Dried 1 tsp (0.6g)	2	0	0	0	0	0.1	0	0	1
Coriander Seed 1 tsp (1.8g)	5	0	0	0	1	0.8	--	0	1
Corn Salad, Raw 1 cup (56g)	12	0	--	0	2	--	--	1	2
Corn, Sweet, White 1 ear, medium (6-3/4" to 7-1/2" long) (90g)	77	1	0	0	17	2.4	3	3	14
Corn, Sweet, White, Canned, Cream Style, No Salt 1 can (303 x 406) (482g)	347	2	0	0	87	5.8	11	8	14
Corn, Sweet, White, Canned, Cream Style, Regular Pack 1 can (303 x 406) (482g)	347	2	0	0	87	5.8	11	8	1374
Corn, Sweet, White, Canned, Vacuum Pack, No Salt 1 can (303 x 406) (340g)	269	2	0	0	66	6.8	--	8	10
Corn, Sweet, White, Canned, Vacuum Pack, Regular Pack 1 can (303 x 406) (340g)	269	2	0	0	66	6.8	--	8	925
Corn, Sweet, White, Canned, Whole Kernel, Drained, Solids 1 can (303 x 406) (298g)	241	3	0	0	55	6.0	7	8	963
Corn, Sweet, White, Canned, Whole Kernel, No Salt, Solids and Liquids 1 can (303 x 406) (482g)	308	2	0	0	74	3.4	--	9	58
Corn, Sweet, White, Canned, Whole Kernel, Regular Pack, Solids and Liquids 1 can (303 x 406) (482g)	308	2	0	0	74	8.2	--	9	1027
Corn, Sweet, White, Cooked, Boiled, Drained, with Salt 1 ear, medium (6-3/4" to 7-1/2" long) (103g)	100	1	0	0	22	2.8	8	3	261
Corn, Sweet, White, Cooked, Boiled, Drained, Without Salt 1 ear, medium (6-3/4" to 7-1/2" long) (103g)	100	1	0	0	22	2.8	8	3	3
Corn, Sweet, White, Frozen, Kernels Cut Off Cob, Boiled, Drained, with Salt 1 pkg (10 oz), yields (284g)	227	1	0	0	56	6.8	9	8	696
Corn, Sweet, White, Frozen, Kernels Cut Off Cob, Boiled, Drained, Without Salt 1 pkg (10 oz), yields (284g)	227	1	0	0	56	6.8	9	8	14
Corn, Sweet, White, Frozen, Kernels Cut Off Cob, Unprepared 1 pkg (10 oz) (284g)	250	2	0	0	59	6.8	--	9	9

Food Serving size	Cal.	(g) Total Fat	(g) Sat. Fat	(mg) Chol.	(g) Carb.	(g) Fiber	(g) Sug.	(g) Prot.	(mg) Sod.
Corn, Sweet, White, Frozen, Kernels On Cob, Cooked, Boiled, Drained, with Salt 1 ear, yields (63g)	59	0	0	0	14	1.8	--	2	151
Corn, Sweet, White, Frozen, Kernels On Cob, Cooked, Boiled, Drained, Without Salt 1 ear, yields (63g)	59	0	0	0	14	1.3	--	2	3
Corn, Sweet, White, Frozen, Kernels On Cob, Unprepared 1 ear, yields (125g)	123	1	0	0	29	3.5	--	4	6
Corn, Sweet, Yellow, Canned, Brine, Regular Packed, Solids and Liquids 1 can (303 x 406) (482g)	308	2	0	0	74	8.2	14	9	1027
Corn, Sweet, Yellow, Canned, Cream Style, No Salt 1 can (303 x 406) (482g)	347	2	0	0	87	5.8	16	8	14
Corn, Sweet, Yellow, Canned, Cream Style, Regular Packed 1 can (303 x 406) (482g)	347	2	0	0	87	5.8	16	8	1374
Corn, Sweet, Yellow, Canned, No Salt, Solids and Liquids 1 can (303 x 406) (482g)	308	2	0	0	74	8.2	14	9	58
Corn, Sweet, Yellow, Canned, Vacuum Pack, No Salt 1 can (303 x 406) (340g)	269	2	0	0	66	6.8	12	8	10
Corn, Sweet, Yellow, Canned, Vacuum Packed, Regular Packed 1 can, 15 oz (303 x 406) (425g)	336	2	0	0	83	8.5	15	10	1156
Corn, Sweet, Yellow, Canned, Whole Kernel, Drained Solid 1 can (12 oz), yields (211g)	171	2	0	0	40	4.0	6	6	629
Corn, Sweet, Yellow, Cooked, Boiled, Drained, with Salt 1 ear, medium (6-3/4" to 7-1/2" long) (103g)	99	2	0	0	22	2.5	5	4	261
Corn, Sweet, Yellow, Cooked, Boiled, Drained, Without Salt 1 ear, medium (6-3/4" to 7-1/2" long) (103g)	99	2	0	0	22	2.5	5	4	1
Corn, Sweet, Yellow, Frozen, Kernels Cut Off Cob, Boiled, Drained, Without Salt 1 pkg (10 oz), yields (284g)	230	2	0	0	55	6.8	9	7	3
Corn, Sweet, Yellow, Frozen, Kernels Cut Off Cob, Unprepared 1 pkg (284g)	250	2	0	0	59	6.0	7	9	9
Corn, Sweet, Yellow, Frozen, Kernels On Cob, Cooked, Boiled, Drained, with Salt 1 ear, yields (63g)	59	0	0	0	14	1.8	2	2	151

Food Serving size	Cal.	(g) Total Fat	(g) Sat. Fat	(mg) Chol.	(g) Carb.	(g) Fiber	(g) Sug.	(g) Prot.	(mg) Sod.
Corn, Sweet, Yellow, Frozen, Kernels On Cob, Cooked, Boiled, Drained, Without Salt									
1 ear, yields (63g)	59	0	0	0	14	1.8	2	2	3
Corn, Sweet, Yellow, Frozen, Kernels On Cob, Unprepared									
1 ear, yields (125g)	123	1	0	0	29	3.5	5	4	6
Corn, Sweet, Yellow, Frozen, Kernels, Cut Off Cob, Boiled, Drained, with Salt									
1 pkg (10 oz), yields (284g)	224	2	0	0	53	6.8	9	7	696
Corn, Sweet, Yellow, Raw									
1 ear, large (7-3/4" to 9" long), yields (143g)	123	2	0	0	27	2.9	9	5	21
Corn, White									
1 cup (166g)	606	8	1	0	123	--	--	16	58
Corn, with Red and Green Peppers, Canned, Solids and Liquids									
1 cup (227g)	170	1	0	0	41	--	--	5	788
Corn, Yellow									
1 cup (166g)	606	8	1	0	123	12.1	1	16	58
Corn, Yellow, Whole Kernel, Frozen, Microwaved									
1 cup (141g)	185	2	0	0	36	3.7	5	5	6
Cress, Garden, Cooked, Boiled, Drained, with Salt									
1 cup (135g)	31	1	0	0	5	0.9	4	3	329
Cress, Garden, Cooked, Boiled, Drained, Without Salt									
.5 cup (68g)	16	0	0	0	3	0.5	2	1	5
Cress, Garden, Raw									
1 sprig (1g)	0	0	0	0	0	0.0	0	0	0
Cucumber, Peeled, Raw									
1 cup, sliced (119g)	14	0	0	0	3	0.8	2	1	2
Cucumber, with Peel, Raw									
1 cucumber (8-1/4") (301g)	45	0	0	0	11	1.5	5	2	6
Dandelion Greens, Cooked, Boiled, Drained, with Salt									
1 cup, chopped (105g)	35	1	--	0	7	3.0	2	2	294
Dandelion, Greens, Cooked, Boiled, Drained, Without Salt									
1 cup, chopped (105g)	35	1	0	0	7	3.0	1	2	46
Dandelion, Greens, Raw									
1 cup, chopped (55g)	25	0	0	0	5	1.9	0	1	42
Dill Weed, Dried									
1 tsp (1g)	3	0	0	0	1	0.1	--	0	2

Food Serving size	Cal.	(g) Total Fat	(g) Sat. Fat	(mg) Chol.	(g) Carb.	(g) Fiber	(g) Sug.	(g) Prot.	(mg) Sod.
Dill Weed, Fresh 5 sprigs (1g)	0	0	0	0	0	0.0	--	0	1
Eggplant, Cooked, Boiled, Drained, with Salt 1 cup, (1" cubes) (99g)	33	0	0	0	8	2.5	3	1	237
Eggplant, Cooked, Boiled, Drained, Without Salt 1 cup (1" cubes) (99g)	35	0	0	0	9	2.5	3	1	1
Eggplant, Pickled 1 cup (136g)	67	1	0	0	13	3.4	0	1	2277
Eggplant, Raw 1 eggplant, peeled (yield from 1-1/4 lb) (458g)	110	1	0	0	26	15.6	11	5	9
Endive, Raw .5 cup, chopped (25g)	4	0	0	0	1	0.8	0	0	6
Falafel, Home Prepared 1 patty (approx 2-1/4" dia) (17g)	57	3	0	0	5	--	--	2	50
Fennel, Bulb, Raw 1 bulb (234g)	73	0	--	0	17	7.3	--	3	122
Gardenburger, Black Bean Chipotle Burger 1 patty (71g)	95	3	0	0	16	4.5	1	5	387
Gardenburger, Breaded Chik 'N Veggie Patties 1 patty (71g)	155	9	1	0	13	3.6	1	9	493
Gardenburger, California Burger 1 patty (71g)	102	4	0	0	15	2.6	1	4	400
Gardenburger, Flame Grilled Burger 1 patty (71g)	87	3	0	0	6	5.1	0	12	501
Gardenburger, Garden Vegan 1 patty (71g)	75	1	0	0	12	4.3	0	9	273
Gardenburger, Gourmet Baja Steak 1 steak (156g)	192	6	2	6	36	9.7	3	7	688
Gardenburger, Gourmet Fire Dragon Steak 1 steak (156g)	158	8	2	0	28	11.9	7	5	566
Gardenburger, Gourmet Hula Steak 1 steak (156g)	253	8	6	0	48	10.8	12	6	602

Food Serving size	Cal.	(g) Total Fat	(g) Sat. Fat	(mg) Chol.	(g) Carb.	(g) Fiber	(g) Sug.	(g) Prot.	(mg) Sod.
Gardenburger, Gourmet Tuscany Steak									
1 steak (156g)	215	8	4	17	36	12.9	4	12	747
Gardenburger, Herb Crusted Cutlet									
1 patty (71g)	142	7	1	0	13	3.2	1	9	413
Gardenburger, Homestyle Classic Veggie Burger									
1 patty (71g)	121	6	0	0	8	4.5	0	12	493
Gardenburger, Malibu Burger, Made with Organic Whole Grains, Corn and Carrots									
1 patty (91g)	171	8	1	0	21	4.6	2	5	611
Gardenburger, Original									
1 patty (71g)	103	3	1	9	18	4.6	1	5	401
Gardenburger, Savory Portobello Veggie Burger									
1 patty (71g)	99	3	1	3	17	5.0	1	4	493
Gardenburger, Sun-dried Tomato Basil Burger									
1 patty (71g)	97	3	1	3	17	3.7	2	4	275
Gardenburger, Veggie Medley Burger									
1 patty (71g)	96	3	0	0	17	5.2	1	3	376
Gourd, Dishcloth (Towelgourd), Cooked, Boiled, Drained, with Salt									
.5 cup (1" slices) (89g)	48	0	0	0	12	--	--	1	229
Gourd, White-flowered (Calabash), Cooked, Boiled, Drained, with Salt									
1 cup (1" cubes) (146g)	19	0	0	0	5	--	--	1	347
Grape Leaves, Canned									
1 leaf (4g)	3	0	0	0	0	--	--	0	114
Grape Leaves, Raw									
1 leaf (3g)	3	0	0	0	1	0.3	0	0	0
Green Giant, Harvest Burger, Original Flavor, All Vegetable Protein Patty, Frozen									
1 patty (90g)	138	4	1	0	7	5.7	5	18	411
Hearts of Palm, Canned									
1 piece (33g)	9	0	0	0	2	0.8	--	1	141
Horseradish, Prepared									
1 tsp (5g)	2	0	0	0	1	0.2	0	0	16
Horseradish, Tree Leafy Tips, Cooked, Boiled, Drained, Without Salt									
1 cup, chopped (42g)	25	0	0	0	5	0.8	0	2	4
Horseradish, Tree Leafy Tips, Raw									
1 cup, chopped (21g)	13	0	--	0	2	0.4	--	2	2

Food Serving size	Cal.	(g) Total Fat	(g) Sat. Fat	(mg) Chol.	(g) Carb.	(g) Fiber	(g) Sug.	(g) Prot.	(mg) Sod.
Horseradish, Tree, Leafy Tips, Cooked, Boiled, Drained, with Salt									
1 cup, chopped (42g)	25	0	--	0	5	0.8	0	2	103
Horseradish, Tree, Pods, Cooked, Boiled, Drained, with Salt									
1 cup, slices (118g)	42	0	--	0	10	5.0	--	2	329
Horseradish, Tree, Pods, Cooked, Boiled, Drained, Without Salt									
1 cup, slices (118g)	42	0	0	0	10	5.0	--	2	51
Horseradish, Tree, Pods, Raw									
1 pod (15-1/3" long) (11g)	4	0	0	0	1	0.4	--	0	5
Jerusalem Artichokes, Raw									
1 cup, slices (150g)	110	0	0	0	26	2.4	14	3	6
Kale, Cooked, Boiled, Drained, with salt									
1 cup, chopped (130g)	36	1	0	0	7	2.6	2	2	337
Kale, Cooked, Boiled, Drained, Without Salt									
1 cup, chopped (130g)	36	1	0	0	7	2.6	2	2	30
Kale, Frozen, Cooked, Boiled, Drained, with Salt									
1 cup, chopped (130g)	39	1	0	0	7	2.6	2	4	326
Kale, Frozen, Cooked, Boiled, Drained, Without Salt									
.5 cup, chopped or diced (65g)	20	0	0	0	3	1.3	1	2	10
Kale, Frozen, Unprepared									
.333 pkg (10 oz) (94g)	26	0	0	0	5	1.9	--	3	14
Kale, Raw									
1 cup, chopped (67g)	34	0	0	0	7	1.3	--	2	29
Kale, Scotch, Cooked, Boiled, Drained, with Salt									
1 cup, chopped (130g)	36	1	0	0	7	--	--	2	365
Kale, Scotch, Cooked, Boiled, Drained, Without Salt									
1 cup, chopped (130g)	36	1	0	0	7	1.6	--	2	59
Kale, Scotch, Raw									
1 cup, chopped (67g)	28	0	0	0	6	1.1	--	2	47
Kohlrabi, Cooked, Boiled, Drained, with Salt									
1 cup, slices (165g)	48	0	0	0	11	1.8	5	3	424
Kohlrabi, Cooked, Boiled, Drained, Without Salt									
1 slice (16g)	4	0	0	0	1	0.6	0	0	3
Kohlrabi, Cooked, Boiled, Drained, Without Salt									
1 cup, slices (165g)	48	0	0	0	11	1.8	5	3	35

Food Serving size	Cal.	(g) Total Fat	(g) Sat. Fat	(mg) Chol.	(g) Carb.	(g) Fiber	(g) Sug.	(g) Prot.	(mg) Sod.
Leeks (Bulb and Lower Leaf Portion), Cooked, Boiled, Drained, with Salt									
.25 cup, chopped (26g)	8	0	0	0	2	0.3	1	0	64
Leeks (Bulb and Lower Leaf Portion), Cooked, Boiled, Drained, Without Salt									
.25 cup, chopped or diced (26g)	8	0	0	0	2	0.3	1	0	3
Leeks (Bulb and Lower Leaf Portion), Freeze-dried									
.25 cup (0.8g)	3	0	0	0	1	0.1	--	0	0
Leeks (Bulb and Lower Leaf Portion), Raw									
1 leek (89g)	54	0	0	0	13	1.6	3	1	18
Lentils, Mature Seeds, Cooked, Boiled, with Salt									
1 cup (198g)	226	1	0	0	39	15.6	4	18	471
Lima Beans, Immature Seeds, Canned, No Salt, Solids and Liquids									
1 can (303 x 406) (454g)	322	1	0	0	61	16.3	4	18	18
Mixed Vegetable and Fruit Juice Drink, with Added Nutrition									
8 fl oz (247g)	72	0	0	0	18	0.0	5	0	52
Mustard Greens, Frozen, Cooked, Boiled, Drained, with Salt									
1 pkg (10 oz), yields (212g)	40	1	0	0	7	5.9	1	5	553
Mustard Greens, Frozen, Cooked, Boiled, Drained, Without Salt									
1 pkg (10 oz), yields (212g)	40	1	0	0	7	5.9	1	5	53
Mustard Greens, Frozen, Unprepared									
1 pkg (10 oz) (284g)	57	1	0	0	10	9.4	--	7	82
Mustard Spinach (Tendergreen), Cooked, Boiled, Drained, with Salt									
1 cup, chopped (180g)	29	0	--	0	5	3.6	--	3	450
Mustard Spinach (Tendergreen), Cooked, Boiled, Drained, Without Salt									
1 cup, chopped (180g)	29	0	--	0	5	3.6	--	3	25
Onion Rings, Breaded, Partially Fried, Frozen, Prepared, Heated in Oven									
10 rings, large (3-4" dia) (71g)	289	19	6	0	27	0.9	--	4	266
Onions, Canned, Solids and Liquids									
.5 cup, chopped or diced (112g)	21	0	0	0	5	1.3	2	1	416
Onions, Cooked, Boiled, Drained, with Salt									
1 tbsp, chopped (15g)	6	0	0	0	1	0.2	1	0	36
Onions, Cooked, Boiled, Drained, Without Salt									
1 tbsp, chopped (15g)	7	0	0	0	2	0.2	1	0	0
Onions, Dehydrated Flakes									
.25 cup (14g)	49	0	0	0	12	1.3	5	1	3

Food Serving size	Cal.	(g) Total Fat	(g) Sat. Fat	(mg) Chol.	(g) Carb.	(g) Fiber	(g) Sug.	(g) Prot.	(mg) Sod.
Onions, Frozen, Chopped, Cooked, Boiled, Drained, with Salt									
.5 cup, chopped or diced (105g)	27	0	0	0	6	1.8	3	1	260
Onions, Frozen, Chopped, Cooked, Boiled, Drained, Without Salt									
.5 cup, chopped or diced (105g)	29	0	0	0	7	1.9	3	1	13
Onions, Frozen, Chopped, Unprepared									
1 pkg (10 oz) (284g)	82	0	0	0	19	5.1	--	2	34
Onions, Frozen, Whole, Cooked, Boiled, Drained, with Salt									
1 cup (210g)	55	0	0	0	13	2.9	6	1	512
Onions, Frozen, Whole, Cooked, Boiled, Drained, Without Salt									
1 cup (210g)	59	0	0	0	14	2.9	6	1	17
Onions, Frozen, Whole, Unprepared									
1 pkg (10 oz) (284g)	99	0	0	0	24	4.8	11	3	28
Onions, Yellow, Sauteed									
1 cup, chopped (87g)	115	9	1	--	7	1.5	--	1	10
Parsley, Freeze-dried									
.25 cup (1.4g)	4	0	--	0	1	0.5	--	0	5
Peas and Carrots, Canned, No Salt, Solids and Liquids									
1 cup (255g)	97	1	0	0	22	8.4	7	6	10
Peas and Carrots, Canned, Regular Pkg, Solids and Liquids									
1 cup (255g)	97	1	0	0	22	5.1	--	6	663
Peas and Carrots, Frozen, Cooked, Boiled, Drained, with Salt									
.5 cup (80g)	38	0	0	0	8	2.5	3	2	243
Peas and Carrots, Frozen, Cooked, Boiled, Drained, Without Salt									
.5 cup (80g)	38	0	0	0	8	2.5	3	2	54
Peas and Carrots, Frozen, Unprepared									
1 pkg (10 oz) (284g)	151	1	0	0	32	9.7	--	10	224
Peas and Onions, Canned, Solids and Liquids									
1 cup (120g)	61	0	0	0	10	2.8	--	4	530
Peas and Onions, Frozen, Cooked, Boiled, Drained, Without Salt									
1 cup (180g)	81	0	0	0	16	4.0	7	5	67
Peas and Onions, Frozen, Unprepared									
1 pkg (10 oz) (284g)	199	1	0	0	38	9.9	--	11	173
Peas, Edible-podded, Boiled, Drained, Without Salt									
1 cup (160g)	67	0	0	0	11	4.5	6	5	6

Food Serving size	Cal.	(g) Total Fat	(g) Sat. Fat	(mg) Chol.	(g) Carb.	(g) Fiber	(g) Sug.	(g) Prot.	(mg) Sod.
Peas, Edible-podded, Cooked, Boiled, Drained, with Salt									
1 cup (160g)	64	0	0	0	10	4.5	6	5	384
Peas, Edible-podded, Frozen, Cooked, Boiled, Drained, with Salt									
1 pkg (10 oz), yields (253g)	127	1	0	0	21	7.8	12	9	610
Peas, Edible-podded, Frozen, Cooked, Boiled, Drained, Without Salt									
1 pkg (10 oz), yields (253g)	132	1	0	0	23	7.8	12	9	13
Peas, Edible-podded, Frozen, Unprepared									
1 pkg (10 oz) (284g)	119	1	0	0	20	8.8	--	8	11
Peas, Green (Includes Baby and Lesuer Types), Canned, Drained Solids, Unprepared									
1 can (303 x 406) (313g)	216	2	0	0	36	15.3	9	14	911
Peas, Green, Canned, No Salt, Drained Solids									
1 can (303 x 406) (313g)	216	1	0	0	39	12.8	13	14	6
Peas, Green, Canned, No Salt, Solids and Liquids									
1 can (303 x 406) (482g)	255	1	0	0	47	15.9	15	15	43
Peas, Green, Canned, Regular Pkg, Solids and Liquids									
1 can (303 x 406) (482g)	255	1	0	0	47	15.9	15	15	1205
Peas, Green, Canned, Seasoned, Solids and Liquids									
.5 cup (114g)	57	0	0	0	11	2.3	--	4	290
Peas, Green, Cooked, Boiled, Drained, with Salt									
1 cup (160g)	134	0	0	0	25	8.8	9	9	382
Peas, Green, Cooked, Boiled, Drained, Without Salt									
1 cup (160g)	134	0	0	0	25	8.8	9	9	5
Peas, Green, Frozen, Cooked, Boiled, Drained, with Salt									
1 pkg (10 oz), yields (253g)	197	1	0	0	36	13.9	12	13	817
Peas, Green, Frozen, Cooked, Boiled, Drained, Without Salt									
1 pkg (10 oz), yields (253g)	197	1	0	0	36	13.9	12	13	182
Peas, Split, Mature Seeds, Cooked, Boiled, with Salt									
1 cup (196g)	227	1	0	0	40	16.3	6	16	466
Peas, Split, Mature Seeds, Cooked, Boiled, Without Salt									
1 tbsp (12.2g)	14	0	0	0	3	1.0	0	1	0
Peas, Split, Mature Seeds, Raw									
1 lb (453.6g)	1547	5	1	0	274	115.7	36	111	68
Peppers, Chili, Ground, Canned									
1 cup (139g)	29	0	0	0	6	2.4	--	1	552

Food Serving size	Cal.	(g) Total Fat	(g) Sat. Fat	(mg) Chol.	(g) Carb.	(g) Fiber	(g) Sug.	(g) Prot.	(mg) Sod.
Peppers, Hot Chili, Green, Canned, Pods, Excluding Seeds, Solids and Liquids									
.5 cup, chopped or diced (68g)	14	0	0	0	3	0.9	2	1	798
Peppers, Hot Chili, Green, Raw									
.5 cup, chopped or diced (75g)	30	0	0	0	7	1.1	4	2	5
Peppers, Hot Chili, Red, Canned, Excluding Seeds, Solids and Liquids									
.5 cup, chopped or diced (68g)	14	0	0	0	3	0.9	2	1	798
Peppers, Hot Chili, Sun-dried									
1 pepper (0.5g)	2	0	0	0	0	0.1	0	0	0
Peppers, Jalapeno, Canned, Solids and Liquids									
1 cup, sliced (104g)	28	1	0	0	5	2.7	2	1	1738
Peppers, Pasilla, Dried									
1 pepper (7g)	24	1	--	0	4	1.9	--	1	6
Peppers, Sweet, Green, Canned, Solids and Liquids									
1 cup, halves (140g)	25	0	0	0	5	1.7	--	1	1917
Peppers, Sweet, Green, Cooked, Boiled, Drained, with Salt									
1 pepper (73g)	19	0	0	0	4	0.9	2	1	174
Peppers, Sweet, Green, Cooked, Boiled, Drained, Without Salt									
1 tablespoon, chopped (11.6g)	3	0	0	0	1	0.1	0	0	0
Peppers, Sweet, Green, Freeze-dried									
.25 cup (1.6g)	5	0	0	0	1	0.3	1	0	3
Peppers, Sweet, Green, Frozen, Chopped, Cooked, Boiled, Drained, with Salt									
1 tablespoon, chopped (11.6g)	2	0	0	0	0	--	--	0	28
Peppers, Sweet, Green, Frozen, Chopped, Unprepared									
1 pkg (10 oz) (284g)	57	1	0	0	13	4.5	--	3	14
Peppers, Sweet, Red, Canned, Solids and Liquids									
.5 cup, halves (70g)	13	0	0	0	3	0.8	--	1	958
Peppers, Sweet, Red, Cooked, Boiled, Drained, with Salt									
1 pepper (73g)	19	0	0	0	4	0.9	3	1	174
Peppers, Sweet, Red, Cooked, Boiled, Drained, Without Salt									
1 tbsp (11.6g)	3	0	0	0	1	0.1	1	0	0
Peppers, Sweet, Red, Freeze-dried									
.25 cup (1.6g)	5	0	0	0	1	0.3	1	0	3
Peppers, Sweet, Red, Frozen, Chopped, Cooked, Boiled, Drained, with Salt									
1 tbsp, chopped (11.6g)	2	0	0	0	0	--	--	0	28

Food Serving size	Cal.	(g) Total Fat	(g) Sat. Fat	(mg) Chol.	(g) Carb.	(g) Fiber	(g) Sug.	(g) Prot.	(mg) Sod.
Peppers, Sweet, Red, Frozen, Chopped, Cooked, Boiled, Drained, Without Salt									
1 tbsp, chopped (11.6g)	2	0	0	0	0	--	0	0	0
Peppers, Sweet, Red, Frozen, Chopped, Unprepared									
.1 pkg (10 oz) (28g)	6	0	0	0	1	0.4	1	0	1
Peppers, Sweet, Red, Raw									
1 cup, sliced (92g)	29	0	0	0	6	1.9	4	1	4
Pickle Relish, Hamburger									
.5 cup (122g)	157	1	0	0	42	3.9	--	1	1337
Pickle Relish, Hot Dog									
.5 cup (122g)	111	1	0	0	28	1.8	--	2	1331
Pickle Relish, Sweet									
1 tbsp (15g)	20	0	0	0	5	0.2	4	0	122
Pickles, Chowchow, with Cauliflower Onion Mustard, Sweet									
1 cup (245g)	296	2	0	0	65	3.7	59	4	1291
Pickles, Cucumber, Dill or Kosher Dill									
1 cup (about 23 slices) (155g)	19	0	0	0	4	1.7	2	1	1356
Pickles, Cucumber, Dill, Low Sodium									
1 slice (6g)	1	0	0	0	0	0.1	0	0	1
Pickles, Cucumber, Sour									
1 large (4" long) (135g)	15	0	0	0	3	1.6	1	0	1631
Pickles, Cucumber, Sour, Low Sodium									
1 cup (about 23 slices) (155g)	17	0	0	0	4	1.9	2	1	28
Pickles, Cucumber, Sweet (Includes Bread and Butter Pickles)									
1 cup (153g)	139	1	0	0	32	1.5	28	1	699
Pickles, Cucumber, Sweet, Low Sodium (Includes Bread and Butter Pickles)									
1 cup, sliced (170g)	207	0	0	0	57	1.9	45	1	31
Pimiento, Canned									
1 tbsp (12g)	3	0	0	0	1	0.2	0	0	2
Potato Flour									
1 cup (160g)	571	1	0	0	133	9.4	6	11	88
Potato Pancakes									
1 medium, 3-1/4 in. x 3-5/8 in., 5/8 in. thick (37g)	99	5	1	35	10	1.2	1	2	283
Potato Puffs, Frozen, Oven-heated									
1 puff (8.4g)	16	1	0	0	2	0.2	0	0	40

Food Serving size	Cal.	(g) Total Fat	(g) Sat. Fat	(mg) Chol.	(g) Carb.	(g) Fiber	(g) Sug.	(g) Prot.	(mg) Sod.
Potato Puffs, Frozen, Unprepared 1 cup (128g)	224	10	2	0	33	2.4	0	3	585
Potato Salad, Home-prepared 1 cup (250g)	358	21	4	170	28	3.3	--	7	1323
Potato Soup, Instant, Dry, Mix 1 serving, 1/3 cup (39g)	134	1	0	5	30	3.0	4	4	239
Potato Sticks .5 cup (18g)	94	6	2	0	10	0.6	0	1	45
Potatoes, au Gratin, Dry Mix, Prepared with Water, Whole Milk and Butter 1 pkg, yield, 5.5 oz (822g)	764	34	21	123	106	7.4	--	19	3609
Potatoes, au Gratin, Dry Mix, Unprepared .167 pkg (5.5 oz) (26g)	82	1	1	--	19	1.1	--	2	545
Potatoes, au Gratin, Home-prepared from Recipe Using Butter 1 cup (245g)	323	19	12	56	28	4.4	--	12	1061
Potatoes, au Gratin, Home-prepared from Recipe Using Margarine 1 cup (245g)	323	19	9	37	28	4.4	--	12	1061
Potatoes, Baked, Flesh and Skin, with Salt 1 potato, medium (2-1/4" to 3-1/4" dia) (173g)	161	0	0	0	37	3.8	2	4	17
Potatoes, Baked, Flesh, with Salt 1 potato (2-1/3" x 4-3/4") (156g)	145	0	0	0	34	2.3	3	3	376
Potatoes, French Fries, All Types, Salt Added in Process, Frozen, Oven-heated 1 pkg (9 oz), yields (198g)	325	10	2	0	55	5.5	1	5	768
Potatoes, French Fries, All Types, Salt Added in Process, Frozen, Unprepared 1 pkg (9 oz) (255g)	375	12	3	0	63	4.8	1	6	847
Potatoes, French Fries, All Types, Salt Not Added in Processing, Frozen 1 pkg (9 oz) (255g)	383	12	2	0	63	4.8	1	6	59
Potatoes, French Fries, All Types, Salt Not Added in Processing, Frozen, Oven-heated 10 strips (74g)	127	4	1	0	21	1.9	0	2	24
Potatoes, French Fries, Crinkle/Regular Cut, Salt Added in Process, Frozen 10 strips (82g)	143	4	1	0	25	2.2	0	2	294

Food Serving size	Cal.	(g) Total Fat	(g) Sat. Fat	(mg) Chol.	(g) Carb.	(g) Fiber	(g) Sug.	(g) Prot.	(mg) Sod.
Potatoes, French Fries, Crinkle/Regular Cut, Salt Added in Process, Frozen, Oven-heated									
10 strips (69g)	115	4	1	0	19	1.6	0	2	270
Potatoes, French Fries, Shoestring, Salt Added in Process, Frozen									
10 strips (30g)	50	2	0	0	8	0.7	0	1	97
Potatoes, French Fries, Shoestring, Salt Added in Process, Frozen, Oven-heated									
10 strips (21g)	42	1	0	0	7	0.6	0	1	84
Potatoes, French Fries, Steak Fries, Salt Added in Process, Frozen									
10 strips (153g)	203	5	1	0	36	2.9	0	3	485
Potatoes, French Fries, Steak Fries, Salt Added in Process, Frozen, Oven-heated									
10 strips (133g)	202	5	1	0	36	3.5	0	3	496
Potatoes, Frozen, French Fries, Partially Fried, Cottage-cut, Prepared, Heated in Oven, Without Salt									
1 pkg (9 oz), yields (198g)	432	16	8	0	67	6.3	--	7	89
Potatoes, Frozen, French Fries, Partially Fried, Cottage-cut, Prepared, Heated in Oven, with Salt									
1 pkg (9 oz), yields (198g)	432	16	8	0	67	6.3	--	7	556
Potatoes, Frozen, French Fries, Partially Fried, Cottage-cut, Unprepared									
1 pkg (9 oz) (255g)	390	15	7	0	61	7.7	--	6	82
Potatoes, Frozen, French Fries, Partially Fried, Extruded, Prepared, Heated in Oven, Without Salt									
1 pkg (9 oz), yields (198g)	659	37	12	0	79	6.3	--	7	1214
Potatoes, Frozen, French Fries, Partially Fried, Extruded, Unprepared									
1 pkg (9 oz) (255g)	663	38	12	0	77	11.5	--	7	1250
Potatoes, Frozen, Whole, Unprepared									
1 cup (182g)	142	0	0	0	32	2.2	1	4	46
Potatoes, Hashed Brown, Frozen, Plain, Prepared									
.5 cup (78g)	170	9	4	0	22	1.6	1	2	27
Potatoes, Hashed Brown, Frozen, Plain, Unprepared									
1 pkg (12 oz) (340g)	279	2	1	--	60	4.8	--	7	75
Potatoes, Hashed Brown, Frozen, with Butter Sauce, Unprepared									
1 pkg (6 oz) (170g)	230	11	4	--	31	4.9	--	3	131
Potatoes, Hashed Brown, Home-prepared									
1 cup (156g)	413	20	3	0	55	5.0	2	5	534
Potatoes, Mashed, Dehydrated, Flakes Without Milk, Dry Form									
1 cup (60g)	212	0	0	0	49	4.0	2	5	62

Food Serving size	Cal.	Total Fat (g)	Sat. Fat (g)	Chol. (mg)	Carb. (g)	Fiber (g)	Sug. (g)	Prot. (g)	Sod. (mg)
Potatoes, Mashed, Dehydrated, Granules with Milk, Dry Form 1 cup (200g)	714	2	1	4	155	13.2	7	22	164
Potatoes, Mashed, Dehydrated, Granules Without Milk, Dry Form 1 cup (200g)	744	1	0	0	171	14.2	7	16	134
Potatoes, Mashed, Dehydrated, Prepared from Flakes Without Milk, Whole Milk and Butter 1 cup (210g)	204	11	7	29	23	1.7	3	4	344
Potatoes, Mashed, Dehydrated, Prepared from Granules with Milk, Water and Margarine Added 1 cup (210g)	244	10	2	4	34	2.7	4	4	361
Potatoes, Mashed, Dehydrated, Prepared from Granules Without Milk, Whole Milk and Butter 1 cup (210g)	227	10	6	29	30	4.6	--	4	540
Potatoes, Mashed, Home-prepared, Whole Milk and Butter Added 1 cup (210g)	237	9	5	23	35	3.2	3	4	666
Potatoes, Mashed, Home-prepared, Whole Milk and Margarine Added 1 cup (210g)	233	9	2	2	36	3.2	3	4	699
Potatoes, Mashed, Home-prepared, Whole Milk, Added 1 cup (210g)	174	1	1	4	37	3.2	3	4	634
Potatoes, Mashed, Prepared from Flakes, Without Milk, Whole Milk and Margarine 1 cup (210g)	237	12	3	8	32	4.8	--	4	697
Potatoes, Mashed, Prepared from Granules, Without Milk, Whole Milk and Margarine 1 cup (210g)	227	10	3	6	30	4.6	--	4	552
Potatoes, Microwaved, Cooked in Skin, Flesh and Skin, Without Salt 1 potato (2-3/4" dia by 4-3/4" long) (202g)	212	0	0	0	49	4.6	--	5	16
Potatoes, Microwaved, Cooked in Skin, Flesh, with Salt 1 potato (2-1/3" x 4-3/4") (156g)	156	0	0	0	36	2.5	--	3	379
Potatoes, Microwaved, Cooked in Skin, Flesh, Without Salt 1 potato (2-1/3" x 4-3/4") (156g)	156	0	0	0	36	2.5	--	3	11
Potatoes, Microwaved, Cooked in Skin, Without Salt 1 skin (58g)	77	0	0	0	17	3.2	--	3	9

Food Serving size	Cal.	(g) Total Fat	(g) Sat. Fat	(mg) Chol.	(g) Carb.	(g) Fiber	(g) Sug.	(g) Prot.	(mg) Sod.
Potatoes, Microwaved, Cooked, in Skin, Flesh and Skin, with Salt 1 potato (2-1/3" x 4-3/4") (202g)	212	0	0	0	49	4.6	--	5	493
Potatoes, Microwaved, Cooked, in Skin, with Salt 1 skin (58g)	77	0	0	0	17	3.2	--	3	146
Potatoes, O'Brien, Home-prepared 1 recipe, yields (1162g)	941	15	9	46	180	--	--	27	2522
Potatoes, Scalloped, Dry Mix, Prepared with Water, Whole Milk and Butter .167 pkg (5.5 oz), yields (137g)	127	6	4	15	17	1.5	--	3	467
Potatoes, Scalloped, Dry Mix, Unprepared .167 pkg (5.5 oz) (26g)	93	1	0	1	19	2.2	--	2	410
Potatoes, Scalloped, Home-prepared with Butter 1 cup (245g)	216	9	6	29	26	4.7	--	7	821
Potatoes, Scalloped, Home-prepared with Margarine 1 cup (245g)	216	9	3	15	26	4.7	--	7	821
Pumpkin and Squash Seed Kernels, Dried 1 oz (28.35g)	158	14	2	0	3	1.7	0	9	2
Pumpkin and Squash Seed Kernels, Roasted, with Salt 1 oz (28.35g)	163	14	2	0	4	1.8	0	8	73
Pumpkin and Squash Seed Kernels, Roasted, Without Salt 1 oz (28.35g)	163	14	2	0	4	1.8	0	8	5
Pumpkin and Squash Seeds, Whole, Roasted, with Salt 1 oz (85 seeds) (28.35g)	126	5	1	0	15	5.2	--	5	720
Pumpkin and Squash Seeds, Whole, Roasted, Without Salt 1 oz, (85 seeds) (28.35g)	126	5	1	0	15	5.2	--	5	5
Pumpkin Flowers, Cooked, Boiled, Drained, Without Salt 1 cup (134g)	20	0	0	0	4	1.2	3	1	8
Pumpkin Flowers, Raw 1 flower (2g)	0	0	0	0	0	--	--	0	0
Pumpkin Leaves, Cooked, Boiled, Drained, with Salt 1 cup (71g)	15	0	0	0	2	1.9	0	2	173
Pumpkin Leaves, Cooked, Boiled, Drained, Without Salt 1 cup (71g)	15	0	0	0	2	1.9	0	2	6
Pumpkin Leaves, Raw 1 cup (39g)	7	0	0	0	1	--	--	1	4

Food Serving size	Cal.	(g) Total Fat	(g) Sat. Fat	(mg) Chol.	(g) Carb.	(g) Fiber	(g) Sug.	(g) Prot.	(mg) Sod.
Pumpkin Pie Mix, Canned 1 cup (270g)	281	0	0	0	71	22.4	--	3	562
Pumpkin, Canned, with Salt 1 cup (245g)	83	1	0	0	20	7.1	8	3	590
Pumpkin, Canned, Without salt 1 cup (245g)	83	1	0	0	20	7.1	8	3	12
Pumpkin, Cooked, Boiled, Drained, with Salt 1 cup, mashed (245g)	49	0	0	0	12	2.7	2	2	581
Pumpkin, Cooked, Boiled, Drained, Without Salt 1 cup, mashed (245g)	49	0	0	0	12	2.7	2	2	2
Pumpkin, Flowers, Cooked, Boiled, Drained, with Salt 1 cup (134g)	20	0	0	0	4	1.2	3	1	324
Sauerkraut, Canned, Low Sodium 1 cup (142g)	31	0	0	0	6	3.6	1	1	437
Sauerkraut, Canned, Solids and Liquids 1 cup, undrained (236g)	45	0	0	0	10	6.8	4	2	1560
Spinach Souffle 1 recipe, yields (813g)	1398	105	50	959	48	5.7	15	64	4602
Tomatoes, Red, Ripe, Canned, Packed in Tomato Juice 1 tbsp (15g)	3	0	0	0	1	0.2	0	0	21
Tomatoes, Red, Ripe, Canned, Packed in Tomato Juice, No Salt Added 1 tbsp (15g)	3	0	0	0	1	0.2	0	0	2
Tomatoes, Red, Ripe, Canned, Stewed 1 cup (255g)	66	0	0	0	16	2.6	9	2	564
Tomatoes, Red, Ripe, Canned, with Green Chilies 1 cup (241g)	36	0	0	0	9	--	--	2	966
Turnips, Frozen, Cooked, Boiled, Drained, Without Salt 1 cup (156g)	36	0	0	0	7	3.1	4	2	56
Vegetable Juice Cocktail, Canned 6 fl oz (182g)	35	0	0	0	8	1.5	6	1	360
Vegetable Oil Spread, Unspecified Oils, Approximately 37% Fat, with Salt 1 cup (232g)	786	88	20	0	2	0.0	0	1	1366
Vegetable Oil, Palm Kernel 1 cup (218g)	1879	218	178	0	0	0.0	0	0	0
Vegetable Oil-butter Spread, Reduced Calorie 1 cup (207g)	963	110	37	112	0	0.0	--	0	1203

Food Serving size	Cal.	(g) Total Fat	(g) Sat. Fat	(mg) Chol.	(g) Carb.	(g) Fiber	(g) Sug.	(g) Prot.	(mg) Sod.
Vegetables, Mixed (Corn, Lima Beans, Peas, Green Beans, Carrots) Canned, No Salt 1 cup (182g)	67	0	0	0	13	5.6	1	3	47
Vegetables, Mixed, Canned, Drained, Solids 1 cup (163g)	80	0	0	0	15	4.9	4	4	243
Vegetables, Mixed, Canned, Solids and Liquids 1 cup (245g)	88	1	0	0	17	9.3	--	3	549
Vegetables, Mixed, Frozen, Cooked, Boiled, Drained, with Salt .5 cup (91g)	55	0	0	0	12	4.0	3	3	247
Vegetables, Mixed, Frozen, Cooked, Boiled, Drained, Without Salt .5 cup (91g)	59	0	0	0	12	4.0	3	3	32
Vegetables, Mixed, Frozen, Unprepared 1pkg (2-1/2 lb) (1134g)	726	6	1	0	153	45.4	--	38	533
Vegetarian Fillets 1 fillet (85g)	247	15	2	0	8	5.2	0	20	417
Vegetarian Meatloaf or Patties 1 slice (56g)	110	5	1	0	4	2.6	0	12	308
Vegetarian Stew 1 cup (247g)	304	7	1	0	17	2.7	35	42	988
Veggie Burgers or Soy Burgers, Unprepared 1 pattie (70g)	124	4	1	4	10	3.4	1	11	398
Worthington Vegetable Scallops, Canned, Unprepared .5 cup (85g)	93	1	0	0	4	2.9	0	17	391
Worthington Veja-links, Canned, Unprepared 1 link (31g)	48	3	0	1	1	1.0	0	5	164

Spices/Seasonings

Allspice, Ground 1 tsp (1.9g)	5	0	0	0	1	0.4	--	0	1
Anise Seed 1 tsp, whole (2.1g)	7	0	0	0	1	0.3	--	0	0
Bread Crumbs, Dry, Grated, Plain 1 cup (108g)	427	6	1	0	78	4.9	7	14	791

Food Serving size	Cal.	(g) Total Fat	(g) Sat. Fat	(mg) Chol.	(g) Carb.	(g) Fiber	(g) Sug.	(g) Prot.	(mg) Sod.
Bread Crumbs, Dry, Grated, Seasoned									
1 cup (120g)	460	7	2	1	82	5.9	7	17	2111
Capers, Canned									
1 tbsp, drained (8.6g)	2	0	0	0	0	0.3	0	0	255
Celery Seed									
1 tsp (2g)	8	1	0	0	1	0.2	0	0	3
Chervil, Dried									
1 tsp (0.6g)	1	0	0	0	0	0.1	--	0	0
Chili Powder									
1 tsp (2.7g)	8	0	0	0	1	0.9	0	0	44
Cinnamon, Ground									
1 tsp (2.6g)	6	0	0	0	2	1.4	0	0	0
Cloves, Ground									
1 tsp (2.1g)	7	0	0	0	1	0.7	0	0	5
Curry Powder									
1 tsp (2g)	7	0	0	0	1	0.7	0	0	1
Dill Seed									
1 tsp (2.1g)	6	0	0	0	1	0.4	--	0	0
Fennel Seed									
1 tsp, whole (2g)	7	0	0	0	1	0.8	--	0	2
Fenugreek Seed									
1 tsp (3.7g)	12	0	0	0	2	0.9	--	1	2
Garlic Powder									
1 tsp (3.1g)	10	0	0	0	2	0.3	0	1	2
George Weston Bakeries, Brownberry Sage and Onion Stuffing Mix, Dry									
1 serving (67g)	261	3	1	--	49	3.6	--	9	1126
Ginger, Ground									
1 tsp (1.8g)	6	0	0	0	1	0.3	0	0	0
Mace, Ground									
1 tsp (1.7g)	8	1	0	0	1	0.3	--	0	1
Marjoram, Dried									
1 tsp (0.6g)	2	0	0	0	0	0.2	0	0	0
Mustard, Prepared, Yellow									
1 cup (249g)	167	10	1	0	13	8.2	2	11	2826

Food Serving size	Cal.	(g) Total Fat	(g) Sat. Fat	(mg) Chol.	(g) Carb.	(g) Fiber	(g) Sug.	(g) Prot.	(mg) Sod.
Nutmeg, Ground 1 tsp (2.2g)	12	1	1	0	1	0.5	1	0	0
Onion Powder 1 tsp (2.4g)	8	0	0	0	2	0.4	0	0	2
Paprika 1 tsp (2.3g)	6	0	0	0	1	0.8	0	0	2
Parsley, Dried 1 tbsp (1.6g)	5	0	0	0	1	0.4	0	0	7
Pepper, Ancho, Dried 1 pepper (17g)	48	1	0	0	9	3.7	--	2	7
Pepper, Banana, Raw 1 small (4" long) (33g)	9	0	0	0	2	1.1	1	1	4
Pepper, Black 1 tsp, ground (2.3g)	6	0	0	0	1	0.6	0	0	0
Pepper, Red or Cayenne 1 tsp (1.8g)	6	0	0	0	1	0.5	0	0	1
Pepper, Serrano, Raw 1 pepper (6.1g)	2	0	0	0	0	0.2	0	0	1
Pepper, White 1 tsp, ground (2.4g)	7	0	0	0	2	0.6	--	0	0
Peppermint, Fresh 2 leaves (0.1g)	0	0	0	0	0	0.0	--	0	0
Poppy Seed 1 tsp (2.8g)	15	1	0	0	1	0.5	0	1	1
Poultry Seasoning 1 tsp (1.5g)	5	0	0	0	1	0.2	0	0	0
Pumpkin Pie Spice 1 tsp (1.7g)	6	0	0	0	1	0.3	0	0	1
Rosemary, Dried 1 tsp (1.2g)	4	0	0	0	1	0.5	--	0	1
Rosemary, Fresh 1 tsp (0.7g)	1	0	0	0	0	0.1	--	0	0
Saffron 1 tsp (0.7g)	2	0	0	0	0	0.0	--	0	1

Food Serving size	Cal.	(g) Total Fat	(g) Sat. Fat	(mg) Chol.	(g) Carb.	(g) Fiber	(g) Sug.	(g) Prot.	(mg) Sod.
Sage, Ground 1 tsp (0.7g)	2	0	0	0	0	0.3	0	0	0
Salt, Table 1 tbsp (18g)	0	0	0	0	0	0.0	0	0	6976
Savory, Ground 1 tsp (1.4g)	4	0	0	0	1	0.6	--	0	0
Spearmint, Dried 1 tsp (0.5g)	1	0	0	0	0	0.1	--	0	2
Spearmint, Fresh 2 leaves (0.3g)	0	0	0	0	0	0.0	--	0	0
Spices, Basil, Dried 1 tbsp, leaves (2.1g)	5	0	0	0	1	0.8	0	0	2
Spices, Bay Leaf 1 tsp, crumbled (0.6g)	2	0	0	0	0	0.2	--	0	0
Spices, Cardamom 1 tsp, ground (2g)	6	0	0	0	1	0.6	--	0	0
Spices, Mustard Seed, Ground 1 tsp (2g)	10	1	0	0	1	0.2	0	1	0
Spices, Oregano, Dried 1 tsp, ground (1.8g)	5	0	0	0	1	0.8	0	0	0
Spices, Tarragon, Dried 1 tbsp, leaves (1.8g)	5	0	0	0	1	0.1	--	0	1
Spices, Thyme, Dried 1 tbsp, leaves (2.7g)	7	0	0	0	2	1.0	0	0	1
Thyme, Fresh .5 tsp (0.4g)	0	0	0	0	0	0.1	--	0	0
Turmeric, Ground 1 tsp (2.2g)	8	0	0	0	1	0.5	0	0	1

Fruits

ChooseMyPlate.gov

Why Eat Fruits?

Fruits provide nutrients vital for health and maintenance of your body. Most fruits are naturally low in fat, sodium, and calories. None have cholesterol. Fruits are sources of many essential nutrients that are under-consumed, including potassium, dietary fiber, vitamin C, and folate (folic acid). Diets rich in potassium may help to maintain healthy blood pressure. Dietary fiber from fruits, as part of an overall healthy diet, helps reduce blood cholesterol levels and may lower risk of heart disease. Vitamin C is important for growth and repair of all body tissues, helps heal cuts and wounds, and keeps teeth and gums healthy.

Daily Goal

Two cups for an adult on a 2000-calorie diet
One-cup equivalents:

1 two-and-a-half-inch whole fruit	8 oz fruit juice (100%)
1 cup chopped or sliced fruit	32 seedless grapes
½ cup dried fruit	8 large strawberries

Shopping Tips

- Eat a variety of fruits.
- Choose fresh in season.
- Buy locally grown fruits when available.
- Buy fruits that are frozen and canned in water or 100% juice.
- Refrigerate or freeze cut-up fruit to store for later use.

Shopping List Essentials

Apples	Berries	Grapes	Grapefruits
Bananas	Melon	Oranges	

Red Flags

Fruit juice concentrates calories and sugar and eliminates fiber. Eat the whole fruit for all the nutrients. Make sure that fruit drinks are 100% fruit and not sugar water with a little fruit juice. When purchasing frozen or canned fruit, be aware of extra sugar and calories in added sauces.

Food Serving size	Cal.	(g) Total Fat	(g) Sat. Fat	(mg) Chol.	(g) Carb.	(g) Fiber	(g) Sug.	(g) Prot.	(mg) Sod.
Fruits									
Apples, Canned, Sweetened, Sliced, Drained, Heated									
1 cup, slices (204g)	137	1	0	0	34	4.1	30	0	6
Apples, Canned, Sweetened, Sliced, Drained, Unheated									
1 cup, slices (204g)	137	1	0	0	34	3.5	31	0	6
Apples, Dehydrated (Low Moisture), Sulfured, Stewed									
1 cup (193g)	143	0	0	0	38	5.0	--	1	50
Apples, Dehydrated (Low Moisture), Sulfured, Uncooked									
1 cup (60g)	208	0	0	0	56	7.4	49	1	74
Apples, Dried, Sulfured, Stewed, with Sugar									
1 cup (280g)	232	0	0	0.	58	5.3	--	1	53
Apples, Dried, Sulfured, Stewed, Without Sugar									
1 cup (255g)	145	0	0	0	39	5.1	34	1	51
Apples, Dried, Sulfured, Uncooked									
1 ring (6.4g)	16	0	0	0	4	0.6	4	0	6
Apples, Frozen, Unsweetened, Heated									
1 cup, slices (206g)	97	1	0	0	25	2.7	--	1	6
Apples, Frozen, Unsweetened, Unheated									
1 cup, slices (173g)	83	1	0	0	21	2.2	--	0	5
Apples, Raw, with Skin									
1 cup, slices (109g)	57	0	0	0	15	2.6	11	0	1
Apples, Raw, Without Skin									
1 large (3-1/4" dia) (216g)	104	0	0	0	28	2.8	22	1	0
Apples, Raw, Without Skin, Cooked, Boiled									
1 cup, slices (171g)	91	1	0	0	23	4.1	19	0	2
Apples, Raw, Without Skin, Cooked, Microwave									
1 cup, slices (170g)	95	1	0	0	24	4.8	20	0	2
Applesauce, Canned, Sweetened, with Salt									
1 cup (255g)	194	0	0	0	51	3.1	--	0	71
Applesauce, Canned, Sweetened, Without Salt									
1 cup (246g)	167	0	0	0	43	3.0	36	0	5
Applesauce, Canned, Unsweetened, with Vitamin C									
1 cup (244g)	102	0	0	0	27	2.7	23	0	5

Food Serving size	Cal.	(g) Total Fat	(g) Sat. Fat	(mg) Chol.	(g) Carb.	(g) Fiber	(g) Sug.	(g) Prot.	(mg) Sod.
Applesauce, Canned, Unsweetened, Without Added Vitamin C									
1 cup (244g)	102	0	0	0	27	2.7	23	0	5
Apricots, Canned, Extra Heavy Syrup Packed, Without Skin, Solids and Liquids									
1 cup, whole, without pits (246g)									
	236	0	0	0	61	3.9	--	1	32
Apricots, Canned, Extra Light Syrup Packed, with Skin, Solids and Liquids									
1 cup, halves (247g)	121	0	0	0	31	4.0	--	1	5
Apricots, Canned, Heavy Syrup Packed, with Skin, Solids and Liquids									
1 cup, whole (240g)	199	0	0	0	52	3.8	48	1	10
Apricots, Canned, Heavy Syrup Packed, Without Skin, Solids and Liquids									
1 cup, whole, without pits (258g)									
	214	0	0	0	55	4.1	--	1	28
Apricots, Canned, Heavy Syrup, Drained									
1 cup, whole (182g)	151	0	0	0	39	4.9	34	1	7
Apricots, Canned, Juice Packed, with Skin, Solids and Liquids									
1 apricot, half with liquid (36g)	17	0	0	0	4	0.6	4	0	1
Apricots, Canned, Light Syrup Packed, with Skin, Solids and Liquids									
1 apricot, half with liquid (40g)	25	0	0	0	7	0.6	6	0	2
Apricots, Canned, Water Packed, Without Skin, Solids and Liquids									
1 cup, whole, without pits (227g)	50	0	0	0	12	2.5	--	2	25
Apricots, Dehydrated (Low-Moisture), Sulfured, Stewed									
1 cup (249g)	314	1	0	0	81	--	--	5	12
Apricots, Dehydrated (Low-Moisture), Sulfured, Uncooked									
1 cup (119g)	381	1	0	0	99	--	--	6	15
Apricots, Dried, Sulfured, Stewed, with Sugar									
1 cup, halves (270g)	305	0	0	0	79	11.1	--	3	8
Apricots, Dried, Sulfured, Stewed, Without Sugar									
1 cup, halves (250g)	213	0	0	0	55	6.5	49	3	10
Apricots, Dried, Sulfured, Uncooked									
1 half (3.5g)	8	0	0	0	2	0.3	2	0	0
Apricots, Frozen, Sweetened									
1 cup (242g)	237	0	0	0	61	5.3	--	2	10
Apricots, Raw									
1 cup, sliced (165g)	79	1	0	0	18	3.3	15	2	2

Food Serving size	Cal.	(g) Total Fat	(g) Sat. Fat	(mg) Chol.	(g) Carb.	(g) Fiber	(g) Sug.	(g) Prot.	(mg) Sod.
Bananas, Dehydrated, or Banana Powder 1 tbsp (6.2g)	21	0	0	0	5	0.6	3	0	0
Bananas, Raw 1 cup, sliced (150g)	134	0	0	0	34	3.9	18	2	2
Blackberries, Canned, Heavy Syrup, Solids and Liquids 1 cup (256g)	236	0	0	0	59	8.7	50	3	8
Blackberries, Frozen, Unsweetened 1 pkg (18 oz) (510g)	326	2	0	0	80	25.5	54	6	5
Blackberries, Raw 1 cup (144g)	62	1	0	0	14	7.6	7	2	1
Blueberries, Canned, Heavy Syrup, Solids and Liquids 1 cup (256g)	225	1	0	0	56	4.1	52	2	8
Blueberries, Canned, Light Syrup, Drained 1 cup (244g)	215	1	0	0	55	6.3	43	3	7
Blueberries, Frozen, Sweetened 1 pkg (10 oz) (284g)	230	0	0	0	62	6.2	56	1	3
Blueberries, Frozen, Unsweetened 1 pkg (20 oz) (567g)	289	4	0	0	69	15.3	48	2	6
Blueberries, Raw 50 berries (68g)	39	0	0	0	10	1.6	7	1	1
Blueberries, Wild, Canned, Heavy Syrup, Drained 1 cup (319g)	341	1	--	--	90	15.6	62	2	3
Blueberries, Wild, Frozen 1 cup, frozen (140g)	71	0	0	--	19	6.2	--	0	4
Boysenberries, Canned, Heavy Syrup 1 cup (256g)	225	0	0	0	57	6.7	--	3	8
Boysenberries, Frozen, Unsweetened 1 pkg (10 oz) (284g)	142	1	0	0	35	15.1	20	3	3
Carambola, (Starfruit), Raw 1 cup, sliced (108g)	33	0	0	0	7	3.0	4	1	2
Carissa, (Natal-plum), Raw 1 fruit, without skin and seeds (20g)	12	0	--	0	3	--	--	0	1
Chayote, Fruit, Cooked, Boiled, Drained, Without Salt 1 cup (1" pieces) (160g)	38	1	0	0	8	4.5	--	1	2

Food Serving size	Cal.	(g) Total Fat	(g) Sat. Fat	(mg) Chol.	(g) Carb.	(g) Fiber	(g) Sug.	(g) Prot.	(mg) Sod.
Chayote, Fruit, Raw 1 chayote (5-3/4") (203g)	39	0	0	0	9	3.5	3	2	4
Cherimoya, Raw 1 cup, pieces (160g)	120	1	0	0	28	4.8	21	3	11
Cherries, Sour, Red, Canned, Extra Heavy Syrup Packed, Solids and Liquids 1 cup (261g)	298	0	0	0	76	2.1	--	2	18
Cherries, Sour, Red, Canned, Heavy Syrup Packed, Solids and Liquids 1 cup (256g)	233	0	0	0	60	2.8	57	2	18
Cherries, Sour, Red, Canned, Light Syrup Packed, Solids and Liquids 1 cup (252g)	189	0	0	0	49	2.0	--	2	18
Cherries, Sour, Red, Canned, Water Packed, Solids and Liquids 1 cup (244g)	88	0	0	0	22	2.7	19	2	17
Cherries, Sour, Red, Frozen, Unsweetened 1 pkg (18 oz) (510g)	235	2	1	0	56	8.2	46	5	5
Cherries, Sour, Red, Raw 1 cup, with pits yields (103g)	52	0	0	0	13	1.6	9	1	3
Cherries, Sweet, Canned, Extra Heavy Syrup Packed, Solids and Liquids 1 cup, pitted (261g)	266	0	0	0	68	3.9	--	2	8
Cherries, Sweet, Canned, Juice Packed, Solids and Liquids 1 cup, pitted (250g)	135	0	0	0	35	3.8	31	2	8
Cherries, Sweet, Canned, Light Syrup Packed, Solids and Liquids 1 cup, pitted (252g)	169	0	0	0	44	3.8	40	2	8
Cherries, Sweet, Canned, Pitted, Heavy Syrup Packed, Solids and Liquids 1 cup (253g)	210	0	0	0	54	3.5	41	2	8
Cherries, Sweet, Canned, Water Packed, Solids and Liquids 1 cup, pitted (248g)	114	0	0	0	29	3.7	25	2	2
Cherries, Sweet, Frozen, Sweetened 1 pkg (10 oz) (284g)	253	0	0	0	64	6.0	58	3	3
Cherries, Sweet, Raw 1 cup, without pits (154g)	97	0	0	0	25	3.2	20	2	0
Cherries, Sweetened, Canned, Pitted, Heavy Syrup, Drained 1 cup (179g)	149	0	0	0	38	4.1	29	1	5
Clementines, Raw 1 fruit (74g)	35	0	--	--	9	1.3	7	1	1

Food Serving size	Cal.	(g) Total Fat	(g) Sat. Fat	(mg) Chol.	(g) Carb.	(g) Fiber	(g) Sug.	(g) Prot.	(mg) Sod.
Crabapples, Raw 1 cup, slices (110g)	84	0	0	0	22	--	--	0	1
Cranberries, Dried, Sweetened .33 cup (40g)	123	1	0	0	33	2.3	26	0	1
Cranberries, Raw 1 cup, whole (100g)	46	0	0	0	12	4.6	4	0	2
Currants, European Black, Raw 1 cup (112g)	71	0	0	0	17	--	--	2	2
Currants, Red and White, Raw 1 cup (112g)	63	0	0	0	15	4.8	8	2	1
Currants, Zante, Dried 1 cup (144g)	408	0	0	0	107	9.8	97	6	12
Dates, Deglet Noor 1 date, pitted (7.1g)	20	0	0	0	5	0.6	4	0	0
Dates, Medjool 1 date, pitted (24g)	66	0	--	--	18	1.6	16	0	0
Elderberries, Raw 1 cup (145g)	106	1	0	0	27	10.2	--	1	9
Figs, Canned, Extra Heavy Syrup Packed, Solids and Liquids 1 cup (261g)	279	0	0	0	73	--	--	1	3
Figs, Canned, Heavy Syrup Packed, Solids and Liquids 1 fig, with liquid (28g)	25	0	0	0	6	0.6	6	0	0
Figs, Canned, Light Syrup Packed, Solids and Liquids 1 fig, with liquid (28g)	19	0	0	0	5	0.5	5	0	0
Figs, Canned, Water Packed, Solids and Liquids 1 fig, with liquid (27g)	14	0	0	0	4	0.6	3	0	0
Figs, Dried, Stewed 1 cup (259g)	277	1	0	0	71	10.9	60	4	10
Figs, Dried, Uncooked 1 fig (8.4g)	21	0	0	0	5	0.8	4	0	1
Figs, Raw 1 medium (2-1/4" dia) (50g)	37	0	0	0	10	1.5	8	0	1
Fruit Butters, Apple 1 tbsp (17g)	29	0	0	0	7	0.3	6	0	3

Food Serving size	Cal.	(g) Total Fat	(g) Sat. Fat	(mg) Chol.	(g) Carb.	(g) Fiber	(g) Sug.	(g) Prot.	(mg) Sod.
Fruit Cocktail, Canned, Extra Heavy Syrup, Solids and Liquids									
.5 cup (130g)	114	0	0	0	30	1.4	--	1	8
Fruit Cocktail, Canned, Extra Light Syrup, Solids and Liquids									
.5 cup (123g)	55	0	0	0	14	1.4	--	0	5
Fruit Cocktail, Canned, Heavy Syrup, Drained									
1 cup (214g)	150	0	0	0	40	3.6	37	1	13
Fruit Cocktail, Canned, Heavy Syrup, Solids and Liquids									
1 cup (248g)	181	0	0	0	47	2.5	44	1	15
Fruit Cocktail, Canned, Juice Packed, Solids and Liquids									
1 cup (237g)	109	0	0	0	28	2.4	26	1	9
Fruit Cocktail, Canned, Light Syrup, Solids and Liquids									
1 cup (242g)	138	0	0	0	36	2.4	34	1	15
Fruit Cocktail, Canned, Water Packed, Solids and Liquids									
1 cup (237g)	76	0	0	0	20	2.4	18	1	9
Fruit Leather, Pieces									
1 pkg (27g)	97	1	0	0	22	0.0	16	0	109
Fruit Leather, Rolls									
1 small (14g)	52	0	0	0	12	0.0	7	0	44
Fruit Salad, Canned, Extra Heavy Syrup, Solids and Liquids									
1 cup (259g)	228	0	0	0	59	2.6	--	1	13
Fruit Salad, Canned, Heavy Syrup, Solids and Liquids									
1 cup (255g)	186	0	0	0	49	2.6	46	1	15
Fruit Salad, Canned, Juice Packed, Solids and Liquids									
1 cup (249g)	125	0	0	0	32	2.5	--	1	12
Fruit Salad, Canned, Light Syrup, Solids and Liquids									
1 cup (252g)	146	0	0	0	38	2.5	--	1	15
Fruit Salad, Canned, Water Packed, Solids and Liquids									
1 cup (245g)	74	0	0	0	19	2.5	--	1	7
Fruit Salad, Tropical, Canned, with Heavy Syrup, Solids and Liquids									
1 cup (257g)	221	0	0	0	57	3.3	--	1	5
Fruit, Mixed (Peach and Pear and Pineapple), Canned, Heavy Syrup, Solids and Liquids									
1 cup (255g)	184	0	0	0	48	2.6	--	1	10

Food Serving size	Cal.	(g) Total Fat	(g) Sat. Fat	(mg) Chol.	(g) Carb.	(g) Fiber	(g) Sug.	(g) Prot.	(mg) Sod.
Fruit, Mixed (Peach, Cherry-Sweetened and Sour, Raspberry, Grape, Boysenberry) Frozen, Sweetened									
1 pkg (10 oz) (284g)	278	1	0	0	69	5.4	--	4	9
Fruit, Mixed (Prune and Apricot and Pear), Dried									
1 pkg (11 oz) (293g)	712	1	0	0	188	22.9	--	7	53
Gooseberries, Canned, Light Syrup Packed, Solids and Liquids									
1 cup (252g)	184	1	0	0	47	6.0	--	2	5
Gooseberries, Raw									
1 cup (150g)	66	1	0	0	15	6.5	--	1	2
Grapefruit, Raw, Pink and Red and White, All Areas									
.5 large (approx 4-1/2" dia) (166g)	53	0	0	0	13	1.8	12	1	0
Grapefruit, Raw, Pink and Red, All Areas									
.5 fruit (3-3/4" dia) (123g)	52	0	0	0	13	2.0	8	1	0
Grapefruit, Raw, Pink and Red, California and Arizona									
.5 fruit (3-3/4" dia) (123g)	46	0	0	0	12	--	--	1	1
Grapefruit, Raw, Pink and Red, Florida									
.5 fruit (3-3/4" dia) (123g)	37	0	0	0	9	1.4	--	1	0
Grapefruit, Raw, White, All Areas									
.5 fruit (3-3/4" dia) (118g)	39	0	0	0	10	1.3	9	1	0
Grapefruit, Raw, White, California									
.5 fruit (3-3/4" dia) (118g)	44	0	0	0	11	--	--	1	0
Grapefruit, Raw, White, Florida									
.5 fruit (3-3/4" dia) (118g)	38	0	0	0	10	--	--	1	0
Grapefruit, Sections, Canned, Juice Packed, Solids and Liquids									
1 cup (249g)	92	0	0	0	23	1.0	22	2	17
Grapefruit, Sections, Canned, Light Syrup Packed, Solids and Liquids									
1 cup (254g)	152	0	0	0	39	1.0	38	1	5
Grapefruit, Sections, Canned, Water Packed, Solids and Liquids									
1 cup (244g)	88	0	0	0	22	1.0	21	1	5
Grapes, American Type (Slip Skin), Raw									
1 grape (2.4g)	2	0	0	0	0	0.0	0	0	0
Grapes, Canned, Thompson Seedless, Heavy Syrup Packed, Solids and Liquids									
1 cup (256g)	195	0	0	0	50	1.5	49	1	13

Food Serving size	Cal.	(g) Total Fat	(g) Sat. Fat	(mg) Chol.	(g) Carb.	(g) Fiber	(g) Sug.	(g) Prot.	(mg) Sod.
Grapes, Canned, Thompson Seedless, Water Packed, Solids and Liquids									
1 cup (245g)	98	0	0	0	25	1.5	24	1	15
Grapes, Muscadine, Raw									
1 grape (6g)	3	0	--	--	1	0.2	--	0	0
Grapes, Red or Green (European Type, Such as Thompson Seedless), Raw									
10 grapes (49g)	34	0	0	0	9	0.4	8	0	1
Guava Nectar, Canned									
1 cup (251g)	143	0	--	--	37	2.5	31	0	18
Guavas, Common, Raw									
1 fruit, without refuse (55g)	37	1	0	0	8	3.0	5	1	1
Guavas, Strawberry, Raw									
1 fruit, without refuse (6g)	4	0	0	0	1	0.3	--	0	2
Jackfruit, Raw									
1 cup, 1" pieces (151g)	143	1	0	0	35	2.3	29	3	3
Java-plum, (Jambolan), Raw									
3 fruit (9g)	5	0	--	0	1	--	--	0	1
Kiwifruit, Gold, Raw									
1 fruit (86g)	52	0	0	--	12	1.7	9	1	3
Kiwifruit, Green, Raw									
1 fruit (2" dia) (69g)	42	0	0	0	10	2.1	6	1	2
Kumquats, Raw									
1 fruit, without refuse (19g)	13	0	0	0	3	1.2	2	0	2
Lemon Peel, Raw									
1 tsp (2g)	1	0	0	0	0	0.2	0	0	0
Lemons, Raw, Without Peel									
1 fruit (2-1/8" dia) (58g)	17	0	0	0	5	1.6	1	1	1
Litchis, Dried									
1 fruit (2.5g)	7	0	0	0	2	0.1	2	0	0
Litchis, Raw									
1 fruit, without refuse (9.6g)	6	0	0	0	2	0.1	1	0	0
Loganberries, Frozen									
1 cup, unthawed (147g)	81	0	0	0	19	7.8	11	2	1
Longans, Raw									
1 fruit, without refuse (3.2g)	2	0	--	0	0	0.0	--	0	0

Food Serving size	Cal.	(g) Total Fat	(g) Sat. Fat	(mg) Chol.	(g) Carb.	(g) Fiber	(g) Sug.	(g) Prot.	(mg) Sod.
Loquats, Raw 1 large (20g)	9	0	0	0	2	0.3	--	0	0
Mammy-apple, (Mamey), Raw 1 fruit, without refuse (846g)	431	4	1	0	106	25.4	--	4	127
Mango Nectar, Canned 1 cup (251g)	128	0	0	0	33	0.8	31	0	13
Mangos, Raw 1 fruit, without refuse (336g)	202	1	0	0	50	5.4	46	3	3
Mangosteen, Canned, Syrup Packed 1 cup (216g)	158	1	--	0	39	3.9	--	1	15
Maraschino Cherries, Canned, Drained 1 cherry (NLEA serving) (5g)	8	0	0	0	2	0.2	2	0	0
Melon Balls, Frozen 1 cup, unthawed (173g)	57	0	0	0	14	1.2	--	1	54
Melon, Cantaloupe, Raw 1 cup, cubes (160g)	54	0	0	0	13	1.4	13	1	26
Melon, Casaba, Raw 1 melon (1640g)	459	2	0	0	108	14.8	93	18	148
Melon, Honeydew, Raw 1 cup, diced (approx 20 pieces per cup) (170g)	61	0	0	0	15	1.4	14	1	31
Mulberries, Raw 10 fruit (15g)	6	0	0	0	1	0.3	1	0	2
Nectarines, Raw 1 small (2-1/3" dia) (129g)	57	0	0	0	14	2.2	10	1	0
Oheloberries, Raw 10 fruit (11g)	3	0	--	0	1	--	--	0	0
Orange Peel, raw 1 tsp (2g)	2	0	0	0	1	0.2	--	0	0
Orange, Raw, California, Valencia 1 fruit (2-5/8" dia) (121g)	59	0	0	0	14	3.0	--	1	0
Oranges, Raw, All Commercial Varieties 1 large (3-1/16" dia) (184g)	86	0	0	0	22	4.4	17	2	0
Oranges, Raw, Florida 1 fruit (2-5/8" dia) (141g)	65	0	0	0	16	3.4	13	1	0

Food Serving size	Cal.	(g) Total Fat	(g) Sat. Fat	(mg) Chol.	(g) Carb.	(g) Fiber	(g) Sug.	(g) Prot.	(mg) Sod.
Oranges, Raw, Navels 1 fruit (2-7/8" dia) (140g)	69	0	0	0	18	3.1	12	1	1
Oranges, Raw, with Peel 1 fruit, without seeds (159g)	100	0	0	0	25	7.2	--	2	3
Orange-strawberry-banana Juice 1 fl oz (29.2g)	15	0	0	0	4	0.1	--	0	1
Papaya Nectar, Canned 1 fl oz (31.2g)	18	0	0	0	5	0.2	4	0	2
Papaya, Canned, Heavy Syrup, Drained 1 piece (39g)	80	0	0	--	22	0.6	20	0	4
Papayas, Raw 1 cup, mashed (230g)	99	1	0	0	25	3.9	18	1	18
Passion-fruit (Granadilla), Purple, Raw 1 fruit, without refuse (18g)	17	0	0	0	4	1.9	2	0	5
Passion-fruit Juice, Purple, Raw 1 fl oz (30.9g)	16	0	0	0	4	0.1	4	0	2
Peaches, Canned, Extra Heavy Syrup Pack, Solids and Liquids 1 cup, halves or slices (262g)	252	0	0	0	68	2.6	--	1	21
Peaches, Canned, Extra Light Syrup, Solids and Liquids 1 cup, halves or slices (247g)	104	0	0	0	27	2.5	--	1	12
Peaches, Canned, Heavy Syrup Pack, Solids and Liquids 1 half, with liquid (98g)	73	0	0	0	20	1.3	18	0	6
Peaches, Canned, Heavy Syrup, Drained 1 half (73g)	53	0	0	0	13	0.9	11	0	4
Peaches, Canned, Juice Packed, Solids and Liquids 1 cup, halves or slices (248g)	109	0	0	0	29	3.2	25	2	10
Peaches, Canned, Light Syrup Pack, Solids and Liquids 1 half, with liquid (98g)	53	0	0	0	14	1.3	13	0	5
Peaches, Canned, Water Packed, Solids and Liquids 1 half, with liquid (98g)	24	0	0	0	6	1.3	5	0	3
Peaches, Dehydrated (Low-moisture), Sulfured, Stewed 1 cup (242g)	322	1	0	0	83	--	--	5	10
Peaches, Dehydrated (Low-moisture), Sulfured, Uncooked 1 cup (116g)	377	1	0	0	96	--	--	6	12

Food Serving size	Cal.	(g) Total Fat	(g) Sat. Fat	(mg) Chol.	(g) Carb.	(g) Fiber	(g) Sug.	(g) Prot.	(mg) Sod.
Peaches, Dried, Sulfured, Stewed, with Sugar 1 cup (270g)	278	1	0	0	72	6.5	--	3	5
Peaches, Dried, Sulfured, Stewed, Without Sugar 1 cup (258g)	199	1	0	0	51	7.0	44	3	5
Peaches, Dried, Sulfured, Uncooked 1 half (13g)	31	0	0	0	8	1.1	5	0	1
Peaches, Frozen, Sliced, Sweetened 10 slices (155g)	146	0	0	0	37	2.8	34	1	9
Peaches, Raw 1 small (2-1/2" dia) (130g)	51	0	0	0	12	2.0	11	1	0
Peaches, Spiced, Canned, Heavy Syrup Pack, Solids and Liquids 1 cup, whole (242g)	182	0	0	0	49	3.1	45	1	10
Pears, Asian, Raw 1 fruit, 3-3/8" high x 3" diameter (275g)	116	1	0	0	29	9.9	19	1	0
Pears, Canned, Extra Heavy Syrup Pack, Solids and Liquids 1 half, with liquid (79g)	77	0	0	0	20	1.3	--	0	4
Pears, Canned, Extra Light Syrup Pack, Solids and Liquids 1 half, with liquid (76g)	36	0	0	0	9	1.2	--	0	2
Pears, Canned, Heavy Syrup Pack, Solids and Liquids 1 half, with liquid (76g)	56	0	0	0	15	1.2	12	0	4
Pears, Canned, Heavy Syrup, Drained 1 half (48g)	36	0	0	0	9	1.3	8	0	2
Pears, Canned, Juice Packed, Solids and Liquids 1 half, with liquid (76g)	38	0	0	0	10	1.2	7	0	3
Pears, Canned, Light Syrup Pack, Solids and Liquids 1 half, with liquid (76g)	43	0	0	0	12	1.2	9	0	4
Pears, Canned, Water Packed, Solids and Liquids 1 half, with liquid (76g)	22	0	0	0	6	1.2	5	0	2
Pears, Dried, Sulfured, Stewed, with Sugar 1 cup, halves (280g)	392	1	0	0	104	16.2	--	2	8
Pears, Dried, Sulfured, Stewed, Without Sugar 1 cup, halves (255g)	324	1	0	0	86	16.3	70	2	8
Pears, Dried, Sulfured, Uncooked 1 half (18g)	47	0	0	0	13	1.4	11	0	1

Food Serving size	Cal.	(g) Total Fat	(g) Sat. Fat	(mg) Chol.	(g) Carb.	(g) Fiber	(g) Sug.	(g) Prot.	(mg) Sod.
Pears, Raw									
1 medium (178g)	103	0	0	0	28	5.5	17	1	2
Persimmons, Japanese, Dried									
1 fruit, without refuse (34g)	93	0	--	0	25	4.9	--	0	1
Persimmons, Japanese, Raw									
1 fruit (2-1/2" dia) (168g)	118	0	0	0	31	6.0	21	1	2
Persimmons, Native, Raw									
1 fruit, without refuse (25g)	32	0	--	0	8	--	--	0	0
Pineapple, Canned, Extra Heavy Syrup Packed, Solids and Liquids									
1 cup, crushed, sliced, or chunks (260g)	216	0	0	0	56	2.1	--	1	3
Pineapple, Canned, Heavy Syrup Packed, Solids and Liquids									
1 slice, or ring (3" dia) with liquid (49g)	38	0	0	0	10	0.4	8	0	0
Pineapple, Canned, Juice Packed, Drained									
1 cup, crushed (195g)	117	0	0	0	30	2.5	28	1	2
Pineapple, Canned, Juice Packed, Solids and Liquids									
1 slice, or ring (3" dia) with liquid (47g)	28	0	0	0	7	0.4	7	0	0
Pineapple, Canned, Light Syrup Packed, Solids and Liquids									
1 slice, or ring (3" dia) with liquid (48g)	25	0	0	0	6	0.4	6	0	0
Pineapple, Canned, Water Packed, Solids and Liquids									
1 slice, or ring (3" dia) with liquid (47g)	15	0	0	0	4	0.4	4	0	0
Pineapple, Frozen, Chunks, Sweetened									
1 cup, chunks (245g)	211	0	0	0	54	2.7	52	1	5
Pineapple, Raw, All Varieties									
1 fruit (905g)	453	1	0	0	119	12.7	89	5	9
Pineapple, Raw, Extra Sweet Variety									
1 slice (4-2/3" dia x 3/4" thick) (166g)	85	0	--	--	22	2.3	17	1	2
Pineapple, Raw, Traditional Variety									
1 slice (4-2/3" dia x 3/4" thick) (175g)	79	0	--	--	21	--	15	1	2

Food Serving size	Cal.	(g) Total Fat	(g) Sat. Fat	(mg) Chol.	(g) Carb.	(g) Fiber	(g) Sug.	(g) Prot.	(mg) Sod.
Plantains, Cooked 1 cup, slices (154g)	179	0	0	0	48	3.5	22	1	8
Plantains, Green, Fried 10 slices (1/4" thick) (53g)	164	6	2	--	26	1.9	2	1	1
Plantains, Raw 1 medium (179g)	218	1	0	0	57	4.1	27	2	7
Plantains, Yellow, Fried, Latino Restaurant 1 cup (169g)	399	13	3	--	69	5.4	37	2	10
Plums, Canned, Heavy Syrup, Drained 1 cup, with pits yields (183g)	163	0	0	0	42	2.7	39	1	35
Plums, Canned, Purple, Extra Heavy Syrup Packed, Solids and Liquids 1 cup, pitted (261g)	264	0	0	0	69	2.6	--	1	50
Plums, Canned, Purple, Heavy Syrup Packed, Solids and Liquids 1 plum, with liquid (46g)	41	0	0	0	11	0.4	10	0	9
Plums, Canned, Purple, Juice Packed, Solids and Liquids 1 plum, with liquid (46g)	27	0	0	0	7	0.4	7	0	0
Plums, Canned, Purple, Light Syrup Packed, Solids and Liquids 1 plum, with liquid (46g)	29	0	0	0	7	0.4	7	0	9
Plums, Canned, Purple, Water Packed, Solids and Liquids 1 plum, with liquid (46g)	19	0	0	0	5	0.4	5	0	0
Plums, Dried (Prunes), Sweetened, with Added Sugar 1 cup, pitted (248g)	308	1	0	0	82	9.4	--	3	5
Plums, Dried (Prunes), Sweetened, Without Added Sugar 1 cup, pitted (248g)	265	0	0	0	70	7.7	62	2	2
Plums, Dried (Prunes), Uncooked 1 prune, pitted (9.5g)	23	0	0	0	6	0.7	4	0	0
Plums, Raw 1 fruit (2-1/8" dia) (66g)	30	0	0	0	8	0.9	7	0	0
Pomegranates, Raw .5 cup, arils (seed/juice sacs) (87g)	72	1	0	0	16	3.5	12	1	3
Prickly Pears, Raw 1 fruit, without refuse (103g)	42	1	0	0	10	3.7	--	1	5
Prune Puree 2 tbsp (36g)	93	0	0	0	23	1.2	14	1	8

Food Serving size	Cal.	(g) Total Fat	(g) Sat. Fat	(mg) Chol.	(g) Carb.	(g) Fiber	(g) Sug.	(g) Prot.	(mg) Sod.
Prunes, Canned, Heavy Syrup Packed, Solids and Liquids									
5 prunes, with liquid (86g)	90	0	0	0	24	3.3	--	1	3
Prunes, Dehydrated (Low-moisture), Sweetened									
1 cup (280g)	316	1	0	0	83	--	--	3	6
Prunes, Dehydrated (Low-moisture), Uncooked									
1 cup (132g)	447	1	0	0	118	--	--	5	7
Pummelo, Raw									
1 fruit, without refuse (609g)	231	0	--	0	59	6.1	--	5	6
Quinces, Raw									
1 fruit, without refuse (92g)	52	0	0	0	14	1.7	--	0	4
Raisins, Golden, Seedless									
1 cup (not packed) (145g)	438	1	0	0	115	5.8	86	5	17
Raisins, Seeded									
1 cup (not packed) (145g)	429	1	0	0	114	9.9	--	4	41
Raisins, Seedless									
1 cup (not packed) (145g)	434	1	0	0	115	5.4	86	4	16
Rambutan, Canned, Syrup Packed									
1 cup (214g)	175	0	--	0	45	1.9	--	1	24
Raspberries, Canned, Red, Heavy Syrup Packed, Solids and Liquids									
1 cup (256g)	233	0	0	0	60	8.4	51	2	8
Raspberries, Frozen, Red, Sweetened									
1 pkg (10 oz) (284g)	293	0	0	0	74	12.5	62	2	3
Raspberries, Raw									
1 pint, as purchased, yields (312g)	162	2	0	0	37	20.3	14	4	3
Squash, Summer, All Varieties, Cooked, Boiled, Drained, with Salt									
1 cup, sliced (180g)	36	1	0	0	8	2.5	5	2	427
Squash, Summer, All Varieties, Cooked, Boiled, Drained, Without Salt									
1 cup, sliced (180g)	36	1	0	0	8	2.5	5	2	2
Squash, Summer, All Varieties, Raw									
1 large (323g)	52	1	0	0	11	3.6	7	4	6
Squash, Summer, Crookneck and Straightneck, Canned, Drained, Solid, Without Salt									
1 cup, mashed (240g)	31	0	0	0	7	3.4	3	1	12

Food Serving size	Cal.	(g) Total Fat	(g) Sat. Fat	(mg) Chol.	(g) Carb.	(g) Fiber	(g) Sug.	(g) Prot.	(mg) Sod.
Squash, Summer, Crookneck and Straightneck, Cooked, Boiled, Drained, with Salt 1 cup, sliced (180g)	34	1	0	0	7	2.0	4	2	427
Squash, Summer, Crookneck and Straightneck, Cooked, Boiled, Drained, Without Salt .5 cup, sliced (90g)	21	0	0	0	3	1.0	2	1	1
Squash, Summer, Crookneck and Straightneck, Frozen, Cooked, Boiled, Drained, with Salt 1 cup, sliced (192g)	48	0	0	0	11	2.7	4	2	465
Squash, Summer, Crookneck and Straightneck, Frozen, Cooked, Boiled, Drained, Without Salt 1 cup, sliced (192g)	48	0	0	0	11	2.7	4	2	12
Squash, Summer, Crookneck and Straightneck, Frozen, Unprepared 1 cup, sliced (130g)	26	0	0	0	6	1.6	--	1	7
Squash, Summer, Crookneck and Straightneck, Raw 1 cup, sliced (127g)	24	0	0	0	5	1.3	4	1	3
Squash, Summer, Scallop, Cooked, Boiled, Drained, with Salt .5 cup, mashed (120g)	19	0	0	0	4	2.3	2	1	284
Squash, Summer, Scallop, Cooked, Boiled, Drained, Without Salt 1 cup, sliced (180g)	29	0	0	0	6	3.4	3	2	2
Squash, Summer, Scallop, Raw 1 cup, sliced (130g)	23	0	0	0	5	--	--	2	1
Squash, Summer, Zucchini, Including Skin, Cooked, Boiled, Drained, with Salt .5 cup, mashed (120g)	18	0	0	0	3	1.2	2	1	287
Squash, Summer, Zucchini, Including Skin, Cooked, Boiled, Drained, Without Salt .5 cup, mashed (120g)	18	0	0	0	3	1.2	2	1	4
Squash, Summer, Zucchini, Including Skin, Frozen, Cooked, Boiled, Drained, with Salt 1 cup (223g)	31	0	0	0	7	2.9	4	3	531
Squash, Summer, Zucchini, Including Skin, Frozen, Cooked, Boiled, Drained, Without Salt 1 cup (223g)	38	0	0	0	8	2.9	4	3	4
Squash, Summer, Zucchini, Including Skin, Frozen, Unprepared 1 pkg (3 lb) (1361g)	231	2	0	0	49	17.7	23	16	27

Food Serving size	Cal.	(g) Total Fat	(g) Sat. Fat	(mg) Chol.	(g) Carb.	(g) Fiber	(g) Sug.	(g) Prot.	(mg) Sod.
Squash, Summer, Zucchini, Including Skin, Raw									
1 cup, sliced (113g)	19	0	0	0	4	1.1	3	1	9
Squash, Summer, Zucchini, Italian Style, Canned									
1 cup (227g)	66	0	0	0	16	--	--	2	849
Squash, Winter, Acorn, Cooked, Baked, with Salt									
1 cup, cubes (205g)	115	0	0	0	30	9.0	--	2	492
Squash, Winter, Acorn, Cooked, Baked, Without Salt									
1 cup, cubes (205g)	115	0	0	0	30	9.0	--	2	8
Squash, Winter, Acorn, Cooked, Boiled, Mashed, with Salt									
1 cup, mashed (245g)	83	0	0	0	22	6.4	--	2	586
Squash, Winter, Acorn, Cooked, Boiled, Mashed, Without Salt									
1 cup, mashed (245g)	83	0	0	0	22	6.4	--	2	7
Squash, Winter, Acorn, Raw									
1 squash (4 inch dia) (431g)	172	0	0	0	45	6.5	--	3	13
Squash, Winter, All Varieties, Cooked, Baked, with Salt									
1 cup, cubes (205g)	80	1	0	0	18	5.7	7	2	486
Squash, Winter, All Varieties, Cooked, Baked, Without Salt									
1 cup, cubes (205g)	76	1	0	0	18	5.7	7	2	2
Squash, Winter, All Varieties, Raw									
1 cup, cubes (116g)	39	0	0	0	10	1.7	3	1	5
Squash, Winter, Butternut, Cooked, Baked, with Salt									
1 cup, cubes (205g)	82	0	0	0	22	6.6	4	2	492
Squash, Winter, Butternut, Cooked, Baked, Without Salt									
1 cup, cubes (205g)	82	0	0	0	22	6.6	4	2	8
Squash, Winter, Butternut, Frozen, Cooked, Boiled, with Salt									
1 cup, mashed (240g)	94	0	0	0	24	--	--	3	571
Squash, Winter, Butternut, Frozen, Cooked, Boiled, Without Salt									
1 cup, mashed (240g)	94	0	0	0	24	--	--	3	5
Squash, Winter, Butternut, Frozen, Unprepared									
1 pkg (4 lb) (1814g)	1034	2	0	0	261	23.6	51	32	36
Squash, Winter, Butternut, Raw									
1 cup, cubes (140g)	63	0	0	0	16	2.8	3	1	6
Squash, Winter, Hubbard, Cooked, Baked, with Salt									
1 cup, cubes (205g)	103	1	0	0	22	--	--	5	500

Food Serving size	Cal.	(g) Total Fat	(g) Sat. Fat	(mg) Chol.	(g) Carb.	(g) Fiber	(g) Sug.	(g) Prot.	(mg) Sod.
Squash, Winter, Hubbard, Cooked, Baked, Without Salt									
1 cup, cubes (205g)	103	1	0	0	22	--	--	5	16
Squash, Winter, Hubbard, Cooked, Boiled, Mashed, with Salt									
1 cup, mashed (236g)	71	1	0	0	15	6.8	7	3	569
Squash, Winter, Hubbard, Cooked, Boiled, Mashed, Without Salt									
1 cup, mashed (236g)	71	1	0	0	15	6.8	7	3	12
Squash, Winter, Hubbard, Raw									
1 cup, cubes (116g)	46	1	0	0	10	--	--	2	8
Squash, Winter, Spaghetti, Cooked, Boiled, Drained or Baked, with Salt									
1 cup (155g)	42	0	0	0	10	2.2	4	1	394
Squash, Winter, Spaghetti, Cooked, Boiled, Drained or Baked, Without Salt									
1 cup (155g)	42	0	0	0	10	2.2	4	1	28
Squash, Winter, Spaghetti, Raw									
1 cup, cubes (101g)	31	1	0	0	7	--	--	1	17
Squash, Zucchini, Baby, Raw									
1 medium (11g)	2	0	0	0	0	0.1	--	0	0
Strawberries, Canned, Heavy Syrup Packed, Solids and Liquids									
1 cup (254g)	234	1	0	0	60	4.3	55	1	10
Strawberries, Frozen, Sweetened, Sliced									
1 pkg (10 oz) (284g)	273	0	0	0	74	5.4	68	2	9
Strawberries, Frozen, Sweetened, Whole									
1 pkg (10 oz) (284g)	222	0	0	0	60	5.4	53	1	3
Strawberries, Frozen, Unsweetened									
1 cup, unthawed (149g)	52	0	0	0	14	3.1	7	1	3
Strawberries, Raw									
1 cup, pureed (232g)	74	1	0	0	18	4.6	11	2	2
Tamarinds, Raw									
1 fruit (3" x 1") (2g)	5	0	0	0	1	0.1	1	0	1
Tangerines (Mandarin Oranges), Canned, Juice Packed									
1 cup (249g)	92	0	0	0	24	1.7	22	2	12
Tangerines (Mandarin Oranges), Canned, Juice Packed, Drained									
1 cup (189g)	72	0	0	0	18	2.3	16	1	9
Tangerines (Mandarin Oranges), Canned, Light Syrup Packed									
1 cup (252g)	154	0	0	0	41	1.8	39	1	15

Food Serving size	Cal.	(g) Total Fat	(g) Sat. Fat	(mg) Chol.	(g) Carb.	(g) Fiber	(g) Sug.	(g) Prot.	(mg) Sod.
Tangerines (Mandarin Oranges), Raw									
1 small (2-1/4" dia) (76g)	40	0	0	0	10	1.4	8	1	2
Tomatillos, Raw									
.5 cup, chopped or diced (66g)	21	1	0	0	4	1.3	3	1	1
Watermelon, Raw									
1 cup, diced (152g)	46	0	0	0	11	0.6	9	1	2

Fruit Juice Drinks/Juice Cocktails

Food Serving size	Cal.	(g) Total Fat	(g) Sat. Fat	(mg) Chol.	(g) Carb.	(g) Fiber	(g) Sug.	(g) Prot.	(mg) Sod.
Apple Cider-flavored Drink, Powder, Low Calorie, with Vitamin C, Prepared									
1 fl oz (30g)	0	0	0	0	0	0.0	0	0	4
Apple Cider-flavored Drink, Powder, Vitamin C and Sugar									
1 packet (21g)	83	0	0	0	21	0.0	1	0	20
Apple Juice, Canned or Bottled, Unsweetened, with Added Vitamin C									
1 fl oz (31g)	14	0	0	0	4	0.1	3	0	1
Apple Juice, Canned or Bottled, Unsweetened, Without Added Vitamin C									
1 fl oz (31g)	14	0	0	0	4	0.1	3	0	1
Apple Juice, Frozen Concentrate, Unsweetened, Diluted with 3 Volumes Water, with Vitamin C									
1 fl oz (29.9g)	14	0	0	0	3	0.0	--	0	2
Apple Juice, Frozen Concentrate, Unsweetened, Diluted, with 3 Volumes Water, Without Vitamin C									
1 fl oz (29.9g)	14	0	0	0	3	0.0	3	0	2
Apple Juice, Frozen Concentrate, Unsweetened, Undiluted, with Vitamin C									
1 can (6 fl oz) (211g)	350	1	0	0	87	--	82	1	53
Apple Juice, Frozen Concentrate, Unsweetened, Undiluted, Without Vitamin C									
1 can (6 fl oz) (211g)	350	1	0	0	87	0.8	82	1	53
Apricot Nectar, Canned, with Vitamin C									
1 fl oz (31.4g)	18	0	0	0	5	0.2	--	0	1
Apricot Nectar, Canned, Without Vitamin C									
1 fl oz (31.4g)	18	0	0	0	5	0.2	4	0	1
Apricots, Canned, Water Packed, with Skin, Solids and Liquids									
1 apricot, half with liquid (36g)	10	0	0	0	2	0.6	2	0	1
Blackberry Juice, Canned									
1 cup (250g)	95	2	0	0	20	0.3	19	1	3

Food Serving size	Cal.	(g) Total Fat	(g) Sat. Fat	(mg) Chol.	(g) Carb.	(g) Fiber	(g) Sug.	(g) Prot.	(mg) Sod.
Citrus Fruit Juice Drink, Frozen Concentrate 1 can (12 fl oz) (423g)	685	0	0	0	170	0.8	121	5	13
Citrus Fruit Juice Drink, Frozen Concentrate, Prepared with Water 1 fl oz (31g)	14	0	0	0	4	0.0	3	0	1
Cranberry Juice Cocktail, Bottled 1 fl oz (31.6g)	17	0	0	0	4	0.0	4	0	1
Cranberry Juice Cocktail, Bottled, Low Calorie, with Calcium, Saccharin and Corn Sweetener 1 fl oz (29.6g)	6	0	0	0	1	0.0	1	0	1
Cranberry Juice Cocktail, Frozen Concentrate 1 can (12 fl oz) (435g)	874	0	0	0	224	0.9	185	0	17
Cranberry Juice Cocktail, Frozen Concentrate, Prepared with Water 1 fl oz (29.6g)	14	0	0	0	3	0.0	3	0	1
Cranberry Juice, Unsweetened 1 fl oz (31.6g)	15	0	0	0	4	0.0	--	0	1
Cranberry Sauce, Canned, Sweetened 1 slice (1/2" thick, approx 8 slices per can) (57g)	86	0	0	0	22	0.6	22	0	17
Cranberry-apple Juice Drink, Bottled 1 fl oz (30.6g)	19	0	0	0	5	0.0	4	0	1
Cranberry-apple Juice Drink, Low-calorie, with Vitamin C 1 fl oz (30g)	6	0	0	0	1	0.0	0	0	2
Cranberry-apricot Juice Drink, Bottled 1 fl oz (30.6g)	20	0	0	0	5	0.0	--	0	1
Cranberry-grape Juice Drink, Bottled 1 fl oz (30.6g)	17	0	0	0	4	0.0	--	0	1
Fruit Punch Drink, Frozen Concentrate 1 can (12 fl oz) (418g)	677	0	0	0	173	1.7	--	1	33
Grape Juice Cocktail, Frozen Concentrate, Diluted with 3 Volumes Water with Added Vitamin C 1 fl oz (31.2g)	16	0	0	0	4	0.0	4	0	1
Grape Juice Cocktail, Frozen Concentrate, Undiluted, with Added Vitamin C 1 can (6 fl oz) (216g)	387	1	0	0	96	0.6	95	1	15
Grape Juice Drink, Canned 1 fl oz (31.3g)	18	0	0	0	5	0.0	4	0	3

Food Serving size	Cal.	(g) Total Fat	(g) Sat. Fat	(mg) Chol.	(g) Carb.	(g) Fiber	(g) Sug.	(g) Prot.	(mg) Sod.
Grape Juice, Canned or Bottled, Unsweetened, with Added Vitamin C									
1 fl oz (31.6g)	19	0	0	0	5	0.1	4	0	2
Grape Juice, Canned or Bottled, Unsweetened, Without Added Vitamin C									
1 fl oz (31.6g)	19	0	0	0	5	0.1	4	0	2
Grapefruit Juice, Pink, Raw									
1 fruit, yields (196g)	76	0	0	0	18	--	--	1	2
Grapefruit Juice, White, Canned, Sweetened									
1 fl oz (31.2g)	14	0	0	0	3	0.0	3	0	1
Grapefruit Juice, White, Canned, Unsweetened									
1 fl oz (30.9g)	12	0	0	0	3	0.0	3	0	0
Grapefruit Juice, White, Frozen Concentrate, Unsweetened, Diluted with 3 Volumes Water									
1 fl oz (30.9g)	13	0	0	0	3	0.0	3	0	0
Grapefruit Juice, White, Frozen Concentrate, Unsweetened, Undiluted									
1 can (6 fl oz) (207g)	302	1	0	0	72	0.8	71	4	6
Grapefruit Juice, White, Raw									
1 fl oz (30.9g)	12	0	0	0	3	0.0	3	0	0
Juice, Apple and Grape Blend, with Added Vitamin C									
8 fl oz (250g)	125	0	--	--	31	--	27	0	18
Juice, Apple, Grape and Pear Blend, with Added Ascorbic Acid and Calcium									
8 fl oz (250g)	130	0	0	0	32	0.5	25	0	13
Lemon Juice, Canned or Bottled									
1 tbsp (15g)	3	0	0	0	1	0.1	0	0	3
Lemon Juice, Frozen, Unsweetened, Single Strength									
1 fl oz (30.5g)	7	0	0	0	2	0.1	1	0	0
Lemon Juice, Raw									
1 fl oz (30.5g)	7	0	0	0	2	0.1	1	0	0
Lemonade, Frozen Concentrate, Pink, Prepared with Water									
1 fl oz (30.9g)	13	0	0	0	3	0.0	3	0	1
Lemonade, Frozen Concentrate, White									
1 can (12 fl oz) (438g)	858	3	0	0	219	1.3	195	1	31
Lemonade, Frozen Concentrate, White, Prepared with Water									
1 fl oz (30.9g)	12	0	0	0	3	0.0	3	0	1
Lemonade, Low Calorie, with Aspartame, Powder									
1 serving (2g)	7	0	0	0	2	0.0	0	0	0

Food Serving size	Cal.	(g) Total Fat	(g) Sat. Fat	(mg) Chol.	(g) Carb.	(g) Fiber	(g) Sug.	(g) Prot.	(mg) Sod.
Lemonade, Low Calorie, with Aspartame, Powder, Prepared with Water									
1 fl oz (29.8g)	1	0	0	0	0	0.0	0	0	1
Lime Juice, Canned or Bottled, Unsweetened									
1 fl oz (30.8g)	6	0	0	0	2	0.1	0	0	5
Lime Juice, Raw									
1 fl oz (30.8g)	8	0	0	0	3	0.1	1	0	1
Limeade, Frozen Concentrate									
1 can (12 fl oz) (437g)	1079	0	0	0	272	0.0	262	0	0
Limeade, Frozen Concentrate, Prepared with Water									
1 fl oz (30.9g)	16	0	0	0	4	0.0	4	0	1
Limes, Raw									
1 NLEA serving (67g)	20	0	0	0	7	1.9	1	0	1
Orange and Apricot Juice Drink, Canned									
1 fl oz (31.2g)	16	0	0	0	4	0.0	4	0	1
Orange Breakfast Drink, Ready-to-drink									
1 fl oz (31.3g)	13	0	0	0	3	0.1	2	0	1
Orange Breakfast Drink, Ready-to-drink, with Added Nutrients									
1 cup (8 fl oz) (253g)	134	0	0	0	33	0.3	20	0	137
Orange Drink, Breakfast Type, with Juice and Pulp, Frozen Concentrate									
1 can (12 fl oz) (436g)	667	0	0	0	170	0.4	166	2	113
Orange Drink, Breakfast Type, with Juice and Pulp, Frozen Concentrate, Prepared with Water									
1 fl oz (31.3g)	14	0	0	0	4	0.0	3	0	3
Orange Drink, Canned, with Added Vitamin C									
1 fl oz (31g)	15	0	0	0	4	0.0	3	0	1
Orange Juice Drink									
1 fl oz (31.1g)	17	0	0	0	4	0.1	--	0	1
Orange Juice, Canned, Unsweetened									
1 fl oz (31.1g)	15	0	0	0	3	0.1	3	0	1
Orange Juice, Chilled, Including from Concentrate									
1 fl oz (31.1g)	15	0	0	0	4	0.1	3	0	1
Orange Juice, Chilled, Including from Concentrate, Fortified with Calcium									
1 fl oz (31.1g)	15	0	0	0	4	0.1	3	0	1
Orange Juice, Chilled, Including from Concentrate, Fortified with Calcium and Vitamin D									
1 fl oz (31.1g)	15	0	0	0	4	0.1	3	0	1

Food Serving size	Cal.	(g) Total Fat	(g) Sat. Fat	(mg) Chol.	(g) Carb.	(g) Fiber	(g) Sug.	(g) Prot.	(mg) Sod.
Orange Juice, Frozen Concentrate, Unsweetened, Diluted with 3 Volumes of Water									
1 fl oz (31.1g)	14	0	0	0	3	0.1	3	0	0
Orange Juice, Frozen Concentrate, Unsweetened, Undiluted									
1 fl oz (35.5g)	56	0	0	0	14	0.3	13	1	1
Orange Juice, Raw									
1 fl oz (31g)	14	0	0	0	3	0.1	3	0	0
Orange-flavor Drink, Breakfast Type, Low Calorie, Powder									
1 portion, amount of dry mix to make 8 fl oz prepared (2.5g)	5	0	0	0	2	0.1	0	0	2
Orange-flavor Drink, Breakfast Type, Powder									
1 serving, 2 tbsp (26g)	100	0	0	0	26	0.1	24	0	4
Orange-flavor Drink, Breakfast Type, Powder, Prepared with Water									
1 fl oz (33.9g)	17	0	0	0	4	0.0	4	0	2
Orange-flavor Drink, Breakfast Type, with Pulp, Frozen Concentrate									
1 can (12 fl oz) (424g)	729	2	0	0	182	0.8	177	0	102
Orange-flavor Drink, Breakfast Type, with Pulp, Frozen Concentrate Prepared with Water									
1 fl oz (31g)	15	0	0	0	4	0.0	4	0	3
Orange-grapefruit Juice, Canned, Unsweetened									
1 fl oz (30.9g)	13	0	0	0	3	0.0	3	0	1
Passion-fruit Juice, Yellow, Raw									
1 fl oz (30.9g)	19	0	0	0	4	0.1	4	0	2
Peach Nectar, Canned with Vitamin C									
1 fl oz (31.1g)	17	0	0	0	4	0.2	--	0	2
Peach Nectar, Canned, Without Vitamin C									
1 fl oz (31.1g)	17	0	0	0	4	0.2	4	0	2
Pear Nectar, Canned, with Vitamin C									
1 fl oz (31.2g)	19	0	0	0	5	0.2	--	0	1
Pear Nectar, Canned, Without Vitamin C									
1 fl oz (31.2g)	19	0	0	0	5	0.2	5	0	1
Pineapple and Grapefruit Juice Drink, Canned									
1 fl oz (31.3g)	15	0	0	0	4	0.0	4	0	4
Pineapple and Orange Juice Drink, Canned									
1 fl oz (31.3g)	16	0	0	0	4	0.0	4	0	1

Food Serving size	Cal.	(g) Total Fat	(g) Sat. Fat	(mg) Chol.	(g) Carb.	(g) Fiber	(g) Sug.	(g) Prot.	(mg) Sod.
Pineapple Juice, Canned, Unsweetened, with Added Vitamin C									
1 fl oz (31.3g)	17	0	0	0	4	0.1	3	0	1
Pineapple Juice, Canned, Unsweetened, Without Vitamin C									
1 fl oz (31.3g)	17	0	0	0	4	0.1	3	0	1
Pineapple Juice, Frozen Concentrate, Unsweetened, Diluted with 3 Volumes Water									
1 fl oz (31.2g)	16	0	0	0	4	0.1	4	0	0
Pineapple Juice, Frozen Concentrate, Unsweetened, Undiluted									
1 can (6 fl oz) (216g)	387	0	0	0	96	1.5	94	3	6
Pomegranate Juice, Bottled									
1 fl oz (31.4g)	17	0	0	0	4	0.0	4	0	3
Prune Juice, Canned									
1 fl oz (32g)	23	0	0	0	6	0.3	5	0	1
Tangerine Juice, Canned, Sweetened									
1 fl oz (31.1g)	16	0	0	0	4	0.1	4	0	0
Tangerine Juice, Frozen Concentrate, Sweetened, Diluted with 3 Volumes Water									
1 fl oz (30.1g)	14	0	0	0	3	--	--	0	0
Tangerine Juice, Frozen Concentrate, Sweetened, Undiluted									
1 can (6 fl oz) (214g)	345	1	0	0	83	1.3	--	3	6
Tangerine Juice, Raw									
1 fl oz (30.9g)	13	0	0	0	3	0.1	3	0	0
Tomato and Vegetable Juice, Low Sodium									
1 fl oz (30.2g)	7	0	0	0	1	0.2	0	0	21
Tomato Juice, Canned, with Salt									
6 fl oz (182g)	31	0	0	0	8	0.7	6	1	490
Tomato Juice, Canned, Without Salt									
1 fl oz (30.4g)	5	0	0	0	1	0.1	1	0	3

Dairy

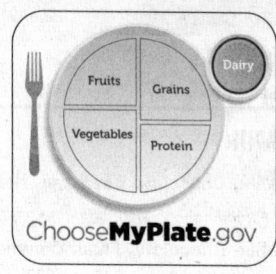

ChooseMyPlate.gov

Why Eat Dairy?

Consuming dairy products provides health benefits, especially improved bone health. Intake of dairy products is also associated with a reduced risk of cardiovascular disease and type 2 diabetes, and with lower blood pressure in adults. Foods in the dairy group provide nutrients that are vital for health and maintenance of your body. These nutrients include calcium, potassium, vitamin D, and protein. Calcium is used for building bones and teeth and in maintaining bone mass. Diets rich in potassium may help to maintain healthy blood pressure. Vitamin D functions in the body to maintain proper levels of calcium and phosphorous, thereby helping to build and maintain bones.

Daily Goal

Three cups for an adult on a 2000-calorie diet
One-cup equivalents:

1 cup milk	⅓ cup shredded cheese
1 cup yogurt	2 oz processed cheese
1½ oz hard cheese	2 cups cottage cheese

Shopping Tips

- Choose low-fat or fat-free dairy products.
- If you don't or can't consume milk, choose lactose-free products or milk alternatives.
- Look for good sources of calcium: 10% DV or higher.
- Use fat-free or low-fat yogurt as a snack or to make dips or smoothies.

Shopping List Essentials

Milk, low-fat or fat-free
Yogurt, low-fat or fat-free
Cottage cheese, low-fat or fat-free

Soy milk, calcium-fortified
Cheese, reduced-fat
Lactose-free milk, if needed

Red Flags

The fat in dairy products is highly saturated, so the lower the fat content the better. Move from whole milk to reduced-fat, to low-fat, to skim or fat-free gradually to let your taste buds adjust.

Food Serving size	Cal.	(g) Total Fat	(g) Sat. Fat	(mg) Chol.	(g) Carb.	(g) Fiber	(g) Sug.	(g) Prot.	(mg) Sod.

Milk

Milk, Chocolate Beverage, Hot Cocoa, Homemade

| 1 fl oz (31.2g) | 24 | 1 | 0 | 2 | 3 | 0.3 | 3 | 1 | 14 |

Milk, Chocolate, Fluid, Commercial, Low Fat, with Added Vitamins A and D

| 1 quart (1000g) | 630 | 10 | 6 | 30 | 104 | 5.0 | 99 | 32 | 610 |

Milk, Chocolate, Fluid, Commercial, Reduced Fat, with Added Calcium

| 1 fl oz (31.2g) | 24 | 1 | 0 | 2 | 4 | 0.2 | 3 | 1 | 21 |

Milk, Chocolate, Fluid, Commercial, Reduced Fat, with Added Vitamins A and D

| 1 fl oz (31.2g) | 24 | 1 | 0 | 2 | 4 | 0.2 | 3 | 1 | 21 |

Milk, Chocolate, Fluid, Commercial, Whole, with Added Vitamins A and D

| 1 fl oz (31.2g) | 26 | 1 | 1 | 4 | 3 | 0.2 | 3 | 1 | 19 |

Milk, Condensed, Evaporated, Non-fat, with Added Vitamins A and D

| 1 fl oz (31.9g) | 25 | 0 | 0 | 1 | 4 | 0.0 | 4 | 2 | 37 |

Milk, Condensed, Evaporated, with Added Vitamin D, No Added Vitamin A

| 1 ff oz (31.5g) | 42 | 2 | 1 | 9 | 3 | 0.0 | 3 | 2 | 33 |

Milk, Condensed, Evaporated, with Vitamin A

| .5 cup (126g) | 169 | 10 | 6 | 37 | 13 | 0.0 | -- | 9 | 134 |

Milk, Condensed, Evaporated, Without Added Vitamins A and D

| 1 fl oz (31.5g) | 43 | 2 | 1 | 9 | 3 | 0.0 | 3 | 2 | 33 |

Milk, Condensed, Sweetened

| 1 fl oz (38.2g) | 123 | 3 | 2 | 13 | 21 | 0.0 | 21 | 3 | 49 |

Milk, Dry, Non-fat, Calcium Reduced

| .25 lb (113g) | 400 | 0 | 0 | 2 | 59 | 0.0 | -- | 40 | 2576 |

Milk, Dry, Whole, with Added Vitamin D

| .25 cup (32g) | 159 | 9 | 5 | 31 | 12 | 0.0 | 12 | 8 | 119 |

Milk, Dry, Whole, Without Added Vitamin D

| .25 cup (32g) | 159 | 9 | 5 | 31 | 12 | 0.0 | 12 | 8 | 119 |

Milk, Fluid, Non-fat, Calcium Fortified (Fat Free or Skim)

| 1 fl oz (30.9g) | 11 | 0 | 0 | 1 | 1 | 0.0 | 0 | 1 | 16 |

Milk, Human, Mature, Fluid

| 1 fl oz (30.8g) | 22 | 1 | 1 | 4 | 2 | 0.0 | 2 | 0 | 5 |

Milk, Low Fat, Fluid, 1% Milk Fat, Protein Fortified, with Added Vitamins A and D

| 1 quart (984g) | 472 | 12 | 7 | 39 | 54 | 0.0 | -- | 39 | 571 |

Food Serving size	Cal.	(g) Total Fat	(g) Sat. Fat	(mg) Chol.	(g) Carb.	(g) Fiber	(g) Sug.	(g) Prot.	(mg) Sod.
Milk, Low Fat, Fluid, 1% Milk Fat, with Added Non-fat Milk Solids, with Vitamins A and D									
1 quart (980g)	421	10	6	39	49	0.0	--	34	510
Milk, Low Fat, Fluid, 1% Milk Fat, with Added Vitamins A and D									
1 fl oz (30.5g)	13	0	0	2	2	0.0	2	1	13
Milk, Low Sodium, Fluid, Whole									
1 fl oz (30.5g)	19	1	1	4	1	0.0	1	1	1
Milk, Non-fat, Fluid, Protein Fortified, with Added Vitamins A and D (Fat Free or Skim)									
1 quart (984g)	403	2	2	20	55	0.0	--	39	581
Milk, Non-fat, Fluid, with Added Non fat Milk Solids, Vitamins A and D									
1 fl oz (30.6g)	11	0	0	1	2	0.0	2	1	16
Milk, Non-fat, Fluid, with Added Vitamins A and D (Fat Free or Skim)									
1 fl oz (30.6g)	10	0	0	1	2	0.0	2	1	13
Milk, Non-fat, Fluid, Without Added Vitamins A and D (Fat Free or Skim)									
1 quart (980g)	333	1	0	20	49	0.0	50	33	412
Milk, Producer, Fluid, 3.7% Milk Fat									
1 quart (976g)	625	36	22	137	45	0.0	--	32	478
Milk, Reduced Fat, Fluid, 2% Milk Fat, Protein Fortified, with Added Vitamins A and D									
1 quart (984g)	551	19	12	79	54	0.0	52	39	581
Milk, Reduced Fat, Fluid, 2% Milk Fat, with Added Non-fat Milk Solids and Vitamins A and D									
1 quart (980g)	500	19	12	78	49	0.0	--	34	510
Milk, Reduced Fat, Fluid, 2% Milk Fat, with Added Vitamins A and D									
1 fl oz (30.5g)	15	1	0	2	1	0.0	2	1	14
Milk, Reduced Fat, Fluid, 2% Milk Fat, with Non-fat Milk Solids, Without Vitamin A									
1 quart (980g)	549	19	12	78	54	0.0	--	39	578
Milk, Reduced Fat, Ready-to-drink, Flavored and Sweetened, with Calcium, Vitamins A and D									
1 cup (244g)	188	4	3	20	29	1.0	28	7	120
Milk, Whole, 3.25% Milk Fat, with Added Vitamin D									
1 tbsp (15g)	9	0	0	2	1	0.0	1	0	6
Milk, Whole, 3.25% Milk Fat, Without Added Vitamins A and D									
1 tbsp (15g)	9	0	0	2	1	0.0	1	0	6

Food Serving size	Cal.	(g) Total Fat	(g) Sat. Fat	(mg) Chol.	(g) Carb.	(g) Fiber	(g) Sug.	(g) Prot.	(mg) Sod.

Milk Based Desserts (Puddings, Frozen Yogurts, Ice Cream)

Food Serving size	Cal.	Total Fat	Sat. Fat	Chol.	Carb.	Fiber	Sug.	Prot.	Sod.
Corn Pudding, Home Prepared .667 cup (#6 scoop) (167g)	219	8	4	120	28	2.0	11	7	471
Cream, Fluid, Heavy Whipping 1 cup, fluid (yields 2 cups whipped) (238g)	821	88	55	326	7	0.0	0	5	90
Cream, Fluid, Light Whipping 1 cup, fluid (yields 2 cups whipped) (239g)	698	74	46	265	7	0.0	0	5	81
Dessert Topping, Powder 1 portion, amount to make 1 tbsp (1.3g)	8	1	0	0	1	0.0	1	0	2
Dessert Topping, Powder, 1.5 oz Prepared with 1/2 Cup Milk 1 tbsp (4g)	8	1	0	0	1	0.0	1	0	3
Dessert Topping, Pressurized 1 tbsp (4g)	11	1	1	0	1	0.0	1	0	2
Dessert Topping, Semi Solid, Frozen 1 tbsp (4g)	13	1	1	0	1	0.0	1	0	1
Desserts, Mousse, Chocolate, Prepared from Recipe 1 recipe, yield (808g)	1818	129	74	1131	130	4.8	120	33	307
Desserts, Pudding, Chocolate, Dry Mix, Regular 1 portion, amount to make 1/2 cup (25g)	91	1	0	0	22	1.1	11	1	88
Desserts, Rennin, Chocolate, Dry Mix 1 pkg (2 oz) (57g)	207	2	1	0	52	2.9	--	1	40
Desserts, Rennin, Tablets, Unsweetened 1 pkg (0.35 oz) (9.9g)	8	0	0	0	2	0.0	--	0	2579
Desserts, Rennin, Vanilla, Dry Mix 1 pkg (1.5 oz) (43g)	165	0	--	0	43	0.0	--	0	3
Egg Custard, Dry Mix 1 portion, amount to make 1/2 cup (21g)	86	1	0	54	17	0.0	--	1	59
Flan, Caramel Custard, Dry Mix 1 portion, amount to make 1/2 cup (21g)	73	0	--	0	19	0.0	--	0	91

Food Serving size	Cal.	(g) Total Fat	(g) Sat. Fat	(mg) Chol.	(g) Carb.	(g) Fiber	(g) Sug.	(g) Prot.	(mg) Sod.
Frozen Novelites, Ice Cream, Chocolate or Caramel Covered, with Nuts									
1 bar (54g)	171	11	7	1	17	0.3	--	2	50
Frozen Novelites, Juice Type, Juice with Cream									
2.5 oz (71g)	82	1	1	5	17	0.1	0	1	30
Frozen Novelties, Fat Free Fudgesicle Bars									
1 serving, 1 pop (51g)	65	0	0	2	14	0.9	10	3	48
Ice Cream, Breyers, 98% Fat Free Chocolate									
1 serving, 1/2 cup (68g)	92	1	1	5	21	3.9	14	3	51
Ice Cream, Breyers, 98% Fat Free Vanilla									
1 serving, 1/2 cup (68g)	93	1	1	5	21	3.7	14	2	50
Ice Cream, Breyers, All Natural Light French Chocolate									
1 serving, 1/2 cup (68g)	137	5	3	28	20	0.7	16	4	51
Ice Cream, Breyers, All Natural Light French Vanilla									
1 serving, 1/2 cup (68g)	118	4	2	36	18	0.1	14	3	50
Ice Cream, Breyers, All Natural Light Mint Chocolate Chip									
1 serving, 1/2 cup (68g)	133	5	3	10	19	0.4	17	3	46
Ice Cream, Breyers, All Natural Light Vanilla									
1 serving, 1/2 cup (68g)	110	3	2	10	17	0.1	15	3	48
Ice Cream, Breyers, All Natural Light Vanilla/Chocolate/Strawberry									
1 serving, 1/2 cup (68g)	109	3	2	10	18	0.3	15	3	47
Ice Cream, Breyers, No Sugar Added, Butter Pecan									
1 serving, 1/2 cup (68g)	122	7	3	12	14	0.6	4	3	112
Ice Cream, Breyers, No Sugar Added, Chocolate Caramel									
1 serving, 1/2 cup (71g)	107	4	3	11	18	0.7	4	3	55
Ice Cream, Breyers, No Sugar Added, French Vanilla									
1 serving, 1/2 cup (68g)	105	5	3	36	14	0.3	5	3	59
Ice Cream, Breyers, No Sugar Added, Vanilla									
1 serving, 1/2 cup (69g)	99	4	3	12	15	0.3	4	3	46
Ice Cream, Breyers, No Sugar Added, Vanilla Fudge Twirl									
1 serving, 1/2 cup (72g)	110	4	3	12	18	0.6	4	3	52
Ice Cream, Breyers, No Sugar Added, Vanilla/Chocolate/Strawberry									
1 serving, 1/2 cup (68g)	97	4	3	12	15	0.5	4	3	46
Ice Cream, Chocolate									
.5 cup (4 fl oz) (66g)	143	7	4	22	19	0.8	17	3	50

Food Serving size	Cal.	(g) Total Fat	(g) Sat. Fat	(mg) Chol.	(g) Carb.	(g) Fiber	(g) Sug.	(g) Prot.	(mg) Sod.
Ice Cream, Chocolate, Light 1 unit (100g)	187	7	4	28	26	0.8	25	5	71
Ice Cream, Chocolate, Light, No Sugar Added 1 serving, 1/2 cup (72g)	125	4	3	12	19	0.6	4	3	54
Ice Cream, Chocolate, Rich 1 cubic inch (10.2g)	26	2	1	6	2	0.1	5	0	6
Ice Cream, French Vanilla, Soft-serve .5 cup (4 fl oz) (86g)	191	11	6	78	19	0.6	18	4	52
Ice Cream, Regular, Low Carbohydrate, Chocolate 1 individual (3.5 fl oz) (58g)	137	7	4	20	16	2.8	4	2	44
Ice Cream, Regular, Low Carbohydrate, Vanilla .5 cup (4 fl oz) (66g)	143	8	4	21	15	3.2	4	2	32
Ice Cream, Strawberry .5 cup (4 fl oz) (66g)	127	6	3	19	18	0.6	--	2	40
Ice Cream, Vanilla 1 serving, 1/2 cup (66g)	137	7	4	29	16	0.5	14	2	53
Ice Cream, Vanilla, Light 1 serving, 1/2 cup (76g)	137	4	2	21	22	0.2	17	4	56
Ice Cream, Vanilla, Light, No Sugar Added 1 serving, 1/2 cup (68g)	115	5	3	18	15	0.0	4	3	65
Ice Cream, Vanilla, Light, Soft-serve 1 serving, 1/2 cup (88g)	111	2	1	11	19	0.0	16	4	62
Ice Cream, Vanilla, Rich .5 cup (107g)	266	17	11	98	24	0.0	22	4	65
Kraft Cheeze Whiz, Light Pasteurized Process Cheese Product 2 tbsp (33g)	71	3	2	12	5	0.1	3	5	563
Kraft Free Singles American Non-fat Pasteurized Process Cheese Product 2 tbsp (35g)	52	0	0	6	4	0.1	2	8	454
Kraft Velveeta Light Reduced Fat Pasteurized Process Cheese Product 1 oz (28g)	62	3	2	12	3	0.0	2	5	444
Light Ice Cream, Soft-serve, Blended with Cookie Pieces 12 fl oz, cup (337g)	570	19	9	51	86	0.3	0	13	253
Light Ice Cream, Soft-serve, Blended with Milk Chocolate Candies 12 fl oz, cup (348g)	633	22	13	56	93	0.7	13	14	188

Food Serving size	Cal.	(g) Total Fat	(g) Sat. Fat	(mg) Chol.	(g) Carb.	(g) Fiber	(g) Sug.	(g) Prot.	(mg) Sod.
Milk Dessert, Frozen, Milk Fat Free, Chocolate									
1 cup (137g)	229	1	1	0	52	0.0	--	6	133
Milk Shakes, Thick Chocolate									
1 container (10.6 oz) (300g)	357	8	5	33	63	0.9	63	9	333
Milk Shakes, Thick Vanilla									
1 container (11 oz) (313g)	351	9	6	38	56	0.0	56	12	297
Puddings, All Flavors Except Chocolate, Low Calorie, Instant, Dry Mix									
1 pkg, 4 servings (32g)	112	0	0	0	27	0.3	0	0	1360
Puddings, Banana, Dry Mix, Instant									
1 portion, amount to make 1/2 cup (25g)	92	0	0	0	23	0.0	19	0	375
Puddings, Banana, Dry Mix, Instant, with Added Oil									
1 portion, amount to make 1/2 cup (25g)	97	1	0	0	22	0.0	--	0	375
Puddings, Banana, Dry Mix, Regular									
1 portion, amount to make 1/2 cup (22g)	81	0	0	0	20	0.1	16	0	173
Puddings, Banana, Dry Mix, Regular with Added Oil									
1 portion, amount to make 1/2 cup (22g)	85	1	0	0	19	0.1	--	0	173
Puddings, Chocolate Flavor, Low Calorie, Instant, Dry Mix									
1 pkg, 1.4 oz box, 4 servings (40g)	142	1	0	0	31	2.4	1	2	1135
Puddings, Chocolate Flavor, Low Calorie, Regular, Dry Mix									
1 pkg (40g)	146	1	1	0	30	4.0	5	4	1330
Puddings, Chocolate, Dry Mix, Instant									
1 portion, amount to make 1/2 cup (25g)	95	0	0	0	22	0.9	17	1	357
Puddings, Chocolate, Dry Mix, Instant, Prepared with Whole Milk									
1 pkg, yield (2 cups) (570g)	684	18	10	51	112	4.6	68	18	559
Puddings, Chocolate, Dry Mix, Instant, Prepared with Whole Milk									
1 pkg, yield (2 cups) (587g)	652	18	11	65	110	5.9	--	18	1667
Puddings, Chocolate, Ready-to-eat									
1 container, refrigerated, 4 oz container (108g)	153	5	1	1	25	0.0	19	2	164

Food Serving size	Cal.	(g) Total Fat	(g) Sat. Fat	(mg) Chol.	(g) Carb.	(g) Fiber	(g) Sug.	(g) Prot.	(mg) Sod.
Puddings, Coconut Cream, Dry Mix, Instant									
1 portion, amount to make 1/2 cup (25g)									
	97	1	1	0	23	1.0	16	0	260
Puddings, Coconut Cream, Dry Mix, Instant, Prepared with 2% Milk									
1 pkg, yield (2 cups) (587g)	628	14	8	35	113	0.6	--	17	1444
Puddings, Coconut Cream, Dry Mix, Instant, Prepared with Whole Milk									
1 pkg, yield (2 cups) (587g)	687	21	12	65	112	0.6	--	17	1444
Puddings, Coconut Cream, Dry Mix, Regular									
1 portion, amount to make 1/2 cup (25g)									
	109	3	3	0	20	0.4	20	0	171
Puddings, Coconut Cream, Dry Mix, Regular, Prepared with 2% Milk									
1 pkg, yield (2 cups) (559g)	581	14	10	39	100	1.1	--	17	911
Puddings, Coconut Cream, Dry Mix, Regular, Prepared with Whole Milk									
1 pkg, yield (2 cups) (559g)	637	21	14	67	99	1.1	--	17	906
Puddings, Lemon, Dry Mix, Instant									
1 portion, amount to make 1/2 cup (25g)									
	95	0	0	0	24	0.0	--	0	333
Puddings, Lemon, Dry Mix, Instant, Prepared with Whole Milk									
1 pkg, yield (2 cups) (587g)	675	17	10	65	118	0.0	--	16	1567
Puddings, Lemon, Dry Mix, Regular									
1 portion, amount to make 1/2 cup (21g)									
	76	0	--	0	19	0.0	--	0	106
Puddings, Lemon, Dry Mix, Regular with Added Oil, Phosphorus, Sodium									
1 portion, amount to make 1/2 cup (21g)									
	77	0	0	0	19	0.0	--	0	178
Puddings, Rice, Dry Mix									
1 portion, amount to make 1/2 cup (27g)									
	102	0	--	0	25	0.2	--	1	99
Puddings, Rice, Ready-to-eat									
1 serving, 4 oz refrigerated (113g)	133	3	2	20	22	1.0	16	4	139
Puddings, Tapioca, Dry Mix									
1 portion, amount to make 1/2 cup (23g)									
	85	0	--	0	22	0.0	15	0	110
Puddings, Tapioca, Dry Mix, with No Added Salt									
1 portion, amount to make 1/2 cup (23g)									
	85	0	--	0	22	0.0	--	0	2

Food Serving size	Cal.	(g) Total Fat	(g) Sat. Fat	(mg) Chol.	(g) Carb.	(g) Fiber	(g) Sug.	(g) Prot.	(mg) Sod.
Puddings, Tapioca, Ready-to-eat 1 container, refrigerated 4 oz (110g)	143	4	1	1	24	0.0	16	2	160
Puddings, Tapioca, Ready-to-eat, Fat Free 1 container, refrigerated 4 oz (112g)	105	0	0	1	24	0.0	16	2	209
Puddings, Vanilla, Dry Mix, Instant 1 portion, amount to make 1/2 cup (25g)	94	0	0	0	23	0.0	23	0	360
Puddings, Vanilla, Dry Mix, Instant, Prepared with Whole Milk 1 pkg, yield (2 cups) (569g)	649	17	10	63	112	0.0	103	15	1627
Puddings, Vanilla, Dry Mix, Regular 1 portion, amount to make 1/2 cup (22g)	83	0	0	0	21	0.1	17	0	140
Puddings, Vanilla, Dry Mix, Regular with Added Oil 1 portion, amount to make 1/2 cup (22g)	81	0	0	0	20	0.0	--	0	166
Puddings, Vanilla, Dry Mix, regular, Prepared with Whole Milk 1 pkg, yield (2 cups) (559g)	632	16	9	50	106	0.6	96	16	872
Puddings, Vanilla, Ready-to-eat 1 container, refrigerated 4 oz (110g)	143	4	1	1	25	0.0	19	2	156
Puddings, Vanilla, Ready-to-eat, Fat Free 1 serving, 3.5 oz shelf stable (99g)	88	0	0	0	20	0.0	15	2	189
Sherbet, Orange 1 bar (2.75 fl oz) (66g)	95	1	1	1	20	0.9	16	1	30
Sour Cream, Imitation, Cultured 1 oz (28.35g)	59	6	5	0	2	0.0	2	1	29
Sour Dressing, Non-butterfat, Cultured, Filled Cream-type 1 tbsp (12g)	21	2	2	1	1	0.0	1	0	6

Cheeses

Food Serving size	Cal.	(g) Total Fat	(g) Sat. Fat	(mg) Chol.	(g) Carb.	(g) Fiber	(g) Sug.	(g) Prot.	(mg) Sod.
Cheese Fondue .5 cup (108g)	247	15	9	49	4	0.0	--	15	143
Cheese Food, Cold Pack, American 1 pkg (8 oz) (227g)	751	56	35	145	19	0.0	--	45	2193

Food Serving size	Cal.	(g) Total Fat	(g) Sat. Fat	(mg) Chol.	(g) Carb.	(g) Fiber	(g) Sug.	(g) Prot.	(mg) Sod.
Cheese Food, Pasteurized Process, American									
1 oz (28.35g)	94	7	4	23	2	0.0	2	5	359
Cheese Food, Pasteurized Process, American									
1 pkg (8 oz) (227g)	745	56	35	145	17	0.0	17	45	3623
Cheese Food, Pasteurized Process, Swiss									
1 pkg (8 oz) (227g)	733	55	35	186	10	0.0	--	50	3523
Cheese Product, Pasteurized Process, American, Reduced Fat, Fortified with Vitamin D									
1 cup (128g)	307	18	11	68	14	0.0	10	23	2031
Cheese Sauce, Prepared from Recipe									
2 tbsp (30g)	59	4	2	11	2	0.0	0	3	148
Cheese Spread, Cream Cheese Base									
1 oz (28.35g)	84	8	5	26	1	0.0	3	2	191
Cheese Spread, Pasteurized Process, American									
1 cup (244g)	708	52	33	134	21	0.0	18	40	3282
Cheese Spread, Pasteurized Process, American									
1 jar (5 oz) (142g)	412	30	19	78	12	0.0	--	23	2308
Cheese, American Cheddar, Imitation									
1 cubic inch (18g)	43	3	2	6	2	0.0	--	3	242
Cheese, Blue									
1 cubic inch (17g)	60	5	3	13	0	0.0	0	4	237
Cheese, Brick									
1 cup, shredded (113g)	419	34	21	106	3	0.0	1	26	633
Cheese, Brie									
1 cup, sliced (144g)	481	40	25	144	1	0.0	1	30	906
Cheese, Camembert									
1 oz (28.35g)	85	7	4	20	0	0.0	0	6	239
Cheese, Caraway									
1 oz (28.35g)	107	8	5	26	1	0.0	--	7	196
Cheese, Cheddar									
1 cup, melted (244g)	983	81	51	256	3	0.0	1	61	1515
Cheese, Cheshire									
1 oz (28.35g)	110	9	6	29	1	0.0	--	7	198
Cheese, Colby									
1 cup, shredded (113g)	445	36	23	107	3	0.0	1	27	683

Food Serving size	Cal.	(g) Total Fat	(g) Sat. Fat	(mg) Chol.	(g) Carb.	(g) Fiber	(g) Sug.	(g) Prot.	(mg) Sod.
Cheese, Cottage, Creamed, Large or Small Curd									
1 cup, large curd (not packed) (210g)	206	9	4	36	7	0.0	6	23	764
Cheese, Cottage, Creamed, with Fruit									
4 oz (113g)	110	4	3	15	5	0.2	3	12	389
Cheese, Cottage, Low Fat, 1 % Milk Fat, with Vegetables									
1 cup (226g)	151	2	1	7	7	0.0	2	25	911
Cheese, Cottage, Low Fat, 1% Milk Fat									
4 oz (113g)	81	1	1	5	3	0.0	3	14	459
Cheese, Cottage, Low Fat, 1% Milk Fat, Lactose Reduced									
1 cup (227g)	168	2	1	9	7	1.4	--	28	499
Cheese, Cottage, Low Fat, 1% Milk Fat, No Sodium									
1 cup (226g)	163	2	1	9	6	0.0	1	28	29
Cheese, Cottage, Low Fat, 2% Milk Fat									
4 oz (113g)	97	3	1	11	4	0.0	4	13	373
Cheese, Cottage, Non-fat, Uncreamed, Dry, Large or Small Curd									
4 oz (113g)	81	0	0	8	8	0.0	2	12	373
Cheese, Cottage, with Vegetables									
1 cup (226g)	215	9	6	32	7	0.2	6	25	911
Cheese, Cream									
1 tbsp (14.5g)	50	5	3	16	1	0.0	0	1	47
Cheese, Cream, Low Fat									
1 tbsp (15g)	30	2	1	8	1	0.0	1	1	71
Cheese, Edam									
1 pkg (7 oz) (198g)	707	55	35	176	3	0.0	3	49	1911
Cheese, Feta									
1 oz (28.35g)	75	6	4	25	1	0.0	1	4	316
Cheese, Fontina									
1 cup, shredded (108g)	420	34	21	125	2	0.0	2	28	864
Cheese, Gjetost									
1 pkg (8 oz) (227g)	1058	67	43	213	97	0.0	--	22	1362
Cheese, Goat, Hard Type									
1 oz (28.35g)	128	10	7	30	1	0.0	1	9	98
Cheese, Goat, Semisoft Type									
1 oz (28.35g)	103	8	6	22	1	0.0	1	6	146

Food Serving size	Cal.	(g) Total Fat	(g) Sat. Fat	(mg) Chol.	(g) Carb.	(g) Fiber	(g) Sug.	(g) Prot.	(mg) Sod.
Cheese, Goat, Soft Type 1 oz (28.35g)	76	6	4	13	0	0.0	0	5	104
Cheese, Gouda 1 pkg (7 oz) (198g)	705	54	35	226	4	0.0	4	49	1622
Cheese, Gruyere 1 cup, shredded (108g)	446	35	20	119	0	0.0	0	32	363
Cheese, Limburger 1 oz (28.35g)	93	8	5	26	0	0.0	0	6	227
Cheese, Low Fat, Cheddar or Colby 1 cup, shredded (113g)	195	8	5	24	2	0.0	1	28	692
Cheese, Low-sodium, Cheddar or Colby 1 cup, shredded (113g)	450	37	23	113	2	0.0	1	28	24
Cheese, Mexican, Blend, Reduced Fat 1 cup, diced (132g)	372	26	15	82	5	0.0	1	33	1024
Cheese, Mexican, Queso Anejo 1 oz (28.35g)	106	8	5	30	1	0.0	1	6	321
Cheese, Mexican, Queso Asadero 1 cup, shredded (113g)	402	32	20	119	3	0.0	3	26	740
Cheese, Mexican, Queso Chihuahua 1 cup, shredded (113g)	423	34	21	119	6	0.0	6	24	697
Cheese, Monterey 1 cup, shredded (113g)	421	34	22	101	1	0.0	1	28	606
Cheese, Monterey, Low Fat 1 cup, shredded (113g)	350	24	16	73	1	0.0	--	32	637
Cheese, Mozzarella, Low Sodium 1 cup, shredded (113g)	316	19	12	61	4	0.0	0	31	18
Cheese, Mozzarella, Non-fat 1 cup, shredded (113g)	159	0	0	20	4	2.0	4	36	840
Cheese, Mozzarella, Part Skim Milk 1 oz (28.35g)	72	5	3	18	1	0.0	0	7	175
Cheese, Mozzarella, Part Skim Milk, Low Moisture 1 cup, shredded (113g)	341	23	12	61	4	0.0	1	29	737
Cheese, Mozzarella, Whole Milk 1 oz (28.35g)	85	6	4	22	1	0.0	0	6	178

Food Serving size	Cal.	(g) Total Fat	(g) Sat. Fat	(mg) Chol.	(g) Carb.	(g) Fiber	(g) Sug.	(g) Prot.	(mg) Sod.
Cheese, Mozzarella, Whole Milk, Low Moisture									
1 cubic inch (18g)	57	4	3	16	0	0.0	0	4	75
Cheese, Muenster									
1 cup, shredded (113g)	416	34	22	108	1	0.0	1	26	710
Cheese, Muenster, Low Fat									
1 cubic inch (18g)	49	3	2	11	1	0.0	0	4	108
Cheese, Neufchatel									
1 pkg (3 oz) (85g)	215	19	11	63	3	0.0	3	8	284
Cheese, Parmesan, Dry Grated, Reduced Fat									
1 tbsp (5g)	13	1	1	4	0	0.0	0	1	76
Cheese, Parmesan, Grated									
1 tbsp (5g)	22	1	1	4	0	0.0	0	2	76
Cheese, Parmesan, Hard									
1 cubic inch (10.3g)	40	3	2	7	0	0.0	0	4	165
Cheese, Parmesan, Low Sodium									
1 tbsp (5g)	23	1	1	4	0	0.0	--	2	3
Cheese, Parmesan, Shredded									
1 tbsp (5g)	21	1	1	4	0	0.0	0	2	85
Cheese, Pasteurized Process, American									
1 cup, melted (244g)	915	76	48	229	4	0.0	1	54	3060
Cheese, Pasteurized Process, American									
1 cubic inch (18g)	68	6	4	17	0	0.0	0	4	117
Cheese, Pasteurized Process, American, Low Fat									
1 cup, shredded (113g)	203	8	5	40	4	0.0	0	28	1616
Cheese, Pasteurized Process, Cheddar or American, Fat Free									
1 slice (3/4 oz) (21g)	31	0	0	2	3	0.0	--	5	321
Cheese, Pasteurized Process, Cheddar or American, Low Sodium									
1 cup, shredded (113g)	425	35	22	106	2	0.0	0	25	8
Cheese, Pasteurized Process, Pimiento									
1 cup, melted (244g)	915	76	48	229	4	0.2	2	54	3484
Cheese, Pasteurized Process, Swiss									
1 cup, shredded (113g)	377	28	18	96	2	0.0	1	28	1548
Cheese, Pasteurized Process, Swiss									
1 cubic inch (18g)	60	5	3	15	0	0.0	--	4	123

Food Serving size	Cal.	(g) Total Fat	(g) Sat. Fat	(mg) Chol.	(g) Carb.	(g) Fiber	(g) Sug.	(g) Prot.	(mg) Sod.
Cheese, Pasteurized Process, Swiss, Low Fat 1 cup, shredded (113g)	186	6	4	40	5	0.0	3	29	1616
Cheese, Port de Salut 1 cup, shredded (113g)	398	32	19	139	1	0.0	1	27	603
Cheese, Provolone 1 oz (28.35g)	100	8	5	20	1	0.0	0	7	248
Cheese, Provolone, Reduced Fat 1 cup, shredded (113g)	310	20	13	62	4	0.0	1	28	990
Cheese, Ricotta, Part Skim Milk 1 oz (28.35g)	39	2	1	9	1	0.0	0	3	35
Cheese, Ricotta, Whole Milk .5 cup (124g)	216	16	10	63	4	0.0	0	14	104
Cheese, Romano 5 pkg (5 oz) (142g)	550	38	24	148	5	0.0	1	45	1704
Cheese, Roquefort 1 pkg (3 oz) (85g)	314	26	16	77	2	0.0	--	18	1538
Cheese, Substitute, Mozzarella 1 oz (28.35g)	70	3	1	0	7	0.0	7	3	194
Cheese, Swiss 1 cup, melted (244g)	927	68	43	224	13	0.0	3	66	468
Cheese, Swiss, Low Fat 1 cup, shredded (108g)	187	6	4	38	4	0.0	0	31	281
Cheese, Swiss, Low Sodium 1 cup, shredded (108g)	404	30	19	99	4	0.0	1	31	15
Cheese, Tilsit 1 pkg (6 oz) (170g)	578	44	29	173	3	0.0	--	41	1280
Imitation Cheese, American or Cheddar, Low Cholesterol 1 cubic inch (18g)	70	6	1	3	0	0.0	--	5	121
Kraft Velveeta Pasteurized Process Cheese Spread 1 slice (21g)	64	5	3	17	2	0.0	2	3	315

Yogurt

Kraft Breyers Light n' Lively Low Fat Strawberry Yogurt (1% Milk Fat) 1 container (8 oz) (227g)	245	2	1	20	50	0.5	44	7	102

Food Serving size	Cal.	(g) Total Fat	(g) Sat. Fat	(mg) Chol.	(g) Carb.	(g) Fiber	(g) Sug.	(g) Prot.	(mg) Sod.
Kraft Breyers Light Non-fat Strawberry Yogurt (with Aspartame and Fructose Sweetener)									
1 container (8 oz) (227g)	125	0	0	11	22	0.0	17	8	102
Kraft Breyers Low Fat Strawberry Yogurt (1% Milk Fat)									
2 tbsp (32g)	31	0	0	3	6	0.1	6	1	17
Kraft Breyers Smooth and Creamy Low Fat Strawberry Yogurt (1% Milk Fat)									
1 container (4.4 oz) (125g)	128	1	1	11	25	0.4	22	5	69

Dairy Alternatives (Soy Milk and Yogurts, Coconut Milk, Almond Milk, etc.)

Food Serving size	Cal.	(g) Total Fat	(g) Sat. Fat	(mg) Chol.	(g) Carb.	(g) Fiber	(g) Sug.	(g) Prot.	(mg) Sod.
Cream Substitute, Flavored, Liquid									
1 cup (100g)	251	14	3	0	35	1.1	33	1	80
Cream Substitute, Fluid with Hydrogenated Vegetable Oils and Soy Protein									
1 fl oz (30g)	41	3	1	0	3	0.0	3	0	24
Cream Substitute, Liquid, Light									
1 fl oz (30g)	21	1	0	0	3	0.0	--	0	18
Cream Substitute, Powder, Light									
1 packet (3g)	13	0	0	0	2	0.0	--	0	7
Cream Substitute, with Lauric Acid Oil									
.5 cup (120g)	163	12	11	0	14	0.0	--	1	95
Cream, Fluid, Half and Half									
1 tbsp (15g)	20	2	1	6	1	0.0	0	0	6
Cream, Fluid, Light Coffee or Table									
1 tbsp (15g)	29	3	2	10	1	0.0	0	0	6
Cream, Half and Half, Fat Free									
1 container (8 oz) (227g)	134	3	2	11	20	0.0	11	6	327
Cream, Sour, Cultured									
1 tbsp (12g)	23	2	1	6	0	0.0	0	0	10
Cream, Sour, Reduced Fat, Cultured									
1 tbsp (15g)	20	2	1	6	1	0.0	0	0	6
Cream, Substitute, Powder									
1 tsp (2g)	11	1	1	0	1	0.0	1	0	4
Cream, Whipped, Cream Topping, Pressurized									
1 tbsp (3g)	8	1	0	2	0	0.0	0	0	4

Food Serving size	Cal.	(g) Total Fat	(g) Sat. Fat	(mg) Chol.	(g) Carb.	(g) Fiber	(g) Sug.	(g) Prot.	(mg) Sod.
Dairy Drink Mix, Chocolate, Reduced Calorie, with Aspartame, Powder, Prepared with Water and Ice 1 serving (243g)	70	1	0	5	11	1.9	7	5	148
Dairy Drink Mix, Chocolate, Reduced Calorie, with Low-calorie Sweeteners, Powder 1 packet (.75 oz) (21g)	69	1	0	5	11	2.0	7	5	138
Frozen Novelties, Fruit and Juice Bars 1 bar (3 fl oz) (92g)	80	0	0	0	19	0.9	16	1	4
Frozen Novelties, Ice Type, Fruit, No Sugar Added 1 bar (51g)	12	0	0	0	3	0.0	--	0	3
Frozen Novelties, Ice Type, Italian, Restaurant Prepared .5 cup (116g)	61	0	0	0	16	0.0	--	0	5
Frozen Novelties, Ice Type, Lime .5 cup (4 fl oz) (99g)	127	0	0	0	32	0.0	32	0	22
Frozen Novelties, Ice Type, Pineapple-coconut .5 cup (4 fl oz) (99g)	112	3	2	0	24	0.7	--	0	35
Frozen Novelties, Ice Type, Pop 1 serving, 1.75 fl oz pop (52g)	41	0	0	0	10	0.0	7	0	4
Frozen Novelties, Ice Type, Pop, with Low-calorie Sweetener 1 serving, 1.75 fl oz pop (55g)	13	0	0	0	3	0.0	--	0	6
Frozen Novelties, Ice Type, Sugar Free, Orange, Cherry and Grape Popsicle 1 serving, 1.75 fl oz pop (55g)	12	0	0	0	3	0.0	1	0	6
Frozen Novelties, Juice Type, Orange 1 fl oz (29.8g)	28	0	0	0	7	0.0	--	0	2
Frozen Novelties, Juice Type, Popsicle Scribblers 1 serving, 1.2 fl oz pop (33g)	27	0	--	--	6	0.0	5	0	4
Frozen Novelties, Klondike, Slim-a-Bear Chocolate Cone 1 serving, 1 cone (79g)	177	3	1	2	36	3.4	19	3	126
Frozen Novelties, Klondike, Slim-a-Bear Chocolate Sandwich 1 serving, 1 sandwich (64g)	136	2	1	3	28	3.1	14	4	120
Frozen Novelties, Klondike, Slim-a-Bear Fudge Brownie, 98% Fat Free, No Sugar Added 1 serving, 3.5 fl oz bar (74g)	92	1	1	5	22	4.4	5	3	89
Frozen Novelties, Klondike, Slim-a-Bear Mint Sandwich 1 serving, 1 sandwich (64g)	134	1	0	3	28	2.8	14	4	122

Food Serving size	Cal.	(g) Total Fat	(g) Sat. Fat	(mg) Chol.	(g) Carb.	(g) Fiber	(g) Sug.	(g) Prot.	(mg) Sod.
Frozen Novelties, Klondike, Slim-a-Bear Vanilla Cone									
1 serving, 1 cone (79g)	175	3	1	2	35	3.0	20	3	126
Frozen Novelties, Klondike, Slim-a-Bear Vanilla Sandwich									
1 serving, 1 sandwich (64g)	135	1	0	3	28	2.8	14	4	122
Frozen Novelties, No Sugar Added, Creamsicle Pops									
1 serving, 1 pop (44g)	25	0	0	1	6	0.1	1	1	18
Frozen Novelties, No Sugar Added, Fudgesicle Pops									
1 serving (84g)	88	1	0	2	19	1.3	3	3	86
Frozen Novelties, Sugar Free, Creamsicle Pops									
1 serving, 2 pops (80g)	39	2	2	0	10	6.0	0	1	5
Frozen Yogurt, Chocolate									
1 cup (174g)	221	6	4	23	38	4.0	--	5	110
Frozen Yogurt, Chocolate, Soft-serve									
.5 cup (4 fl oz) (72g)	115	4	3	4	18	1.6	--	3	71
Frozen Yogurt, Flavors Other than Chocolate									
1 cup (174g)	221	6	4	23	38	0.0	--	5	110
Frozen Yogurt, Vanilla, Soft-serve									
.5 cup (72g)	114	4	2	1	17	0.0	17	3	63
Kraft Breakstone's Fat-free Sour Cream									
2 tbsp (31g)	28	0	0	3	5	0.0	2	1	22
Kraft Breakstone's Reduced Fat Sour Cream									
1 oz (28g)	43	3	2	14	2	0.0	2	1	17
Milk Substitute, Fluid, with Lauric Acid Oil									
1 quart (976g)	595	33	30	0	60	0.0	--	17	761
Milk, Buttermilk, Dried									
1 tbsp (6.5g)	25	0	0	4	3	0.0	3	2	34
Milk, Buttermilk, Fluid, Cultured, Low Fat									
1 fl oz (30.6g)	12	0	0	1	1	0.0	1	1	32
Milk, Buttermilk, Fluid, Cultured, Reduced Fat									
1 fl oz (30.6g)	17	1	0	2	2	0.0	--	1	26
Milk, Dry, Non-fat, Instant, with Added Vitamins A and D									
1 envelope (1-1/3 cup) (91g)	326	1	0	16	47	0.0	47	32	500
Milk, Dry, Non-fat, Instant, Without Added Vitamins A and D									
1 envelope (1-1/3 cup) (91g)	326	1	0	16	47	0.0	47	32	500

Food Serving size	Cal.	(g) Total Fat	(g) Sat. Fat	(mg) Chol.	(g) Carb.	(g) Fiber	(g) Sug.	(g) Prot.	(mg) Sod.
Milk, Dry, Non-fat, Regular, with Added Vitamins A and D .25 cup (30g)	109	0	0	6	16	0.0	16	11	161
Milk, Dry, Non-fat, Regular, Without Added Vitamins A and D .25 cup (30g)	109	0	0	6	16	0.0	16	11	161
Milk, Filled, Fluid, with Blend of Hydrogenated Vegetable Oils 1 quart (976g)	615	34	7	20	46	0.0	--	33	556
Milk, Filled, Fluid, with Lauric Acid Oil 1 fl oz (30.5g)	19	1	1	1	1	0.0	1	1	17
Milk, Goat, Fluid, with Added Vitamin D 1 fl oz (30.5g)	21	1	1	3	1	0.0	1	1	15
Milk, Imitation, Non-soy 1 fl oz (30.5g)	14	1	0	0	2	0.0	0	0	17
Milk, Indian Buffalo, Fluid 1 quart (976g)	947	67	45	185	51	0.0	--	37	508
Milk, Sheep, Fluid 1 quart (980g)	1058	69	45	265	53	0.0	--	59	431
Silk Banana-strawberry Soy Yogurt 1 container (170g)	150	2	0	0	29	1.0	18	4	26
Silk Black Cherry Soy Yogurt 1 container (170g)	150	2	0	0	29	1.0	20	4	20
Silk Blueberry Soy Yogurt 1 container (170g)	150	2	0	0	29	1.0	21	4	26
Silk Chai, Soy Milk 1 cup (243g)	129	3	1	0	19	0.0	14	6	100
Silk Chocolate, Soy Milk 1 cup (243g)	141	3	1	0	23	1.9	19	5	100
Silk Coffee, Soy Milk 1 cup (243g)	151	3	1	0	25	0.0	23	5	100
Silk French Vanilla Creamer 1 tbsp (15g)	20	1	0	0	3	0.0	3	0	10
Silk Hazelnut Creamer 1 tbsp (15g)	20	1	0	0	3	0.0	3	0	10
Silk Key Lime Soy Yogurt 1 container (170g)	150	2	0	0	30	1.0	21	4	26

Food Serving size	Cal.	(g) Total Fat	(g) Sat. Fat	(mg) Chol.	(g) Carb.	(g) Fiber	(g) Sug.	(g) Prot.	(mg) Sod.
Silk Light Chocolate, Soy Milk 1 cup (243g)	119	2	0	0	22	1.9	19	5	100
Silk Light Plain, Soy Milk 1 cup (243g)	70	2	0	0	8	1.0	6	6	119
Silk Light Vanilla, Soy Milk 1 cup (243g)	80	2	0	0	10	1.0	7	6	95
Silk Mocha, Soy Milk 1 cup (243g)	141	3	1	0	22	0.0	18	5	100
Silk Nog, Soy Milk .5 cup (122g)	90	2	0	0	15	0.0	12	3	74
Silk Original Creamer 1 tbsp (15g)	15	1	0	0	1	0.0	0	0	10
Silk Peach, Soy Yogurt 1 container (170g)	160	2	0	0	32	1.0	25	4	26
Silk Plain, Soy Milk 1 cup (243g)	100	4	1	0	8	1.0	6	7	119
Silk Plain, Soy Yogurt 1 container (227g)	150	4	0	0	22	0.9	12	6	30
Silk Plus Fiber, Soy Milk 1 cup (243g)	100	3	1	0	14	5.1	7	6	95
Silk Plus for Bone Health, Soy Milk 1 cup (243g)	100	3	1	0	11	1.9	7	6	95
Silk Plus Omega-3 DHA, Soy Milk 1 cup (243g)	109	5	1	0	8	1.0	6	7	119
Silk Raspberry, Soy Yogurt 1 container (170g)	150	2	0	0	30	1.0	22	4	26
Silk Strawberry, Soy Yogurt 1 container (170g)	160	2	0	0	31	1.0	22	4	26
Silk Unsweetened, Soy Milk 1 cup (243g)	80	4	1	0	4	1.0	1	7	85
Silk Vanilla, Soy Milk 1 cup (243g)	100	3	1	0	10	1.0	7	6	95
Silk Vanilla, Soy Yogurt (Family Size) 1 container (227g)	179	4	0	0	31	0.9	24	6	30

Food Serving size	Cal.	(g) Total Fat	(g) Sat. Fat	(mg) Chol.	(g) Carb.	(g) Fiber	(g) Sug.	(g) Prot.	(mg) Sod.
Silk Vanilla, Soy Yogurt (Single Serving Size) 1 container (170g)	150	3	0	0	25	1.0	18	5	20
Silk Very Vanilla, Soy Milk 1 cup (243g)	129	4	1	0	19	1.0	16	6	141
Soy Milk (All Flavors), Enhanced 1 cup (243g)	109	5	1	0	8	1.0	6	7	122
Soy Milk (All Flavors), Low Fat, with Added Calcium and Vitamins A and D 1 cup (243g)	104	2	0	0	17	1.9	9	4	90
Soy Milk (All Flavors), Non-fat, with Added Calcium and Vitamins A and D 1 cup (243g)	68	0	0	0	10	0.5	9	6	139
Soy Milk (All Flavors), Unsweetened, with Added Calcium with Added Vitamins A and D 1 cup (243g)	80	4	1	0	4	1.2	1	7	90
Soy Milk, Chocolate and Other Flavors, Light with Added Calcium and Vitamins A and D 1 cup (243g)	114	2	0	0	20	1.7	17	5	112
Soy Milk, Chocolate, Non-fat, with Added Calcium and Vitamins A and D 1 cup (243g)	107	0	0	0	21	0.5	9	6	139
Soy Milk, Chocolate, Unfortified 1 fl oz (30.6g)	19	0	0	0	3	0.1	2	1	16
Soy Milk, Chocolate, with Added Calcium and Vitamins A and D 1 fl oz (30.6g)	19	0	0	0	3	0.1	2	1	16
Soy Milk, Original and Vanilla, Light with Added Calcium and Vitamins A and D 1 cup (243g)	73	2	0	0	9	0.7	6	6	117
Soy Milk, Original and Vanilla, Light, Unsweetened, with Added Calcium and Vitamins A and D 1 cup (243g)	83	2	0	0	9	1.5	1	6	153
Soy Milk, Original and Vanilla, Unfortified 1 fl oz (30.6g)	17	1	0	0	2	0.2	1	1	16
Soy Milk, Original and Vanilla, with Added Calcium and Vitamins A and D 1 fl oz (30.6g)	13	0	0	0	2	0.1	1	1	14
Tofu Yogurt 1 cup (262g)	246	5	1	0	42	0.5	6	9	92
Whipped Cream Substitute, Dietetic, Made from Powder Mix 1 cup (80g)	80	5	3	0	8	0.0	4	1	85

Food Serving size	Cal.	(g) Total Fat	(g) Sat. Fat	(mg) Chol.	(g) Carb.	(g) Fiber	(g) Sug.	(g) Prot.	(mg) Sod.
Whipped Topping, Frozen, Low Fat									
1 cup (75g)	168	10	8	2	18	0.0	--	2	54
Yogurt Parfait, Low Fat, with Fruit and Granola									
1 item (149g)	125	2	1	4	24	1.6	--	5	73
Yogurt, Frozen, Chocolate, Non-fat Milk, with Low Calorie Sweetener									
1 cup (186g)	199	1	1	7	37	3.7	--	8	151
Yogurt, Fruit Variety, Non-fat, Fortified with Vitamin D									
1 container (4.4 oz) (125g)	119	0	0	3	24	0.0	24	6	73
Yogurt, Fruit, Low Fat, 10 Grams Protein per 8 oz									
1 container (6 oz) (170g)	173	2	1	7	32	0.0	32	7	99
Yogurt, Fruit, Low Fat, 10 Grams Protein per 8 oz, Fortified with Vitamin D									
1 container (6 oz) (170g)	173	2	1	7	32	0.0	32	7	99
Yogurt, Fruit, Low Fat, 11 Grams Protein per 8 oz									
.5 container (4 oz) (113g)	119	2	1	7	21	0.0	--	5	73
Yogurt, Fruit, Low Fat, 9 Grams Protein per 8 oz									
1 container,(4.4 oz) (125g)	124	1	1	6	23	0.0	23	5	66
Yogurt, Fruit, Low Fat, 9 Grams Protein per 8 oz, Fortified with Vitamin D									
1 container (4.4 oz) (125g)	124	1	1	6	23	0.0	23	5	66
Yogurt, Fruit, Low Fat, with Low Calorie Sweetener									
1 cup (8 fl oz) (245g)	257	3	2	15	46	0.0	7	12	142
Yogurt, Fruit, Low Fat, with Low Calorie Sweetener, Fortified with Vitamin D									
1 cup (8 fl oz) (245g)	257	3	2	15	46	0.0	7	12	142
Yogurt, Fruit, Variety, Non-fat									
1 container (4.4 oz) (125g)	119	0	0	3	24	0.0	1	6	73
Yogurt, Plain, Low Fat, 12 Grams Protein per 8 oz									
1 container (8 oz) (227g)	143	4	2	14	16	0.0	16	12	159
Yogurt, Plain, Skim Milk, 13 Grams Protein per 8 oz									
1 container (8 oz) (227g)	127	0	0	5	17	0.0	17	13	175
Yogurt, Plain, Whole Milk, 8 Grams Protein per 8 oz									
1 container (8 oz) (227g)	138	7	5	30	11	0.0	11	8	104
Yogurt, Vanilla, Low Fat, 11 Grams Protein per 8 oz									
1 container (8 oz) (227g)	193	3	2	11	31	0.0	31	11	150
Yogurt, Vanilla, Low Fat, 11 Grams Protein per 8 oz, Fortified with Vitamin D									
1 container (8 oz) (227g)	193	3	2	11	31	0.0	31	11	150

Protein Foods

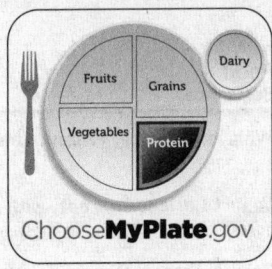

ChooseMyPlate.gov

Why Eat Proteins?

Protein foods are meat, poultry, fish, eggs, nuts, and seed. They provide nutrients that are vital for health and maintenance of your body. These include protein, B vitamins (niacin, thiamin, riboflavin, and B_6), vitamin E, iron, zinc, and magnesium. Proteins function as building blocks for bones, muscles, cartilage, skin, and blood. B vitamins help the body release energy, play a vital role in the function of the nervous system, aid in the formation of red blood cells, and help build tissues. Iron is used to carry oxygen in the blood. Seafood contains a range of nutrients, notably the omega-3 fatty acids, EPA and DHA. Eating about 8 ounces per week of a variety of seafood contributes to the prevention of heart disease.

Daily Goal

5 ½ ounces for an adult on a 2000-calorie diet
8 ounces of fish per week
One-ounce equivalents:

1 ounce lean meat, poultry, or fish	1 tablespoon peanut butter
1 egg	¼ cup cooked dried beans or peas
½ ounce nuts or seeds	¼ cup tofu/roasted soybeans

Shopping Tips

- Choose low fat or lean cuts of meat.
- Cook low fat—bake, broil, or grill.
- Vary your meals with more fish, beans, peas, nuts, and seeds.
- Select fish rich in omega-3 fats: salmon, trout, or herring.
- Trim visible fat and skin from meat before cooking.

Shopping List Essentials

Lean beef	Turkey	Eggs	Beans
Chicken	Fish	Almonds	

Red Flags

Choosing proteins that are high in saturated fat and cholesterol may increase your risk for coronary heart disease. These include fatty cuts of beef, pork, and lamb; regular (75% to 85% lean) ground beef; regular sausages, hot dogs, and bacon; some luncheon meats, such as regular bologna and salami; and some poultry, such as duck.

Food Serving size	Cal.	(g) Total Fat	(g) Sat. Fat	(mg) Chol.	(g) Carb.	(g) Fiber	(g) Sug.	(g) Prot.	(mg) Sod.
Meats (Beef, Lamb, Pork, Game, Organ)									
Bacon Bits, Meatless 1 tbsp (7g)	33	2	0	0	2	0.7	0	2	124
Bacon, Meatless 1 oz, cooked yield (16g)	50	5	1	0	1	0.4	0	2	234
Beef Jerky, Chopped and Formed 1 piece, large (20g)	82	5	2	10	2	0.4	2	7	416
Beef, Bologna, Reduced Sodium 1 slice, medium (28g)	87	8	3	16	1	0.0	0	3	191
Beef, Bottom Round, Roast, Lean Only, 0" Fat, Choice, Roasted 1 roast (yield from 627g raw meat) (515g)	953	39	14	402	0	0.0	0	140	185
Beef, Bottom Sirloin, Tri-tip Roast, Lean and Fat, 0" Fat, All Grades, Cooked, Roasted 1 roast (yield from 690g raw meat) (569g)	1201	63	23	472	0	0.0	0	148	302
Beef, Bottom Sirloin, Tri-tip Roast, Lean and Fat, 0" Fat, Choice, Cooked, Roasted 1 roast (yield from 714g raw meat) (591g)	1306	73	27	502	0	0.0	0	152	296
Beef, Bottom Sirloin, Tri-tip Roast, Lean and Fat, 0" Fat, Select, Cooked, Roasted 1 roast (yield from 666g raw meat) (547g)	1099	53	20	443	0	0.0	0	145	306
Beef, Bottom Sirloin, Tri-tip Roast, Lean, 0" Fat, Choice, Cooked, Roasted 1 roast (591g)	1141	58	21	473	0	0.0	0	156	319
Beef, Bottom Sirloin, Tri-tip Roast, Lean, 0" Fat, Select, Cooked, Roasted 1 roast (yield from 666g raw meat) (547g)	979	38	14	416	0	0.0	0	149	317
Beef, Bottom Sirloin, Tri-tip Steak, Lean, 0" fat, All Grades, Cooked, Broiled 1 lb (453.6g)	1134	60	22	485	0	0.0	0	139	331
Beef, Brisket, Flat Half, Lean and Fat, 0" Fat, All Grades, Cooked, Braised 1 steak (yield from 418g raw meat) (270g)	575	22	9	248	0	0.0	0	89	146
Beef, Brisket, Flat Half, Lean and Fat, 0" Fat, Select, Cooked, Braised 1 steak (yield from 388g raw meat) (247g)	506	17	7	230	0	0.0	0	83	141

Food Serving size	Cal.	(g) Total Fat	(g) Sat. Fat	(mg) Chol.	(g) Carb.	(g) Fiber	(g) Sug.	(g) Prot.	(mg) Sod.
Beef, Brisket, Flat Half, Lean and Fat, 1/8" Fat, All Grades, Cooked, Braised									
3 oz (85g)	246	16	6	90	0	0.0	0	24	41
Beef, Brisket, Flat Half, Lean and Fat, 1/8" Fat, Choice, Cooked, Braised									
1 steak, (yield from 593 g raw meat) (409g)	1219	80	34	438	0	0.0	0	117	188
Beef, Brisket, Flat Half, Lean, 0" Fat, All Grades, Cooked, Braised									
3 oz (85g)	174	6	2	85	0	0.0	0	28	46
Beef, Brisket, Flat Half, Lean, 1/8" Fat, All Grades, Cooked, Braised									
1 lb (453.6g)	889	27	10	440	0	0.0	0	150	245
Beef, Brisket, Flat Half, Lean, 1/8" Fat, Choice, Cooked, Braised									
1 lb (453.6g)	921	31	12	440	0	0.0	0	150	240
Beef, Brisket, Flat Half, Lean, 1/8" Fat, Select, Cooked, Braised									
1 lb (453.6g)	857	24	9	445	0	0.0	0	151	249
Beef, Brisket, Point Half, Lean and Fat, 0" Fat, All Grades, Cooked, Braised									
3 oz (85g)	304	24	10	78	0	0.0	0	20	58
Beef, Brisket, Point Half, Lean and Fat, 1/8" Fat, All Grades, Cooked, Braised									
3 oz (85g)	297	23	9	78	0	0.0	0	21	59
Beef, Brisket, Point Half, Lean, 0" Fat, All Grades, Cooked, Braised									
3 oz (85g)	207	12	4	77	0	0.0	0	24	65
Beef, Brisket, Whole, Lean and Fat, 0" Fat, All Grades, Cooked, Braised									
1 piece, cooked, excluding refuse (yield from 1 lb raw meat with refuse) (314g)	914	61	24	292	0	0.0	0	84	204
Beef, Brisket, Whole, Lean and Fat, 1/8" Fat, All Grades, Cooked, Braised									
3 oz (85g)	281	21	8	79	0	0.0	0	22	54
Beef, Brisket, Whole, Lean, 0" Fat, All Grades, Cooked, Braised									
1 piece, cooked, excluding refuse (yield from 1 lb raw meat with refuse) (264g)	576	27	10	246	0	0.0	0	79	185
Beef, Chuck Eye Country-style Ribs, Boneless, Lean, 0" Fat, All Grades, Cooked, Braised									
1 piece (227g)	518	26	12	227	0	0.0	0	71	157
Beef, Chuck Eye Country-style Ribs, Boneless, Lean, 0" Fat, Choice, Cooked									
1 piece (224g)	524	27	12	224	0	0.0	8	69	155
Beef, Chuck Eye Country-style Ribs, Boneless, Lean, 0" Fat, Select, Cooked, Braised									
1 piece (231g)	511	24	12	229	0	0.0	8	74	162

Food Serving size	Cal.	(g) Total Fat	(g) Sat. Fat	(mg) Chol.	(g) Carb.	(g) Fiber	(g) Sug.	(g) Prot.	(mg) Sod.
Beef, Chuck Eye Roast, Boneless, America's Beef Roast, Lean, 0" Fat, All Grades, Cooked									
1 roast (609g)	1114	52	21	512	0	0.0	0	162	487
Beef, Chuck Eye Roast, Boneless, America's Beef Roast, Lean, 0" Fat, Choice, Cooked									
1 roast (586g)	1113	55	22	498	0	0.0	0	155	463
Beef, Chuck Eye Roast, Boneless, America's Beef Roast, Lean, 0" Fat, Select, Cooked									
1 roast (645g)	1109	46	19	522	0	0.0	0	174	522
Beef, Chuck Eye Steak, Boneless, Lean, 0" Fat, All Grades, Cooked, Grilled									
1 steak (308g)	644	33	15	271	0	0.0	17	86	231
Beef, Chuck Eye Steak, Boneless, Lean, 0" Fat, Choice, Cooked, Grilled									
1 steak (307g)	660	35	15	267	0	0.0	15	86	230
Beef, Chuck Eye Steak, Boneless, Lean, 0" Fat, Select, Cooked, Grilled									
1 steak (309g)	615	30	15	281	0	0.0	16	86	229
Beef, Chuck for Stew, Lean and Fat, All Grades, Cooked, Braised									
1 lb (453.6g)	866	31	13	449	0	0.0	61	147	304
Beef, Chuck for Stew, Lean and Fat, Choice, Cooked, Braised									
1 lb (453.6g)	880	32	14	435	0	0.0	0	147	295
Beef, Chuck for Stew, Lean and Fat, Select, Cooked, Braised									
1 lb (453.6g)	844	29	11	463	0	0.0	0	146	308
Beef, Chuck, Arm Pot Roast, Lean and Fat, 0" Fat, All Grades, Cooked, Braised									
1 roast (yield from 1601 g raw meat) (1166g)	3463	224	88	1353	0	0.0	0	337	548
Beef, Chuck, Arm Pot Roast, Lean and Fat, 0" Fat, Select, Cooked, Braised									
1 roast (yield from 1675 g raw meat) (1236g)	3498	217	85	1421	0	0.0	0	361	593
Beef, Chuck, Arm Pot Roast, Lean and Fat, 1/8" Fat, All Grades, Cooked, Braised									
3 oz (85g)	257	16	6	102	0	0.0	0	26	43
Beef, Chuck, Arm Pot Roast, Lean and Fat, 1/8" Fat, Choice, Cooked, Braised									
3 oz (85g)	263	17	7	103	0	0.0	0	26	42
Beef, Chuck, Arm Pot Roast, Lean and Fat, 1/8" Fat, Select, Cooked, Braised									
3 oz (85g)	251	16	6	101	0	0.0	0	26	43

Food Serving size	Cal.	(g) Total Fat	(g) Sat. Fat	(mg) Chol.	(g) Carb.	(g) Fiber	(g) Sug.	(g) Prot.	(mg) Sod.
Beef, Chuck, Arm Pot Roast, Lean, 0" Fat, Choice, Cooked, Braised 1 roast (yield from 1528g raw meat) (1095g)									
	2321	84	32	1095	0	0.0	0	365	591
Beef, Chuck, Arm Pot Roast, Lean, 0" Fat, Select, Cooked, Braised 1 roast (yield from 1675 g raw meat) (1236g)									
	2410	72	27	1211	0	0.0	0	412	680
Beef, Chuck, Arm Pot Roast, Lean, 1/8" Fat, All Grades, Cooked, Braised 1 lb (453.6g)									
	971	33	13	472	0	0.0	0	157	254
Beef, Chuck, Arm Pot Roast, Lean, 1/8" Fat, Choice, Cooked, Braised 1 lb (453.6g)									
	1016	38	14	481	0	0.0	0	157	254
Beef, Chuck, Blade Boast, Lean, 0" Fat, All Grades, Cooked, Braised 1 piece, cooked, excluding refuse (yield from 1 lb raw meat with refuse) (191g)									
	483	25	10	202	0	0.0	0	59	136
Beef, Chuck, Blade Roast, Lean and Fat, 1/8" Fat, All Grades, Cooked, Braised 3 oz (85g)									
	290	21	9	88	0	0.0	0	23	55
Beef, Chuck, Blade Roast, Lean and Fat, 1/8" Fat, Choice, Cooked, Braised 3 oz (85g)									
	305	23	9	88	0	0.0	0	22	54
Beef, Chuck, Blade Roast, Lean and Fat, 1/8" Fat, Select, Cooked, Braised 3 oz (85g)									
	270	19	8	88	0	0.0	0	23	56
Beef, Chuck, Clod Roast, Lean and Fat, 0" Fat, All Grades, Cooked, Roasted 1 lb (453.6g)									
	939	49	18	313	0	0.0	6	117	322
Beef, Chuck, Clod Roast, Lean and Fat, 0" Fat, Choice, Cooked, Roasted 1 lb (453.6g)									
	980	56	19	304	0	0.0	13	112	322
Beef, Chuck, Clod Roast, Lean and Fat, 0" Fat, Select, Cooked, Roasted 1 lb (453.6g)									
	889	40	15	331	0	0.0	2	124	327
Beef, Chuck, Clod Roast, Lean Only, to 1/4" Fat, All Grades, Cooked, Roasted 1 lb (453.6g)									
	785	31	10	322	0	0.0	--	120	322
Beef, Chuck, Clod Roast, Lean, 0" Fat, All Grades, Cooked, Roasted 1 lb (453.6g)									
	780	29	9	304	0	0.0	--	122	336
Beef, Chuck, Clod Roast, Lean, 0" Fat, Choice, Cooked, Roasted 3 oz (1 serving) (85g)									
	145	6	2	74	0	0.0	0	22	63
Beef, Chuck, Clod Roast, Lean, 0" Fat, Select, Cooked, Roasted 3 oz (1 serving) (85g)									
	146	5	2	77	0	0.0	0	24	63
Beef, Chuck, Clod Steak, Lean Only, to 1/4" Fat, All Grades, Cooked, Braised 1 lb (453.6g)									
	857	32	10	426	0	0.0	4	133	272

Food Serving size	Cal.	(g) Total Fat	(g) Sat. Fat	(mg) Chol.	(g) Carb.	(g) Fiber	(g) Sug.	(g) Prot.	(mg) Sod.
Beef, Chuck, Clod, Shoulder Tender, Medium, Lean and Fat, 0" Fat, All Grades, Cooked, Grilled									
1 serving (3 oz) (85g)	150	6	2	66	0	0.0	4	22	50
Beef, Chuck, Clod, Shoulder Tender, Medium, Lean and Fat, 0" Fat, Choice, Cooked, Grilled									
1 serving (3 oz) (85g)	154	7	2	65	0	0.0	2	22	51
Beef, Chuck, Clod, Shoulder Tender, Medium, Lean and Fat, 0" Fat, Select, Cooked, Grilled									
1 serving (3 oz) (85g)	146	5	1	68	0	0.0	4	22	49
Beef, Chuck, Clod, Shoulder Top and Center Steak, Lean and Fat, 0", All Grades, Grilled									
1 serving (3 oz) (85g)	155	7	2	65	0	0.0	8	22	51
Beef, Chuck, Clod, Top and Center, Steak, Lean and Fat, 0" Fat, Select, Cooked, Grilled									
1 serving (3 oz) (85g)	150	6	2	65	0	0.0	8	23	53
Beef, Chuck, Clod, Top Blade, Steak, Lean and Fat, 0" Fat, All Grades, Cooked, Grilled									
1 serving (3 oz) (85g)	189	11	4	71	0	0.0	15	21	65
Beef, Chuck, Clod, Top Blade, Steak, Lean and Fat, 0" Fat, Choice, Cooked, Grilled									
1 serving (3 oz) (85g)	194	12	5	71	0	0.0	17	21	66
Beef, Chuck, Clod, Top Blade, Steak, Lean and Fat, 0" Fat, Select, Cooked, Grilled									
1 serving (3 oz) (85g)	180	10	4	71	0	0.0	11	21	65
Beef, Chuck, Eye Country-style Ribs, Boneless, Lean and Fat, 0" Fat, All Grades, Cooked									
1 piece (227g)	672	47	20	218	0	0.0	0	63	148
Beef, Chuck, Eye Country-style Ribs, Boneless, Lean and Fat, 0" Fat, Choice, Cooked									
1 piece (224g)	679	48	21	215	0	0.0	0	61	146
Beef, Chuck, Eye Country-style Ribs, Boneless, Lean and Fat, 0" Fat, Select, Cooked									
1 piece (231g)	658	44	20	222	0	0.0	--	66	152
Beef, Chuck, Eye Roast, Boneless, America's Beef Roast, Lean and Fat, 0", All Grades, Cooked, Roasted									
1 roast (609g)	1437	93	39	505	0	0.0	--	150	463

Food Serving size	Cal.	(g) Total Fat	(g) Sat. Fat	(mg) Chol.	(g) Carb.	(g) Fiber	(g) Sug.	(g) Prot.	(mg) Sod.
Beef, Chuck, Eye Roast, Boneless, America's Beef Roast, Lean and Fat, 0", Choice, Cooked, Roasted									
1 roast (586g)	1412	93	38	498	0	0.0	--	143	440
Beef, Chuck, Eye Roast, Boneless, America's Beef Roast, Lean and Fat, 0", Select, Cooked, Roasted									
1 roast (645g)	1477	93	40	522	0	0.0	--	160	490
Beef, Chuck, Eye Steak, Boneless, Lean and Fat, 0" Fat, All Grades, Cooked, Grilled									
1 steak (308g)	853	60	27	268	0	0.0	16	77	219
Beef, Chuck, Eye Steak, Boneless, Lean and Fat, 0" Fat, Choice, Cooked, Grilled									
1 steak (307g)	869	62	27	264	0	0.0	--	77	218
Beef, Chuck, Eye Steak, Boneless, Lean and Fat, 0" Fat, Select, Cooked, Grilled									
1 steak (309g)	825	57	27	275	0	0.0	15	77	216
Beef, Chuck, Mock Tender Steak, Boneless, Lean and Fat, 0" Fat, All Grades, Cooked									
1 steak (141g)	310	14	5	159	0	0.0	--	45	94
Beef, Chuck, Mock Tender Steak, Boneless, Lean and Fat, 0" Fat, All Grades, Cooked									
1 steak (198g)	253	9	4	135	0	0.0	--	42	158
Beef, Chuck, Mock Tender Steak, Boneless, Lean and Fat, 0" Fat, Choice, Cooked									
1 steak (141g)	317	15	5	155	0	0.0	--	45	93
Beef, Chuck, Mock Tender Steak, Boneless, Lean and Fat, 0" Fat, Select, Cooked									
1 steak (141g)	298	13	5	165	0	0.0	--	45	97
Beef, Chuck, Mock Tender Steak, Boneless, Lean, 0" Fat, All Grades, Cooked, Braised									
1 steak (141g)	268	9	4	161	0	0.0	15	47	96
Beef, Chuck, Mock Tender Steak, Boneless, Lean, 0" Fat, Choice, Cooked, Braised									
1 steak (141g)	278	10	4	157	0	0.0	0	47	94
Beef, Chuck, Mock Tender Steak, Boneless, Lean, 0" Fat, Select, Cooked, Braised									
1 steak (141g)	255	8	3	166	0	0.0	4	46	99
Beef, Chuck, Mock Tender Steak, Lean and Fat, 0" Fat, All Grades, Cooked, Broiled									
1 lb (453.6g)	726	25	8	286	0	0.0	10	117	322

Food Serving size	Cal.	(g) Total Fat	(g) Sat. Fat	(mg) Chol.	(g) Carb.	(g) Fiber	(g) Sug.	(g) Prot.	(mg) Sod.
Beef, Chuck, Mock Tender Steak, Lean and Fat, 0" Fat, USDA Choice, Cooked, Broiled									
1 lb (453.6g)	730	26	8	295	0	0.0	--	117	331
Beef, Chuck, Mock Tender Steak, Lean and Fat, 0" Fat, USDA Select, Cooked, Broiled									
1 lb (453.6g)	721	24	9	272	0	0.0	--	118	308
Beef, Chuck, Mock Tender Steak, Lean, 0" Fat, All Grades, Cooked, Broiled									
1 lb (453.6g)	721	25	8	286	0	0.0	12	117	322
Beef, Chuck, Mock Tender Steak, Lean, 0" Fat, Choice, Cooked, Broiled									
3 oz (1 serving) (85g)	137	5	1	80	0	0.0	0	22	62
Beef, Chuck, Mock Tender Steak, Lean, 0" Fat, Select, Cooked, Broiled									
3 oz (1 serving) (85g)	133	4	2	84	0	0.0	0	22	58
Beef, Chuck, Pot Roast, Lean, 1/8" Fat, Select, Cooked, Braised									
1 lb (453.6g)	930	29	11	467	0	0.0	0	157	259
Beef, Chuck, Short Ribs, Boneless, 0" Fat, Choice, Cooked, Broiled									
1 piece (272g)	680	41	19	277	0	0.0	0	78	204
Beef, Chuck, Short Ribs, Boneless, Lean and Fat, 0" Fat, All Grades, Cooked, Braised									
1 piece (289g)	881	65	29	289	0	0.0	14	74	202
Beef, Chuck, Short Ribs, Boneless, Lean and Fat, 0" Fat, Choice, Cooked, Braised									
1 piece (272g)	862	65	29	267	0	0.0	32	69	190
Beef, Chuck, Short Ribs, Boneless, Lean and Fat, 0" Fat, Select, Cooked, Braised									
1 piece (315g)	904	64	29	324	0	0.0	0	81	224
Beef, Chuck, Short Ribs, Boneless, Lean, 0" Fat, All Grades, Cooked, Braised									
1 piece (289g)	694	40	19	303	0	0.0	0	83	217
Beef, Chuck, Short Ribs, Boneless, Lean, 0" Fat, Select, Cooked, Braised									
1 piece (315g)	706	38	18	340	0	0.0	0	91	236
Beef, Chuck, Shoulder Clod, Top and Center, Steak, Lean and Fat, 0" Fat, Choice, Cooked, Grilled									
1 serving (3 oz) (85g)	156	7	3	63	0	0.0	2	22	50
Beef, Chuck, Top Blade, Lean and Fat, 0" Fat, All Grades, Cooked, Broiled									
1 lb (453.6g)	980	53	18	277	0	0.0	16	117	304
Beef, Chuck, Top Blade, Lean and Fat, 0" Fat, Choice, Cooked, Broiled									
1 lb (453.6g)	1030	59	19	263	0	0.0	8	117	308

Food Serving size	Cal.	(g) Total Fat	(g) Sat. Fat	(mg) Chol.	(g) Carb.	(g) Fiber	(g) Sug.	(g) Prot.	(mg) Sod.
Beef, Chuck, Top Blade, Lean and Fat, 0" Fat, Select, Cooked, Broiled									
1 lb (453.6g)	907	45	16	304	0	0.0	17	116	304
Beef, Chuck, Top Blade, Lean Only, to 0" Fat, All Grades, Cooked, Broiled									
1 lb (453.6g)	921	46	15	272	0	0.0	14	119	308
Beef, Chuck, Top Blade, Lean, 0" Fat, Choice, Cooked, Broiled									
3 oz (1 serving) (85g)	184	10	3	79	0	0.0	0	22	58
Beef, Chuck, Top Blade, Lean, 0" Fat, Select, Cooked, Broiled									
3 oz (1 serving) (85g)	156	7	2	80	0	0.0	0	22	58
Beef, Chuck, Under Blade Center Steak, Boneless, Denver Cut, Lean and Fat, All Grades, Cooked									
1 steak (353g)	801	48	20	332	1	0.0	--	92	258
Beef, Chuck, Under Blade Center Steak, Boneless, Denver Cut, Lean, 0" Fat									
1 steak (353g)	777	45	19	332	0	0.0	0	94	258
Beef, Chuck, Under Blade Center Steak, Boneless, Denver Cut, Lean, 0" Fat									
1 steak (356g)	812	48	20	328	1	0.0	0	94	260
Beef, Chuck, Under Blade Center Steak, Boneless, Denver Cut, Lean, 0" Fat, Select, Cooked									
1 steak (349g)	729	40	17	335	0	0.0	0	93	258
Beef, Chuck, Under Blade Pot Roast, Boneless, Lean and Fat, 0" Fat, Choice, Cooked, Braised									
1 roast (658g)	2013	141	56	658	0	0.0	0	174	401
Beef, Chuck, Under Blade Pot Roast, Boneless, Lean and Fat, 0" Fat, Select, Cooked, Braised									
1 roast (629g)	1812	120	49	616	0	0.0	0	171	403
Beef, Chuck, Under Blade Pot Roast, Boneless, Lean, 0" Fat, All Grades, Cooked									
1 roast (647g)	1398	68	26	673	0	0.0	0	198	421
Beef, Chuck, Under Blade Pot Roast, Boneless, Lean, 0" Fat, All Grades, Cooked, Braised									
1 roast (960g)	1344	58	26	634	3	0.0	0	203	778
Beef, Chuck, Under Blade Pot Roast, Boneless, Lean, 0" Fat, Choice, Cooked, Braised									
1 roast (658g)	1520	73	29	691	0	0.0	0	200	415
Beef, Chuck, Under Blade Pot Roast, Boneless, Lean, 0" Fat, Select, Cooked, Braised									
1 roast (629g)	1359	59	22	642	0	0.0	0	193	421

Food Serving size	Cal.	(g) Total Fat	(g) Sat. Fat	(mg) Chol.	(g) Carb.	(g) Fiber	(g) Sug.	(g) Prot.	(mg) Sod.
Beef, Chuck, Under Blade Steak, Boneless, Lean and Fat, 0" Fat, All Grades									
1 steak (449g)	1235	81	33	431	0	0.0	0	127	292
Beef, Chuck, Under Blade Steak, Boneless, Lean and Fat, 0" Fat, Choice, Cooked									
1 steak (445g)	1264	86	34	436	0	0.0	--	123	285
Beef, Chuck, Under Blade Steak, Boneless, Lean and Fat, 0" Fat, Select, Cooked									
1 steak (454g)	1185	73	30	427	0	0.0	--	132	300
Beef, Chuck, Under Blade Steak, Boneless, Lean, 0" Fat, All Grades, Cooked, Braised									
1 steak (449g)	983	47	18	480	0	0.0	--	141	292
Beef, Chuck, Under Blade Steak, Boneless, Lean, 0" Fat, Choice, Cooked, Braised									
1 steak (445g)	988	49	19	472	0	0.0	--	138	289
Beef, Chuck, Under Blade Steak, Boneless, Lean, 0" Fat, Select, Cooked, Braised									
1 steak (454g)	976	44	16	490	0	0.0	--	145	300
Beef, Chuck, Under Blade, Pot Roast, Boneless, Lean and Fat, 0" Fat, All Grades, Cooked, Broiled									
1 roast (647g)	1883	133	53	641	0	0.0	0	173	401
Beef, Composite of Retail Cuts, Lean and Fat, 0" Fat, All Grades, Cooked									
1 piece, cooked, excluding refuse (yield from 1 lb raw meat with refuse) (279g)	762	48	19	243	0	0.0	0	76	173
Beef, Composite of Retail Cuts, Lean and Fat, 0" Fat, Choice, Cooked									
3 oz (85g)	241	16	6	74	0	0.0	0	23	53
Beef, Composite of Retail Cuts, Lean and Fat, 0" Fat, Select, Cooked									
3 oz (85g)	222	14	5	73	0	0.0	0	23	54
Beef, Composite of Retail Cuts, Lean and Fat, 1/8" Fat, All Grades, Cooked									
3 oz (85g)	247	17	7	74	0	0.0	0	22	54
Beef, Composite of Retail Cuts, Lean and Fat, 1/8" Fat, Choice, Cooked									
3 oz (85g)	256	18	7	74	0	0.0	0	22	53
Beef, Composite of Retail Cuts, Lean and Fat, 1/8" Fat, Prime, Cooked									
3 oz (85g)	254	18	7	71	0	0.0	0	22	54
Beef, Composite of Retail Cuts, Lean and Fat, 1/8" Fat, Select, Cooked									
3 oz (85g)	236	15	6	73	0	0.0	0	23	54
Beef, Composite of Retail Cuts, Lean, 0" Fat, All Grades, Cooked									
3 oz (85g)	179	8	3	73	0	0.0	0	25	56

Food Serving size	Cal.	(g) Total Fat	(g) Sat. Fat	(mg) Chol.	(g) Carb.	(g) Fiber	(g) Sug.	(g) Prot.	(mg) Sod.
Beef, Composite of Retail Cuts, Lean, 0" Fat, Choice, Cooked									
3 oz (85g)	186	9	3	73	0	0.0	0	25	56
Beef, Composite of Retail Cuts, Lean, 0" Fat, Select, Cooked									
3 oz (85g)	171	7	3	73	0	0.0	0	25	56
Beef, Cured, Breakfast Strips, Cooked									
1 pkg, cooked (yield from 12 oz raw product) (170g)	763	58	24	202	2	0.0	0	53	3830
Beef, Cured, Breakfast Strips, Raw or Unheated									
1 pkg, (net weight, 12 oz) (340g)	1380	132	54	279	2	0.0	--	43	3247
Beef, Cured, Corned Beef, Brisket, Cooked									
3 oz (85g)	213	16	5	83	0	0.0	0	15	964
Beef, Cured, Corned beef, Canned									
1 slice (3/4 oz) (21g)	53	3	1	18	0	0.0	0	6	211
Beef, Cured, Dried									
10 slices (28g)	43	1	0	22	1	0.0	1	9	781
Beef, Cured, Luncheon Meat, Jellied									
1 slice (1 oz) (4" x 4" x 3/32" thick) (28g)	31	1	0	10	0	0.0	--	5	370
Beef, Cured, Pastrami									
1 slice (1 oz) (28g)	41	2	1	19	0	0.0	0	6	248
Beef, Cured, Sausage, Cooked, Smoked									
1 oz (28.35g)	88	8	3	19	1	0.0	--	4	321
Beef, Cured, Smoked, Chopped Beef									
1 slice (1 oz) (28g)	37	1	1	13	1	0.0	--	6	352
Beef, Cured, Thin-sliced Beef									
5 slices (21g)	37	1	0	9	1	0.0	0	6	302
Beef, Flank, Steak, Lean and Fat, 0" Fat, All Grades, Cooked, Broiled									
1 steak (yield from 475 g raw meat) (383g)	735	32	13	303	0	0.0	0	106	214
Beef, Flank, Steak, Lean and Fat, 0" Fat, Choice, Cooked, Braised									
3 oz (85g)	224	14	6	61	0	0.0	0	23	60
Beef, Flank, Steak, Lean and Fat, 0" Fat, Choice, Cooked, Broiled									
1 steak (yield from 483 g raw meat) (387g)	782	36	15	313	0	0.0	0	107	205

Food Serving size	Cal.	(g) Total Fat	(g) Sat. Fat	(mg) Chol.	(g) Carb.	(g) Fiber	(g) Sug.	(g) Prot.	(mg) Sod.
Beef, Flank, Steak, Lean and Fat, 0" Fat, Select, Cooked, Broiled 1 steak (yield from 467 g raw meat) (379g)	694	27	11	296	0	0.0	0	105	220
Beef, Flank, Steak, Lean, 0" Fat, All Grades, Cooked, Broiled 1 steak (383g)	712	28	12	299	0	0.0	0	107	218
Beef, Flank, Steak, Lean, 0" Fat, Choice, Ccooked, Braised 1 piece, cooked, excluding refuse (yield from 1 lb raw meat with refuse) (246g)	583	32	14	175	0	0.0	0	69	177
Beef, Flank, Steak, Lean, 0" Fat, Choice, Cooked, Broiled 1 steak (387g)	751	32	13	310	0	0.0	0	108	217
Beef, Flank, Steak, Lean, 0" Fat, Select, Cooked, Broiled 1 steak (yield from 467 g raw meat) (379g)	675	25	10	288	0	0.0	0	106	224
Beef, Ground, 70% Lean Meat/30% Fat, Crumbles, Cooked, Pan-browned 1 portion (yield from 1/2 lb raw meat) (139g)	375	25	10	122	0	0.0	0	36	133
Beef, Ground, 70% Lean Meat/30% Fat, Loaf, Cooked, Baked 1 loaf (yield from 1 lb raw meat) (284g)	684	44	18	187	0	0.0	0	68	207
Beef, Ground, 70% Lean Meat/30% Fat, Patty, Cooked, Broiled 1 patty (70g)	191	13	5	57	0	0.0	0	18	57
Beef, Ground, 70% Lean Meat/30% Fat, Patty, Cooked, Pan-broiled 1 patty (77g)	183	12	5	60	0	0.0	0	18	71
Beef, Ground, 75% Lean Meat, 25% Fat, Crumbles, Cooked, Pan-browned 1 portion (yield from 1/2 lb raw meat) (139g)	385	25	10	124	0	0.0	8	37	129
Beef, Ground, 75% Lean Meat, 25% Fat, Loaf, Cooked, Baked 1 loaf (yield from 1 lb raw meat) (284g)	721	47	18	233	0	0.0	19	70	199
Beef, Ground, 75% Lean Meat, 25% Fat, Patty, Cooked, Broiled 1 patty (yield from 1/4 lb raw meat) (70g)	195	13	5	62	0	0.0	1	18	55
Beef, Ground, 75% Lean Meat, 25% Fat, Patty, Cooked, Pan-broiled 1 patty (yield from 1/4 lb raw meat) (77g)	191	13	5	64	0	0.0	4	18	67

Food Serving size	Cal.	(g) Total Fat	(g) Sat. Fat	(mg) Chol.	(g) Carb.	(g) Fiber	(g) Sug.	(g) Prot.	(mg) Sod.
Beef, Ground, 80% Lean Meat, 20% Fat, Crumbles, Cooked, Pan-browned 1 portion (yield from 1/2 lb raw meat) (149g)									
	405	26	10	133	0	0.0	7	40	136
Beef, Ground, 80% Lean Meat, 20% Fat, Loaf, Cooked, Baked 1 loaf (yield from 1 lb raw meat) (309g)									
	785	50	19	278	0	0.0	11	78	207
Beef, Ground, 80% Lean Meat, 20% Fat, Patty, Cooked, Broiled 1 patty (yield from 1/4 lb raw meat) (77g)									
	209	14	5	70	0	0.0	2	20	58
Beef, Ground, 80% Lean Meat, 20% Fat, Patty, Cooked, Pan-broiled 1 patty (yield from 1/4 lb raw meat) (83g)									
	204	13	5	71	0	0.0	4	20	69
Beef, Ground, 85% Lean Meat, 15% Fat, Crumbles, Cooked, Pan-browned 1 portion (yield from 1/2 lb raw meat) (149g)									
	381	23	9	134	0	0.0	4	41	133
Beef, Ground, 85% Lean Meat, 15% Fat, Loaf, Cooked, Baked 1 loaf (yield from 1 lb raw meat) (309g)									
	742	44	17	281	0	0.0	21	80	198
Beef, Ground, 85% Lean Meat, 15% Fat, Patty, Cooked, Broiled 1 patty (yield from 1/4 lb raw meat) (77g)									
	193	12	5	69	0	0.0	2	20	55
Beef, Ground, 85% Lean Meat, 15% Fat, Patty, Cooked, Pan-broiled 1 patty (yield from 1/4 lb raw meat) (83g)									
	193	12	4	71	0	0.0	4	20	66
Beef, Ground, 90% Lean Meat, 10% Fat, Crumbles, Cooked, Pan-browned 1 portion (yield from 1/2 lb raw meat) (154g)									
	354	19	7	137	0	0.0	5	44	134
Beef, Ground, 90% Lean Meat, 10% Fat, Loaf, Cooked, Baked 1 loaf (yield from 1 lb raw meat) (323g)									
	691	36	14	278	0	0.0	10	86	197
Beef, Ground, 90% Lean Meat, 10% Fat, Patty, Cooked, Broiled 1 patty (yield from 1/4 lb raw meat) (82g)									
	178	10	4	70	0	0.0	4	21	56
Beef, Ground, 90% Lean Meat, 10% Fat, Patty, Cooked, Pan-broiled 1 patty (yield from 1/4 lb raw meat) (86g)									
	175	9	4	71	0	0.0	4	22	65

Food Serving size	Cal.	(g) Total Fat	(g) Sat. Fat	(mg) Chol.	(g) Carb.	(g) Fiber	(g) Sug.	(g) Prot.	(mg) Sod.
Beef, Ground, 95% Lean Meat, 5% Fat, Crumbles, Cooked, Pan-browned 1 portion (yield from 1/2 lb raw meat) (154g)									
	297	12	5	137	0	0.0	8	45	131
Beef, Ground, 95% Lean Meat, 5% Fat, Loaf, Cooked, Baked 1 loaf (yield from 1 lb raw meat) (323g)									
	562	21	9	236	0	0.0	14	88	187
Beef, Ground, 95% Lean Meat, 5% Fat, Patty, Cooked, Broiled 1 patty (yield from 1/4 lb raw meat) (82g)									
	140	5	2	62	0	0.0	1	22	53
Beef, Ground, 95% Lean Meat, 5% Fat, Patty, Cooked, Pan-broiled 1 patty (yield from 1/4 lb raw meat) (86g)									
	141	5	2	65	0	0.0	5	22	61
Beef, Ground, Patties, Frozen, Cooked, Broiled 3 oz (85g)									
	251	19	7	71	0	0.0	0	20	65
Beef, Loin, Lottom Sirloin Butt, Tri-tip, Lean, 0" Fat, All Grades, Cooked, Roasted 1 roast (569g)									
	1036	47	18	444	0	0.0	0	152	313
Beef, Loin, Porterhouse Steak, Lean and Fat, 0" Fat, USDA Choice, Cooked, Broiled 1 lb (453.6g)									
	1284	91	34	313	0	0.0	0	107	295
Beef, Loin, T-bone Steak, Lean & Fat, 0" Fat, USDA Choice, Cooked, Broiled 1 lb (453.6g)									
	1170	78	29	277	0	0.0	0	109	304
Beef, Plate, Inside Skirt Steak, Lean, 0" Fat, All Grades, Cooked, Broiled 3 oz (1 serving) (85g)									
	174	9	3	72	0	0.0	0	23	65
Beef, Plate, Outside Skirt Steak, Lean and Fat, 0" Fat, All Grades, Cooked Broiled 1 lb (453.6g)									
	1157	78	32	268	0	0.0	22	107	417
Beef, Plate, Outside Skirt Steak, Lean, 0" Fat, All Grades, Cooked, Broiled 3 oz (1 serving) (85g)									
	198	12	5	77	0	0.0	0	21	80
Beef, Plate, Skirt Steak, Lean and Fat, 0" Fat, All Grades, Cooked, Broiled 1 lb (453.6g)									
	998	55	21	272	0	0.0	--	119	340
Beef, Retail Cuts, Fat, Cooked 3 oz (85g)									
	578	60	24	81	0	0.0	0	9	20
Beef, Rib Eye, Small End (Ribs 10- 12) Lean, 0" Fat, Select, Cooked, Broiled 1 steak (231g)									
	420	14	5	219	0	0.0	0	69	146

Food Serving size	Cal.	(g) Total Fat	(g) Sat. Fat	(mg) Chol.	(g) Carb.	(g) Fiber	(g) Sug.	(g) Prot.	(mg) Sod.
Beef, Rib Eye, Small End (Ribs 10-12), Lean and Fat, 0" Fat, All Grades, Cooked, Broiled									
1 steak (yield from 295g raw meat) (233g)	580	34	13	207	0	0.0	0	64	130
Beef, Rib Eye, Small End (Ribs 10-12), Lean and Fat, 0" Fat, Choice, Cooked, Broiled									
1 steak (yield from 297g raw meat) (236g)	625	40	15	208	0	0.0	0	63	125
Beef, Rib Eye, Small End (Ribs 10-12), Lean and Fat, 0" Fat, Select, Cooked, Broiled									
1 steak (yield from 294g raw meat) (231g)	541	29	11	213	0	0.0	0	65	136
Beef, Rib Eye, Small End (Ribs 10-12), Lean, 0" Fat, Choice, Cooked, Broiled									
3 oz (85g)	174	8	3	77	0	0.0	0	25	51
Beef, Rib, Large End (Ribs 6-9), Lean and Fat, 0" Fat, Choice, Cooked, Roasted									
3 oz (85g)	316	26	10	72	0	0.0	--	19	54
Beef, Rib, Large End (Ribs 6-9), Lean and Fat, 0" Fat, Select, Cooked, Roasted									
3 oz (85g)	281	22	9	71	0	0.0	--	20	55
Beef, Rib, Large End (Ribs 6-9), Lean and Fat, 1/8" Fat, All Grades, Cooked, Broiled									
3 oz (85g)	287	23	9	68	0	0.0	--	18	54
Beef, Rib, Large End (Ribs 6-9), Lean and Fat, 1/8" Fat, All Grades, Cooked, Roasted									
3 oz (85g)	302	24	10	72	0	0.0	0	20	54
Beef, Rib, Large End (Ribs 6-9), Lean and Fat, 1/8" Fat, Choice, Cooked, Broiled									
3 oz (85g)	315	27	11	69	0	0.0	--	18	54
Beef, Rib, Large End (Ribs 6-9), Lean and Fat, 1/8" Fat, Choice, Cooked, Roasted									
3 oz (85g)	321	27	11	72	0	0.0	--	19	54
Beef, Rib, Large End (Ribs 6-9), Lean and Fat, 1/8" Fat, Prime, Cooked, Broiled									
3 oz (85g)	343	30	12	73	0	0.0	--	18	53
Beef, Rib, Large End (Ribs 6-9), Lean and Fat, 1/8" Fat, Prime, Cooked, Roasted									
3 oz (85g)	334	28	12	72	0	0.0	--	19	54
Beef, Rib, Large End (Ribs 6-9), Lean and Fat, 1/8" Fat, Select, Cooked, Broiled									
3 oz (85g)	275	22	9	68	0	0.0	--	18	54
Beef, Rib, Large End (Ribs 6-9), Lean and Fat, 1/8" Fat, Select, Cooked, Roasted									
3 oz (85g)	283	22	9	71	0	0.0	--	20	55

Food Serving size	Cal.	(g) Total Fat	(g) Sat. Fat	(mg) Chol.	(g) Carb.	(g) Fiber	(g) Sug.	(g) Prot.	(mg) Sod.
Beef, Rib, Large End (Ribs 6-9), Lean, 0" Fat, All Grades, Cooked, Roasted									
3 oz (85g)	202	11	5	69	0	0.0	0	23	62
Beef, Rib, Large End (Ribs 6-9), Lean, 0" Fat, Choice, Cooked, Roasted									
3 oz (85g)	215	13	5	69	0	0.0	--	23	62
Beef, Rib, Large End (Ribs 6-9), Lean, 0" Fat, Select, Cooked, Roasted									
3 oz (85g)	187	10	4	69	0	0.0	--	23	62
Beef, Rib, Short Ribs, Lean and Fat, Choice, Cooked, Braised									
1 piece, cooked, excluding refuse (yield from 1 lb raw meat with refuse) (225g)	1060	94	40	212	0	0.0	0	49	113
Beef, Rib, Short Ribs, Lean, Choice, Cooked, Braised									
3 oz (85g)	251	15	7	79	0	0.0	0	26	49
Beef, Rib, Small End (Ribs 10-12), Lean and Fat, 0" Fat, All Grades, Cooked, Broiled									
3 oz (85g)	212	13	5	76	0	0.0	0	23	48
Beef, Rib, Small End (Ribs 10-12), Lean and Fat, 0" Fat, Choice, Cooked, Broiled									
3 oz (85g)	265	19	8	71	0	0.0	--	21	54
Beef, Rib, Small End (Ribs 10-12), Lean and Fat, 0" Fat, Select, Cooked, Broiled									
3 oz (85g)	242	17	7	71	0	0.0	--	21	54
Beef, Rib, Small End (Ribs 10-12), Lean and Fat, 1/8" Fat, All Grades, Cooked, Broiled									
3 oz (85g)	247	17	7	82	0	0.0	0	22	45
Beef, Rib, Small End (Ribs 10-12), Lean and Fat, 1/8" Fat, All Grades, Cooked, Roasted									
3 oz (85g)	290	23	9	71	0	0.0	--	19	54
Beef, Rib, Small End (Ribs 10-12), Lean and Fat, 1/8" Fat, Choice, Cooked, Broiled									
3 oz (85g)	258	19	7	80	0	0.0	0	21	42
Beef, Rib, Small End (Ribs 10-12), Lean and Fat, 1/8" Fat, Choice, Cooked, Roasted									
3 oz (85g)	305	25	10	71	0	0.0	--	19	54
Beef, Rib, Small End (Ribs 10-12), Lean and Fat, 1/8" Fat, Prime, Cooked, Broiled									
3 oz (85g)	301	24	10	71	0	0.0	--	21	54
Beef, Rib, Small End (Ribs 10-12), Lean and Fat, 1/8" Fat, Prime, Cooked, Roasted									
3 oz (85g)	349	30	12	71	0	0.0	--	19	55

Food Serving size	Cal.	(g) Total Fat	(g) Sat. Fat	(mg) Chol.	(g) Carb.	(g) Fiber	(g) Sug.	(g) Prot.	(mg) Sod.
Beef, Rib, Small End (Ribs 10-12), Lean and Fat, 1/8" Fat, Select, Cooked, Broiled									
3 oz (85g)	236	15	6	88	0	0.0	0	23	49
Beef, Rib, Small End (Ribs 10-12), Lean and Fat, 1/8" Fat, Select, Cooked, Roasted									
3 oz (85g)	275	21	9	71	0	0.0	--	19	54
Beef, Rib, Small End (Ribs 10-12), Lean, 0" Fat, All Grades, Cooked, Broiled									
3 oz (85g)	164	6	2	77	0	0.0	0	25	52
Beef, Rib, Small End (Ribs 10-12), Lean, 0" Fat, Choice, Cooked, Broiled									
3 oz (85g)	191	10	4	68	0	0.0	--	24	59
Beef, Rib, Small End (Ribs 10-12), Lean, 0" Fat, Select, Cooked, Broiled									
3 oz (85g)	168	7	3	68	0	0.0	--	24	59
Beef, Rib, Small End (Ribs 10-12), Lean, 1/8" Fat, All Grades, Cooked, Broiled									
1 lb (453.6g)	885	35	13	395	0	0.0	0	134	281
Beef, Rib, Small End (Ribs 10-12), Lean, 1/8" Fat, Choice, Cooked, Broiled									
1 lb (453.6g)	916	41	16	399	0	0.0	0	128	263
Beef, Rib, Small End (Ribs 10-12), Lean, 1/8" Fat, Select, Cooked, Broiled									
1 lb (453.6g)	853	28	11	445	0	0.0	25	140	299
Beef, Rib, Whole (Ribs 6-12), Lean and Fat, 1/8" Fat, All Grades, Cooked, Broiled									
3 oz (85g)	286	23	9	70	0	0.0	--	19	54
Beef, Rib, Whole (Ribs 6-12), Lean and Fat, 1/8" Fat, All Grades, Cooked, Roasted									
3 oz (85g)	298	24	10	71	0	0.0	--	19	54
Beef, Rib, Whole (Ribs 6-12), Lean and Fat, 1/8" Fat, Choice, Cooked, Broiled									
3 oz (85g)	299	24	10	70	0	0.0	--	19	54
Beef, Rib, Whole (Ribs 6-12), Lean and Fat, 1/8" Fat, Choice, Cooked, Roasted									
3 oz (85g)	310	25	10	71	0	0.0	0	19	54
Beef, Rib, Whole (Ribs 6-12), Lean and Fat, 1/8" Fat, Prime, Cooked, Broiled									
3 oz (85g)	328	28	11	72	0	0.0	--	19	53
Beef, Rib, Whole (Ribs 6-12), Lean and Fat, 1/8" Fat, Prime, Cooked, Roasted									
3 oz (85g)	340	29	12	72	0	0.0	--	19	55
Beef, Rib, Whole (Ribs 6-12), Lean and Fat, 1/8" Fat, Select, Cooked, Broiled									
3 oz (85g)	268	21	8	69	0	0.0	--	19	54
Beef, Rib, Whole (Ribs 6-12), Lean and Fat, 1/8" Fat, Select, Cooked, Roasted									
3 oz (85g)	281	22	9	71	0	0.0	--	20	55

Food Serving size	Cal.	(g) Total Fat	(g) Sat. Fat	(mg) Chol.	(g) Carb.	(g) Fiber	(g) Sug.	(g) Prot.	(mg) Sod.
Beef, Round, Bottom Round Roast, Lean, 0" Fat, Select, Cooked, Roasted 1 roast (yield from 572 g raw meat) (464g)									
	784	25	9	353	0	0.0	0	131	176
Beef, Round, Bottom Round Roast, Lean, 1/8" Fat, Select, Cooked, Roasted 1 lb (453.6g)	744	21	7	336	0	0.0	19	129	172
Beef, Round, Bottom Round, Roast, Lean and Fat, 0" Fat, All Grades, Cooked, Roasted 1 roast (yield from 600 g raw meat) (489g)									
	914	38	14	386	0	0.0	0	134	176
Beef, Round, Bottom Round, Roast, Lean and Fat, 0" Fat, Choice, Cooked, Roasted 1 roast (yield from 627 g raw meat) (515g)									
	1025	48	17	417	0	0.0	0	138	180
Beef, Round, Bottom Round, Roast, Lean and Fat, 0" Fat, Select, Cooked, Roasted 1 roast (yield from 572 g raw meat) (464g)									
	812	28	10	357	0	0.0	0	130	172
Beef, Round, Bottom Round, Roast, Lean and Fat, 1/8" Fat, All Grades, Cooked, Roasted 1 piece, cooked, excluding refuse (yield from 1 lb raw meat with refuse) (338g)									
	737	39	15	287	0	0.0	0	89	118
Beef, Round, Bottom Round, Roast, Lean and Fat, 1/8" Fat, Choice, Cooked, Roasted 1 piece, cooked, excluding refuse (yield from 1 lb raw meat with refuse) (338g)									
	754	42	16	291	0	0.0	0	88	115
Beef, Round, Bottom Round, Roast, Lean and Fat, 1/8" Fat, Select, Cooked, Roasted 1 piece, cooked, excluding refuse (yield from 1 lb raw meat with refuse) (338g)									
	717	37	14	284	0	0.0	0	90	118
Beef, Round, Bottom Round, Roast, Lean, 0" Fat, All Grades, Cooked, Roasted 1 roast (yield from 600 g raw meat) (489g)									
	866	32	11	377	0	0.0	0	136	176
Beef, Round, Bottom Round, Roast, Lean, 1/8" Fat, All Grades, Cooked 1 oz (28.35g)	46	2	1	22	0	0.0	0	8	10
Beef, Round, Bottom Round, Roast, Lean, 1/8" Fat, Choice, Cooked, Roasted 1 lb (453.6g)	812	31	11	349	0	0.0	0	125	163

Food Serving size	Cal.	(g) Total Fat	(g) Sat. Fat	(mg) Chol.	(g) Carb.	(g) Fiber	(g) Sug.	(g) Prot.	(mg) Sod.
Beef, Round, Bottom Round, Steak, Lean and Fat, 0" Fat, All Grades, Cooked, Braised 3 oz (85g)	190	8	3	81	0	0.0	0	29	37
Beef, Round, Bottom Round, Steak, Lean and Fat, 0" Fat, Choice, Cooked, Braised 1 steak (yield from 299g raw meat) (191g)	439	19	7	183	0	0.0	0	63	80
Beef, Round, Bottom Round, Steak, Lean and Fat, 0" Fat, Select, Cooked, Braised 1 steak (yield from 281 g raw meat) (179g)	388	14	5	166	0	0.0	0	62	81
Beef, Round, Bottom Round, Steak, Lean and Fat, 1/8" Fat, All Grades, Cooked, Braised 3 oz (85g)	210	10	4	85	0	0.0	0	28	37
Beef, Round, Bottom Round, Steak, Lean and Fat, 1/8" Fat, Choice, Cooked, Braised 1 steak (yield from 341 g raw meat) (227g)	577	29	11	229	0	0.0	0	75	95
Beef, Round, Bottom Round, Steak, Lean and Fat, 1/8" Fat, Select, Cooked, Braised 3 oz (85g)	204	10	4	83	0	0.0	0	28	37
Beef, Round, Bottom Round, Steak, Lean, 0" Fat, All Grades, Cooked, Braised 3 oz (85g)	182	7	2	79	0	0.0	0	29	37
Beef, Round, Bottom Round, Steak, Lean, 0" Fat, Choice, Cooked, Braised 3 oz (85g)	190	8	3	81	0	0.0	0	28	37
Beef, Round, Bottom Round, Steak, Lean, 0" Fat, Select, Cooked, Braised 3 oz (85g)	175	5	2	77	0	0.0	0	30	39
Beef, Round, Bottom Round, Steak, Lean, 1/8" Fat, All Grades, Cooked, Braised 1 lb (453.6g)	980	35	12	426	0	0.0	0	156	204
Beef, Round, Bottom Round, Steak, Lean, 1/8" Fat, Choice, Cooked, Braised 1 lb (453.6g)	1034	41	14	440	0	0.0	0	155	204
Beef, Round, Bottom Round, Steak, Lean, 1/8" Fat, Select, Cooked, Braised 1 lb (453.6g)	930	29	10	417	0	0.0	0	156	209
Beef, Round, Eye of Round, Roast, Lean and Fat, 0" Fat, All Grades, Cooked, Roasted 1 roast (yield from 436 g raw meat) (346g)	581	17	6	263	0	0.0	0	101	131

Food Serving size	Cal.	(g) Total Fat	(g) Sat. Fat	(mg) Chol.	(g) Carb.	(g) Fiber	(g) Sug.	(g) Prot.	(mg) Sod.
Beef, Round, Eye of Round, Roast, Lean and Fat, 0" Fat, Choice, Cooked, Roasted 1 roast (yield from 445g raw meat) (355g)	589	17	6	266	0	0.0	0	101	131
Beef, Round, Eye of Round, Roast, Lean and Fat, 0" Fat, Select, Cooked, Roasted 1 roast (yield from 426g raw meat) (337g)	570	16	6	256	0	0.0	0	100	131
Beef, Round, Eye of Round, Roast, Lean and Fat, 1/8" Fat, All Grades, Cooked, Roasted 3 oz (85g)	177	8	3	71	0	0.0	0	24	31
Beef, Round, Eye of Round, Roast, Lean and Fat, 1/8" Fat, Choice, Cooked, Roasted 3 oz (85g)	180	9	3	73	0	0.0	0	24	31
Beef, Round, Eye of Round, Roast, Lean and Fat, 1/8" Fat, Select, Cooked, Roasted 1 roast (yield from 530g raw meat) (417g)	851	39	15	346	0	0.0	0	117	154
Beef, Round, Eye of Round, Roast, Lean, 0" Fat, All Grades, Cooked, Roasted 1 roast (yield from 436g raw meat) (346g)	561	14	5	256	0	0.0	0	101	131
Beef, Round, Eye of Round, Roast, Lean, 0" Fat, Choice, Cooked, Roasted 1 roast (yield from 445g raw meat) (355g)	575	15	5	263	0	0.0	0	102	135
Beef, Round, Eye of Round, Roast, Lean, 0" Fat, Select, Cooked, Roasted 1 roast (yield from 42g raw meat) (337g)	549	13	5	249	0	0.0	0	101	131
Beef, Round, Eye of Round, Roast, Lean, 1/8" Fat, All Grades, Cooked, Roasted 1 lb (453.6g)	767	21	7	345	0	0.0	0	135	172
Beef, Round, Eye of Round, Roast, Lean, 1/8" Fat, Choice, Cooked, Roasted 1 lb (453.6g)	794	24	8	354	0	0.0	0	135	177
Beef, Round, Eye of Round, Roast, Lean, 1/8" Fat, Select, Cooked, Roasted 1 lb (453.6g)	739	19	6	340	0	0.0	15	134	177
Beef, Round, Full Cut, Lean and Fat, 1/8" Fat, Choice, Cooked, Broiled 3 oz (85g)	200	11	4	67	0	0.0	0	23	53
Beef, Round, Full Cut, Lean and Fat, 1/8" Fat, Select, Cooked, Broiled 3 oz (85g)	185	9	4	67	0	0.0	0	23	53

Food Serving size	Cal.	(g) Total Fat	(g) Sat. Fat	(mg) Chol.	(g) Carb.	(g) Fiber	(g) Sug.	(g) Prot.	(mg) Sod.
Beef, Round, Full Cut, Lean, 1/4" Fat, Choice, Cooked, Broiled 3 oz (85g)	162	6	2	66	0	0.0	0	25	54
Beef, Round, Full Cut, Lean, 1/4" Fat, Select, Cooked, Broiled 3 oz (85g)	146	4	2	66	0	0.0	--	25	54
Beef, Round, Knuckle, Tip Center, Steak, Lean and Fat, 0" Fat, All Grades, Cooked, Grilled 1 steak (150g)	266	10	4	116	0	0.0	6	41	78
Beef, Round, Knuckle, Tip Center, Steak, Lean and Fat, 0" Fat, Choice, Cooked, Grilled 1 steak (156g)	293	13	4	117	0	0.0	2	42	80
Beef, Round, Knuckle, Tip Center, Steak, Lean and Fat, 0" Fat, Select, Cooked, Grilled 1 steak (160g)	259	9	3	118	0	0.0	3	43	85
Beef, Round, Knuckle, Tip Side, Steak, Lean and Fat, 0" Fat, All Grades, Cooked, Grilled 1 serving (3 oz) (85g)	143	4	2	68	0	0.0	3	25	46
Beef, Round, Knuckle, Tip Side, Steak, Lean and Fat, 0" Fat, Choice, Cooked, Grilled 1 serving (3 oz) (85g)	148	5	2	70	0	0.0	3	24	47
Beef, Round, Knuckle, Tip Side, Steak, Lean and Fat, 0" Fat, Select, Cooked, Grilled 1 serving (3 oz) (85g)	136	3	1	66	0	0.0	4	25	44
Beef, Round, Out Round, Bottom Round, Steak, Lean and Fat, 0" Fat, All Grades, Cooked, Grilled 1 serving (3 oz) (85g)	155	6	2	65	0	0.0	--	23	49
Beef, Round, Out Round, Bottom Round, Steak, Lean and Fat, 0" Fat, Choice, Cooked, Grilled 1 serving (3 oz) (85g)	162	7	3	66	0	0.0	2	23	48
Beef, Round, Out Round, Bottom Round, Steak, Lean and Fat, 0" Fat, Select, Cooked, Grilled 1 serving (3 oz) (85g)	141	4	1	64	0	0.0	11	24	51
Beef, Round, Tip Round, Roast, Lean and Fat, 0" Fat, All Grades, Cooked, Roasted 3 oz (85g)	160	7	3	66	0	0.0	0	23	30
Beef, Round, Tip Round, Roast, Lean and Fat, 0" Fat, Choice, Cooked, Roasted 1 roast (yield from 1405 g raw meat) (1138g)	2230	101	37	910	0	0.0	0	307	398

Food Serving size	Cal.	(g) Total Fat	(g) Sat. Fat	(mg) Chol.	(g) Carb.	(g) Fiber	(g) Sug.	(g) Prot.	(mg) Sod.
Beef, Round, Tip Round, Roast, Lean and Fat, 0" Fat, Select, Cooked, Roasted									
1 roast (yield from 1388 g raw meat) (1141g)	2065	86	31	867	0	0.0	0	303	399
Beef, Round, Tip Round, Roast, Lean and Fat, 1/8" Fat, All Grades, Cooked, Roasted									
3 oz (85g)	186	10	4	70	0	0.0	0	23	54
Beef, Round, Tip Round, Roast, Lean and Fat, 1/8" Fat, Choice, Cooked, Roasted									
3 oz (85g)	194	10	4	70	0	0.0	0	23	54
Beef, Round, Tip Round, Roast, Lean and Fat, 1/8" Fat, Select, Cooked, Roasted									
3 oz (85g)	179	9	3	70	0	0.0	0	23	54
Beef, Round, Tip Round, Roast, Lean, 0" Fat, All Grades, Cooked, Roasted									
3 oz (85g)	148	5	2	63	0	0.0	0	23	31
Beef, Round, Tip Round, Roast, Lean, 0" Fat, Choice, Cooked, Roasted									
1 roast (yield from 1405 g raw meat) (1138g)	2003	73	26	865	0	0.0	0	315	410
Beef, Round, Tip Round, Roast, Lean, 0" Fat, Select, Cooked, Roasted									
1 roast (yield from 1388 g raw meat) (1141g)	1700	50	18	810	0	0.0	0	312	411
Beef, Round, Top Round, Lean and Fat, 0" Fat, All Grades, Cooked, Braised									
3 oz (85g)	178	5	2	77	0	0.0	0	30	38
Beef, Round, Top Round, Lean and Fat, 0" Fat, Choice, Cooked, Braised									
3 oz (85g)	184	6	2	77	0	0.0	0	30	38
Beef, Round, Top Round, Lean and Fat, 0" Fat, Select, Cooked, Braised									
3 oz (85g)	170	5	2	77	0	0.0	0	30	38
Beef, Round, Top Round, Lean and Fat, 1/8" Fat, All Grades, Cooked, Braised									
3 oz (85g)	202	9	3	77	0	0.0	0	29	38
Beef, Round, Top Round, Lean and Fat, 1/8" Fat, Choice, Cooked, Braised									
3 oz (85g)	213	10	4	77	0	0.0	0	29	38
Beef, Round, Top Round, Lean and Fat, 1/8" Fat, Choice, Cooked, Pan-fried									
3 oz (85g)	226	12	4	82	0	0.0	0	28	58
Beef, Round, Top Round, Lean and Fat, 1/8" Fat, Select, Cooked, Braised									
3 oz (85g)	191	7	3	77	0	0.0	0	29	38
Beef, Round, Top Round, Lean, 0" Fat, All Grades, Cooked, Braised									
3 oz (85g)	169	4	1	77	0	0.0	0	31	38
Beef, Round, Top Round, Lean, 0" Fat, Choice, Cooked, Braised									
3 oz (85g)	176	5	2	77	0	0.0	0	31	38

Food Serving size	Cal.	(g) Total Fat	(g) Sat. Fat	(mg) Chol.	(g) Carb.	(g) Fiber	(g) Sug.	(g) Prot.	(mg) Sod.
Beef, Round, Top Round, Lean, 0" Fat, Select, Cooked, Braised									
3 oz (85g)	162	3	1	77	0	0.0	0	31	38
Beef, Round, Top Round, Lean, 1/8" Fat, Choice, Cooked, Pan-fried									
3 oz (85g)	194	7	2	87	2	0.0	0	29	55
Beef, Round, Top Round, Steak, Lean and Fat, 0" Fat, All Grades, Cooked, Broiled									
1 steak (yield from 381g raw meat) (277g)	521	16	6	235	0	0.0	0	88	114
Beef, Round, Top Round, Steak, Lean and Fat, 0" Fat, Choice, Cooked, Broiled									
1 steak (yield from 396g raw meat) (284g)	568	20	7	253	0	0.0	0	90	119
Beef, Round, Top Round, Steak, Lean and Fat, 0" Fat, Select, Cooked, Broiled									
1 steak (yield from 368 g meat) (269g)	476	12	4	215	0	0.0	0	85	113
Beef, Round, Top Round, Steak, Lean and Fat, 1/8" Fat, All Grades, Cooked, Broiled									
3 oz (85g)	173	8	3	77	0	0.0	0	26	35
Beef, Round, Top Round, Steak, Lean and Fat, 1/8" Fat, Choice, Cooked, Broiled									
3 oz (85g)	190	9	3	78	0	0.0	0	26	34
Beef, Round, Top Round, Steak, Lean and Fat, 1/8" Fat, Prime, Cooked, Broiled									
3 oz (85g)	191	9	3	71	0	0.0	0	27	52
Beef, Round, Top Round, Steak, Lean and Fat, 1/8" Fat, Select, Cooked, Broiled									
3 oz (85g)	171	7	2	74	0	0.0	0	26	35
Beef, Round, Top Round, Steak, Lean, 0" Fat, All Grades, Cooked, Broiled									
1 steak (277g)	515	16	5	233	0	0.0	0	88	116
Beef, Round, Top Round, Steak, Lean, 0" Fat, Choice, Cooked, Broiled									
1 steak (284g)	559	19	7	250	0	0.0	0	90	122
Beef, Round, Top Round, Steak, Lean, 0" Fat, Select, Cooked, Broiled									
1 steak (269g)	473	12	4	215	0	0.0	0	85	113
Beef, Round, Top Round, Steak, Lean, 1/8" Fat, All Grades, Cooked, Broiled									
1 lb (453.6g)	839	25	9	381	0	0.0	0	144	191
Beef, Round, Top Round, Steak, Lean, 1/8" Fat, Choice, Cooked, Broiled									
1 lb (453.6g)	875	28	10	390	0	0.0	0	145	191
Beef, Round, Top Round, Steak, Lean, 1/8" Fat, Select, Cooked, Broiled									
1 lb (453.6g)	803	21	7	372	0	0.0	0	143	195
Beef, Shank Crosscuts, Lean, 1/4" Fat, Choice, Cooked, Simmered									
3 oz (85g)	171	5	2	66	0	0.0	--	29	54

Food Serving size	Cal.	(g) Total Fat	(g) Sat. Fat	(mg) Chol.	(g) Carb.	(g) Fiber	(g) Sug.	(g) Prot.	(mg) Sod.
Beef, Short Loin, Porterhouse Steak, Lean and Fat, 0" Fat, All Grades, Cooked, Broiled									
1 lb (453.6g)	1252	87	33	304	0	0.0	0	109	295
Beef, Short Loin, Porterhouse Steak, Lean and Fat, 0" Fat, USDA Select, Cooked, Broiled									
1 lb (453.6g)	1211	82	32	290	0	0.0	0	111	295
Beef, Short Loin, Porterhouse Steak, Lean and Fat, 1/8" Fat, All Grades, Cooked, Broiled									
3 oz (85g)	252	19	7	60	0	0.0	3	20	54
Beef, Short Loin, Porterhouse Steak, Lean and Fat, 1/8" Fat, Choice, Cooked, Broiled									
3 oz (85g)	254	19	7	63	0	0.0	0	20	54
Beef, Short Loin, Porterhouse Steak, Lean and Fat, 1/8" Fat, Select, Cooked, Broiled									
3 oz (85g)	250	18	7	55	0	0.0	3	20	54
Beef, Short Loin, Porterhouse Steak, Lean, 0" Fat, All Grades, Cooked, Broiled									
1 lb (453.6g)	962	51	18	281	0	0.0	0	118	313
Beef, Short Loin, Porterhouse Steak, Lean, 0" Fat, Choice, Cooked, Broiled									
1 serving (85g)	190	11	4	77	0	0.0	0	22	59
Beef, Short Loin, Porterhouse Steak, Lean, 0" Fat, Select, Cooked, Broiled									
1 serving (85g)	165	7	3	71	0	0.0	0	23	59
Beef, Short Loin, T-bone Steak, Lean and Fat, 0" Fat, All Grades, Cooked, Broiled									
1 lb (453.6g)	1120	72	28	272	0	0.0	0	110	304
Beef, Short Loin, T-bone Steak, Lean and Fat, 0" Fat, USDA Select, Cooked, Broiled									
1 lb (453.6g)	1043	64	25	268	0	0.0	0	111	308
Beef, Short Loin, T-bone Steak, Lean and Fat, 1/8" Fat, All Grades, Cooked, Broiled									
3 oz (85g)	238	17	6	53	0	0.0	6	21	56
Beef, Short Loin, T-bone Steak, Lean and Fat, 1/8" Fat, Choice, Cooked, Broiled									
3 oz (85g)	243	17	7	55	0	0.0	0	20	56
Beef, Short Loin, T-bone Steak, Lean and Fat, 1/8" Fat, Select, Cooked, Broiled									
3 oz (85g)	225	15	6	48	0	0.0	3	21	56
Beef, Short Loin, T-bone Steak, Lean, 0" Fat, All Grades, Cooked, Broiled									
1 lb (453.6g)	857	39	14	249	0	0.0	0	118	322

Food Serving size	Cal.	(g) Total Fat	(g) Sat. Fat	(mg) Chol.	(g) Carb.	(g) Fiber	(g) Sug.	(g) Prot.	(mg) Sod.
Beef, Short Loin, T-bone Steak, Lean, 0" Fat, Choice, Cooked, Broiled 1 serving (85g)	168	8	3	71	0	0.0	0	22	60
Beef, Short Loin, T-bone Steak, Lean, 0" Fat, Select, Cooked, Broiled 1 serving (85g)	150	6	2	68	0	0.0	0	22	60
Beef, Short Loin, T-bone Steak, Lean, 1/4" Fat, All Grades, Cooked, Broiled 1 lb (453.6g)	916	44	16	259	0	0.0	0	123	340
Beef, Short Loin, Top Loin, Lean and Fat, 1/8" Fat, Prime, Cooked, Broiled 1 steak, excluding refuse (yield from 1 raw steak, with refuse, weighing 242g)	518	37	15	132	0	0.0	0	43	107
Beef, Short Loin, Top Loin, Steak, Lean and Fat, 0" Fat, All Grades, Cooked, Broiled 1 steak, excluding refuse (yield from 1 raw steak, with refuse, weighing 223g)	299	12	5	126	0	0.0	0	45	91
Beef, Short Loin, Top Loin, Steak, Lean and Fat, 0" Fat, Choice, Cooked, Broiled 3 oz (85g)	174	8	3	71	0	0.0	0	24	48
Beef, Short Loin, Top Loin, Steak, Lean and Fat, 0" Fat, Select, Cooked, Broiled 1 steak (yield from 186 g raw meat) (150g)	270	9	4	119	0	0.0	0	44	92
Beef, Short Loin, Top Loin, Steak, Lean and Fat, 1/8" Fat, All Grades, Cooked, Broiled 1 steak, excluding refuse (yield from 1 raw steak, with refuse, weighing 242g)	436	28	11	158	0	0.0	0	44	89
Beef, Short Loin, Top Loin, Steak, Lean and Fat, 1/8" Fat, Choice, Cooked, Broiled 3 oz (1 serving) (85g)	236	16	6	85	0	0.0	0	22	44
Beef, Short Loin, Top Loin, Steak, Lean and Fat, 1/8" Fat, Select, Cooked, Broiled 3 oz (85g)	213	13	5	79	0	0.0	0	23	48
Beef, Short Loin, Top Loin, Steak, Lean, 0" Fat, All Grades, Cooked, Broiled 3 oz (85g)	155	5	2	67	0	0.0	0	25	51
Beef, Short Loin, Top Loin, Steak, Lean, 0" Fat, Choice, Cooked, Broiled 3 oz (85g)	163	6	2	69	0	0.0	0	25	50
Beef, Short Loin, Top Loin, Steak, Lean, 0" Fat, Select, Cooked, Broiled 3 oz (85g)	146	4	2	65	0	0.0	0	25	53
Beef, Short Loin, Top Loin, Steak, Lean, 1/8" Fat, All Grades, Cooked, Broiled 1 lb (453.6g)	857	32	12	367	0	0.0	0	133	277

Food Serving size	Cal.	(g) Total Fat	(g) Sat. Fat	(mg) Chol.	(g) Carb.	(g) Fiber	(g) Sug.	(g) Prot.	(mg) Sod.
Beef, Short Loin, Top Loin, Steak, Lean, 1/8" Fat, Choice, Cooked, Broiled									
1 lb (453.6g)	912	38	15	381	0	0.0	0	132	272
Beef, Short Loin, Top Loin, Steak, Lean, 1/8" Fat, Select, Cooked, Broiled									
1 lb (453.6g)	803	26	10	354	0	0.0	40	134	281
Beef, Shoulder Pot Roast, Boneless, Lean and Fat, 0" Fat, All Grades, Cooked, Braised									
1 roast (787g)	1605	70	24	763	0	0.0	0	244	480
Beef, Shoulder Pot Roast, Boneless, Lean and Fat, 0" Fat, Choice, Cooked, Braised									
1 roast (793g)	1642	73	26	769	0	0.0	0	245	476
Beef, Shoulder Pot Roast, Boneless, Lean and Fat, 0" Fat, Select, Cooked, Braised									
1 roast (779g)	1558	66	22	763	0	0.0	0	243	483
Beef, Shoulder Pot Roast, Boneless, Lean, 0" Fat, All Grades, Cooked, Braised									
1 roast (787g)	1543	61	20	771	0	0.0	167	248	480
Beef, Shoulder Pot Roast, Boneless, Lean, 0" Fat, Choice, Cooked, Braised									
1 roast (793g)	1586	66	22	769	0	0.0	24	248	476
Beef, Shoulder Pot Roast, Boneless, Lean, 0" Fat, Select, Cooked, Braised									
1 roast (779g)	1480	55	17	771	0	0.0	190	247	491
Beef, Shoulder Steak, Boneless, Lean and Fat, 0" Fat, All Grades, Cooked, Grilled									
1 steak (287g)	522	20	8	232	0	0.0	4	81	192
Beef, Shoulder Steak, Boneless, Lean and Fat, 0" Fat, Choice, Cooked, Grilled									
1 steak (280g)	521	20	9	227	0	0.0	12	79	188
Beef, Shoulder Steak, Boneless, Lean and Fat, 0" Fat, Select, Cooked, Grilled									
1 steak (297g)	526	18	8	244	0	0.0	--	84	199
Beef, Shoulder Steak, Boneless, Lean Only, 0" Fat, Choice, Cooked, Grilled									
3 oz (1 serving) (85g)	151	5	2	67	0	0.0	0	24	58
Beef, Shoulder Steak, Boneless, Lean, 0" Fat, All Grades, Cooked, Grilled									
3 oz (1 serving) (85g)	149	5	2	69	0	0.0	6	24	58
Beef, Shoulder Steak, Boneless, Lean, 0" Fat, Select, Cooked, Grilled									
3 oz (1 serving) (85g)	144	4	2	70	0	0.0	0	24	58
Beef, Shoulder Top Blade Steak, Boneless, Lean and Fat, 0" Fat, All Grades, Cooked, Grilled									
1 steak (186g)	391	21	8	177	0	0.0	0	51	158

Food Serving size	Cal.	(g) Total Fat	(g) Sat. Fat	(mg) Chol.	(g) Carb.	(g) Fiber	(g) Sug.	(g) Prot.	(mg) Sod.
Beef, Shoulder Top Blade Steak, Boneless, Lean and Fat, 0" Fat, Choice, Cooked, Grilled 1 steak (177g)	389	22	9	165	0	0.0	0	49	149
Beef, Shoulder Top Blade Steak, Boneless, Lean and Fat, 0" Fat, Select, Cooked, Grilled 1 steak (199g)	386	18	8	195	0	0.0	0	55	175
Beef, Shoulder Top Blade Steak, Boneless, Lean, 0" Fat, All Grades, Cooked, Grilled 1 steak (186g)	365	17	7	177	0	0.0	0	52	162
Beef, Shoulder Top Blade Steak, Boneless, Lean, 0" Fat, Choice, Cooked, Grilled 1 steak (177g)	358	17	7	165	0	0.0	0	50	150
Beef, Shoulder Top Blade Steak, Boneless, Lean, 0" Fat, Select, Cooked, Grilled 1 steak (199g)	372	17	7	195	0	0.0	0	56	177
Beef, Sirloin, Tri-tip Steak, Lean and Fat, 0" Fat, All Grades, Cooked, Broiled 1 lb (453.6g)	1202	69	26	308	0	0.0	--	136	327
Beef, Tenderloin, Lean and Fat, 0" Fat, Select, Cooked, Broiled 1 steak (yield from 136 g raw meat) (108g)	221	11	4	90	0	0.0	0	29	63
Beef, Tenderloin, Lean and Fat, 1/8" Fat, All Grades, Cooked, Roasted 3 oz (85g)	275	21	8	72	0	0.0	0	20	48
Beef, Tenderloin, Lean and Fat, 1/8" Fat, Choice, Cooked, Roasted 3 oz (85g)	281	22	9	72	0	0.0	0	20	55
Beef, Tenderloin, Lean and Fat, 1/8" Fat, Prime, Cooked, Roasted 3 oz (85g)	292	23	9	75	0	0.0	0	20	47
Beef, Tenderloin, Lean and Fat, 1/8" Fat, Select, Cooked, Roasted 3 oz (85g)	269	20	8	72	0	0.0	0	20	48
Beef, Tenderloin, Steak, Lean and Fat, 1/8" Fat, Select, Cooked, Broiled 3 oz (85g)	223	14	6	82	0	0.0	0	23	48
Beef, Tenderloin, Steak, Lean and Fat, 0" Fat, All Grades, Cooked, Broiled 1 steak, excluding refuse (yield from 1 raw steak, with refuse, weighing 135g)	203	10	4	80	0	0.0	0	26	52
Beef, Tenderloin, Steak, Lean and Fat, 0" Fat, Choice, Cooked, Broiled 1 steak (yield from 161 g raw meat) (126g)	291	16	6	113	0	0.0	0	35	69

Food Serving size	Cal.	(g) Total Fat	(g) Sat. Fat	(mg) Chol.	(g) Carb.	(g) Fiber	(g) Sug.	(g) Prot.	(mg) Sod.
Beef, Tenderloin, Steak, Lean and Fat, 1/8" Fat, All Grades, Cooked, Broiled									
1 steak, excluding refuse (yield from 1 raw steak, with refuse, weighing 154g)	278	18	7	101	0	0.0	0	28	56
Beef, Tenderloin, Steak, Lean and Fat, 1/8" Fat, Choice, Cooked, Broiled									
3 oz (85g)	232	15	6	84	0	0.0	0	22	44
Beef, Tenderloin, Steak, Lean and Fat, 1/8" Fat, Prime, Cooked, Broiled									
1 steak, excluding refuse (yield from 1 raw steak, with refuse, weighing 154g)	326	24	9	91	0	0.0	0	27	63
Beef, Tenderloin, Steak, Lean, 0" Fat, All Grades, Coked, Broiled									
3 oz (85g)	164	7	3	69	0	0.0	0	24	50
Beef, Tenderloin, Steak, Lean, 0" Fat, Select, Cooked, Broiled									
3 oz (85g)	152	6	2	65	0	0.0	0	24	50
Beef, Tenderloin, Steak, Lean, 1/8" Fat, All Grades, Cooked, Broiled									
1 lb (453.6g)	907	38	14	372	0	0.0	0	132	272
Beef, Tenderloin, Steak, Lean, 1/8" Fat, Choice, Cooked, Broiled									
1 lb (453.6g)	934	41	16	386	0	0.0	0	132	268
Beef, Tenderloin, Steak, Lean, 1/8" Fat, Select, Cooked, Broiled									
1 lb (453.6g)	880	35	13	376	0	0.0	35	132	281
Beef, Tenderloin, Steak, Lean, 0" Fat, Choice, Cooked, Broiled									
3 oz (85g)	175	8	3	72	0	0.0	0	25	50
Beef, Top Sirloin, Steak, Lean and Fat, 0" Fat, All Grades, Cooked, Broiled									
3 oz (85g)	180	8	3	75	0	0.0	0	25	52
Beef, Top Sirloin, Steak, Lean and Fat, 0" Fat, Choice, Cooked, Broiled									
1 steak (yield from 532 g raw meat) (393g)	861	41	16	350	0	0.0	0	114	228
Beef, Top Sirloin, Steak, Lean and Fat, 0" Fat, Select, Cooked, Broiled									
1 steak (yield from 505 g raw meat) (375g)	773	33	13	326	0	0.0	0	111	236
Beef, Top Sirloin, Steak, Lean and Fat, 1/8" Fat, All Grades, Cooked, Broiled									
3 oz (85g)	207	12	5	78	0	0.0	0	23	48
Beef, Top Sirloin, Steak, Lean and Fat, 1/8" Fat, Choice, Cooked, Broiled									
3 oz (85g)	218	13	5	82	0	0.0	0	23	46
Beef, Top Sirloin, Steak, Lean and Fat, 1/8" Fat, Choice, Cooked, Pan-fried									
3 oz (85g)	266	18	7	83	0	0.0	0	24	60

Food Serving size	Cal.	(g) Total Fat	(g) Sat. Fat	(mg) Chol.	(g) Carb.	(g) Fiber	(g) Sug.	(g) Prot.	(mg) Sod.
Beef, Top Sirloin, Steak, Lean and Fat, 1/8" Fat, Select, Cooked, Broiled									
3 oz (85g)	196	11	4	76	0	0.0	0	23	48
Beef, Top Sirloin, Steak, Lean, 0" Fat, All Grades, Cooked, Broiled									
3 oz (85g)	156	5	2	70	0	0.0	0	26	54
Beef, Top Sirloin, Steak, Lean, 0" Fat, Choice, Cooked, Broiled									
3 oz (85g)	160	6	2	71	0	0.0	0	26	54
Beef, Top Sirloin, Steak, Lean, 0" Fat, Select, Cooked, Broiled									
3 oz (85g)	150	4	2	69	0	0.0	0	26	56
Beef, Top Sirloin, Steak, Lean, 1/8" Fat, All Grades, Cooked, Broiled									
1 lb (453.6g)	807	26	10	358	0	0.0	0	133	277
Beef, Top Sirloin, Steak, Lean, 1/8" Fat, Choice, Cooked, Broiled									
1 lb (453.6g)	848	30	12	367	0	0.0	0	134	277
Beef, Top Sirloin, Steak, Lean, 1/8" Fat, Select, Cooked, Broiled									
1 lb (453.6g)	771	22	9	349	0	0.0	--	133	281
Beef, Variety Meats and By-products, Brain, Cooked, Pan-fried									
3 oz (85g)	167	13	3	1696	0	0.0	--	11	134
Beef, Variety Meats and By-products, Brain, Cooked, Simmered									
3 oz (85g)	128	9	2	2635	1	0.0	0	10	92
Beef, Variety Meats and By-products, Heart, Cooked, Simmered									
3 oz (85g)	140	4	1	180	0	0.0	0	24	50
Beef, Variety Meats and By-products, Kidneys, Cooked, Simmered									
3 oz (85g)	134	4	1	609	0	0.0	0	23	80
Beef, Variety Meats and By-products, Liver, Cooked, Braised									
1 slice (68g)	130	4	1	269	3	0.0	0	20	54
Beef, Variety Meats and By-products, Liver, Cooked, Pan-fried									
1 slice (82g)	144	4	1	312	4	0.0	0	22	63
Beef, Variety Meats and By-products, Lungs, Cooked, Braised									
3 oz (85g)	102	3	1	235	0	0.0	--	17	86
Beef, Variety Meats and By-products, Pancreas, Cooked, Braised									
3 oz (85g)	230	15	5	223	0	0.0	--	23	51
Beef, Variety Meats and By-products, Spleen, Cooked, Braised									
3 oz (85g)	123	4	1	295	0	0.0	--	21	48
Beef, Variety Meats and By-products, Thymus, Cooked, Braised									
3 oz (85g)	271	21	7	250	0	0.0	--	19	99

Food Serving size	Cal.	(g) Total Fat	(g) Sat. Fat	(mg) Chol.	(g) Carb.	(g) Fiber	(g) Sug.	(g) Prot.	(mg) Sod.
Beef, Variety Meats and By-products, Tongue, Cooked, Simmered									
3 oz (85g)	241	19	7	112	0	0.0	0	16	55
Bison, Ground, Grass-fed, Cooked									
3 oz (85g)	152	7	3	60	0	0.0	0	22	65
Carl Buddig, Cooked Corned Beef, Chopped, Pressed									
1 serving, 2 oz (57g)	81	4	2	37	1	0.0	--	11	765
Carl Buddig, Cooked, Smoked, Beef Pastrami, Chopped, Pressed									
1 pkg (71g)	100	5	2	46	1	0.0	--	14	750
Carl Buddig, Smoked Sliced Beef									
1 pkg (71g)	99	5	2	48	0	0.0	--	14	1016
Carl Buddig, Smoked Sliced Chicken, Light and Dark Meat									
1 pkg (71g)	117	7	2	38	0	0.0	--	13	677
Carl Buddig, Smoked Sliced Ham									
1 pkg (71g)	116	7	2	39	1	0.0	--	13	981
Carl Buddig, Smoked Sliced Turkey, Light and Dark Meat									
1 pkg (71g)	114	6	2	40	1	0.0	--	12	778
Game Meat, Antelope, Cooked, Roasted									
3 oz (85g)	128	2	1	107	0	0.0	--	25	46
Game Meat, Bear, Cooked, Simmered									
3 oz (85g)	220	11	3	83	0	0.0	0	28	60
Game Meat, Beaver, Cooked, Roasted									
3 oz (85g)	180	6	2	99	0	0.0	0	30	50
Game Meat, Beefalo, Composite of Cuts, Cooked, Roasted									
3 oz (85g)	160	5	2	49	0	0.0	--	26	70
Game Meat, Bison, Chuck, Shoulder Clod, Lean, 3-5 lb. Roasted, Cooked, Braised									
1 serving (3 oz) (85g)	164	5	2	94	0	0.0	0	29	48
Game Meat, Bison, Ground, Cooked, Pan-broiled									
1 serving (3 oz) (85g)	202	13	--	71	0	0.0	0	20	62
Game Meat, Bison, Lean, Cooked, Roasted									
3 oz (85g)	122	2	1	70	0	0.0	0	24	48
Game Meat, Bison, Rib Eye, Lean, 1" Steak, Cooked, Broiled									
1 serving (3 oz) (85g)	150	5	2	67	0	0.0	0	25	44
Game Meat, Bison, Top Round, Lean, 1" Steak, Cooked, Broiled									
1 serving (3 oz) (85g)	148	4	2	72	0	0.0	0	26	35

Food Serving size	Cal.	(g) Total Fat	(g) Sat. Fat	(mg) Chol.	(g) Carb.	(g) Fiber	(g) Sug.	(g) Prot.	(mg) Sod.
Game Meat, Bison, Top Sirloin, Lean, 1" Steak, Cooked, Broiled									
1 serving (3 oz) (85g)	145	5	2	73	0	0.0	0	24	45
Game Meat, Boar, Wild, Cooked, Roasted									
3 oz (85g)	136	4	1	65	0	0.0	0	24	51
Game Meat, Buffalo, Water, Cooked, Roasted									
3 oz (85g)	111	2	1	52	0	0.0	--	23	48
Game Meat, Caribou, Cooked, Roasted									
3 oz (85g)	142	4	1	93	0	0.0	0	25	51
Game Meat, Deer, Cooked, Roasted									
3 oz (85g)	134	3	1	95	0	0.0	--	26	46
Game Meat, Deer, Ground, Cooked, Pan-broiled									
1 serving (3 oz) (85g)	159	7	3	83	0	0.0	0	22	66
Game Meat, Deer, Loin, Lean, 1" Steak, Cooked, Broiled									
1 serving (3 oz) (85g)	128	2	1	67	0	0.0	0	26	48
Game Meat, Deer, Shoulder Clod, Lean, 3-5 lb. Roasted, Cooked, Braised									
1 serving (3 oz) (85g)	162	3	2	96	0	0.0	0	31	44
Game Meat, Deer, Tenderloin, Lean, 0.5-1 lb. Roasted, Cooked, Broiled									
1 serving (3 oz) (85g)	127	2	1	75	0	0.0	0	25	48
Game Meat, Deer, Top Round, Lean, 1" Steak, Cooked, Broiled									
1 serving (3 oz) (85g)	129	2	1	72	0	0.0	0	27	38
Game Meat, Elk, Cooked, Roasted									
3 oz (85g)	124	2	1	62	0	0.0	--	26	52
Game Meat, Elk, Ground, Cooked, Pan-broiled									
1 serving (3 oz) (85g)	164	7	3	66	0	0.0	0	23	72
Game Meat, Elk, Loin, Lean, Cooked, Broiled									
1 serving (3 oz) (85g)	142	3	1	64	0	0.0	0	26	46
Game Meat, Elk, Round, Lean, Cooked, Broiled									
1 serving (3 oz) (85g)	133	2	1	66	0	0.0	0	26	43
Game Meat, Elk, Tenderloin, Lean, Cooked, Broiled									
1 serving (3 oz) (85g)	138	3	1	61	0	0.0	0	26	43
Game Meat, Goat, Cooked, Roasted									
3 oz (85g)	122	3	1	64	0	0.0	0	23	73
Game Meat, Moose, Cooked, Roasted									
3 oz (85g)	114	1	0	66	0	0.0	0	25	59

Food Serving size	Cal.	(g) Total Fat	(g) Sat. Fat	(mg) Chol.	(g) Carb.	(g) Fiber	(g) Sug.	(g) Prot.	(mg) Sod.
Game Meat, Muskrat, Cooked, Roasted									
3 oz (85g)	199	10	--	103	0	0.0	--	26	81
Game Meat, Rabbit, Domesticated, Composite of Cuts, Cooked, Roasted									
3 oz (85g)	167	7	2	70	0	0.0	--	25	40
Game Meat, Rabbit, Domesticated, Composite of Cuts, Cooked, Stewed									
3 oz (85g)	175	7	2	73	0	0.0	0	26	31
Game Meat, Rabbit, Wild, Cooked, Stewed									
3 oz (85g)	147	3	1	105	0	0.0	0	28	38
Game Meat, Raccoon, Cooked, Roasted									
3 oz (85g)	217	12	3	82	0	0.0	0	25	67
Game Meat, Squirrel, Cooked, Roasted									
3 oz (85g)	147	4	1	103	0	0.0	0	26	101
Goose, Domesticated, Meat and Skin, Cooked, Roasted									
1 unit (yield from 1 lb ready-to-cook goose) (188g)	573	41	13	171	0	0.0	0	47	132
Goose, Domesticated, Meat Only, Cooked, Roasted									
.5 goose (591g)	1407	75	27	567	0	0.0	--	171	449
Lamb, Australian, Imported, Fresh, Composite of Retail Cuts, Lean and Fat, 1/8" Fat, Cooked									
3 oz (85g)	218	14	7	74	0	--	--	21	65
Lamb, Australian, Imported, Fresh, Composite of Retail Cuts, Lean, 1/8" Fat, Cooked									
3 oz (85g)	171	8	3	74	0	--	--	23	68
Lamb, Australian, Imported, Fresh, Fat, Cooked									
3 oz (85g)	543	56	30	71	0	--	--	8	43
Lamb, Australian, Imported, Fresh, Foreshank, Lean and Fat, 1/8" Fat, Cooked, Braised									
3 oz (85g)	201	12	6	77	0	--	--	21	79
Lamb, Australian, Imported, Fresh, Foreshank, Lean, 1/8" Fat, Cooked, Braised									
3 oz (85g)	140	4	2	78	0	--	--	23	85
Lamb, Australian, Imported, Fresh, Leg, Center Slice, Bone-in, Lean and Fat, 1/8" Fat, Cooked, Broiled									
3 oz (85g)	183	10	5	72	0	--	--	22	55
Lamb, Australian, Imported, Fresh, Leg, Center Slice, Bone-in, Lean, 1/8" Fat, Cooked, Broiled									
3 oz (85g)	156	7	3	72	0	--	--	23	56

Food Serving size	Cal.	(g) Total Fat	(g) Sat. Fat	(mg) Chol.	(g) Carb.	(g) Fiber	(g) Sug.	(g) Prot.	(mg) Sod.
Lamb, Australian, Imported, Fresh, Leg, Shank Half, Lean and Fat, 1/8" Fat, Cooked, Roasted									
3 oz (85g)	196	12	5	71	0	--	--	21	57
Lamb, Australian, Imported, Fresh, Leg, Shank Half, Lean, 1/8" Fat, Cooked, Roasted									
3 oz (85g)	155	6	2	71	0	--	--	23	59
Lamb, Australian, Imported, Fresh, Leg, Sirloin Chops, Boneless, Lean and Fat, 1/8" Fat, Cooked, Broiled									
3 oz (85g)	200	12	5	72	0	--	--	22	54
Lamb, Australian, Imported, Fresh, Leg, Sirloin Chops, Boneless, Lean, 1/8" Fat, Cooked, Broiled									
3 oz (85g)	160	7	3	72	0	--	--	23	56
Lamb, Australian, Imported, Fresh, Leg, Sirloin Half, Boneless, Lean and Fat, 1/8" Fat, Cooked, Roasted									
3 oz (85g)	239	16	8	87	0	--	--	21	66
Lamb, Australian, Imported, Fresh, Leg, Sirloin Half, Boneless, Lean, 1/8" Fat, Cooked, Roasted									
3 oz (85g)	183	9	4	89	0	--	--	24	71
Lamb, Australian, Imported, Fresh, Leg, Whole (Shank and Sirloin), Lean and Fat, 1/8" Fat, Cooked, Roasted									
3 oz (85g)	207	13	6	75	0	--	--	21	60
Lamb, Australian, Imported, Fresh, Leg, Whole (Shank and Sirloin), Lean, 1/8" Fat, Cooked, Roasted									
3 oz (85g)	162	7	3	76	0	--	--	23	61
Lamb, Australian, Imported, Fresh, Loin, Lean and Fat, 1/8" Fat, Cooked, Broiled									
3 oz (85g)	186	10	5	70	0	--	--	22	66
Lamb, Australian, Imported, Fresh, Loin, Lean, 1/8" Fat, Cooked, Broiled									
3 oz (85g)	163	7	3	69	0	--	--	23	68
Lamb, Australian, Imported, Fresh, Rib, Lean and Fat, 1/8" Fat, Cooked, Roasted									
3 oz (85g)	235	17	8	68	0	--	--	19	65
Lamb, Australian, Imported, Fresh, Rib, Lean, 1/8" Fat, Cooked, Roasted									
3 oz (85g)	179	10	4	68	0	--	--	21	70
Lamb, Australian, Imported, Fresh, Shoulder, Arm, Lean and Fat, 1/8" Fat, Cooked, Braised									
3 oz (85g)	264	17	8	90	0	--	--	25	62

Food Serving size	Cal.	(g) Total Fat	(g) Sat. Fat	(mg) Chol.	(g) Carb.	(g) Fiber	(g) Sug.	(g) Prot.	(mg) Sod.
Lamb, Australian, Imported, Fresh, Shoulder, Arm, Lean, 1/8" Fat, Cooked, Braised									
3 oz (85g)	202	9	4	94	0	--	--	29	66
Lamb, Australian, Imported, Fresh, Shoulder, Blade, Lean and Fat, 1/8" Fat, Cooked, Broiled									
3 oz (85g)	247	19	9	71	0	--	--	18	75
Lamb, Australian, Imported, Fresh, Shoulder, Blade, Lean, 1/8" Fat, Cooked, Broiled									
3 oz (85g)	196	12	5	72	0	--	--	20	80
Lamb, Australian, Imported, Fresh, Shoulder, Whole (Arm and Boiled), Lean and Fat, 1/8" Fat, Cooked									
3 oz (85g)	252	18	9	76	0	--	--	20	72
Lamb, Australian, Imported, Fresh, Shoulder, Whole (Arm and Boiled), Lean, 1/8" Fat, Cooked									
3 oz (85g)	198	11	5	77	0	--	--	22	77
Lamb, Domestic, Composite of Retail Cuts, Fat, 1/4" Fat, Choice, Cooked									
3 oz (85g)	498	50	23	97	0	0.0	0	10	49
Lamb, Domestic, Composite of Retail Cuts, Lean and Fat, 1/4" Fat, Choice, Cooked									
3 oz (85g)	250	18	8	82	0	0.0	0	21	61
Lamb, Domestic, Composite of Retail Cuts, Lean and Fat, 1/8" Fat, Choice, Cooked									
3 oz (85g)	230	15	6	82	0	0.0	--	22	61
Lamb, Domestic, Composite of Retail Cuts, Lean, 1/4" Fat, Choice, Cooked									
3 oz (85g)	175	8	3	78	0	0.0	--	24	65
Lamb, Domestic, Cubed for Stew (Leg and Shoulder), Lean, 1/4" Fat, Cooked, Braised									
3 oz (85g)	190	7	3	92	0	0.0	0	29	60
Lamb, Domestic, Cubed for Stew (Leg and Shoulder), Lean, 1/4" Fat, Cooked, Broiled									
3 oz (85g)	158	6	2	77	0	0.0	--	24	65
Lamb, Domestic, Foreshank, Lean and Fat, 1/4" Fat, Choice, Cooked, Braised									
3 oz (85g)	207	11	5	90	0	0.0	0	24	61
Lamb, Domestic, Foreshank, Lean and Fat, 1/8" Fat, Cooked, Braised									
3 oz (85g)	207	11	5	90	0	0.0	--	24	61

Food Serving size	Cal.	(g) Total Fat	(g) Sat. Fat	(mg) Chol.	(g) Carb.	(g) Fiber	(g) Sug.	(g) Prot.	(mg) Sod.
Lamb, Domestic, Foreshank, Lean, 1/4" Fat, Choice, Cooked, Braised									
3 oz (85g)	159	5	2	88	0	0.0	--	26	63
Lamb, Domestic, Leg, Shank Half, Lean and Fat, 1/4" Fat, Choice, Cooked, Roasted									
3 oz (85g)	191	11	4	77	0	0.0	--	22	55
Lamb, Domestic, Leg, Shank Half, Lean and Fat, 1/8" Fat, Choice, Cooked, Roasted									
3 oz (85g)	184	10	4	77	0	0.0	--	23	55
Lamb, Domestic, Leg, Shank Half, Lean, 1/4" Fat, Choice, Cooked, Roasted									
3 oz (85g)	153	6	2	74	0	0.0	--	24	56
Lamb, Domestic, Leg, Sirloin Half, Lean and Fat, 1/4" Fat, Choice, Cooked, Roasted									
3 oz (85g)	248	18	7	82	0	0.0	--	21	58
Lamb, Domestic, Leg, Sirloin Half, Lean and Fat, 1/8" Fat, Choice, Cooked, Roasted									
3 oz (85g)	241	17	7	82	0	0.0	--	21	58
Lamb, Domestic, Leg, Sirloin Half, Lean, 1/4" Fat, Choice, Cooked, Roasted									
3 oz (85g)	173	8	3	78	0	0.0	--	24	60
Lamb, Domestic, Leg, Whole (Shank and Sirloin), Lean and Fat, 1/4" Fat, Choice, Cooked, Roasted									
3 oz (85g)	219	14	6	79	0	0.0	0	22	56
Lamb, Domestic, Leg, Whole (Shank and Sirloin), Lean and Fat, 1/8" Fat, Choice, Cooked, Roasted									
3 oz (85g)	206	12	5	78	0	0.0	--	22	57
Lamb, Domestic, Leg, Whole (Shank and Sirloin), Lean, 1/4" Fat, Choice, Cooked, Roasted									
3 oz (85g)	162	7	2	76	0	0.0	0	24	58
Lamb, Domestic, Loin, Lean and Fat, 1/4" Fat, Choice, Cooked, Broiled									
1 chop, excluding refuse (yield from 1 raw chop, with refuse, weighing 120g)									
	202	15	6	64	0	0.0	0	16	49
Lamb, Domestic, Loin, Lean and Fat, 1/4" Fat, Choice, Cooked, Roasted									
3 oz (85g)	263	20	9	81	0	0.0	0	19	54
Lamb, Domestic, Loin, Lean and Fat, 1/8" Fat, Choice, Cooked, Broiled									
1 steak, excluding refuse (yield from 1 raw steak, with refuse, weighing 102g)									
	157	11	5	52	0	0.0	--	14	41
Lamb, Domestic, Loin, Lean and Fat, 1/8" Fat, Choice, Cooked, Roasted									
3 oz (85g)	247	18	8	79	0	0.0	--	20	54

Food Serving size	Cal.	(g) Total Fat	(g) Sat. Fat	(mg) Chol.	(g) Carb.	(g) Fiber	(g) Sug.	(g) Prot.	(mg) Sod.
Lamb, Domestic, Loin, Lean, 1/4" Fat, Choice, Cooked, Broiled									
1 chop, excluding refuse (yield from 1 raw chop, with refuse, weighing 120g)									
	99	4	2	44	0	0.0	0	14	39
Lamb, Domestic, Loin, Lean, 1/4" Fat, Choice, Cooked, Roasted									
3 oz (85g)	172	8	3	74	0	0.0	--	23	56
Lamb, Domestic, Rib, Lean and Fat, 1/4" Fat, Choice, Cooked, Broiled									
3 oz (85g)	307	25	11	84	0	0.0	0	19	65
Lamb, Domestic, Rib, Lean and Fat, 1/4" Fat, Choice, Cooked, Roasted									
3 oz (85g)	305	25	11	82	0	0.0	--	18	62
Lamb, Domestic, Rib, Lean and Fat, 1/8" Fat, Choice, Cooked, Broiled									
3 oz (85g)	289	23	10	83	0	0.0	--	20	65
Lamb, Domestic, Rib, Lean and Fat, 1/8" Fat, Choice, Cooked, Roasted									
3 oz (85g)	290	23	10	82	0	0.0	--	19	63
Lamb, Domestic, Rib, Lean, 1/4" Fat, Choice, Cooked, Broiled									
3 oz (85g)	200	11	4	77	0	0.0	0	24	72
Lamb, Domestic, Rib, Lean, 1/4" Fat, Choice, Cooked, Roasted									
3 oz (85g)	197	11	4	75	0	0.0	--	22	69
Lamb, Domestic, Shoulder, Arm, Lean and Fat, 1/4" Fat, Choice, Cooked, Braised									
1 chop, excluding refuse (yield from 1 raw chop, with refuse, weighing 160g)									
	242	17	7	84	0	0.0	--	21	50
Lamb, Domestic, Shoulder, Arm, Lean and Fat, 1/4" Fat, Choice, Cooked, Broiled									
1 chop, excluding refuse (yield from 1 raw chop, with refuse, weighing 160g)									
	261	18	8	89	0	0.0	--	23	72
Lamb, Domestic, Shoulder, Arm, Lean and Fat, 1/4" Fat, Choice, Cooked, Roasted									
3 oz (85g)	237	17	7	78	0	0.0	--	19	55
Lamb, Domestic, Shoulder, Arm, Lean and Fat, 1/8" Fat, Choice, Cooked, Braised									
1 steak, excluding refuse (yield from 1 raw steak, with refuse, weighing 102g)									
	152	10	4	54	0	0.0	--	14	32
Lamb, Domestic, Shoulder, Arm, Lean and Fat, 1/8" Fat, Choice, Roasted									
3 oz (85g)	227	16	7	77	0	0.0	--	19	55
Lamb, Domestic, Shoulder, Arm, Lean and Fat, 1/8" Fat, Cooked, Broiled									
1 steak, excluding refuse (yield from 1 raw steak, with refuse, weighing 102g)									
	159	11	5	57	0	0.0	--	15	46

Food Serving size	Cal.	(g) Total Fat	(g) Sat. Fat	(mg) Chol.	(g) Carb.	(g) Fiber	(g) Sug.	(g) Prot.	(mg) Sod.
Lamb, Domestic, Shoulder, Arm, Lean, 1/4" Fat, Choice, Cooked, Braised 1 chop, excluding refuse (yield from 1 raw chop, with refuse, weighing 160g)									
	153	8	3	67	0	0.0	--	20	42
Lamb, Domestic, Shoulder, Arm, Lean, 1/4" Fat, Choice, Cooked, Broiled 1 chop, excluding refuse (yield from 1 raw chop, with refuse, weighing 160g)									
	148	7	3	68	0	0.0	--	21	61
Lamb, Domestic, Shoulder, Arm, Lean, 1/4" Fat, Choice, Cooked, Roasted 3 oz (85g)									
	163	8	3	73	0	0.0	--	22	57
Lamb, Domestic, Shoulder, Blade, Lean and Fat, 1/4" Fat, Choice, Cooked, Braised 3 oz (85g)									
	293	21	9	99	0	0.0	--	24	64
Lamb, Domestic, Shoulder, Blade, Lean and Fat, 1/4" Fat, Choice, Cooked, Broiled 3 oz (85g)									
	236	17	7	81	0	0.0	0	20	70
Lamb, Domestic, Shoulder, Blade, Lean and Fat, 1/4" Fat, Choice, Cooked, Roasted 3 oz (85g)									
	239	18	7	78	0	0.0	--	19	56
Lamb, Domestic, Shoulder, Blade, Lean and Fat, 1/8" Fat, Choice, Cooked, Braised 3 oz (85g)									
	288	20	8	99	0	0.0	--	25	64
Lamb, Domestic, Shoulder, Blade, Lean and Fat, 1/8" Fat, Choice, Cooked, Broiled 3 oz (85g)									
	227	16	6	81	0	0.0	--	20	71
Lamb, Domestic, Shoulder, Blade, Lean, 1/4" Fat, Choice, Cooked, Braised 3 oz (85g)									
	245	14	5	99	0	0.0	--	27	67
Lamb, Domestic, Shoulder, Blade, Lean, 1/4" Fat, Choice, Cooked, Broiled 3 oz (85g)									
	179	10	3	77	0	0.0	--	22	75
Lamb, Domestic, Shoulder, Blade, Lean, 1/4" Fat, Choice, Cooked, Roasted 3 oz (85g)									
	178	10	4	74	0	0.0	--	21	58
Lamb, Domestic, Shoulder, Whole (Arm and Boiled), Lean and Fat, 1/4" Fat, Choice, Cooked, Braised 3 oz (85g)									
	292	21	9	99	0	0.0	--	24	64
Lamb, Domestic, Shoulder, Whole (Arm and Boiled), Lean and Fat, 1/4" Fat, Choice, Cooked, Broiled 3 oz (85g)									
	236	16	7	82	0	0.0	--	21	66

Food Serving size	Cal.	(g) Total Fat	(g) Sat. Fat	(mg) Chol.	(g) Carb.	(g) Fiber	(g) Sug.	(g) Prot.	(mg) Sod.
Lamb, Domestic, Shoulder, Whole (Arm and Boiled), Lean and Fat, 1/4" Fat, Choice, Cooked, Roasted									
3 oz (85g)	235	17	7	78	0	0.0	0	19	56
Lamb, Domestic, Shoulder, Whole (Arm and Boiled), Lean and Fat, 1/8" Fat, Choice, Cooked, Braised									
3 oz (85g)	287	20	8	99	0	0.0	--	25	63
Lamb, Domestic, Shoulder, Whole (Arm and Boiled), Lean and Fat, 1/8" Fat, Choice, Cooked, Broiled									
3 oz (85g)	228	16	6	81	0	0.0	--	20	70
Lamb, Domestic, Shoulder, Whole (Arm and Boiled), Lean and Fat, 1/8" Fat, Choice, Cooked, Roasted									
3 oz (85g)	229	16	7	77	0	0.0	--	19	56
Lamb, Domestic, Shoulder, Whole (Arm and Boiled), Lean, 1/4" Fat, Choice, Cooked, Braised									
3 oz (85g)	241	14	5	99	0	0.0	--	28	67
Lamb, Domestic, Shoulder, Whole (Arm and Boiled), Lean, 1/4" Fat, Choice, Cooked, Broiled									
3 oz (85g)	179	9	3	79	0	0.0	0	23	71
Lamb, Domestic, Shoulder, Whole (Arm and Boiled), Lean, 1/4" Fat, Choice, Cooked, Roasted									
3 oz (85g)	173	9	3	74	0	0.0	0	21	58
Lamb, Ground, Cooked, Broiled									
3 oz (85g)	241	17	7	82	0	0.0	0	21	69
Lamb, New Zealand, Imported, Frozen, Composite of Retail Cuts, Fat, Cooked									
3 oz (85g)	498	51	27	93	0	0.0	--	8	30
Lamb, New Zealand, Imported, Frozen, Composite of Retail Cuts, Lean and Fat, 1/8" Fat, Cooked									
3 oz (85g)	230	15	7	90	0	0.0	--	21	39
Lamb, New Zealand, Imported, Frozen, Composite of Retail Cuts, Lean and Fat, Cooked									
3 oz (85g)	259	19	9	93	0	0.0	--	21	39
Lamb, New Zealand, Imported, Frozen, Composite of Retail Cuts, Lean, Cooked									
3 oz (85g)	175	8	3	93	0	0.0	--	25	43
Lamb, New Zealand, Imported, Frozen, Foreshank, Lean and Fat, 1/8" Fat, Cooked, Braised									
3 oz (85g)	219	13	7	87	0	0.0	--	23	40

Food Serving size	Cal.	(g) Total Fat	(g) Sat. Fat	(mg) Chol.	(g) Carb.	(g) Fiber	(g) Sug.	(g) Prot.	(mg) Sod.
Lamb, New Zealand, Imported, Frozen, Foreshank, Lean and Fat, Cooked, Braised									
3 oz (85g)	219	13	7	87	0	0.0	--	23	40
Lamb, New Zealand, Imported, Frozen, Foreshank, Lean, Cooked, Braised									
3 oz (85g)	158	5	2	86	0	0.0	--	26	42
Lamb, New Zealand, Imported, Frozen, Leg, Whole (Shank and Sirloin), Lean and Fat, 1/8" Fat, Cooked, Roasted									
3 oz (85g)	199	12	6	86	0	0.0	--	22	37
Lamb, New Zealand, Imported, Frozen, Leg, Whole (Shank and Sirloin), Lean and Fat, Cooked, Roasted									
3 oz (85g)	209	13	6	86	0	0.0	--	21	37
Lamb, New Zealand, Imported, Frozen, Leg, Whole (Shank and Sirloin), Lean, Looked, Roasted									
3 oz (85g)	154	6	3	85	0	0.0	--	24	38
Lamb, New Zealand, Imported, Frozen, Loin, Lean and Fat, 1/8" Fat, Cooked, Broiled									
1 chop, excluding refuse (yield from 1 raw chop, with refuse, weighing 85g) (42g)	124	9	4	47	0	0.0	--	10	21
Lamb, New Zealand, Imported, Frozen, Loin, Lean and Fat, Cooked, Broiled									
1 chop, excluding refuse (yield from 1 raw chop, with refuse, weighing 85g) (43g)	135	10	5	48	0	0.0	0	10	21
Lamb, New Zealand, Imported, Frozen, Loin, Lean, Cooked, Broiled									
1 chop, excluding refuse (yield from 1 raw chop, with refuse, weighing 85g) (30g)	60	2	1	34	0	0.0	--	9	17
Lamb, New Zealand, Imported, Frozen, Rib, Lean and Fat, 1/8" Fat, Cooked, Roasted									
3 oz (85g)	269	22	11	84	0	0.0	--	17	37
Lamb, New Zealand, Imported, Frozen, Rib, Lean and Fat, Cooked, Roasted									
3 oz (85g)	289	24	12	85	0	0.0	0	16	37
Lamb, New Zealand, Imported, Frozen, Rib, Lean, Cooked, Roasted									
3 oz (85g)	167	9	4	80	0	0.0	0	21	41
Lamb, New Zealand, Imported, Frozen, Shoulder, Whole (Arm and Boiled), Lean and Fat, 1/8" Fat, Cooked, Braised									
3 oz (85g)	291	20	10	105	0	0.0	--	25	44
Lamb, New Zealand, Imported, Frozen, Shoulder, Whole (Arm and Boiled), Lean and Fat, Cooked, Braised									
3 oz (85g)	303	22	11	105	0	0.0	--	24	43

Food Serving size	Cal.	(g) Total Fat	(g) Sat. Fat	(mg) Chol.	(g) Carb.	(g) Fiber	(g) Sug.	(g) Prot.	(mg) Sod.
Lamb, New Zealand, Imported, Frozen, Shoulder, Whole (Arm and Boiled), Lean, Cooked, Braised									
3 oz (85g)	242	13	6	108	0	0.0	--	29	48
Lamb, Variety Meats and By-products, Brain, Cooked, Braised									
3 oz (85g)	123	9	2	1737	0	0.0	--	11	114
Lamb, Variety Meats and By-products, Brain, Cooked, Pan-fried									
3 oz (85g)	232	19	5	2128	0	0.0	--	14	133
Lamb, Variety Meats and By-products, Heart, Cooked, Braised									
3 oz (85g)	157	7	3	212	2	0.0	--	21	54
Lamb, Variety Meats and By-products, Kidneys, Cooked, Braised									
3 oz (85g)	116	3	1	480	1	0.0	--	20	128
Lamb, Variety Meats and By-products, Liver, Cooked, Braised									
3 oz (85g)	187	7	3	426	2	0.0	--	26	48
Lamb, Variety Meats and By-products, Liver, Cooked, Pan-fried									
3 oz (85g)	202	11	4	419	3	0.0	--	22	105
Lamb, Variety Meats and By-products, Lungs, Cooked, Braised									
3 oz (85g)	96	3	1	241	0	0.0	--	17	71
Lamb, Variety Meats and By-products, Pancreas, Cooked, Braised									
3 oz (85g)	199	13	6	340	0	0.0	--	19	44
Lamb, Variety Meats and By-products, Spleen, Cooked, Braised									
3 oz (85g)	133	4	1	327	0	0.0	--	22	49
Lamb, Variety Meats and By-products, Tongue, Cooked, Braised									
3 oz (85g)	234	17	7	161	0	0.0	--	18	57
Lamb,Domestic, Shoulder, Blade, Lean and Fat, 1/8" Fat, Choice, Cooked, Roasted									
3 oz (85g)	230	16	7	78	0	0.0	--	19	57
Lambs, Quarters, Cooked, Boiled, Drained, with Salt									
1 cup, chopped (180g)	58	1	0	0	9	3.8	1	6	477
Loma Linda Redi-burger, Canned, Unprepared									
1 slice 5/8" (85g)	124	2	0	0	7	3.7	1	19	432
Loma Linda Swiss Steak with Gravy, Canned, Unprepared									
1 piece (92g)	127	6	1	1	10	2.9	1	9	433
Loma Linda Tender Bits, Canned, Unprepared									
6 pieces (85g)	115	4	1	0	7	3.7	1	13	521

Food Serving size	Cal.	(g) Total Fat	(g) Sat. Fat	(mg) Chol.	(g) Carb.	(g) Fiber	(g) Sug.	(g) Prot.	(mg) Sod.
Loma Linda Tender Rounds with Gravy, Canned, Unprepared 6 pieces (80g)	116	4	1	1	6	2.8	1	13	354
Pastrami, Beef, 98% Fat Free 1 serving, 6 slices (57g)	54	1	0	27	1	0.0	0	11	576
Pork Skins, Barbecue Flavor .5 oz (14.2g)	76	5	2	16	0	--	--	8	379
Pork Skins, Plain .5 oz (14.2g)	77	4	2	13	0	0.0	0	9	258
Pork, Cured, Bacon, Cooked, Baked 1 slice, cooked (8.1g)	44	4	1	9	0	0.0	0	3	178
Pork, Cured, Bacon, Cooked, Broiled, Pan-fried or Roasted 1 slice, cooked (8g)	43	3	1	9	0	0.0	0	3	185
Pork, Cured, Bacon, Cooked, Broiled, Pan-fried or Roasted, Reduced Sodium 1 slice, cooked (8g)	43	3	1	9	0	0.0	--	3	82
Pork, Cured, Bacon, Cooked, Microwaved 1 slice, cooked (5g)	25	2	1	6	0	0.0	0	2	104
Pork, Cured, Bacon, Cooked, Pan-fried 1 slice, cooked (7.9g)	42	3	1	9	0	0.0	0	3	192
Pork, Cured, Breakfast Strips, Cooked 3 slices, cooked (raw product packed 15 per 12-oz bag) (34g)	156	12	4	36	0	0.0	0	10	714
Pork, Cured, Canadian-style Bacon, Grilled 2 slices (6 per 6-oz pkg.) (47g)	87	4	1	27	1	0.0	0	11	727
Pork, Cured, Canadian-style Bacon, Unheated 2 slices (6 per 6-oz pkg.) (57g)	89	4	1	29	1	0.0	0	12	803
Pork, Cured, Fat (from Ham and Arm Picnic), Roasted 3 oz (85g)	502	53	19	73	0	0.0	--	6	530
Pork, Cured, Fat (from Ham and Arm Picnic), Unheated 3 oz (85g)	492	52	19	58	0	0.0	0	5	429
Pork, Cured, Feet, Pickled 1 lb (453.6g)	635	45	13	376	0	0.0	0	53	2540
Pork, Cured, Ham – Water Added, Rump, Bone-in, Lean and Fat, Heated, Roasted 1 serving (3 oz) (85g)	137	7	2	54	1	0.0	1	17	936
Pork, Cured, Ham – Water Added, Rump, Bone-in, Lean and Fat, Unheated 1 lb (453.6g)	780	57	19	245	4	0.0	3	63	4849

Food Serving size	Cal.	(g) Total Fat	(g) Sat. Fat	(mg) Chol.	(g) Carb.	(g) Fiber	(g) Sug.	(g) Prot.	(mg) Sod.
Pork, Cured, Ham – Water Added, Rump, Bone-in, Lean, Heated, Roasted									
1 serving (3 oz) (85g)	103	3	1	53	1	0.0	1	18	978
Pork, Cured, Ham – Water Added, Rump, Bone-in, Lean, Unheated									
1 lb, rump (453.6g)	431	16	6	240	3	0.0	3	70	5307
Pork, Cured, Ham – Water Added, Shank, Bone-in, Lean and Fat, Heated, Roasted									
1 serving (3 oz) (85g)	170	11	4	56	1	0.0	1	16	840
Pork, Cured, Ham – Water Added, Shank, Bone-in, Lean and Fat, Unheated									
1 lb (453.6g)	758	50	16	236	1	0.0	3	76	4373
Pork, Cured, Ham – Water Added, Shank, Bone-in, Lean, Heated, Roasted									
1 serving (3 oz) (85g)	109	4	1	55	1	0.0	1	18	901
Pork, Cured, Ham – Water Added, Shank, Bone-in, Lean, Unheated									
1 oz, shank (28.35g)	26	1	0	14	0	0.0	0	5	295
Pork, Cured, Ham – Water Added, Slice, Bone-in, Lean and Fat, Heated, Pan-broiled									
1 serving (3 oz) (85g)	141	7	2	56	1	0.0	1	18	1113
Pork, Cured, Ham – Water Added, Slice, Bone-in, Lean and Fat, Unheated									
1 lb (453.6g)	735	49	16	249	3	0.0	5	71	4586
Pork, Cured, Ham – Water Added, Slice, Bone-in, Lean, Heated, Pan-broiled									
1 serving (3 oz) (85g)	111	4	1	55	1	0.0	1	19	1168
Pork, Cured, Ham – Water Added, Slice, Bone-in, Lean, Unheated									
1 lb (453.6g)	413	10	3	245	1	0.0	6	79	4944
Pork, Cured, Ham – Water Added, Slice, Boneless, Lean and Fat, Heated, Pan-broiled									
1 serving (3 oz) (85g)	106	4	1	46	1	0.0	1	16	1030
Pork, Cured, Ham – Water Added, Slice, Boneless, Lean, Heated, Pan-broiled									
1 serving (3 oz) (85g)	99	3	1	46	1	0.0	1	16	1040
Pork, Cured, Ham – Water Added, Whole, Boneless, Lean and Fat, Heated, Roasted									
1 serving (3 oz) (85g)	107	5	2	46	1	0.0	1	15	1004
Pork, Cured, Ham – Water Added, Whole, Boneless, Lean and Fat, Unheated									
1 lb, whole (453.6g)	549	24	9	227	5	0.0	6	77	5108
Pork, Cured, Ham – Water Added, Whole, Boneless, Lean, Heated, Roasted									
1 roast, whole (1867g)	2184	82	27	990	26	0.0	29	336	22273
Pork, Cured, Ham – Water Added, Whole, Boneless, Lean, Unheated									
1 lb (453.6g)	499	18	6	227	5	0.0	7	79	5176

Food Serving size	Cal.	(g) Total Fat	(g) Sat. Fat	(mg) Chol.	(g) Carb.	(g) Fiber	(g) Sug.	(g) Prot.	(mg) Sod.
Pork, Cured, Ham and Water Product, Rump, Bone-in, Lean and Fat, Heated, Roasted									
1 serving (3 oz) (85g)	158	10	3	57	1	0.0	1	17	1004
Pork, Cured, Ham and Water Product, Rump, Bone-in, Lean and Fat, Unheated									
1 lb, rump (453.6g)	812	55	18	263	6	0.0	4	73	4491
Pork, Cured, Ham and Water Product, Rump, Bone-in, Lean, Heated, Roasted									
1 serving (3 oz) (85g)	111	4	1	56	1	0.0	1	18	1077
Pork, Cured, Ham and Water Product, Rump, Bone-in, Lean, Unheated									
1 lb (453.6g)	485	15	5	263	6	0.0	4	81	4854
Pork, Cured, Ham and Water Product, Shank, Bone-in, Lean and Fat, Heated, Roasted									
1 serving (3 oz) (85g)	199	15	5	61	1	0.0	1	15	803
Pork, Cured, Ham and Water Product, Shank, Bone-in, Lean and Fat, Unheated									
1 lb, shank (453.6g)	1102	91	30	249	6	0.0	4	65	4246
Pork, Cured, Ham and Water Product, Shank, Bone-in, Lean, Heated, Roasted									
1 serving (3 oz) (85g)	112	4	1	61	1	0.0	1	18	888
Pork, Cured, Ham and Water Product, Shank, Bone-in, Unheated, Lean									
1 oz, shank (28.35g)	32	1	0	15	0	0.0	0	5	309
Pork, Cured, Ham and Water Product, Slice, Bone-in, Lean and Fat, Heated, Pan-broiled									
1 serving (3 oz) (85g)	132	7	2	54	1	0.0	1	17	1010
Pork, Cured, Ham and Water Product, Slice, Bone-in, Lean and Fat, Unheated									
1 lb (453.6g)	676	42	14	227	12	0.0	4	62	4985
Pork, Cured, Ham and Water Product, Slice, Bone-in, Lean, Heated, Pan-broiled									
1 serving (3 oz) (85g)	104	3	1	54	1	0.0	1	18	1051
Pork, Cured, Ham and Water Product, Slice, Bone-in, Lean, Unheated									
1 lb (453.6g)	467	17	6	222	13	0.0	4	66	5262
Pork, Cured, Ham and Water Product, Slice, Boneless, Lean and Fat, Heated, Pan-broiled									
1 serving (3 oz) (85g)	105	4	1	38	4	0.0	4	13	1181
Pork, Cured, Ham and Water Product, Slice, Boneless, Lean, Heated, Pan-broiled									
1 serving (3 oz) (85g)	105	4	1	38	4	0.0	4	13	1182
Pork, Cured, Ham and Water Product, Whole, Boneless, Lean and Fat, Heated, Roasted									
1 serving (3 oz) (85g)	105	5	2	37	4	0.0	4	12	1135

Food Serving size	Cal.	(g) Total Fat	(g) Sat. Fat	(mg) Chol.	(g) Carb.	(g) Fiber	(g) Sug.	(g) Prot.	(mg) Sod.
Pork, Cured, Ham and Water Product, Whole, Boneless, Lean and Fat, Unheated									
1 lb, whole (453.6g)	531	23	7	195	18	0.0	19	64	5933
Pork, Cured, Ham and Water Product, Whole, Boneless, Lean, Heated, Roasted									
1 serving (3 oz) (85g)	105	5	2	37	4	0.0	4	12	1135
Pork, Cured, Ham and Water Product, Whole, Boneless, Lean, Unheated									
1 oz (28.35g)	33	1	0	12	1	0.0	1	4	371
Pork, Cured, Ham with Natural Juices, Rump, Bone-in, Lean and Fat, Heated, Roasted									
1 serving (3 oz) (85g)	150	8	3	61	1	0.0	0	19	715
Pork, Cured, Ham with Natural Juices, Rump, Bone-in, Lean and Fat, Unheated									
1 lb, rump (453.6g)	907	60	20	304	2	0.0	2	89	3801
Pork, Cured, Ham with Natural Juices, Rump, Bone-in, Lean, Heated, Roasted									
1 serving (3 oz) (85g)	116	4	1	61	0	0.0	0	21	732
Pork, Cured, Ham with Natural Juices, Rump, Bone-in, Lean, Unheated									
1 oz, rump (28.35g)	35	1	0	19	0	0.0	0	6	253
Pork, Cured, Ham with Natural Juices, Shank, Bone-in, Lean and Fat, Heated, Roasted									
1 serving (3 oz) (85g)	162	9	3	63	0	0.0	0	19	681
Pork, Cured, Ham with Natural Juices, Shank, Bone-in, Lean and Fat, Unheated									
1 lb, shank (453.6g)	866	50	16	281	1	0.0	1	101	3534
Pork, Cured, Ham with Natural Juices, Shank, Bone-in, Lean, Heated, Roasted									
1 serving (3 oz) (85g)	123	4	1	63	0	0.0	0	21	697
Pork, Cured, Ham with Natural Juices, Shank, Bone-in, Lean, Unheated									
1 oz, shank (28.35g)	37	1	0	18	0	0.0	0	7	229
Pork, Cured, Ham with Natural Juices, Slice, Bone-in, Lean and Fat, Heated, Pan-broiled									
1 serving (3 oz) (85g)	153	7	2	68	0	0.0	0	22	698
Pork, Cured, Ham with Natural Juices, Slice, Bone-in, Lean and Fat, Unheated									
2 slice (468g)	744	35	10	295	1	0.0	0	107	3927
Pork, Cured, Ham with Natural Juices, Slice, Bone-in, Lean, Heated, Pan-broiled									
1 serving (3 oz) (85g)	128	4	1	68	0	0.0	0	24	710
Pork, Cured, Ham with Natural Juices, Slice, Bone-in, Lean, Unheated									
2 slices (468g)	576	13	3	295	0	0.0	0	114	4029

Food Serving size	Cal.	(g) Total Fat	(g) Sat. Fat	(mg) Chol.	(g) Carb.	(g) Fiber	(g) Sug.	(g) Prot.	(mg) Sod.
Pork, Cured, Ham with Natural Juices, Slice, Boneless, Lean and Fat, Heated, Pan-broiled									
1 serving (3 oz) (85g)	100	3	1	49	1	0.0	1	18	986
Pork, Cured, Ham with Natural Juices, Slice, Boneless, Lean, Heated, Pan-broiled									
1 serving (3 oz) (85g)	99	3	1	48	1	0.0	1	18	989
Pork, Cured, Ham with Natural Juices, Spiral Sliced, Boneless, Lean and Fat, Heated, Roasted									
1 roast (920g)	1251	47	4	589	4	0.0	10	204	8988
Pork, Cured, Ham with Natural Juices, Spiral Sliced, Boneless, Lean and Fat, Unheated									
1 lb, spiral slice (453.6g)	585	26	8	259	3	0.0	5	85	3996
Pork, Cured, Ham with Natural Juices, Spiral Sliced, Boneless, Lean, Unheated									
1 lb, spiral slice (453.6g)	494	15	5	259	3	0.0	6	87	4060
Pork, Cured, Ham with Natural Juices, Spiral Sliced, Meat Only, Boneless, Lean, Heated, Roasted									
1 roast (920g)	1159	35	5	580	4	0.0	10	208	9071
Pork, Cured, Ham with Natural Juices, Whole, Boneless, Lean and Fat, Heated, Roasted									
1 serving (3 oz) (85g)	97	3	1	48	1	0.0	1	17	1002
Pork, Cured, Ham with Natural Juices, Whole, Boneless, Lean and Fat, Unheated									
1 lb, whole (453.6g)	508	16	5	240	4	0.0	5	88	4971
Pork, Cured, Ham with Natural Juices, Whole, Boneless, Lean, Heated, Roasted									
1 serving (3 oz) (85g)	96	3	1	48	1	0.0	1	17	1003
Pork, Cured, Ham with Natural Juices, Whole, Boneless, Lean, Unheated									
1 lb (453.6g)	499	15	4	240	4	0.0	5	88	4981
Pork, Cured, Ham, Boneless, Extra Lean (Approximately 5% Fat), Roasted									
3 oz (85g)	123	5	2	45	1	0.0	0	18	1023
Pork, Cured, Ham, Boneless, Extra Lean and Regular, Roasted									
3 oz (85g)	140	7	2	48	0	0.0	0	19	1177
Pork, Cured, Ham, Boneless, Extra Lean and Regular, Unheated									
1 slice (6-1/4" x 4" x 1/16") (1 oz) (28g)	45	2	1	15	1	0.0	0	5	358
Pork, Cured, Ham, Boneless, Low Sodium, Extra Lean and Regular, Roasted									
1 oz, boneless (28.35g)	47	2	1	16	0	0.0	--	6	275
Pork, Cured, Ham, Boneless, Regular (Approximately 11% Fat), Roasted									
3 oz (85g)	151	8	3	50	0	0.0	0	19	1275

Food Serving size	Cal.	(g) Total Fat	(g) Sat. Fat	(mg) Chol.	(g) Carb.	(g) Fiber	(g) Sug.	(g) Prot.	(mg) Sod.
Pork, Cured, Ham, Center Slice, Lean and Fat, Unheated									
4 oz (113g)	229	15	5	61	0	0.0	--	23	1566
Pork, Cured, Ham, Extra Lean (Approximately 4% Fat), Canned, Roasted									
3 oz (85g)	116	4	1	26	0	0.0	--	18	965
Pork, Cured, Ham, Extra Lean (Approximately 4% Fat), Canned, Unheated									
1 oz (28.35g)	34	1	0	11	0	0.0	0	5	356
Pork, Cured, Ham, Extra Lean and Regular, Canned, Roasted									
3 oz (85g)	142	7	2	35	0	0.0	0	18	908
Pork, Cured, Ham, Extra Lean and Regular, Canned, Unheated									
1 oz (28.35g)	41	2	1	11	0	0.0	0	5	362
Pork, Cured, Ham, Low Sodium, Lean and Fat, Cooked									
1 oz, boneless (28.35g)	49	2	1	16	0	0.0	0	6	275
Pork, Cured, Ham, Patties, Grilled									
1 unit, cooked (yield from 1 lb raw meat) (413g)	1412	127	46	297	7	0.0	0	55	4390
Pork, Cured, Ham, Patties, Unheated									
1 patty (65g)	205	18	7	46	1	0.0	--	8	707
Pork, Cured, Ham, Regular (Approximately 13% Fat), Canned, Roasted									
3 oz (85g)	192	13	4	53	0	0.0	--	17	800
Pork, Cured, Ham, Regular (Approximately 13% Fat), Canned, Unheated									
1 oz (28.35g)	54	4	1	11	0	0.0	0	5	352
Pork, Cured, Ham, Rump, Bone-in, Lean and Fat, Heated, Roasted									
1 serving (3 oz) (85g)	150	8	2	60	0	0.0	1	20	702
Pork, Cured, Ham, Rump, Bone-in, Lean and Fat, Unheated									
1 oz, rump (28.35g)	50	3	1	18	0	0.0	0	6	205
Pork, Cured, Ham, Rump, Bone-in, Lean, Heated, Roasted									
1 serving (3 oz) (85g)	112	3	1	60	0	0.0	1	22	719
Pork, Cured, Ham, Rump, Bone-in, Lean, Unheated									
1 lb (453.6g)	567	13	4	286	1	0.0	0	111	3343
Pork, Cured, Ham, Shank, Bone-in, Lean and Fat, Heated, Roasted									
1 serving (3 oz) (85g)	156	8	2	60	0	0.0	1	21	689
Pork, Cured, Ham, Shank, Bone-in, Lean and Fat, Unheated									
1 lb (453.6g)	803	45	14	277	2	0.0	0	98	3701
Pork, Cured, Ham, Shank, Bone-in, Lean, Heated, Roasted									
1 serving (3 oz) (85g)	118	3	1	60	0	0.0	1	23	704

Food Serving size	Cal.	(g) Total Fat	(g) Sat. Fat	(mg) Chol.	(g) Carb.	(g) Fiber	(g) Sug.	(g) Prot.	(mg) Sod.
Pork, Cured, Ham, Shank, Bone-in, Lean, Unheated 1 lb (453.6g)	567	14	4	277	1	0.0	0	108	3837
Pork, Cured, Ham, Slice, Bone-in, Lean and Fat, Heated, Pan-broiled 1 serving (3 oz) (85g)	153	7	1	62	0	0.0	1	22	724
Pork, Cured, Ham, Slice, Bone-in, Lean and Fat, Unheated 1 serving (3 oz) (85g)	147	8	3	55	0	0.0	0	19	632
Pork, Cured, Ham, Slice, Bone-in, Lean, Heated, Pan-broiled 1 serving (3 oz) (85g)	124	3	1	62	0	0.0	1	23	740
Pork, Cured, Ham, Slice, Bone-in, Lean, Unheated 1 serving (3 oz) (85g)	111	3	1	55	0	0.0	0	21	646
Pork, Cured, Ham, Steak, Boneless, Extra Lean, Unheated 1 slice (57g)	70	2	1	26	0	0.0	--	11	723
Pork, Cured, Ham, Whole, Lean and Fat, Roasted 3 oz (85g)	207	14	5	53	0	0.0	0	18	1009
Pork, Cured, Ham, Whole, Lean and Fat, Unheated 1 oz (28.35g)	70	5	2	16	0	0.0	0	5	364
Pork, Cured, Ham, Whole, Lean, Roasted 3 oz (85g)	133	5	2	47	0	0.0	0	21	1128
Pork, Cured, Ham, Whole, Lean, Unheated 1 oz (28.35g)	42	2	1	15	0	0.0	0	6	430
Pork, Cured, Shoulder, Arm Picnic, Lean and Fat, Roasted 3 oz (85g)	238	18	7	49	0	0.0	0	17	911
Pork, Cured, Shoulder, Arm Picnic, Lean, Roasted 3 oz (85g)	145	6	2	41	0	0.0	0	21	1046
Pork, Cured, Shoulder, Blade Roll, Lean and Fat, Roasted 3 oz (85g)	244	20	7	57	0	0.0	--	15	827
Pork, Cured, Shoulder, Blade Roll, Lean and Fat, Unheated 4 oz (113g)	304	25	9	60	0	0.0	--	19	1413
Pork, Fresh, Backribs, Lean and Fat, Cooked, Roasted 1 ribs (yield from 1 lb raw meat with refuse) (878g)	2511	189	68	738	0	0.0	0	202	825
Pork, Fresh, Composite (Leg, Loin, Shoulder and Spareribs), Lean and Fat, Cooked 3 oz (85g)	202	12	4	75	0	0.0	0	22	48

Food Serving size	Cal.	(g) Total Fat	(g) Sat. Fat	(mg) Chol.	(g) Carb.	(g) Fiber	(g) Sug.	(g) Prot.	(mg) Sod.
Pork, Fresh, Composite of Retail Cuts (Leg, Loin and Shoulder), Lean, Cooked									
3 oz (85g)	171	8	3	71	0	0.0	0	23	47
Pork, Fresh, Composite of Retail Cuts (Loin and Shoulder Blade), Lean and Fat, Cooked									
3 oz (85g)	200	12	4	71	0	0.0	0	22	47
Pork, Fresh, Composite of Retail Cuts (Loin and Shoulder Blade), Lean, Cooked									
3 oz (85g)	179	8	3	72	0	0.0	--	25	48
Pork, Fresh, Enhanced, Lean, Top Loin (Chops), Boneless, Lean and Fat, Cooked, Broiled									
1 chop (134g)	190	7	2	71	0	0.0	0	33	314
Pork, Fresh, Enhanced, Loin, Tenderloin, Lean and Fat, Cooked, Roasted									
1 roast (508g)	615	19	6	290	2	0.0	0	109	1168
Pork, Fresh, Enhanced, Loin, Tenderloin, Lean, Cooked, Roasted									
1 roast (508g)	589	16	5	290	2	0.0	0	110	1173
Pork, Fresh, Enhanced, Loin, Top Loin (Chops), Boneless, Lean, Cooked, Broiled									
1 chop (134g)	176	5	2	70	0	0.0	0	33	318
Pork, Fresh, Enhanced, Shoulder (Boston Butt), Blade (Steaks), Lean and Fat, Braised									
1 steak (264g)	694	45	17	256	0	0.0	0	68	399
Pork, Fresh, Enhanced, Shoulder (Boston Butt), Blade (Steaks), Lean, Cooked, Braised									
1 steak (264g)	599	32	12	259	0	0.0	0	73	407
Pork, Fresh, Fat, Cooked									
4 oz (113g)	686	70	28	95	0	0.0	0	12	62
Pork, Fresh, Ground, Cooked									
3 oz (85g)	252	18	7	80	0	0.0	0	22	62
Pork, Fresh, Leg (Ham), Rump Half, Lean and Fat, Cooked, Roasted									
3 oz (85g)	214	12	4	82	0	0.0	0	25	53
Pork, Fresh, Leg (Ham), Rump Half, Lean, Cooked, Roasted									
3 oz (85g)	175	7	2	82	0	0.0	--	26	55
Pork, Fresh, Leg (Ham), Shank Half, Lean and Fat, Cooked, Roasted									
3 oz (85g)	246	17	6	78	0	0.0	--	22	50
Pork, Fresh, Leg (Ham), Shank Half, Lean, Cooked, Roasted									
3 oz (85g)	183	9	3	78	0	0.0	--	24	54
Pork, Fresh, Leg (Ham), Whole, Lean and Fat, Cooked, Roasted									
3 oz (85g)	232	15	5	80	0	0.0	0	23	51

Food Serving size	Cal.	(g) Total Fat	(g) Sat. Fat	(mg) Chol.	(g) Carb.	(g) Fiber	(g) Sug.	(g) Prot.	(mg) Sod.
Pork, Fresh, Leg (Ham), Whole, Lean, Cooked, Roasted 3 oz (85g)	179	8	3	80	0	0.0	0	25	54
Pork, Fresh, Loin, Blade (Chops), Bone-in, Lean and Fat, Cooked, Braised 1 chop (206g)	525	32	9	177	0	0.0	0	55	142
Pork, Fresh, Loin, Blade (Chops), Bone-in, Lean and Fat, Cooked, Broiled 1 chop (219g)	506	31	10	171	0	0.0	0	52	162
Pork, Fresh, Loin, Blade (Chops), Bone-in, Lean and Fat, Cooked, Pan-fried 1 chop (215g)	550	36	10	176	0	0.0	0	54	183
Pork, Fresh, Loin, Blade (Chops), Bone-in, Lean, Cooked, Braised 1 chop (206g)	457	23	5	179	0	0.0	0	58	144
Pork, Fresh, Loin, Blade (Chops), Bone-in, Lean, Cooked, Broiled 1 chop (219g)	423	21	5	171	0	0.0	0	55	166
Pork, Fresh, Loin, Blade (Chops), Bone-in, Lean, Cooked, Pan-fried 1 chop (215g)	477	26	5	176	0	0.0	0	57	189
Pork, Fresh, Loin, Blade (Roasts), Bone-in, Lean and Fat, Cooked, Roasted 1 roast (830g)	2108	139	49	689	0	0.0	0	202	631
Pork, Fresh, Loin, Blade (Roasts), Bone-in, Lean, Cooked, Roasted 1 roast (830g)	1801	99	33	689	0	0.0	0	213	647
Pork, Fresh, Loin, Center Loin (Chops), Bone-in, Lean and Fat, Cooked, Braised 1 chop (187g)	453	25	9	151	0	0.0	0	53	137
Pork, Fresh, Loin, Center Loin (Chops), Bone-in, Lean and Fat, Cooked, Broiled 3 oz (85g)	178	9	3	71	0	0.0	0	22	47
Pork, Fresh, Loin, Center Loin (Chops), Bone-in, Lean, Cooked, Braised 1 chop (187g)	374	15	5	151	0	0.0	0	56	140
Pork, Fresh, Loin, Center Loin (Chops), Bone-in, Lean, Cooked, Broiled 3 oz (85g)	153	6	2	71	0	0.0	0	23	48
Pork, Fresh, Loin, Center Loin (Chops), Bone-in, Lean, Cooked, Pan-fried 1 chop (172g)	335	13	4	134	0	0.0	0	51	170
Pork, Fresh, Loin, Center Loin (Roasts), Bone-in, Lean and Fat, Cooked, Roasted 1 roast (900g)	2079	115	44	684	0	0.0	0	243	747
Pork, Fresh, Loin, Center Loin (Roasts), Bone-in, Lean, Cooked, Roasted 1 roast (900g)	1746	72	26	675	0	0.0	0	257	774
Pork, Fresh, Loin, Center Loin Chops, Bone-in, Lean and Fat, Cooked, Pan-fried 1 chop (172g)	409	23	8	136	0	0.0	0	48	162

Food Serving size	Cal.	(g) Total Fat	(g) Sat. Fat	(mg) Chol.	(g) Carb.	(g) Fiber	(g) Sug.	(g) Prot.	(mg) Sod.
Pork, Fresh, Loin, Center Rib (Chops), Bone-in, Lean and Fat, Cooked, Braised 1 chop (187g)	488	30	10	148	0	0.0	0	50	131
Pork, Fresh, Loin, Center Rib (Chops), Bone-in, Lean and Fat, Cooked, Broiled 3 oz (85g)	189	11	4	57	0	0.0	0	21	47
Pork, Fresh, Loin, Center Rib (Chops), Bone-in, Lean and Fat, Cooked, Pan-fried 1 chop (169g)	433	27	9	132	0	0.0	0	45	142
Pork, Fresh, Loin, Center Rib (Chops), Bone-in, Lean, Cooked, Braised 1 chop (187g)	389	17	5	148	0	0.0	0	54	135
Pork, Fresh, Loin, Center Rib (Chops), Bone-in, Lean, Cooked, Broiled 1 chop, excluding refuse (yield from 1 raw chop, with refuse, weighing 151g)	125	6	2	44	0	0.0	0	17	38
Pork, Fresh, Loin, Center Rib (Chops), Bone-in, Lean, Cooked, Pan-fried 1 chop (169g)	357	16	4	130	0	0.0	0	49	149
Pork, Fresh, Loin, Center Rib (Chops), Boneless, Lean and Fat, Cooked, Braised 1 chop, excluding refuse (yield from 1 raw chop, with refuse, weighing 113g)	207	13	5	59	0	0.0	--	21	32
Pork, Fresh, Loin, Center Rib (Chops), Boneless, Lean and Fat, Cooked, Broiled 1 chop, excluding refuse (yield from 1 raw chop, with refuse, weighing 113g)	208	13	5	66	0	0.0	--	22	50
Pork, Fresh, Loin, Center Rib (Chops), Boneless, Lean and Fat, Cooked, Pan-fried 1 chop, excluding refuse (yield from 1 raw chop, with refuse, weighing 113g)	205	14	5	55	0	0.0	0	19	38
Pork, Fresh, Loin, Center Rib (Chops), Boneless, Lean, Cooked, Braised 1 chop, excluding refuse (yield from 1 raw chop, with refuse, weighing 113g)	152	7	3	51	0	0.0	0	20	30
Pork, Fresh, Loin, Center Rib (Chops), Boneless, Lean, Cooked, Broiled 1 chop, excluding refuse (yield from 1 raw chop, with refuse, weighing 113g)	153	7	3	58	0	0.0	--	21	46
Pork, Fresh, Loin, Center Rib (Chops), Boneless, Lean, Cooked, Pan-fried 1 chop, excluding refuse (yield from 1 raw chop, with refuse, weighing 113g)	148	8	3	46	0	0.0	0	18	34
Pork, Fresh, Loin, Center Rib (Roasts), Bone-in, Lean and Fat, Cooked, Roasted 1 roast (783g)	1942	115	43	611	0	0.0	0	211	713
Pork, Fresh, Loin, Center Rib (Roasts), Bone-in, Lean, Cooked, Roasted 1 roast (783g)	1613	72	25	611	0	0.0	0	226	744

Food Serving size	Cal.	(g) Total Fat	(g) Sat. Fat	(mg) Chol.	(g) Carb.	(g) Fiber	(g) Sug.	(g) Prot.	(mg) Sod.
Pork, Fresh, Loin, Center Rib (Roasts), Boneless, Lean and Fat, Cooked, Roasted									
3 oz (85g)	214	13	5	69	0	0.0	--	23	41
Pork, Fresh, Loin, Center Rib (Roasts), Boneless, Lean, Cooked, Roasted									
3 oz (85g)	182	9	3	71	0	0.0	--	24	43
Pork, Fresh, Loin, Country-style Ribs, Lean and Fat, Cooked, Braised									
3 oz (85g)	232	15	5	88	0	0.0	0	23	49
Pork, Fresh, Loin, Country-style Ribs, Lean and Fat, Cooked, Roasted									
3 oz (85g)	279	22	8	78	0	0.0	--	20	44
Pork, Fresh, Loin, Country-style Ribs, Lean, Cooked, Braised									
3 oz (85g)	210	12	4	89	0	0.0	0	24	51
Pork, Fresh, Loin, Country-style Ribs, Lean, Cooked, Roasted									
3 oz (85g)	210	13	5	79	0	0.0	--	23	25
Pork, Fresh, Loin, Sirloin (Chops), Bone-in, Lean and Fat, Cooked, Braised									
1 chop, excluding refuse (yield from 1 raw chop, with refuse, weighing 151g)									
	196	12	4	66	0	0.0	--	20	41
Pork, Fresh, Loin, Sirloin (Chops), Bone-in, Lean and Fat, Cooked, Broiled									
1 chop, excluding refuse (yield from 1 raw chop, with refuse, weighing 151g)									
	194	12	4	65	0	0.0	0	20	51
Pork, Fresh, Loin, Sirloin (Chops), Bone-in, Lean, Cooked, Braised									
1 chop, excluding refuse (yield from 1 raw chop, with refuse, weighing 151g)									
	142	6	2	58	0	0.0	--	19	38
Pork, Fresh, Loin, Sirloin (Chops), Bone-in, Lean, Cooked, Broiled									
1 chop, excluding refuse (yield from 1 raw chop, with refuse, weighing 151g)									
	143	7	2	57	0	0.0	0	19	48
Pork, Fresh, Loin, Sirloin (Chops), Boneless, Lean and Fat, Cooked, Braised									
1 chop, excluding refuse (yield from 1 raw chop, with refuse, weighing 113g)									
	155	7	2	66	0	0.0	0	22	38
Pork, Fresh, Loin, Sirloin (Chops), Boneless, Lean and Fat, Cooked, Broiled									
1 chop, excluding refuse (yield from 1 raw chop, with refuse, weighing 113g)									
	154	6	2	67	0	0.0	0	23	41
Pork, Fresh, Loin, Sirloin (Chops), Boneless, Lean, Cooked, Braised									
1 chop, excluding refuse (yield from 1 raw chop, with refuse, weighing 113g)									
	140	5	2	65	0	0.0	--	22	37
Pork, Fresh, Loin, Sirloin (Chops), Boneless, Lean, Cooked, Broiled									
1 chop, excluding refuse (yield from 1 raw chop, with refuse, weighing 113g)									
	137	5	2	65	0	0.0	0	22	40

Food Serving size	Cal.	(g) Total Fat	(g) Sat. Fat	(mg) Chol.	(g) Carb.	(g) Fiber	(g) Sug.	(g) Prot.	(mg) Sod.
Pork, Fresh, Loin, Sirloin (Roasts), Bone-in, Lean and Fat, Cooked, Roasted									
3 oz (85g)	196	11	3	76	0	0.0	0	23	48
Pork, Fresh, Loin, Sirloin (Roasts), Bone-in, Lean, Cooked, Roasted									
1 roast, without refuse (985g)	2009	93	28	877	0	0.0	0	274	581
Pork, Fresh, Loin, Sirloin (Roasts), Boneless, Lean and Fat, Cooked, Roasted									
3 oz (85g)	176	8	3	73	0	0.0	0	24	48
Pork, Fresh, Loin, Sirloin (Roasts), Boneless, Lean, Cooked, Roasted									
3 oz (85g)	168	7	3	73	0	0.0	0	25	48
Pork, Fresh, Loin, Tenderloin, Lean and Fat, Cooked, Broiled									
1 chop, excluding refuse (yield from 1 raw chop, with refuse, weighing 113g)	153	6	2	71	0	0.0	--	23	49
Pork, Fresh, Loin, Tenderloin, Lean and Fat, Cooked, Roasted									
3 oz (85g)	125	3	1	62	0	0.0	0	22	48
Pork, Fresh, Loin, Tenderloin, Lean, Cooked, Broiled									
1 chop, excluding refuse (yield from 1 raw chop, with refuse, weighing 113g)	137	5	2	69	0	0.0	--	22	47
Pork, Fresh, Loin, Tenderloin, Lean, Cooked, Roasted									
3 oz (85g)	122	3	1	62	0	0.0	0	22	48
Pork, Fresh, Loin, Top Loin (Chops), Boneless, Enhanced, Lean, Cooked, Pan-broiled									
1 chop, boneless (150g)	254	8	3	113	0	0.0	0	43	314
Pork, Fresh, Loin, Top Loin (Chops), Boneless, Lean and Fat, Cooked, Braised									
1 chop (135g)	270	11	4	97	0	0.0	0	39	89
Pork, Fresh, Loin, Top Loin (Chops), Boneless, Lean and Fat, Cooked, Broiled									
3 oz (85g)	167	8	3	62	0	0.0	0	23	37
Pork, Fresh, Loin, Top Loin (Chops), Boneless, Lean and Fat, Cooked, Pan-fried									
1 chop (142g)	278	11	4	99	0	0.0	0	42	122
Pork, Fresh, Loin, Top Loin (Chops), Boneless, Lean, Cooked, Braised									
1 chop (135g)	230	6	2	96	0	0.0	0	41	90
Pork, Fresh, Loin, Top Loin (Chops), Boneless, Lean, Cooked, Broiled									
1 chop (145g)	251	9	3	104	0	0.0	0	40	65
Pork, Fresh, Loin, Top Loin (Chops), Boneless, Lean, Cooked, Pan-fried									
1 chop (142g)	244	7	3	98	0	0.0	0	43	124
Pork, Fresh, Loin, Top Loin (Roasts), Boneless, Lean and Fat, Cooked, Roasted									
3 oz (85g)	163	7	2	68	0	0.0	0	22	39

Food Serving size	Cal.	(g) Total Fat	(g) Sat. Fat	(mg) Chol.	(g) Carb.	(g) Fiber	(g) Sug.	(g) Prot.	(mg) Sod.
Pork, Fresh, Loin, Top Loin (Roasts), Boneless, Lean, Cooked, Roasted									
3 oz (85g)	147	5	2	67	0	0.0	0	23	40
Pork, Fresh, Loin, Whole, Lean and Fat, Cooked, Braised									
1 chop, excluding refuse (yield from 1 raw chop, with refuse, weighing 151g)									
	213	12	5	71	0	0.0	0	24	43
Pork, Fresh, Loin, Whole, Lean and Fat, Cooked, Broiled									
1 chop, excluding refuse (yield from 1 raw chop, with refuse, weighing 151g)									
	211	12	5	70	0	0.0	0	24	54
Pork, Fresh, Loin, Whole, Lean and Fat, Cooked, Roasted									
1 chop, excluding refuse (yield from 1 raw chop, with refuse, weighing 151g)									
	221	13	5	73	0	0.0	0	24	53
Pork, Fresh, Loin, Whole, Lean, Cooked, Braised									
1 chop, excluding refuse (yield from 1 raw chop, with refuse, weighing 151g)									
	163	7	3	63	0	0.0	0	23	40
Pork, Fresh, Loin, Whole, Lean, Cooked, Broiled									
1 chop, excluding refuse (yield from 1 raw chop, with refuse, weighing 151g)									
	166	8	3	62	0	0.0	0	23	51
Pork, Fresh, Loin, Whole, Lean, Cooked, Roasted									
1 chop, excluding refuse (yield from 1 raw chop, with refuse, weighing 151g)									
	169	8	3	66	0	0.0	0	23	47
Pork, Fresh, Shoulder (Boston Butt), Blade (Steaks), Lean and Fat, Cooked, Braised									
3 oz (85g)	227	15	6	83	0	0.0	0	21	49
Pork, Fresh, Shoulder (Boston Butt), Blade (Steaks), Lean, Cooked, Braised									
1 steak, without refuse (Yield from 1 cooked steak, with refuse, weighing 249g)									
	396	22	9	170	0	0.0	0	45	102
Pork, Fresh, Shoulder, Arm Picnic, Lean and Fat, Cooked, Braised									
3 oz (85g)	280	20	7	93	0	0.0	0	24	75
Pork, Fresh, Shoulder, Arm Picnic, Lean and Fat, Cooked, Roasted									
3 oz (85g)	269	20	7	80	0	0.0	--	20	60
Pork, Fresh, Shoulder, Arm Picnic, Lean, Cooked, Braised									
3 oz (85g)	211	10	4	97	0	0.0	0	27	87
Pork, Fresh, Shoulder, Arm Picnic, Lean, Cooked, Roasted									
3 oz (85g)	194	11	4	81	0	0.0	--	23	68
Pork, Fresh, Shoulder, Blade, Boston (Roasts), Lean and Fat, Cooked, Roasted									
3 oz (85g)	229	16	6	73	0	0.0	0	20	57

Food Serving size	Cal.	(g) Total Fat	(g) Sat. Fat	(mg) Chol.	(g) Carb.	(g) Fiber	(g) Sug.	(g) Prot.	(mg) Sod.
Pork, Fresh, Shoulder, Blade, Boston (Roasts), Lean, Cooked, Roasted									
3 oz (85g)	197	12	4	72	0	0.0	0	21	75
Pork, Fresh, Shoulder, Blade, Boston (Steaks), Lean and Fat, Cooked, Broiled									
1 steak, excluding refuse (yield from 1 raw steak, with refuse, weighing 300g)	438	28	10	161	0	0.0	0	43	117
Pork, Fresh, Shoulder, Blade, Boston (Steaks), Lean, Cooked, Broiled									
1 steak, excluding refuse (yield from 1 raw steak, with refuse, weighing 300g)	334	18	7	138	0	0.0	0	39	109
Pork, Fresh, Shoulder, Whole, Lean and Fat, Cooked, Roasted									
3 oz (85g)	248	18	7	77	0	0.0	0	20	58
Pork, Fresh, Shoulder, Whole, Lean, Cooked, Roasted									
3 oz (85g)	196	12	4	77	0	0.0	0	22	64
Pork, Fresh, Spareribs, Lean and Fat, Cooked, Braised									
3 oz (85g)	337	26	9	103	0	0.0	0	25	79
Pork, Fresh, Spareribs, Lean and Fat, Cooked, Roasted									
1 rack (1533g)	5534	473	142	1610	0	0.0	0	320	1395
Pork, Fresh, Top Loin (Chops), Boneless, Enhanced, Lean and Fat, Cooked, Pan-broiled									
1 chop, boneless (yield from 189g raw meat) (150g)	285	11	4	113	0	0.0	0	43	308
Pork, Fresh, Variety Meats and By-products, Brain, Cooked, Braised									
3 oz (85g)	117	8	2	2169	0	0.0	--	10	77
Pork, Fresh, Variety Meats and By-products, Chitterlings, Cooked, Simmered									
3 oz (85g)	198	17	8	235	0	0.0	0	11	15
Pork, Fresh, Variety Meats and By-products, Ears, Frozen, Cooked, Simmered									
1 unit, cooked (yield from 1 lb raw meat) (422g)	701	46	16	380	1	0.0	--	67	705
Pork, Fresh, Variety Meats and By-products, Feet, Cooked, Simmered									
3 oz (85g)	197	14	4	91	0	0.0	0	19	62
Pork, Fresh, Variety Meats and By-products, Heart, Cooked, Braised									
1 heart (129g)	191	7	2	285	1	0.0	--	30	45
Pork, Fresh, Variety Meats and By-products, Kidneys, Cooked, Braised									
3 oz (85g)	128	4	1	408	0	0.0	--	22	68
Pork, Fresh, Variety Meats and By-products, Liver, Cooked, Braised									
3 oz (85g)	140	4	1	302	3	0.0	--	22	42

Food Serving size	Cal.	(g) Total Fat	(g) Sat. Fat	(mg) Chol.	(g) Carb.	(g) Fiber	(g) Sug.	(g) Prot.	(mg) Sod.
Pork, Fresh, Variety Meats and By-products, Lungs, Cooked, Braised									
3 oz (85g)	84	3	1	329	0	0.0	--	14	69
Pork, Fresh, Variety Meats and By-products, Pancreas, Cooked, Braised									
3 oz (85g)	186	9	3	268	0	0.0	--	24	36
Pork, Fresh, Variety Meats and By-products, Spleen, Cooked, Braised									
3 oz (85g)	127	3	1	428	0	0.0	--	24	91
Pork, Fresh, Variety Meats and By-products, Tail, Cooked, Simmered									
3 oz (85g)	337	30	11	110	0	0.0	--	14	21
Pork, Fresh, Variety Meats and By-products, Tongue, Cooked, Braised									
3 oz (85g)	230	16	5	124	0	0.0	--	20	93
Pork, Leg Sirloin Tip Roast, Boneless, Lean and Fat, Cooked, Braised									
1 piece (609g)	950	16	5	512	0	0.0	0	189	262
Pork, Loin, Leg Cap Steak, Boneless, Lean and Fat, Cooked, Broiled									
1 piece (194g)	307	9	3	157	0	0.0	0	53	147
Pork, Oriental Style, Dehydrated									
1 cup (22g)	135	14	5	15	0	0.0	--	3	151
Pork, Shoulder Breast, Boneless, Lean and Fat, Cooked, Broiled									
1 piece (373g)	604	17	5	291	0	0.0	0	106	201
Pork, Shoulder, Petite Tender, Boneless, Lean and Fat, Cooked, Broiled									
1 piece (92g)	143	4	1	75	0	0.0	0	25	49
Salami Pork Beef, Less Sodium									
3.527 oz (100g)	396	31	11	90	15	0.2	6	15	623
Salami, Cooked, Beef									
1 oz (28.35g)	74	6	3	20	1	0.0	0	4	323
Salami, Cooked, Beef and Pork									
1 slice, round (12.3g)	41	3	1	11	0	0.0	0	3	178
Salami, Cooked, Turkey									
1 serving (28g)	48	3	1	21	0	0.0	0	5	281
Salami, Dry or Hard, Pork									
1 slice (3-1/8" dia x 1/16" thick) (10g)	41	3	1	8	0	0.0	--	2	226
Salami, Dry or Hard, Pork, Beef									
1 oz (28g)	108	8	3	28	1	0.0	0	6	563
Salami, Italian Pork									
1 oz (28g)	119	10	4	22	0	0.0	0	6	529

Food Serving size	Cal.	(g) Total Fat	(g) Sat. Fat	(mg) Chol.	(g) Carb.	(g) Fiber	(g) Sug.	(g) Prot.	(mg) Sod.
Salami, Italian, Pork and Beef, Dry, Sliced, 50% Less Sodium									
1 serving, 5 slices (28g)	98	7	3	25	2	0.0	0	6	262
Scrapple, Pork									
1 oz, cooked (25g)	53	3	1	12	4	0.1	0	2	165
Sheepshead, Cooked, Dry Heat									
3 oz (85g)	107	1	0	54	0	0.0	--	22	62
Veal, Breast, Fat, Cooked									
1 oz (28.35g)	148	15	6	27	0	0.0	--	3	14
Veal, Breast, Plate Half, Boneless, Lean and Fat, Cooked, Braised									
3 oz (85g)	240	16	6	95	0	--	--	22	54
Veal, Breast, Point Half, Boneless, Lean and Fat, Cooked, Braised									
3 oz (85g)	211	12	5	97	0	--	--	24	56
Veal, Breast, Whole, Boneless, Lean and Fat, Cooked, Braised									
3 oz (85g)	226	14	6	96	0	--	--	23	55
Veal, Breast, Whole, Boneless, Lean, Cooked, Braised									
3 oz (85g)	185	8	3	99	0	--	--	26	58
Veal, Composite of Retail Cuts, Fat, Cooked									
3 oz (85g)	546	57	28	62	0	0.0	--	8	48
Veal, Composite of Retail Cuts, Lean and Fat, Cooked									
3 oz (85g)	196	10	4	97	0	0.0	0	26	74
Veal, Composite of Retail Cuts, Lean, Cooked									
3 oz (85g)	167	6	2	100	0	0.0	0	27	76
Veal, Cubed for Stew (Leg and Shoulder), Lean, Cooked, Braised									
3 oz (85g)	160	4	1	123	0	0.0	--	30	79
Veal, Ground, Cooked, Broiled									
3 oz (85g)	146	6	3	88	0	0.0	0	21	71
Veal, Leg (Top Round), Lean and Fat, Cooked, Braised									
3 oz (85g)	179	5	2	114	0	0.0	0	31	57
Veal, Leg (Top Round), Lean and Fat, Cooked, Pan-fried, Breaded									
3 oz (85g)	202	8	3	95	8	0.3	0	23	386
Veal, Leg (Top Round), Lean and Fat, Cooked, Pan-fried, Not Breaded									
3 oz (85g)	179	7	3	89	0	0.0	0	27	65
Veal, Leg (Top Round), Lean and Fat, Cooked, Roasted									
3 oz (85g)	136	4	2	88	0	0.0	0	24	58

Food Serving size	Cal.	(g) Total Fat	(g) Sat. Fat	(mg) Chol.	(g) Carb.	(g) Fiber	(g) Sug.	(g) Prot.	(mg) Sod.
Veal, Leg (Top Round), Lean, Cooked, Braised 3 oz (85g)	173	4	2	115	0	0.0	--	31	57
Veal, Leg (Top Round), Lean, Cooked, Pan-fried, Breaded 3 oz (85g)	184	5	1	96	8	0.2	0	24	387
Veal, Leg (Top Round), Lean, Cooked, Pan-fried, Not Breaded 3 oz (85g)	156	4	1	91	0	0.0	0	28	65
Veal, Leg (Top Round), Lean, Cooked, Roasted 3 oz (85g)	128	3	1	88	0	0.0	--	24	58
Veal, Loin, Lean and Fat, Cooked, Braised 1 chop, excluding refuse (yield from 1 raw chop, with refuse, weighing 195g)	227	14	5	94	0	0.0	0	24	64
Veal, Loin, Lean and Fat, Cooked, Roasted 3 oz (85g)	184	10	4	88	0	0.0	0	21	79
Veal, Loin, Lean, Cooked, Braised 1 chop, excluding refuse (yield from 1 raw chop, with refuse, weighing 195g)	156	6	2	86	0	0.0	0	23	58
Veal, Loin, Lean, Cooked, Roasted 3 oz (85g)	149	6	2	90	0	0.0	0	22	82
Veal, Rib, Lean and Fat, Cooked, Braised 3 oz (85g)	213	11	4	118	0	0.0	0	28	81
Veal, Rib, Lean and Fat, Cooked, Roasted 3 oz (85g)	194	12	5	94	0	0.0	--	20	78
Veal, Rib, Lean, Cooked, Braised 3 oz (85g)	185	7	2	122	0	0.0	0	29	84
Veal, Rib, Lean, Cooked, Roasted 3 oz (85g)	150	6	2	98	0	0.0	--	22	82
Veal, Shank (Fore and Hind), Lean and Fat, Cooked, Braised 3 oz (85g)	162	5	2	105	0	--	--	27	79
Veal, Shank (Fore and Hind), Lean, Cooked, Braised 3 oz (85g)	150	4	1	107	0	0.0	--	27	80
Veal, Shoulder, Arm, Lean and Fat, Cooked, Braised 1 steak, excluding refuse (yield from 1 raw steak, with refuse, weighing 385g)	408	18	7	256	0	0.0	--	58	151
Veal, Shoulder, Arm, Lean and Fat, Cooked, Roasted 3 oz (85g)	156	7	3	92	0	0.0	--	22	77

Food Serving size	Cal.	(g) Total Fat	(g) Sat. Fat	(mg) Chol.	(g) Carb.	(g) Fiber	(g) Sug.	(g) Prot.	(mg) Sod.
Veal, Shoulder, Arm, Lean, Cooked, Braised 1 steak, excluding refuse (yield from 1 raw steak, with refuse, weighing 385g)									
	322	9	2	248	0	0.0	--	57	144
Veal, Shoulder, Arm, Lean, Cooked, Roasted 3 oz (85g)	139	5	2	93	0	0.0	--	22	77
Veal, Shoulder, Blade, Lean and Fat, Cooked, Braised 3 oz (85g)	191	9	3	130	0	0.0	0	27	83
Veal, Shoulder, Blade, Lean and Fat, Cooked, Roasted 3 oz (85g)	158	7	3	99	0	0.0	--	21	85
Veal, Shoulder, Blade, Lean, Cooked, Braised 3 oz (85g)	168	6	2	134	0	0.0	0	28	86
Veal, Shoulder, Blade, Lean, Cooked, Roasted 3 oz (85g)	145	6	2	101	0	0.0	--	22	87
Veal, Shoulder, Whole (Arm and Boiled), Lean and Fat, Cooked, Braised 3 oz (85g)	194	9	3	107	0	0.0	0	27	81
Veal, Shoulder, Whole (Arm and Boiled), Lean and Fat, Cooked, Roasted 3 oz (85g)	156	7	3	96	0	0.0	--	22	82
Veal, Shoulder, Whole (Arm and Boiled), Lean, Cooked, Braised 3 oz (85g)	169	5	1	111	0	0.0	--	29	82
Veal, Shoulder, Whole (Arm and Boiled), Lean, Cooked, Roasted 3 oz (85g)	145	6	2	97	0	0.0	--	22	82
Veal, Sirloin, Lean and Fat, Cooked, Braised 3 oz (85g)	214	11	4	92	0	0.0	--	27	67
Veal, Sirloin, Lean and Fat, Cooked, Roasted 3 oz (85g)	172	9	4	87	0	0.0	0	21	71
Veal, Sirloin, Lean, Cooked, Braised 3 oz (85g)	173	6	2	96	0	0.0	--	29	69
Veal, Sirloin, Lean, Cooked, Roasted 3 oz (85g)	143	5	2	88	0	0.0	--	22	72
Veal, Variety Meats and By-products, Brain, Cooked, Braised 3 oz (85g)	116	8	2	2635	0	0.0	--	10	133
Veal, Variety Meats and By-products, Brain, Cooked, Pan-fried 3 oz (85g)	181	14	3	1802	0	0.0	--	12	150
Veal, Variety Meats and By-products, Heart, Cooked, Braised 3 oz (85g)	158	6	2	150	0	0.0	--	25	49

Food Serving size	Cal.	(g) Total Fat	(g) Sat. Fat	(mg) Chol.	(g) Carb.	(g) Fiber	(g) Sug.	(g) Prot.	(mg) Sod.
Veal, Variety Meats and By-products, Kidneys, Cooked, Braised									
3 oz (85g)	139	5	1	672	0	0.0	--	22	94
Veal, Variety Meats and By-products, Liver, Cooked, Braised									
1 slice (80g)	154	5	2	409	3	0.0	0	23	62
Veal, Variety Meats and By-products, Liver, Cooked, Pan-fried									
1 slice (67g)	129	4	1	325	3	0.0	0	18	57
Veal, Variety Meats and By-products, Lungs, Cooked, Braised									
3 oz (85g)	88	2	1	224	0	0.0	--	16	48
Veal, Variety Meats and By-products, Pancreas, Cooked, Braised									
3 oz (85g)	218	12	4	--	0	0.0	--	25	58
Veal, Variety Meats and By-products, Spleen, Cooked, Braised									
3 oz (85g)	110	2	1	380	0	0.0	--	20	49
Veal, Variety Meats and By-products, Thymus, Cooked, Braised									
3 oz (85g)	106	3	1	298	0	0.0	0	19	50
Veal, Variety Meats and By-products, Tongue, Cooked, Braised									
3 oz (85g)	172	9	4	202	0	0.0	--	22	54
Worthington Choplets, Canned, Unprepared									
2 slices (92g)	95	1	0	0	4	2.6	0	18	420
Worthington Diced Chik, Canned, Unprepared									
.25 cup (55g)	44	0	--	1	2	0.8	0	8	189

Poultry

Food Serving size	Cal.	(g) Total Fat	(g) Sat. Fat	(mg) Chol.	(g) Carb.	(g) Fiber	(g) Sug.	(g) Prot.	(mg) Sod.
Chicken Breast, Fat Free, Mesquite Flavor, Sliced									
1 serving, 2 slices (42g)	34	0	0	15	1	0.0	0	7	437
Chicken Breast, Oven-roasted, Fat Free, Sliced									
1 serving, 2 slices (42g)	33	0	0	15	1	0.0	0	7	457
Chicken, Broilers or Fryers, Light Meat, Meat Only, Cooked, Stewed									
1 unit (yield from 1 lb ready-to-cook chicken) (71g)	113	3	1	55	0	0.0	0	21	46
Chicken, Broilers or Fryers, Back, Meat and Skin, Cooked, Fried, Batter									
.5 back, bone removed (120g)	397	26	7	106	12	--	--	26	380
Chicken, Broilers or Fryers, Back, Meat and Skin, Cooked, Fried, Flour									
.5 back, bone removed (72g)	238	15	4	64	5	--	--	20	65
Chicken, Broilers or Fryers, Back, Meat and Skin, Cooked, Roasted									
.5 back, bone removed (53g)	159	11	3	47	0	0.0	0	14	46

Food Serving size	Cal.	(g) Total Fat	(g) Sat. Fat	(mg) Chol.	(g) Carb.	(g) Fiber	(g) Sug.	(g) Prot.	(mg) Sod.
Chicken, Broilers or Fryers, Back, Meat and Skin, Cooked, Stewed 1 unit (yield from 1 lb ready-to-cook chicken) (36g)	93	7	2	28	0	0.0	0	8	23
Chicken, Broilers or Fryers, Back, Meat Only, Cooked, Fried .5 back, bone and skin removed (58g)	167	9	2	54	3	0.0	--	17	57
Chicken, Broilers or Fryers, Back, Meat Only, Cooked, Stewed .5 back, bone and skin removed (42g)	88	5	1	36	0	0.0	0	11	28
Chicken, Broilers or Fryers, Breast, Meat and Skin, Cooked, Fried, Batter .5 breast, bone removed (140g)	364	18	5	119	13	0.4	0	35	385
Chicken, Broilers or Fryers, Breast, Meat and Skin, Cooked, Fried, Flour .5 breast, bone removed (98g)	218	9	2	87	2	0.1	--	31	74
Chicken, Broilers or Fryers, Breast, Meat and Skin, Cooked, Roasted 1 unit (yield from 1 lb ready-to-cook chicken) (58g)	114	5	1	49	0	0.0	0	17	41
Chicken, Broilers or Fryers, Breast, Meat and Skin, Cooked, Stewed 1 unit (yield from 1 lb ready-to-cook chicken) (66g)	121	5	1	50	0	0.0	0	18	41
Chicken, Broilers or Fryers, Breast, Meat Only, Cooked, Fried .5 breast, bone and skin removed (86g)	161	4	1	78	0	0.0	0	29	68
Chicken, Broilers or Fryers, Breast, Meat Only, Cooked, Roasted 1 unit (yield from 1 lb ready-to-cook chicken) (52g)	86	2	1	44	0	0.0	0	16	38
Chicken, Broilers or Fryers, Breast, Meat Only, Cooked, Stewed 1 unit (yield from 1 lb ready-to-cook chicken) (57g)	86	2	0	44	0	0.0	0	17	36
Chicken, Broilers or Fryers, Dark Meat, Meat and Skin, Cooked, Fried, Batter .5 chicken, bone removed (278g)	828	52	14	247	26	--	--	61	820
Chicken, Broilers or Fryers, Dark Meat, Meat and Skin, Cooked, Fried, Flour .5 chicken, bone removed (184g)	524	31	8	169	8	0.0	0	50	164
Chicken, Broilers or Fryers, Dark Meat, Meat and Skin, Cooked, Roasted .5 chicken, bone removed (167g)	423	26	7	152	0	0.0	--	43	145

Food Serving size	Cal.	(g) Total Fat	(g) Sat. Fat	(mg) Chol.	(g) Carb.	(g) Fiber	(g) Sug.	(g) Prot.	(mg) Sod.
Chicken, Broilers or Fryers, Dark Meat, Meat and Skin, Cooked, Stewed									
.5 chicken, bone removed (184g)	429	27	7	151	0	0.0	--	43	129
Chicken, Broilers or Fryers, Dark Meat, Meat Only, Cooked, Fried									
1 unit (yield from 1 lb ready-to-cook chicken) (91g)	217	11	3	87	2	0.0	--	26	88
Chicken, Broilers or Fryers, Dark Meat, Meat Only, Cooked, Roasted									
1 unit (yield from 1 lb ready-to-cook chicken) (81g)	166	8	2	75	0	0.0	0	22	75
Chicken, Broilers or Fryers, Dark Meat, Meat Only, Cooked, Stewed									
1 unit (yield from 1 lb ready-to-cook chicken) (86g)	165	8	2	76	0	0.0	0	22	64
Chicken, Broilers or Fryers, Drumstick, Meat and Skin, Cooked, Fried, Batter									
1 drumstick, bone removed (72g)	193	11	3	62	6	0.2	--	16	194
Chicken, Broilers or Fryers, Drumstick, Meat and Skin, Cooked, Fried, Flour									
1 drumstick, bone removed (49g)	120	7	2	44	1	0.0	--	13	44
Chicken, Broilers or Fryers, Drumstick, Meat and Skin, Cooked, Roasted									
1 unit (yield from 1 lb ready-to-cook chicken) (31g)	67	3	1	28	0	0.0	0	8	28
Chicken, Broilers or Fryers, Drumstick, Meat and Skin, Cooked, Stewed									
1 unit (yield from 1 lb ready-to-cook chicken) (34g)	69	4	1	28	0	0.0	0	9	26
Chicken, Broilers or Fryers, Drumstick, Meat Only, Cooked, Fried									
1 drumstick, bone and skin removed (42g)	82	3	1	39	0	0.0	--	12	40
Chicken, Broilers or Fryers, Drumstick, Meat Only, Cooked, Roasted									
1 unit (yield from 1 lb ready-to-cook chicken) (26g)	45	1	0	24	0	0.0	0	7	25
Chicken, Broilers or Fryers, Drumstick, Meat Only, Cooked, Stewed									
1 unit (yield from 1 lb ready-to-cook chicken) (28g)	47	2	0	25	0	0.0	0	8	22
Chicken, Broilers or Fryers, Giblets, Cooked, Fried									
1 unit (yield from 1 lb ready-to-cook chicken) (13g)	36	2	0	58	1	0.0	--	4	15

Food Serving size	Cal.	(g) Total Fat	(g) Sat. Fat	(mg) Chol.	(g) Carb.	(g) Fiber	(g) Sug.	(g) Prot.	(mg) Sod.
Chicken, Broilers or Fryers, Giblets, Cooked, Simmered									
1 cup, chopped or dice (145g)	228	7	2	641	0	0.0	0	39	97
Chicken, Broilers or Fryers, Leg, Meat and Skin, Cooked, Fried, Batter									
1 leg, bone removed (158g)	431	26	7	142	14	0.5	--	34	441
Chicken, Broilers or Fryers, Leg, Meat and Skin, Cooked, Fried, Flour									
1 leg, bone removed (112g)	284	16	4	105	3	0.1	--	30	99
Chicken, Broilers or Fryers, Leg, Meat and Skin, Cooked, Roasted									
1 unit (yield from 1 lb ready-to-cook chicken) (69g)	160	9	3	63	0	0.0	0	18	60
Chicken, Broilers or Fryers, Leg, Meat and Skin, Cooked, Stewed									
1 unit (yield from 1 lb ready-to-cook chicken) (75g)	165	10	3	63	0	0.0	0	18	55
Chicken, Broilers or Fryers, Leg, Meat Only, Cooked, Fried									
1 leg, bone and skin removed (94g)	196	9	2	93	1	0.0	--	27	90
Chicken, Broilers or Fryers, Leg, Meat Only, Cooked, Roasted									
1 unit (yield from 1 lb ready-to-cook chicken) (57g)	109	5	1	54	0	0.0	0	15	52
Chicken, Broilers or Fryers, Leg, Meat Only, Cooked, Stewed									
1 unit (yield from 1 lb ready-to-cook chicken) (60g)	111	5	1	53	0	0.0	0	16	47
Chicken, Broilers or Fryers, Light Meat, Meat and Skin, Cooked, Fried, Batter									
.5 chicken, bone removed (188g)	521	29	8	158	18	--	--	44	540
Chicken, Broilers or Fryers, Light Meat, Meat and Skin, Cooked, Fried, Flour									
.5 chicken, bone removed (130g)	320	16	4	113	2	0.1	0	40	100
Chicken, Broilers or Fryers, Light Meat, Meat and Skin, Cooked, Roasted									
.5 chicken, bone removed (132g)	293	14	4	111	0	0.0	--	38	99
Chicken, Broilers or Fryers, Light Meat, Meat and Skin, Cooked, Stewed									
.5 chicken, bone removed (150g)	302	15	4	111	0	0.0	--	39	95
Chicken, Broilers or Fryers, Light Meat, Meat Only, Cooked, Fried									
1 unit (yield from 1 lb ready-to-cook chicken) (64g)	123	4	1	58	0	0.0	--	21	52

Food Serving size	Cal.	(g) Total Fat	(g) Sat. Fat	(mg) Chol.	(g) Carb.	(g) Fiber	(g) Sug.	(g) Prot.	(mg) Sod.
Chicken, Broilers or Fryers, Light Meat, Meat Only, Cooked, Roasted									
1 unit (yield from 1 lb ready-to-cook chicken) (64g)									
	111	3	1	54	0	0.0	0	20	49
Chicken, Broilers or Fryers, Meat and Skin and Giblets and Neck, Fried, Batter									
1 unit (yield from 1 lb ready-to-cook chicken) (308g)									
	896	54	14	317	28	--	--	70	875
Chicken, Broilers or Fryers, Meat and Skin and Giblets and Neck, Fried, Flour									
1 unit (yield from 1 lb ready-to-cook chicken) (212g)									
	577	32	9	237	7	--	--	61	182
Chicken, Broilers or Fryers, Meat and Skin and Giblets and Neck, Roasted									
1 unit (yield from 1 lb ready-to-cook chicken) (205g)									
	480	27	8	219	0	0.0	0	55	162
Chicken, Broilers or Fryers, Meat and Skin and Giblets and Neck, Stewed									
1 unit (yield from 1 lb ready-to-cook chicken) (225g)									
	486	28	8	218	0	0.0	--	55	149
Chicken, Broilers or Fryers, Meat and Skin, Cooked, Fried, Batter									
.5 chicken, bone removed (466g)									
	1347	81	21	405	44	1.4	0	105	1361
Chicken, Broilers or Fryers, Meat and Skin, Cooked, Fried, Flour									
.5 chicken, bone removed (314g)									
	845	47	13	283	10	0.3	0	90	264
Chicken, Broilers or Fryers, Meat and Skin, Cooked, Roasted									
1 unit (yield from 1 lb ready-to-cook chicken) (178g)									
	425	24	7	157	0	0.0	0	49	146
Chicken, Broilers or Fryers, Meat and Skin, Cooked, Stewed									
1 unit (yield from 1 lb ready-to-cook chicken) (200g)									
	438	25	7	156	0	0.0	0	49	134
Chicken, Broilers or Fryers, Meat Only, Cooked, Fried									
1 unit (yield from 1 lb ready-to-cook chicken) (155g)									
	339	14	4	146	3	0.2	0	47	141
Chicken, Broilers or Fryers, Meat Only, Roasted									
1 tbsp (8.7g)	17	1	0	8	0	0.0	0	3	7
Chicken, Broilers or Fryers, Meat Only, Stewed									
1 tbsp (8.7g)	15	1	0	7	0	0.0	0	2	6
Chicken, Broilers or Fryers, Neck, Meat and Skin, Cooked, Fried, Batter									
1 neck, bone removed (52g)	172	12	3	47	5	--	--	10	144

Food Serving size	Cal.	(g) Total Fat	(g) Sat. Fat	(mg) Chol.	(g) Carb.	(g) Fiber	(g) Sug.	(g) Prot.	(mg) Sod.
Chicken, Broilers or Fryers, Neck, Meat and Skin, Cooked, Fried, Flour									
1 neck, bone removed (36g)	120	8	2	34	2	--	--	9	30
Chicken, Broilers or Fryers, Neck, Meat and Skin, Cooked, Simmered									
1 neck, bone removed (38g)	94	7	2	27	0	0.0	0	7	20
Chicken, Broilers or Fryers, Neck, Meat Only, Cooked, Fried									
1 neck, bone and skin removed (22g)	50	3	1	23	0	0.0	--	6	22
Chicken, Broilers or Fryers, Neck, Meat Only, Cooked, Simmered									
1 neck, bone and skin removed (18g)	32	1	0	14	0	0.0	--	4	12
Chicken, Broilers or Fryers, Skin Only, Cooked, Fried, Batter									
.5 chicken, skin only (190g)	749	55	14	141	44	--	--	20	1104
Chicken, Broilers or Fryers, Skin Only, Cooked, Fried, Flour									
.5 chicken, skin only (56g)	281	24	7	41	5	--	--	11	30
Chicken, Broilers or Fryers, Skin Only, Cooked, Roasted									
.5 chicken, skin only (56g)	254	23	6	46	0	0.0	0	11	36
Chicken, Broilers or Fryers, Skin Only, Cooked, Stewed									
.5 chicken, skin only (72g)	261	24	7	45	0	0.0	--	11	40
Chicken, Broilers or Fryers, Thigh, Meat and Skin, Cooked, Fried, Batter									
1 thigh, bone removed (86g)	238	14	4	80	8	0.3	--	19	248
Chicken, Broilers or Fryers, Thigh, Meat and Skin, Cooked, Fried, Flour									
1 thigh, bone removed (62g)	162	9	3	60	2	0.1	--	17	55
Chicken, Broilers or Fryers, Thigh, Meat and Skin, Cooked, Roasted									
1 unit (yield from 1 lb ready-to-cook chicken) (37g)	91	6	2	34	0	0.0	0	9	31
Chicken, Broilers or Fryers, Thigh, Meat and Skin, Cooked, Stewed									
1 thigh, bone removed (68g)	158	10	3	57	0	0.0	0	16	48
Chicken, Broilers or Fryers, Thigh, Meat Only, Cooked, Fried									
1 thigh, bone and skin removed (52g)	113	5	1	53	1	0.0	--	15	49
Chicken, Broilers or Fryers, Thigh, Meat Only, Cooked, Roasted									
1 unit (yield from 1 lb ready-to-cook chicken) (31g)	65	3	1	29	0	0.0	0	8	27
Chicken, Broilers or Fryers, Thigh, Meat Only, Cooked, Stewed									
1 unit (yield from 1 lb ready-to-cook chicken) (33g)	64	3	1	30	0	0.0	0	8	25

Food Serving size	Cal.	(g) Total Fat	(g) Sat. Fat	(mg) Chol.	(g) Carb.	(g) Fiber	(g) Sug.	(g) Prot.	(mg) Sod.
Chicken, Broilers or Fryers, Wing, Meat and Skin, Cooked, Fried, Batter									
1 wing, bone removed (49g)	159	11	3	39	5	0.1	--	10	157
Chicken, Broilers or Fryers, Wing, Meat and Skin, Cooked, Fried, Flour									
1 wing, bone removed (32g)	103	7	2	26	1	0.0	--	8	25
Chicken, Broilers or Fryers, Wing, Meat and Skin, Cooked, Roasted									
1 unit (yield from 1 lb ready-to-cook chicken) (21g)	61	4	1	18	0	0.0	0	6	17
Chicken, Broilers or Fryers, Wing, Meat and Skin, Cooked, Stewed									
1 unit (yield from 1 lb ready-to-cook chicken) (24g)	60	4	1	17	0	0.0	0	5	16
Chicken, Broilers or Fryers, Wing, Meat Only, Cooked, Fried									
1 wing, bone and skin removed (20g)	42	2	1	17	0	0.0	--	6	18
Chicken, Broilers or Fryers, Wing, Meat Only, Cooked, Roasted									
1 wing, bone and skin removed (21g)	43	2	0	18	0	0.0	0	6	19
Chicken, Broilers or Fryers, Wing, Meat Only, Cooked, Stewed									
1 unit (yield from 1 lb ready-to-cook chicken) (14g)	25	1	0	10	0	0.0	0	4	10
Chicken, Canned, Meat Only, with Broth									
1 can (5 oz) (142g)	234	11	3	88	0	0.0	0	31	714
Chicken, Canned, No Broth									
1 can (5 oz) yields (125g)	231	10	3	63	1	0.0	0	32	169
Chicken, Capons, Giblets, Cooked, Simmered									
1 unit (yield from 1 lb ready-to cook capon) (11g)	18	1	0	48	0	0.0	--	3	6
Chicken, Capons, Meat and Skin and Giblets and Neck, Cooked, Roasted									
1 unit (yield from 1 lb ready-to cook capon) (218g)	493	25	7	225	0	0.0	--	62	109
Chicken, Capons, Meat and Skin, Cooked, Roasted									
1 unit (yield from 1 lb ready-to cook capon) (196g)	449	23	6	169	0	0.0	--	57	96
Chicken, Cornish Game Hens, Meat and Skin, Cooked, Roasted									
.5 bird (129g)	334	23	7	169	0	0.0	0	29	83
Chicken, Cornish Game Hens, Meat Only, Cooked, Roasted									
.5 bird (110g)	147	4	1	117	0	0.0	0	26	69

Food Serving size	Cal.	(g) Total Fat	(g) Sat. Fat	(mg) Chol.	(g) Carb.	(g) Fiber	(g) Sug.	(g) Prot.	(mg) Sod.
Chicken, Gizzard, All Classes, Cooked, Simmered									
1 cup, chopped or dice (145g)	223	4	1	537	0	0.0	0	44	81
Chicken, Ground, Crumbles, Cooked, Pan-browned									
3 oz, crumbled (85g)	161	9	3	91	0	0.0	0	20	64
Chicken, Heart, All Classes, Cooked, Simmered									
1 unit (yield from 1 lb ready-to-cook chicken) (1g)	2	0	0	2	0	0.0	--	0	0
Chicken, Meatless									
1 cup (168g)	376	21	3	0	6	6.0	0	40	1191
Chicken, Meatless, Breaded, Fried									
1 cup, pieces (168g)	393	21	2	0	14	7.2	1	36	672
Chicken, Roasting, Dark Meat, Meat Only, Cooked, Roasted									
1 unit (yield from 1 lb ready-to-cook chicken) (94g)	167	8	2	71	0	0.0	--	22	89
Chicken, Roasting, Giblets, Cooked, Simmered									
1 unit (yield from 1 lb ready-to-cook chicken) (15g)	25	1	0	54	0	0.0	--	4	9
Chicken, Roasting, Light Meat, Meat Only, Cooked, Roasted									
1 unit (yield from 1 lb ready-to-cook chicken) (78g)	119	3	1	59	0	0.0	0	21	40
Chicken, Roasting, Meat and Skin and Giblets and Neck, Cooked, Roasted									
1 unit (yield from 1 lb ready-to-cook chicken) (235g)	517	31	9	221	0	0.0	--	56	167
Chicken, Roasting, Meat and Skin, Cooked, Roasted									
.5 chicken, bone removed (480g)	1070	64	18	365	0	0.0	--	115	350
Chicken, Roasting, Meat Only, Cooked, Roasted									
1 unit (yield from 1 lb ready-to-cook chicken) (171g)	286	11	3	128	0	0.0	--	43	128
Chicken, Stewing, Dark Meat, Meat Only, Cooked, Stewed									
1 unit (yield from 1 lb ready-to-cook chicken) (73g)	188	11	3	69	0	0.0	--	21	69
Chicken, Stewing, Giblets, Cooked, Simmered									
1 unit (yield from 1 lb ready-to-cook chicken) (17g)	33	2	0	60	0	0.0	--	4	10

Food Serving size	Cal.	(g) Total Fat	(g) Sat. Fat	(mg) Chol.	(g) Carb.	(g) Fiber	(g) Sug.	(g) Prot.	(mg) Sod.
Chicken, Stewing, Light Meat, Meat Only, Cooked, Stewed 1 unit (yield from 1 lb ready-to-cook chicken) (64g)									
	136	5	1	45	0	0.0	--	21	37
Chicken, Stewing, Meat and Skin and Giblets and Neck, Cooked, Stewed 1 unit (yield from 1 lb ready-to-cook chicken) (202g)									
	432	24	7	216	0	0.0	0	50	135
Chicken, Stewing, Meat and Skin, Cooked, Stewed .5 chicken, bone removed (261g									
	744	49	13	206	0	0.0	--	70	191
Chicken, Stewing, Meat Only, Cooked, Stewed 1 unit (yield from 1 lb ready-to-cook chicken) (137g)									
	325	16	4	114	0	0.0	0	42	107
Chicken, Wing, Frozen, Glazed, Barbecue Flavor, Heated (Microwave) 1 serving (74g)	184	10	3	115	3	0.7	2	19	619
Chicken, Wing, Frozen, Glazed, Barbecue Flavor 1 serving (86g)	181	11	3	108	3	0.5	2	17	529
Chicken, Wing, Frozen, Glazed, Barbecue Flavor, Heated (Conventional Oven) 1 serving (96g)	232	14	4	131	3	0.5	2	21	537
Cooked, Boilers or Fryers, Back, Meat Only, Cooked, Roasted .5 back, bone and skin removed (40g)									
	96	5	1	36	0	0.0	0	11	38
Dove, Cooked (Including Squab) 1 cup, chopped or diced (140g)	298	18	5	162	0	0.0	--	33	80
Duck, Domesticated, Meat and Skin, Cooked, Roasted 1 unit (yield from 1 lb ready-to-cook duck) (173g)									
	583	49	17	145	0	0.0	0	33	102
Duck, Domesticated, Meat Only, Cooked, Roasted 1 unit (yield from 1 lb ready-to-cook duck) (100g)									
	201	11	4	89	0	0.0	0	23	65
Duck, Young Duckling, Domestic, White Peking, Breast, Meat and Skin, Boneless, Cooked, Roasted 3 oz (85g)	172	9	2	116	0	--	--	21	71
Duck, Young Duckling, Domestic, White Peking, Breast, Meat, Boneless, Cooked, Without Skin, Broiled 1 unit (yield from 1 lb ready-to-cook duck) (44g)									
	62	1	0	63	0	--	--	12	46

Food Serving size	Cal.	(g) Total Fat	(g) Sat. Fat	(mg) Chol.	(g) Carb.	(g) Fiber	(g) Sug.	(g) Prot.	(mg) Sod.
Duck, Young Duckling, Domestic, White Peking, Leg, Meat and Skin, Bone-in, Cooked, Roasted 1 unit (yield from 1 lb ready-to-cook duck) (43g)									
	93	5	1	49	0	--	--	12	47
Duck, Young Duckling, Domestic, White Peking, Leg, Meat, Bone-in, Cooked Without Skin, Broasted 1 unit (yield from 1 lb ready-to-cook duck) (35g)									
	62	2	0	37	0	--	--	10	38
Ground Turkey, 85% Lean, 15% Fat, Pan-broiled Crumbles 3 oz (85g)	219	15	4	90	0	0.0	0	21	72
Ground Turkey, 85% Lean, 15% Fat, Patties, Broiled 3 oz (85g)	212	14	4	89	0	0.0	0	22	69
Ground Turkey, 93% Lean, 7% Fat, Pan-broiled Crumbles 3 oz (85g)	181	10	3	88	0	0.0	0	23	77
Ground Turkey, 93% Lean, 7% Fat, Patties, Broiled 3 oz (85g)	176	10	3	90	0	0.0	0	22	77
Ground Turkey, Fat Free, Pan-broiled Crumbles 3 oz (85g)	128	2	1	60	0	0.0	0	27	52
Ground Turkey, Fat Free, Patties, Broiled 3 oz (85g)	117	2	1	55	0	0.0	0	25	50
Pastrami, Turkey 2 slices (57g)	76	4	1	39	1	0.1	2	9	559
Pheasant, Cooked, Total Edible 1 cup, chopped or diced (140g)	335	17	5	125	0	0.0	--	45	60
Poultry Food Poducts, Ground Turkey, Cooked 1 unit, yield from 1 lb raw (330g)									
	670	34	9	307	0	0.0	0	90	257
Poultry Salad Sandwich Spread 1 oz (28.35g)	57	4	1	9	2	0.0	0	3	107
Turkey and Gravy, Frozen 1 pkg (net weight, 5 oz) (142g)	95	4	1	26	7	0.0	--	8	787
Turkey Bacon, Cooked 1 oz (28g)	107	8	2	27	1	0.0	--	8	640
Turkey Breast Meat 1 slice, (3-1/2" square; 8 per 6 oz pkg) (21g)	22	0	0	9	1	0.1	1	4	213

Food Serving size	Cal.	(g) Total Fat	(g) Sat. Fat	(mg) Chol.	(g) Carb.	(g) Fiber	(g) Sug.	(g) Prot.	(mg) Sod.
Turkey Breast, Law Salt, Pepackaged or Deli, Luncheon Meat									
1 slice, NFS (28g)	28	0	0	12	0	0.1	1	6	216
Turkey Breast, Pre-basted, Meat and Skin, Cooked, Roasted									
.5 breast, bone removed (864g)	1089	30	8	363	0	0.0	--	191	3430
Turkey Ham, Cured Turkey Thigh Meat									
1 serving (28g)	35	1	0	20	1	0.1	0	5	312
Turkey Ham, Sliced Especially Lean, Prepackaged or Deli-sliced									
1 cubic inch (20g)	25	1	0	13	1	0.0	--	4	208
Turkey Patties, Breaded, Battered, Fried									
1 thick, slice (approx 3" x 2" x 3/8") (42g)	119	8	2	32	7	0.2	0	6	336
Turkey Roll, Light and Dark Meat									
2 slices (57g)	85	4	1	31	1	0.0	0	10	334
Turkey Roll, Light Meat									
1 slice, rectangle (29g)	28	0	0	10	1	0.0	0	4	302
Turkey Sausage, Reduced Fat, Brown and Serve, Cooked									
1 cup (128g)	261	13	4	74	14	0.4	0	22	790
Turkey Sticks, Breaded, Battered, Fried									
1 stick (2.25 oz) (64g)	179	11	3	41	11	--	--	9	536
Turkey Thigh, Pre-basted, Meat and Skin, Cooked, Roasted									
1 thigh, bone removed (314g)	493	27	8	195	0	0.0	--	59	1372
Turkey, All Classes, Back, Meat and Skin, Cooked, Roasted									
.5 back, bone removed (262g)	639	38	11	238	0	0.0	0	70	191
Turkey, All Classes, Breast, Meat and Skin, Cooked, Roasted									
.5 breast, bone removed (864g)	1633	64	18	639	0	0.0	--	248	544
Turkey, All Classes, Dark Meat, Cooked, Roasted									
1 unit (yield from 1 lb ready-to-cook turkey) (91g)	171	7	2	77	0	0.0	0	26	72
Turkey, All Classes, Dark Meat, Meat and Skin, Cooked, Roasted									
1 unit (yield from 1 lb ready-to-cook turkey) (104g)	230	12	4	93	0	0.0	0	29	79
Turkey, All Classes, Giblets, Cooked, Simmered, Some Giblet Fat									
1 unit (yield from 1 lb ready-to-cook turkey) (10g)	20	1	0	29	0	0.0	0	2	6

Food Serving size	Cal.	(g) Total Fat	(g) Sat. Fat	(mg) Chol.	(g) Carb.	(g) Fiber	(g) Sug.	(g) Prot.	(mg) Sod.
Turkey, All Classes, Leg, Meat and Skin, Cooked, Roasted									
1 leg, bone removed (546g)	1136	54	17	464	1	0.0	0	152	420
Turkey, All Classes, Light Meat, Cooked, Roasted									
1 unit (yield from 1 lb ready-to-cook turkey) (117g)	184	4	1	81	0	0.0	0	35	75
Turkey, All Classes, Light Meat, Meat and Skin, Cooked, Roasted									
1 unit (yield from 1 lb ready-to-cook turkey) (136g)	268	11	3	103	0	0.0	0	39	86
Turkey, All Classes, Meat and Skin and Giblets and Neck, Cooked, Roasted									
1 turkey (4023g)	8247	380	111	3822	3	0.0	--	1126	2695
Turkey, All Classes, Meat and Skin, Cooked, Roasted									
1 unit (yield from 1 lb ready-to-cook turkey) (240g)	499	23	7	197	0	0.0	0	67	163
Turkey, All Classes, Meat Only, Cooked, Roasted									
1 unit (yield from 1 lb ready-to-cook turkey) (208g)	354	10	3	158	0	0.0	0	61	146
Turkey, All Classes, Neck, Meat Only, Cooked, Simmered									
1 neck, bone and skin removed (152g)	274	11	3	185	0	0.0	0	41	85
Turkey, All Classes, Skin Only, Cooked, Roasted									
.5 turkey, skin only (248g)	1099	98	26	280	1	0.0	--	49	131
Turkey, All Classes, Wing, Meat and Skin, Cooked, Roasted									
1 wing, bone removed (186g)	426	23	6	151	0	0.0	0	51	113
Turkey, Breast, Smoked, Lemon Pepper Flavor, 97% Fat Free									
1 slice (28g)	27	0	0	13	0	0.0	0	6	325
Turkey, Canned, Meat Only, with Broth									
1 can (5 oz) (142g)	240	10	3	94	2	0.0	0	34	663
Turkey, Diced, Light and Dark Meat, Seasoned									
.5 lb (227g)	313	14	4	125	2	0.0	--	42	1930
Turkey, Drumstick, Smoked, Cooked, with Skin and Bone Removed									
1 oz, with bone, cooked (yield after bone removed) (21g)	42	2	1	18	0	0.0	0	6	209
Turkey, Fryer-roasters, Back, Meat and Skin, Cooked, Roasted									
1 unit (yield from 1 lb ready-to-cook turkey) (37g)	75	4	1	40	0	0.0	--	10	26

Food Serving size	Cal.	(g) Total Fat	(g) Sat. Fat	(mg) Chol.	(g) Carb.	(g) Fiber	(g) Sug.	(g) Prot.	(mg) Sod.
Turkey, Fryer-roasters, Back, Meat Only, Cooked, Roasted .5 back, bone and skin removed (99g)	168	6	2	94	0	0.0	--	28	72
Turkey, Fryer-roasters, Breast, Meat and Skin, Cooked, Roasted .5 breast, bone removed (344g)	526	11	3	310	0	0.0	--	100	182
Turkey, Fryer-roasters, Breast, Meat Only, Cooked, Roasted .5 breast, bone and skin removed (306g)	413	2	1	254	0	0.0	0	92	159
Turkey, Fryer-roasters, Dark Meat, Meat and Skin, Cooked, Roasted .5 turkey, bone removed (374g)	681	26	8	438	0	0.0	--	104	284
Turkey, Fryer-roasters, Dark Meat, Meat Only, Cooked, Roasted 1 unit (yield from 1 lb ready-to-cook turkey) (91g)	147	4	1	102	0	0.0	--	26	72
Turkey, Fryer-roasters, Leg, Meat and Skin, Cooked, Roasted 1 leg, bone removed (245g)	417	13	4	172	0	0.0	--	70	196
Turkey, Fryer-roasters, Leg, Meat Only, Cooked, Roasted 1 leg, bone and skin removed (224g)	356	8	3	267	0	0.0	--	65	181
Turkey, Fryer-roasters, Light Meat, Meat and Skin, Cooked, Roasted .5 turkey, bone removed (433g)	710	20	5	411	0	0.0	--	125	247
Turkey, Fryer-roasters, Light Meat, Meat Only, Cooked, Roasted 1 unit (yield from 1 lb ready-to-cook turkey) (104g)	146	1	0	89	0	0.0	--	31	58
Turkey, Fryer-roasters, Meat and Skin and Giblets and Neck, Cooked, Roasted 1 turkey (1772g)	3030	100	29	2091	1	0.0	--	498	1152
Turkey, Fryer-roasters, Meat and Skin, Cooked, Roasted .5 turkey, bone removed (808g)	1390	46	13	848	0	0.0	0	228	533
Turkey, Fryer-roasters, Meat Only, Cooked, Roasted 1 unit (yield from 1 lb ready-to-cook turkey) (195g)	293	5	2	191	0	0.0	--	58	131
Turkey, Fryer-roasters, Skin Only, Cooked, Roasted .5 turkey, skin only (121g)	362	28	7	174	0	0.0	--	25	74
Turkey, Fryer-roasters, Wing, Meat and Skin, Cooked, Roasted 1 wing, bone removed (90g)	186	9	2	104	0	0.0	--	25	66
Turkey, Fryer-roasters, Wing, Meat Only, Cooked, Roasted 1 wing, bone and skin removed (60g)	98	2	1	61	0	0.0	0	19	47

Food Serving size	Cal.	(g) Total Fat	(g) Sat. Fat	(mg) Chol.	(g) Carb.	(g) Fiber	(g) Sug.	(g) Prot.	(mg) Sod.
Turkey, Gizzard, All Classes, Cooked, Simmered									
1 gizzard (84g)	108	3	1	171	0	0.0	0	18	56
Turkey, Heart, All Classes, Cooked, Simmered									
10 hearts (207g)	282	10	3	381	1	0.0	0	44	186
Turkey, Light or Dark Meat, Smoked, Cooked, with Skin and Bone Removed									
1 oz, boneless (28.35g)	57	3	1	23	0	0.0	1	8	282
Turkey, Liver, All Classes, Cooked, Simmered									
1 liver (83g)	227	17	6	322	1	0.0	0	17	46
Turkey, Wing, Smoked, Cooked, with Skin and Bone Removed									
1 oz, with bone, cooked (yield after bone removed) (19g)	42	2	1	15	0	0.0	0	5	189
Turkey, Young Hen, Back, Meat and Skin, Cooked, Roasted									
1 unit (yield from 1 lb ready-to-cook turkey) (35g)	89	5	2	30	0	0.0	--	9	24
Turkey, Young Hen, Breast, Meat and Skin, Cooked, Roasted									
.5 breast, bone removed (686g)	1331	54	15	494	0	0.0	--	198	398
Turkey, Young Hen, Dark Meat, Meat and Skin, Cooked, Roasted									
.5 turkey, bone and skin removed (665g)	1543	85	26	559	0	0.0	--	182	479
Turkey, Young Hen, Dark Meat, Meat Only, Cooked, Roasted									
1 unit (yield from 1 lb ready-to-cook turkey) (93g)	179	7	2	74	0	0.0	--	26	70
Turkey, Young Hen, Leg, Meat and Skin, Cooked, Roasted									
1 leg, bone removed (448g)	954	47	15	367	0	0.0	--	124	327
Turkey, Young Hen, Light Meat, Meat and Skin, Cooked, Roasted									
.5 turkey, bone removed (859g)	1778	81	23	636	0	0.0	--	246	498
Turkey, Young Hen, Light Meat, Meat Only, Cooked, Roasted									
1 unit (yield from 1 lb ready-to-cook turkey) (119g)	192	4	1	81	0	0.0	--	36	71
Turkey, Young Hen, Meat and Skin and Giblets and Neck, Cooked, Roasted									
1 turkey (3300g)	7095	348	102	3102	2	0.0	--	924	2079
Turkey, Young Hen, Meat and Skin, Cooked, Roasted									
.5 turkey, bone removed (1524g)	3322	166	48	1189	0	0.0	--	428	975
Turkey, Young Hen, Meat Only, Cooked, Roasted									
1 unit (yield from 1 lb ready-to-cook turkey) (212g)	371	12	4	155	0	0.0	--	62	142

Food Serving size	Cal.	(g) Total Fat	(g) Sat. Fat	(mg) Chol.	(g) Carb.	(g) Fiber	(g) Sug.	(g) Prot.	(mg) Sod.
Turkey, Young Hen, Skin Only, Cooked, Roasted .5 turkey, skin only (196g)	945	87	23	208	0	0.0	--	37	86
Turkey, Young Hen, Wing, Meat and Skin, Cooked, Roasted 1 wing, bone removed (174g)	414	23	6	134	0	0.0	--	48	97
Turkey, Young Tom, Back, Meat and Skin, Cooked, Roasted 1 unit (yield from 1 lb ready-to-cook turkey) (33g)	79	5	1	31	0	0.0	--	9	25
Turkey, Young Tom, Breast, Meat and Skin, Cooked, Roasted .5 breast, bone removed (1329g)	2512	98	28	997	0	0.0	--	380	890
Turkey, Young Tom, Dark Meat, Meat and Skin, Cooked, Roasted .5 turkey, bone removed (1184g)	2557	128	39	1077	0	0.0	--	327	947
Turkey, Young Tom, Dark Meat, Meat Only, Cooked, Roasted 1 unit (yield from 1 lb ready-to-cook turkey) (90g)	167	6	2	79	0	0.0	--	26	74
Turkey, Young Tom, Leg, Meat and Skin, Cooked, Roasted 1 unit (yield from 1 lb ready-to-cook turkey) (70g)	144	7	2	63	0	0.0	--	20	56
Turkey, Young Tom, Light Meat, Meat and Skin, Cooked, Roasted .5 turkey, bone removed (1566g)	2991	121	34	1175	0	0.0	--	446	1049
Turkey, Young Tom, Light Meat, Meat Only, Cooked, Roasted 1 unit (yield from 1 lb ready-to-cook turkey) (117g)	180	3	1	81	0	0.0	--	35	80
Turkey, Young Tom, Meat and Skin, Cooked, Roasted .5 turkey, bone removed (2750g)	5555	249	73	2255	0	0.0	--	772	1980
Turkey, Young Tom, Meat Only, Cooked, Roasted 1 unit (yield from 1 lb ready-to-cook turkey) (206g)	346	10	3	159	0	0.0	--	60	152
Turkey, Young Tom, Meats and Skin and Giblets and Neck, Cooked, Roasted 1 turkey (5957g)	11854	525	154	5719	6	0.0	--	1666	4289
Turkey, Young Tom, Skin Only, Cooked, Roasted .5 turkey, skin only (374g)	1578	139	36	438	0	0.0	--	75	224
Turkey, Young Tom, Wing, Meat and Skin, Cooked, Roasted 1 wing, bone removed (237g)	524	27	7	192	0	0.0	--	65	156

Food Serving size	Cal.	(g) Total Fat	(g) Sat. Fat	(mg) Chol.	(g) Carb.	(g) Fiber	(g) Sug.	(g) Prot.	(mg) Sod.

Sausages and Luncheon Meats

Bacon and Beef Sticks
1 oz (28g) | 145 | 12 | 4 | 29 | 0 | 0.0 | 0 | 8 | 398

Barbecue Loaf, Pork, Beef
1 slice (5-7/8" x 3-1/2" x 1/16") (23g)
| | 40 | 2 | 1 | 9 | 1 | 0.0 | -- | 4 | 307

Beerwurst, Beer Salami, Pork
1 slice (2-3/4" dia x 1/16") (6g)
| | 14 | 1 | 0 | 4 | 0 | 0.0 | -- | 1 | 74

Beerwurst, Beer Salami, Pork and Beef
2 oz (56g) | 155 | 13 | 5 | 35 | 2 | 0.5 | 0 | 8 | 410

Beerwurst, Pork and Beef
1 serving, 2 oz (56g) | 155 | 13 | 5 | 35 | 2 | 0.5 | 0 | 8 | 410

Blood Sausage
4 slices (100g) | 379 | 35 | 13 | 120 | 1 | 0.0 | 1 | 15 | 680

Bologna, Beef
1 slice (28g) | 87 | 8 | 3 | 16 | 1 | 0.0 | 0 | 3 | 302

Bologna, Beef and Pork
3.527 oz (100g) | 308 | 25 | 9 | 60 | 5 | 0.0 | 4 | 15 | 736

Bologna, Beef and Pork, Low Fat
1 cubic inch (14g) | 32 | 3 | 1 | 5 | 0 | 0.0 | -- | 2 | 155

Bologna, Beef, Low Fat
1 cubic inch (14g) | 29 | 2 | 1 | 6 | 1 | 0.0 | 0 | 2 | 165

Bologna, Chicken, Pork
1 slice (28g) | 94 | 9 | 3 | 24 | 1 | 0.0 | 0 | 3 | 347

Bologna, Chicken, Pork, Beef
1 slice (28g) | 76 | 6 | 2 | 23 | 2 | 0.0 | 0 | 3 | 314

Bologna, Chicken, Turkey, Pork
1 slice (28g) | 83 | 7 | 2 | 22 | 2 | 0.0 | 0 | 3 | 258

Bologna, Pork
1 slice (4" dia x 1/8" thick) (23g)
| | 57 | 5 | 2 | 14 | 0 | 0.0 | 0 | 4 | 272

Bologna, Pork and Turkey Lite
1 serving, 2 oz (56g) | 118 | 9 | 3 | 44 | 2 | 0.0 | 0 | 7 | 401

Bologna, Pork, Turkey and Beef
1 oz (28.35g) | 95 | 8 | 3 | 21 | 2 | 0.0 | 0 | 3 | 299

Food Serving size	Cal.	(g) Total Fat	(g) Sat. Fat	(mg) Chol.	(g) Carb.	(g) Fiber	(g) Sug.	(g) Prot.	(mg) Sod.
Bologna, Turkey 1 serving (28g)	59	4	1	21	1	0.1	1	3	351
Bratwurst, Beef and Pork, Smoked 1 serving, 2.33 oz (66g)	196	17	4	51	1	0.0	0	8	560
Bratwurst, Chicken, Cooked 1 serving, 2.96 oz (84g)	148	9	--	60	0	0.0	0	16	60
Bratwurst, Pork, Beef and Turkey, Lite, Smoked 1 serving, 2.33 oz (66g)	123	9	--	37	1	0.0	1	10	648
Bratwurst, Pork, Beef, Link 1 link (70g)	226	19	7	44	2	0.0	2	10	778
Bratwurst, Pork, Cooked 1 link, cooked (85g)	283	25	8	63	2	0.0	0	12	719
Bratwurst, Veal, Cooked 1 serving, 2.96 oz (84g)	286	27	13	66	0	0.0	0	12	50
Braunschweiger (a Liver Sausage), Pork 1 slice, (2-1/2" dia x 1/4" thick) (18g)	59	5	2	32	1	0.0	0	3	209
Butcher Boy Meats, Inc., Turkey Franks 1 serving (56g)	134	10	3	58	3	0.1	1	8	651
Cheesefurter, Cheese Smoky, Pork, Beef 2.33 links (100g)	328	29	10	68	1	0.0	2	14	1082
Chicken Roll, Light Meat 1 pkg (170g)	187	5	1	77	8	0.0	1	28	1800
Chicken Spread 1 serving (1 serving) (56g)	88	10	2	31	2	0.2	0	10	404
Chorizo, Pork and Beef 1 link (4" long) (60g)	273	23	9	53	1	0.0	0	14	741
Corned Beef Loaf, Jellied 2 slices (57g)	87	3	1	27	0	0.0	--	13	543
Dutch Brand Loaf, Chicken, Pork and Beef 1 slice (38g)	104	9	3	23	1	0.1	0	5	401
Frankfurter Meat 1 serving (1 hot dog) (52g)	151	13	--	40	2	0.0	--	5	567
Frankfurter Meat, Heated 1 serving (1 hot dog) (52g)	145	13	--	38	3	0.0	--	5	527

Food Serving size	Cal.	(g) Total Fat	(g) Sat. Fat	(mg) Chol.	(g) Carb.	(g) Fiber	(g) Sug.	(g) Prot.	(mg) Sod.
Frankfurter, Beef 1 frankfurter (5 in long x 7/8 in dia, 8 per lb) (57g)	188	17	7	30	2	0.0	2	6	650
Frankfurter, Beef and Pork 1 frankfurter (45g)	137	12	5	23	1	0.0	0	5	504
Frankfurter, Beef and Pork, Low Fat 1 frankfurter (57g)	87	6	2	25	3	0.0	--	6	716
Frankfurter, Beef, Heated 1 serving (52g)	170	15	6	29	2	0.0	2	6	600
Frankfurter, Beef, Low Fat 1 frankfurter (57g)	131	11	5	23	1	0.0	--	7	593
Frankfurter, Beef, Pork and Turkey, Fat Free 1 frankfurter, 1 NLEA serving (57g)	62	1	0	23	6	0.0	0	7	455
Frankfurter, Chicken 1 link (45g)	100	7	2	43	1	0.2	0	7	380
Frankfurter, Meat and Poultry, Low Fat 1 cup, sliced (143g)	173	4	1	63	12	0.1	3	22	1406
Frankfurter, Meatless 1 frankfurter (70g)	163	10	1	0	5	2.7	--	14	330
Frankfurter, Pork 1 link (76g)	204	18	7	50	0	0.1	0	10	620
Frankfurter, Turkey 1 frankfurter (45g)	100	8	2	35	2	0.0	1	6	485
Frankfurther, Low Sodium 1 frankfurter (57g)	178	16	7	35	1	0.0	--	7	177
Ham and Cheese Loaf or Roll 2 slices (57g)	137	11	4	33	2	0.0	0	8	616
Ham and Cheese Spread 1 oz (28.35g)	69	5	2	17	1	0.0	--	5	339
Ham Salad Spread 1 oz (28.35g)	61	4	1	10	3	0.0	0	2	259
Ham, Chopped, Canned 1 slice (4-1/4" x 4-1/4" x 1/16") (21g)	50	4	1	10	0	0.0	0	3	287

Food Serving size	Cal.	(g) Total Fat	(g) Sat. Fat	(mg) Chol.	(g) Carb.	(g) Fiber	(g) Sug.	(g) Prot.	(mg) Sod.
Ham, Chopped, Not Canned 1 slice (4-1/4" x 4-1/4" x 1/16") (21g)	38	2	1	12	1	0.0	0	3	279
Ham, Honey Smoked, Cooked 1.94 oz (1 serving) (55g)	67	1	1	12	4	0.0	0	10	495
Ham, Minced 1 slice (4-1/4" x 4-1/4" x 1/16") (21g)	55	4	2	15	0	0.0	0	3	261
Ham, Sliced, Extra Lean 1 slice, rectangle (24g)	26	1	0	11	0	0.0	0	5	254
Ham, Sliced, Regular (Approximately 11% Fat) 1 slice (28g)	46	2	1	16	1	0.4	0	5	365
Headcheese, Pork 45g	71	5	2	31	0	0.0	0	6	374
Honey Loaf, Pork, Beef 1 slice (28g)	35	1	0	10	3	0.2	0	3	370
Honey Roll Sausage, Beef 1 oz (28.35g)	52	3	1	14	1	0.0	--	5	375
Hormel, Always Tender, Boneless Pork Loin, Fresh Pork 1 serving (112g)	162	8	3	55	1	--	0	21	401
Hormel, Always Tender, Center Cut Chops, Fresh Pork 1 serving (112g)	187	11	4	58	1	--	0	21	423
Hormel, Always Tender, Pork Loin Filets, Lemon Garlic Flavored 1 serving (112g)	132	5	2	47	2	--	0	20	661
Hormel, Always Tender, Pork Tenderloin, Peppercorn Flavored 4 oz (112g)	123	4	1	53	2	--	0	19	665
Hormel, Always Tender, Pork Tenderloin, Teriyaki Flavored 4 oz (112g)	133	3	1	52	5	--	4	20	463
Hormel, Canadian Style Bacon 1 serving (56g)	68	3	1	27	1	--	1	9	569
Hormel, Cure 81 Ham 1 serving (84g)	89	3	1	43	0	--	0	15	872
Hormel, Pillow Pack, Sliced Turkey Pepperoni 1 serving (30g)	73	3	1	37	1	0.0	0	9	557

Food Serving size	Cal.	(g) Total Fat	(g) Sat. Fat	(mg) Chol.	(g) Carb.	(g) Fiber	(g) Sug.	(g) Prot.	(mg) Sod.
Hormel, Spam, Light Lunch Meat, Pork and Chicken, Minced, Canned, Vitamin C Added 1 oz (28g)	53	4	1	21	0	0.0	0	4	289
Hormel, Spam, Luncheon Meat, Pork with Ham, Minced, Canned 1 serving, 2 oz (56g)	174	15	6	39	2	0.0	--	7	767
Hormel, Wrangler Beef Franks 1 frankfurter (56g)	162	14	6	38	1	0.0	1	7	557
Kielbasa, Kolbassy, Pork, Beef, Non-fat Dry Milk 1 ring (467g)	1443	127	43	308	13	0.0	7	57	4222
Kielbasa, Polish, Turkey and Beef, Smoked 1 serving, 2 oz (56g)	127	10	3	39	2	0.0	0	7	672
Knackwurst, Knockwurst, Pork, Beef 1 oz (28.35g)	87	8	3	17	1	0.0	0	3	264
Lebanon, Bologna, Beef 1 oz (28.35g)	49	3	1	16	0	0.0	0	5	390
Liver Cheese, Pork 1 slice (38g)	116	10	3	66	1	0.0	--	6	466
Liver Sausage, Liverwurst, Pork 1 oz (28.35g)	92	8	3	45	1	0.0	--	4	244
Liverwurst Spread .25 cup (55g)	168	14	5	65	3	1.4	1	7	385
Loma Linda Big Franks, Canned Unprepared 1 link (51g)	111	6	1	0	3	1.8	2	11	217
Loma Linda Linketts, Canned, Unprepared 1 link (35g)	73	4	1	0	2	1.1	0	7	140
Loma Linda Little Links, Canned, Unprepared 2 links (46g)	102	6	1	0	3	1.9	0	9	217
Loma Linda Low Fat Big Franks, Canned, Unprepared 1 link (51g)	79	2	0	0	2	2.1	0	12	245
Loma Linda Vege-burger, Canned, Unprepared .25 cup (55g)	63	1	0	0	2	1.4	0	12	122
Louis Rich, Chicken (White, Oven Roasted) 1 serving (28g)	36	2	0	17	1	0.0	0	5	335
Louis Rich, Chicken Breast (Oven Roasted Deluxe) 1 serving (28g)	28	1	0	14	1	0.0	0	5	333

Food Serving size	Cal.	(g) Total Fat	(g) Sat. Fat	(mg) Chol.	(g) Carb.	(g) Fiber	(g) Sug.	(g) Prot.	(mg) Sod.
Louis Rich, Chicken Breast Classic, Baked, Grilled (Carving Board)									
1 slice (22g)	22	0	0	11	1	0.0	0	4	251
Louis Rich, Franks (Turkey and Chicken Cheese)									
1 serving (45g)	90	7	2	42	2	0.0	1	6	482
Louis Rich, Franks (Turkey and Chicken)									
1 serving (45g)	85	6	2	41	2	0.0	1	5	511
Louis Rich, Turkey (Honey Roasted, Fat Free)									
1 serving (56g)	57	0	0	22	3	0.0	2	11	661
Louis Rich, Turkey Bacon									
1 serving (14g)	35	3	1	13	0	0.0	0	2	170
Louis Rich, Turkey Bologna									
1 serving (28g)	52	4	1	19	1	0.0	0	3	302
Louis Rich, Turkey Breast (Oven Roasted, Fat Free)									
1 serving (28g)	24	0	0	9	1	0.0	0	4	334
Louis Rich, Turkey Breast (Oven Roasted, Portion Fat Free)									
1 serving (56g)	50	0	0	22	1	0.0	0	11	659
Louis Rich, Turkey Breast (Smoked, Carving Board)									
1 slice (22g)	21	0	0	9	0	0.0	0	4	264
Louis Rich, Turkey Breast (Smoked, Portion Fat Free)									
1 serving (56g)	52	0	0	23	1	0.0	0	11	721
Louis Rich, Turkey Breast and White Turkey (Oven Roasted)									
1 serving (28g)	28	1	0	11	1	0.0	0	5	270
Louis Rich, Turkey Breast and White Turkey (Smoked Sliced)									
1 serving (28g)	28	1	0	12	1	0.0	0	5	257
Louis Rich, Turkey Ham (10% Water)									
1 serving (28g)	32	1	0	19	0	0.0	0	5	316
Louis Rich, Turkey Nuggets/Sticks (Breaded)									
1 serving (85g)	235	15	3	34	13	0.4	0	12	577
Louis Rich, Turkey Salami									
1 serving (28g)	41	3	1	21	0	0.0	0	4	281
Louis Rich, Turkey Salami Cotto									
1 serving (28g)	42	3	1	22	0	0.0	0	4	285
Louis Rich, Turkey Smoked Sausage									
1 serving (56g)	90	6	1	37	2	0.0	2	8	530

Food Serving size	Cal.	(g) Total Fat	(g) Sat. Fat	(mg) Chol.	(g) Carb.	(g) Fiber	(g) Sug.	(g) Prot.	(mg) Sod.
Luncheon Meat, Beef, Loaved 2 slices (57g)	176	15	6	36	2	0.0	0	8	758
Luncheon Meat, Beef, Thin Sliced 1 slice, rectangle (13.8g)	16	0	0	7	0	0.0	0	2	154
Luncheon Meat, Pork and Chicken, Minced, Canned, Including Spam Lite 2 oz (1 serving) (56g)	110	8	3	42	1	0.0	1	9	578
Luncheon Meat, Pork, Beef 1 slice (4" x 4" x 3/32" thick) (57g)	201	18	7	31	1	0.0	0	7	737
Luncheon Meat, Pork, Canned 1 slice (4-1/4" x 4-1/4" x 1/16") (21g)	70	6	2	13	0	0.0	0	3	271
Luncheon Meat, Pork, Ham and Chicken, Minced, Canned, Reduced Sodium, Vitamin C (Spam) 2 oz, 1 NLEA serving (56g)	164	14	5	43	2	0.0	0	7	530
Luncheon Meat, Pork, with Ham, Minced, Canned, Including Spam (Hormel) 2 oz, 1 NLEA serving (56g)	176	15	6	40	3	0.0	0	8	745
Luncheon Sausage, Pork and Beef 1 oz (28.35g)	74	6	2	18	0	0.0	--	4	335
Luncheon Slices, Meatless 1 slice, thin (14g)	26	2	0	0	1	0.0	0	2	100
Macaroni and Cheese Loaf, Chicken, Pork and Beef 1 slice (38g)	87	6	2	17	4	0.0	0	4	1
Meatballs, Meatless 1 cup (144g)	284	13	2	0	12	6.6	--	30	792
Mortadella, Beef, Pork 1 slice (15 per 8 oz pkg) (15g)	47	4	1	8	0	0.0	0	2	187
New England Brand, Sausage, Pork, Beef 1 oz (28.35g)	46	2	1	14	1	0.0	--	5	346
Olive Loaf, Pork 2 slices (57g)	134	9	3	22	5	0.0	0	7	846
Oscar Mayer, Bologna (Beef) 1 serving (1 slice) (28g)	88	8	4	18	1	0.0	0	3	330
Oscar Mayer, Bologna (Beef, Light) 1 serving (1 slice) (28g)	56	4	2	12	2	0.0	1	3	322

Food Serving size	Cal.	(g) Total Fat	(g) Sat. Fat	(mg) Chol.	(g) Carb.	(g) Fiber	(g) Sug.	(g) Prot.	(mg) Sod.
Oscar Mayer, Bologna (Chicken, Pork, Beef) 1 serving (28g)	89	8	3	29	1	0.0	0	3	289
Oscar Mayer, Bologna (Fat Free) 1 serving (28g)	22	0	0	7	2	0.0	1	4	274
Oscar Mayer, Bologna (Wisconsin Made Ring) 1 serving (56g)	175	16	6	35	1	0.0	1	7	463
Oscar Mayer, Bologna Light (Pork, Chicken, Beef) 1 serving (1 slice) (28g)	57	4	2	16	2	0.0	1	3	313
Oscar Mayer, Braunschweiger Liver Sausage (Saren Tube) 1 serving (56g)	191	17	6	90	1	0.1	0	8	626
Oscar Mayer, Braunschweiger Liver Sausage (Sliced) 1 serving (1 slice) (28g)	93	8	3	50	1	0.1	0	4	325
Oscar Mayer, Chicken Breast (Honey Glazed) 1 serving (4 slices) (52g)	57	1	0	28	2	0.0	2	10	748
Oscar Mayer, Chicken Breast (Oven Roasted, Fat Free) 1 slice (13g)	11	0	0	6	0	0.0	0	2	161
Oscar Mayer, Ham (40% Ham/Water Product, Smoked, Fat Free) 1 slice (16g)	12	0	0	6	0	0.0	0	2	173
Oscar Mayer, Ham (Chopped with Natural Juice) 1 serving (1 slice) (28g)	50	3	1	17	1	0.0	1	5	350
Oscar Mayer, Ham (Water Added, Baked, Cooked, 96% Fat Free) 1 serving (3 slices) (63g)	66	2	1	30	1	0.0	1	10	782
Oscar Mayer, Ham (Water, Boiled) 1 slice (21g)	22	1	0	10	0	0.0	0	3	283
Oscar Mayer, Ham (Water, Honey) 1 slice (21g)	23	1	0	9	1	0.0	1	4	262
Oscar Mayer, Ham (Water, Smoked, Cooked) 1 slice (21g)	21	1	0	10	0	0.0	0	3	255
Oscar Mayer, Ham and Cheese Loaf 1 serving (28g)	66	5	2	17	1	0.0	1	4	327
Oscar Mayer, Head Cheese 1 serving (28g)	52	4	1	25	0	0.0	0	4	300
Oscar Mayer, Liver Cheese, Pork Fat Wrapped 1 slice (38g)	119	10	4	80	1	0.0	0	6	420

Food Serving size	Cal.	(g) Total Fat	(g) Sat. Fat	(mg) Chol.	(g) Carb.	(g) Fiber	(g) Sug.	(g) Prot.	(mg) Sod.
Oscar Mayer, Luncheon Loaf (Spiced)									
1 serving (28g)	66	5	2	19	2	0.0	1	4	343
Oscar Mayer, Old Fashioned Loaf									
1 serving (28g)	65	5	2	17	2	0.0	1	4	332
Oscar Mayer, Olive Loaf (Chicken, Pork, Turkey)									
1 serving (28g)	74	6	2	20	2	0.0	1	3	369
Oscar Mayer, Pickle, Pimento Loaf (with Chicken)									
1 serving (28g)	75	6	2	22	3	0.0	2	3	357
Oscar Mayer, Pork Sausage Links (Cooked)									
1 link (24g)	82	7	3	18	0	0.0	0	4	201
Oscar Mayer, Salam, Beef Cotto									
1 slice (23g)	47	4	2	19	0	0.0	0	3	301
Oscar Mayer, Salami (for Beer)									
1 slice (23g)	52	4	1	16	0	0.0	0	3	283
Oscar Mayer, Salami (Genoa)									
1 slice (9g)	35	3	1	9	0	0.0	0	2	164
Oscar Mayer, Salami (Hard)									
1 slice (9g)	33	3	1	9	0	0.0	0	2	178
Oscar Mayer, Salami Cotto (Beef, Pork, Chicken)									
1 slice (23g)	56	5	2	18	1	0.0	0	3	252
Oscar Mayer, Sandwich Spread (Pork, Chicken, Beef)									
1 serving (30g)	71	5	2	14	5	0.1	2	2	246
Oscar Mayer, Simmer Sausage, Beef Thuringer Cervalat									
1 slice (23g)	71	6	3	18	0	0.0	0	3	328
Oscar Mayer, Simmer Sausage, Thuringer Cervalat									
1 slice (23g)	70	6	2	19	0	0.0	0	3	329
Oscar Mayer, Smokies (Beef)									
1 serving (1 link) (43g)	127	11	5	27	1	0.0	1	5	416
Oscar Mayer, Smokies (Cheese)									
1 serving (43g)	130	12	4	30	1	0.0	1	6	450
Oscar Mayer, Smokies Links Sausage									
1 serving (43g)	130	12	4	27	1	0.0	1	5	433
Oscar Mayer, Smokies Sausage Little (Pork, Turkey)									
1 serving (57g)	172	15	5	36	1	0.0	1	7	583

Food Serving size	Cal.	(g) Total Fat	(g) Sat. Fat	(mg) Chol.	(g) Carb.	(g) Fiber	(g) Sug.	(g) Prot.	(mg) Sod.
Oscar Mayer, Smokies Sausage Little Cheese (Pork, Turkey)									
1 serving (57g)	180	16	6	38	1	0.0	0	8	591
Oscar Mayer, Turkey Breast (Smoked, Fat Free)									
1 slice (13g)	10	0	0	4	0	0.0	0	2	142
Oscar Mayer, Wieners (Beef Franks Bun Length)									
1 serving (1 link) (57g)	185	17	7	34	2	0.0	1	6	584
Oscar Mayer, Wieners (Beef Franks)									
1 serving (45g)	147	14	6	25	1	0.0	1	5	461
Oscar Mayer, Wieners (Beef Franks, Fat Free)									
1 serving (50g)	39	0	0	15	3	0.0	2	7	464
Oscar Mayer, Wieners (Beef Franks, Light)									
1 serving (57g)	110	8	4	28	2	0.0	1	6	615
Oscar Mayer, Wieners (Cheese Hot Dogs with Turkey)									
1 serving (45g)	143	13	5	33	1	0.0	1	5	514
Oscar Mayer, Wieners (Fat Free Hot Dogs)									
1 serving (50g)	37	0	0	15	2	0.0	1	6	487
Oscar Mayer, Wieners (Light Pork, Turkey, Beef)									
1 serving (57g)	111	8	3	35	2	0.0	1	7	591
Oscar Mayer, Wieners (Pork, Turkey)									
1 serving (1 link) (45g)	147	13	4	32	1	0.0	1	5	445
Oscar Mayer, Wieners Little (Pork, Turkey)									
1 serving (57g)	177	16	6	31	1	0.0	1	6	592
Oven Roasted, Chicken Breast Roll									
1 serving, 2 oz (56g)	75	4	1	22	1	0.0	0	8	494
Pate de Foie Gras, Canned (Goose Liver Pate), Smoked									
1 oz (28.35g)	131	12	4	43	1	0.0	--	3	198
Pate, Chicken Liver, Canned									
1 oz (28.35g)	57	4	1	111	2	0.0	0	4	109
Pate, Goose Liver, Smoked, Canned									
1 oz (28.35g)	131	12	4	43	1	0.0	--	3	198
Pate, Liver, Not Specified, Canned									
1 oz (28.35g)	90	8	3	72	0	0.0	--	4	198
Pate, Truffle Flavor									
1 serving, 2 oz (56g)	183	16	6	59	4	--	--	6	452

Food Serving size	Cal.	(g) Total Fat	(g) Sat. Fat	(mg) Chol.	(g) Carb.	(g) Fiber	(g) Sug.	(g) Prot.	(mg) Sod.
Peppered Loaf, Pork, Beef 3.52 slices (100g)	149	6	2	46	5	0.0	5	17	1523
Pepperoni, Pork, Beef 1 oz (28g)	138	12	4	29	0	0.0	0	6	463
Pickle and Pimento Loaf, Pork 2 slices (57g)	128	9	3	33	5	0.9	5	6	743
Polish Sausage, Pork 1 oz (28.35g)	92	8	3	20	0	0.0	--	4	248
Pork and Beef Sausage, Fresh, Cooked 1 patty, cooked (raw dimensions: 3-7/8" dia x 1/4" thick) (27g)	107	10	3	19	1	0.0	0	4	217
Pork, Sausage Rice Links, Brown and Serve, Cooked 3 links, 1 NLEA serving (60g)	244	23	4	40	1	0.0	--	8	413
Sandwiches and Burgers, Roast Beef Sandwich with Cheese 1 sandwich (176g)	473	18	9	77	45	--	--	32	1633
Sandwiches and Burgers, Steak Sandwich 1 sandwich (204g)	459	14	4	73	52	--	--	30	798
Sausage Berliner Pork, Beef 1 oz (28.35g)	65	5	2	13	1	0.0	1	4	368
Sausage Italian Sweet Links 1 link, 3 oz (84g)	125	7	3	25	2	0.0	0	14	479
Sausage Simmered Pork and Beef Sticks with Cheddar Cheese 1 oz (28.35g)	121	11	3	25	1	0.1	0	6	420
Sausage Turkey Breakfast Links, Mild 2 oz, 2 links (56g)	132	10	2	90	1	0.0	0	9	328
Sausage, Chicken and Beef, Smoked 1 cubic inch (18g)	53	4	1	13	0	0.0	--	3	184
Sausage, Chicken, Beef, Pork, Skinless, Smoked 1 link (84g)	181	12	4	101	7	0.0	2	11	869
Sausage, Italian Turkey, Smoked 1 serving, 2 oz (56g)	88	5	--	30	3	0.5	2	8	520
Sausage, Italian, Pork, Cooked 1 link, 5/lb (67g)	230	18	6	38	3	0.1	1	13	809
Sausage, Italian, Pork, Raw 1 link, 5/lb (91g)	315	29	10	69	1	0.0	--	13	665

Food Serving size	Cal.	(g) Total Fat	(g) Sat. Fat	(mg) Chol.	(g) Carb.	(g) Fiber	(g) Sug.	(g) Prot.	(mg) Sod.
Sausage, Meatless 1 patty (38g)	98	7	1	0	4	1.1	0	7	337
Sausage, Polish Pork and Beef, Smoked 1 serving, 2.67 oz (76g)	229	20	7	54	2	0.0	0	9	644
Sausage, Polish, Beef with Chicken, Hot 5 pieces (55g)	142	11	4	36	2	0.0	0	10	847
Sausage, Pork and Beef with Cheddar Cheese, Smoked 12 oz, serving 2.7 oz (77g)	228	20	7	49	2	0.0	0	10	653
Sausage, Smoked Link Sausage, Pork and Beef 16 oz (454g)	1453	130	44	263	11	0.0	0	54	4136
Sausage, Turkey, Hot, Smoked 2 oz (56g)	88	5	2	30	3	0.5	2	8	520
Sausage, Vienna, Canned, Chicken, Beef, Pork 7 sausages (drained contents from can, net wt 4 oz) (113g)	260	22	8	98	3	0.0	0	12	1095
Smoked Link Sausage, Pork 1 link, little (2" long x 3/4" dia) (16g)	49	5	1	10	0	0.0	0	2	132
Smoked Link Sausage, Pork and Beef, Flavor and Nonfat Dry Milk 2 oz (57g)	153	12	4	37	2	0.0	2	8	725
Smoked Link Sausage, Pork and Beef, Nonfat Dry Milk 1 link, little (2" long x 3/4" dia) (16g)	50	4	2	10	0	0.0	--	2	188
Swiss Wurst Pork and Beef with Swiss Cheese, Smoked 1 serving, 2.7 oz (77g)	236	21	--	47	1	0.0	0	10	637
Thuringer, Cervalat, Simmer Sausage, Beef, Pork 2 oz, 1 serving (56g)	203	17	6	41	2	0.0	0	10	728
Turkey and Pork Sausage, Fresh Bulk, Patty or Link, Cooked 1 oz (28g)	86	6	2	24	0	0.0	--	6	246
Turkey, Pork and Beef Sausage, Low Fat, Smoked 1 lb, 16 oz (453.6g)	458	11	4	95	52	2.7	0	36	3611
Turkey, Pork and Beef, Sausage, Reduced Fat, Smoked 1 cubic inch (14g)	34	2	1	9	0	0.0	--	3	134

Food Serving size	Cal.	(g) Total Fat	(g) Sat. Fat	(mg) Chol.	(g) Carb.	(g) Fiber	(g) Sug.	(g) Prot.	(mg) Sod.
Turkey, White, Rotisserie, Deli Cut									
1.69 oz (1 serving) (48g)	54	1	0	26	4	0.2	2	6	576
Yachtwurst, with Pistachio Nuts, Cooked									
1 serving, 2 oz (56g)	150	13	4	36	1	0.0	0	8	524

Dry Beans and Peas

Food Serving size	Cal.	Total Fat	Sat. Fat	Chol.	Carb.	Fiber	Sug.	Prot.	Sod.
Chickpeas (Garbanzo Beans, Bengal Grams), Mature Seeds, Canned									
1 cup (240g)	286	3	0	0	54	10.6	--	12	718
Chickpeas (Garbanzo Beans, Bengal Grams), Mature Seeds, Raw									
1 tbsp (12.5g)	46	1	0	0	8	2.2	1	2	3
Chickpeas, Mature Seeds, Cooked, Boiled, with Salt									
1 cup (164g)	269	4	0	0	45	12.5	8	15	399
Chickpeas, Mature Seeds, Cooked, Boiled, Without Salt									
1 cup (164g)	269	4	0	0	45	12.5	8	15	11
Cowpeas (Blackeyes), Immature Seeds, Cooked, Boiled, Drained, Without Salt									
1 cup (165g)	160	1	0	0	34	8.3	5	5	7
Cowpeas (Blackeyes), Immature Seeds, Frozen, Cooked, Boiled, Drained, Without Salt									
1 cup (170g)	224	1	0	0	40	10.9	8	14	9
Cowpeas (Blackeyes), Immature Seeds, Frozen, Unprepared									
1 pkg (10 oz) (284g)	395	2	1	0	71	14.2	--	26	17
Cowpeas (Blackeyes), Immature Seeds, Raw									
1 cup (145g)	131	1	0	0	27	7.3	4	4	6
Cowpeas, Cat Jang, Mature Seeds, Cooked, Boiled, with Salt									
1 cup (171g)	200	1	0	0	35	6.2	--	14	436
Cowpeas, Cat Jang, Mature Seeds, Cooked, Boiled, Without Salt									
1 cup (171g)	200	1	0	0	35	6.2	--	14	32
Cowpeas, Cat Jang, Mature Seeds, Raw									
1 cup (167g)	573	3	1	0	100	17.9	--	40	97
Cowpeas, Common (Blackeyes, Crowder, Southern), Mature Seeds, Raw									
1 tbsp (10.5g)	35	0	0	0	6	1.1	1	2	2
Cowpeas, Common (Blackeyes, Crowder, Southern), Mature, Cooked, Boiled, Without Salt									
1 cup (171g)	198	1	0	0	35	11.1	6	13	7

Food Serving size	Cal.	(g) Total Fat	(g) Sat. Fat	(mg) Chol.	(g) Carb.	(g) Fiber	(g) Sug.	(g) Prot.	(mg) Sod.
Cowpeas, Common, Mature Seeds, Canned with Pork									
1 cup (240g)	199	4	1	17	40	7.9	--	7	840
Cowpeas, Common, Mature Seeds, Canned, Plain									
1 cup (240g)	185	1	0	0	33	7.9	--	11	718
Cowpeas, Common, Mature Seeds, Cooked, Boiled, with Salt									
1 cup (171g)	198	1	0	0	35	11.1	6	13	410
Cowpeas, Leafy Tips, Cooked, Boiled, Drained, Without Salt									
1 cup, chopped (53g)	12	0	0	0	1	--	--	2	3
Cowpeas, Leafy Tips, Raw									
1 leaf (3g)	1	0	0	0	0	--	--	0	0
Cowpeas, Young Pods with Seeds, Cooked, Boiled, Drained, Without Salt									
1 cup (95g)	32	0	0	0	7	--	--	2	3
Cowpeas, Young Pods with Seeds, Raw									
1 pod (12g)	5	0	0	0	1	--	--	0	0
Frijoles Rojos Volteados (Refried Beans, Red, Canned)									
1 tbsp (15g)	22	1	0	--	2	0.7	--	1	56
Hummus, Commercial									
1 tbsp (15g)	25	1	0	0	2	0.9	--	1	57
Hummus, Home Prepared									
1 tablespoon (15g)	27	1	0	0	3	0.6	0	1	36
Hyacinth Beans, Immature Seeds, Cooked, Boiled, Drained, with Salt									
1 cup (87g)	44	0	0	0	8	--	--	3	207
Hyacinth Beans, Immature Seeds, Cooked, Boiled, Drained, Without Salt									
1 cup (87g)	44	0	0	0	8	--	--	3	2
Hyacinth Beans, Immature Seeds, Raw									
1 cup (80g)	37	0	0	0	7	--	--	2	2
Hyacinth Beans, Mature Seeds, Cooked, Boiled, with Salt									
1 cup (194g)	227	1	0	0	40	--	--	16	471
Hyacinth Beans, Mature Seeds, Cooked, Boiled, Without Salt									
1 cup (194g)	227	1	0	0	40	--	--	16	14
Hyacinth Beans, Mature Seeds, Raw									
1 cup (210g)	722	4	1	0	128	--	--	50	44
Lupins, Mature Seeds, Cooked, Boiled, with Salt									
1 cup (166g)	193	5	1	0	15	4.6	--	26	398

Food Serving size	Cal.	(g) Total Fat	(g) Sat. Fat	(mg) Chol.	(g) Carb.	(g) Fiber	(g) Sug.	(g) Prot.	(mg) Sod.
Mothbeans, Mature Seeds, Cooked, Boiled, with Salt									
1 cup (177g)	207	1	0	0	37	--	--	14	435
Mung Beans, Mature Seeds, Cooked, Boiled, with Salt									
1 cup (202g)	212	1	0	0	39	15.4	4	14	481
Mung Beans, Mature Seeds, Cooked, Boiled, Without Salt									
1 cup (202g)	212	1	0	0	39	15.4	4	14	4
Mung Beans, Mature Seeds, Raw									
1 tbsp (13g)	45	0	0	0	8	2.1	1	3	2
Mung Beans, Mature Seeds, Sprouted, Cooked, Boiled, Drained, with Salt									
1 cup (124g)	24	0	0	0	4	1.0	4	3	305
Mung Beans, Mature Seeds, Sprouted, Cooked, Boiled, Drained, Without Salt									
1 cup (124g)	26	0	0	0	5	1.0	4	3	12
Mung Beans, Mature Seeds, Sprouted, Cooked, Stir-fried									
1 cup (124g)	62	0	0	0	13	2.4	--	5	11
Mung Beans, Mature Seeds, Sprouted, Raw									
1 pkg (12 oz) (340g)	102	1	0	0	20	6.1	14	10	20
Mungo Beans, Mature Seeds, Cooked, Boiled, with Salt									
1 cup (180g)	189	1	0	0	33	11.5	4	14	437
Mungo Beans, Mature Seeds, Cooked, Boiled, Without Salt									
1 oz, dry, yield after cooking (69g)	72	0	0	0	13	4.4	1	5	5
Mungo Beans, Mature Seeds, Raw									
1 cup (207g)	706	3	0	0	122	37.9	--	52	79
Natto									
1 cup (175g)	371	19	3	0	25	9.5	9	31	12
Pigeon Peas (Reduced Grams), Mature Seeds, Cooked, Boiled, with Salt									
1 cup (168g)	203	1	0	0	39	11.3	--	11	405
Pigeon Peas (Reduced Grams), Mature Seeds, Cooked, Boiled, Without Salt									
1 cup (168g)	203	1	0	0	39	11.3	--	11	8
Pigeon Peas (Reduced Grams), Mature Seeds, Raw									
1 cup (205g)	703	3	1	0	129	30.8	--	44	35
Winged Beans, Mature Seeds, Cooked, Boiled, with Salt									
1 cup (172g)	253	10	1	0	26	--	--	18	428
Winged Beans, Mature Seeds, Cooked, Boiled, Without Salt									
1 cup (172g)	253	10	1	0	26	--	--	18	22

Food Serving size	Cal.	(g) Total Fat	(g) Sat. Fat	(mg) Chol.	(g) Carb.	(g) Fiber	(g) Sug.	(g) Prot.	(mg) Sod.
Winged Beans, Mature Seeds, Raw 1 cup (182g)	744	30	4	0	76	--	--	54	69

Nuts and Seeds

Food Serving size	Cal.	(g) Total Fat	(g) Sat. Fat	(mg) Chol.	(g) Carb.	(g) Fiber	(g) Sug.	(g) Prot.	(mg) Sod.
Acorns, Dried 1 oz (28.35g)	144	9	1	0	15	--	--	2	0
Acorns, Raw 1 oz (28.35g)	110	7	1	0	12	--	--	2	0
Almond Butter, Plain, with Salt 1 tbsp (16g)	98	9	1	0	3	1.6	1	3	34
Almond Butter, Plain, Without Salt 1 tbsp (16g)	98	9	1	0	3	1.6	1	3	1
Almond Paste 1 oz (28.35g)	130	8	1	0	14	1.4	10	3	3
Almonds 1 cup, sliced (92g)	529	45	3	0	20	11.2	4	20	1
Almonds, Blanched 1 tbsp (9.1g)	54	5	0	0	2	0.9	0	2	2
Almonds, Dry Roasted, with Salt 1 oz (22 whole kernels) (28.35g)	169	15	1	0	6	3.1	1	6	96
Almonds, Dry Roasted, Without Salt 1 oz (22 whole kernels) (28.35g)	169	15	1	0	6	3.1	1	6	1
Almonds, Honey Roasted, Unblanched 1 oz (28.35g)	168	14	1	0	8	3.9	--	5	37
Almonds, Oil Roasted, with Salt 1 oz (22 whole kernels) (28.35g)	172	16	1	0	5	3.0	1	6	96
Almonds, Oil Roasted, Without Salt 1 oz (22 whole kernels) (28.35g)	172	16	1	0	5	3.0	1	6	0
Beechnuts, Dried 1 oz (28.35g)	163	14	2	0	9	--	--	2	11
Borage, Raw 1 cup (1" pieces) (89g)	19	1	0	0	3	--	--	2	71
Brazil Nuts, Dried, Unblanched 1 kernel (5g)	33	3	1	0	1	0.4	0	1	0

Food Serving size	Cal.	(g) Total Fat	(g) Sat. Fat	(mg) Chol.	(g) Carb.	(g) Fiber	(g) Sug.	(g) Prot.	(mg) Sod.
Breadfruit Seeds, Boiled 1 oz (28.35g)	48	1	0	0	9	1.4	--	2	7
Breadfruit Seeds, Raw 1 oz (28.35g)	54	2	0	0	8	1.5	--	2	7
Breadfruit Seeds, Roasted 1 oz (28.35g)	59	1	0	0	11	1.7	--	2	8
Breadfruit, Raw .25 fruit, small (96g)	99	0	0	0	26	4.7	11	1	2
Broadbeans (Fava Beans), Mature Seeds, Canned 1 cup (256g)	182	1	0	0	32	9.5	--	14	1160
Broadbeans (Fava Beans), Mature Seeds, Cooked, Boiled, with Salt 1 cup (170g)	187	1	0	0	33	9.2	3	13	410
Broadbeans (Fava Beans), Mature Seeds, Cooked, Boiled, Without Salt 1 cup (170g)	187	1	0	0	33	9.2	3	13	9
Broadbeans (Fava Beans), Mature Seeds, Raw 1 tbsp (9.4g)	32	0	0	0	5	2.4	1	2	1
Broadbeans, Immature Seeds, Raw 1 broadbean (8g)	6	0	0	0	1	0.3	--	0	4
Butternuts, Dried 1 oz (28.35g)	174	16	0	0	3	1.3	--	7	0
Caraway Seeds 1 tsp (2.1g)	7	0	0	0	1	0.8	0	0	0
Cashew Butter, Plain, with Salt 1 oz (28.35g)	166	14	3	0	8	0.6	1	5	174
Cashew Butter, Plain, Without Salt 1 oz (28.35g)	166	14	3	0	8	0.6	--	5	4
Cashew Nuts, Dry Roasted, with Salt 1 oz (28.35g)	163	13	3	0	9	0.9	1	4	181
Cashew Nuts, Dry Roasted, Without Salt 1 tbsp (8.6g)	49	4	1	0	3	0.3	0	1	1
Cashew Nuts, Oil Roasted, with Salt 1 cup, halves and pieces (129g)	749	62	11	0	39	4.3	6	22	397
Cashew Nuts, Oil Roasted, Without Salt 1 cup, halves and pieces (129g)	748	62	11	0	39	4.3	6	22	17

Food Serving size	Cal.	(g) Total Fat	(g) Sat. Fat	(mg) Chol.	(g) Carb.	(g) Fiber	(g) Sug.	(g) Prot.	(mg) Sod.
Chestnuts, Chinese, Boiled and Steamed 1 oz (28.35g)	43	0	0	0	10	--	--	1	1
Chestnuts, Chinese, Dried 1 oz (28.35g)	103	1	0	0	23	--	--	2	1
Chestnuts, Chinese, Raw 1 oz (28.35g)	64	0	0	0	14	--	--	1	1
Chestnuts, Chinese, Roasted 1 oz (28.35g)	68	0	0	0	15	--	--	1	1
Chestnuts, European, Boiled and Steamed 1 oz (28.35g)	37	0	0	0	8	--	--	1	8
Chestnuts, European, Dried, Peeled 1 oz (28.35g)	105	1	0	0	22	--	--	1	10
Chestnuts, European, Dried, Unpeeled 1 oz (28.35g)	106	1	0	0	22	3.3	--	2	10
Chestnuts, European, Raw, Peeled 1 oz (28.35g)	56	0	0	0	13	--	--	0	1
Chestnuts, European, Raw, Unpeeled 1 oz (28.35g)	60	1	0	0	13	2.3	--	1	1
Chestnuts, European, Roasted 1 oz (28.35g)	69	1	0	0	15	1.4	3	1	1
Chestnuts, Japanese, Boiled and Steamed 1 oz (28.35g)	16	0	0	0	4	--	--	0	1
Chestnuts, Japanese, Dried 1 oz (28.35g)	102	0	0	0	23	--	--	1	10
Chestnuts, Japanese, Raw 1 oz (28.35g)	44	0	0	0	10	--	--	1	4
Chestnuts, Japanese, Roasted 1 oz (28.35g)	57	0	0	0	13	--	--	1	5
Chia Seeds, Dried 1 oz (28.35g)	139	9	1	0	12	10.7	--	4	5
Coconut Cream, Raw (Liquid Expressed from Grated Meat) 1 tbsp (15g)	50	5	5	0	1	0.3	--	1	1
Coconut Meat, Dried (Desiccated), Creamed 1 oz (28.35g)	194	20	17	0	6	--	--	2	10

Food Serving size	Cal.	(g) Total Fat	(g) Sat. Fat	(mg) Chol.	(g) Carb.	(g) Fiber	(g) Sug.	(g) Prot.	(mg) Sod.
Coconut Meat, Dried (Desiccated), Not Sweetened									
1 oz (28.35g)	187	18	16	0	7	4.6	2	2	10
Coconut Meat, Dried (Desiccated), Sweetened, Flaked, Canned									
4 oz (114g)	505	36	32	0	47	5.1	--	4	23
Coconut Meat, Dried (Desiccated), Sweetened, Flaked, Packaged									
1 oz (28.35g)	129	8	7	0	15	2.8	10	1	81
Coconut Meat, Dried (Desiccated), Sweetened, Shredded									
1 pkg (7 oz) (199g)	997	71	63	0	95	9.0	86	6	521
Coconut Meat, Dried (Desiccated), Toasted									
1 oz (28.35g)	168	13	12	0	13	--	--	2	10
Coconut Meat, Raw									
1 medium (397g)	1405	133	118	0	60	35.7	25	13	79
Cumin Seed									
1 tsp, whole (2.1g)	8	0	0	0	1	0.2	0	0	4
Ginkgo Nuts, Canned									
1 oz (14 kernels) (28.35g)	31	0	0	0	6	2.6	--	1	87
Ginkgo Nuts, Dried									
1 oz (28.35g)	99	1	0	0	21	--	--	3	4
Ginkgo Nuts, Raw									
1 oz (28.35g)	52	0	0	0	11	--	--	1	2
Hazelnuts or Filberts									
1 cup, ground (75g)	471	46	3	0	13	7.3	3	11	0
Hazelnuts or Filberts, Blanched									
1 oz (28.35g)	178	17	1	0	5	3.1	1	4	0
Hazelnuts or Filberts, Dry Roasted, Without Salt									
1 oz (28.35g)	183	18	1	0	5	2.7	1	4	0
Hickory Nuts, Dried									
1 oz (28.35g)	186	18	2	0	5	1.8	--	4	0
Lotus Seeds, Dried									
1 oz (42 medium seeds) (28.35g)	94	1	0	0	18	--	--	4	1
Lotus Seeds, Raw									
1 oz (28.35g)	25	0	0	0	5	--	--	1	0
Macadamia Nuts, Dry Roasted, with Salt									
1 oz (10-12 kernels) (28.35g)	203	22	3	0	4	2.3	1	2	75

Food Serving size	Cal.	(g) Total Fat	(g) Sat. Fat	(mg) Chol.	(g) Carb.	(g) Fiber	(g) Sug.	(g) Prot.	(mg) Sod.
Macadamia Nuts, Dry Roasted, Without Salt 1 oz (10-12 kernels) (28.35g)	204	22	3	0	4	2.3	1	2	1
Macadamia Nuts, Raw 1 oz (10-12 kernels) (28.35g)	204	21	3	0	4	2.4	1	2	1
Mixed Nuts, Dry Roasted, with Peanuts, with Salt 1 oz (28.35g)	168	15	2	0	7	2.6	1	5	190
Mixed Nuts, Dry Roasted, with Peanuts, Without Salt 1 oz (28.35g)	168	15	2	0	7	2.6	--	5	3
Mixed Nuts, Oil Roasted, with Peanuts, Without Salt 1 tbsp (8.9g)	55	5	1	0	2	0.9	--	1	1
Mixed Nuts, Oil Roasted, Without Peanuts, Without Salt 1 oz (28.35g)	174	16	3	0	6	1.6	--	4	3
Mixed Nuts, Without Peanuts, Oil Roasted, with Salt 1 oz (28.35g)	174	16	3	0	6	1.6	1	4	87
Nuts, Cashew Nuts, Raw 1 oz (28.35g)	157	12	2	0	9	0.9	2	5	3
Nuts, Coconut Cream, Canned, Sweetened 1 tbsp (19g)	68	3	3	0	10	0.0	10	0	7
Nuts, Mixed Nuts, with Peanuts, Oil Roasted, with Salt Added 1 oz (28.35g)	175	16	2	0	6	2.6	1	5	119
Nuts, Pilinuts, Dried 1 oz (15 kernels) (28.35g)	204	23	9	0	1	--	--	3	1
Nuts, Pine Nuts, Dried 1 oz (167 kernels) (28.35g)	191	19	1	0	4	1.0	1	4	1
Peanut Butter with Omega-3, Creamy 1 tbsp (16g)	97	9	2	--	3	1.0	0	4	57
Peanut Butter, Chunk Style, with Salt 2 tbsp (32g)	188	16	3	0	7	2.6	3	8	156
Peanut Butter, Chunk Style, Without Salt 2 tbsp (32g)	188	16	3	0	7	2.6	3	8	5
Peanut Butter, Chunky, Vitamin and Mineral Fortified 1 cup (258g)	1530	133	21	0	46	14.7	28	67	944
Peanut Butter, Reduced Sodium 1 tbsp (16g)	94	8	1	0	3	1.1	0	4	32

Food Serving size	Cal.	(g) Total Fat	(g) Sat. Fat	(mg) Chol.	(g) Carb.	(g) Fiber	(g) Sug.	(g) Prot.	(mg) Sod.
Peanut Butter, Smooth Style, with Salt 2 tbsp (32g)	188	16	3	0	6	1.9	3	8	147
Peanut Butter, Smooth Style, Without Salt 2 tbsp (32g)	188	16	3	0	6	1.9	3	8	5
Peanut Butter, Smooth, Vitamin and Mineral Fortified 2 tbsp (32g)	189	16	3	0	6	1.8	3	8	134
Peanut Flour, Defatted 1 oz (28.35g)	93	0	0	0	10	4.5	2	15	51
Peanut Flour, Low Fat 1 oz (28.35g)	121	6	1	0	9	4.5	--	10	0
Peanut Spread, Reduced Sugar 2 tbsp (31g)	202	17	3	0	4	2.4	1	8	139
Peanuts, All Types, Cooked, Boiled, with Salt 1 cup, shelled (180g)	572	40	5	0	38	15.8	4	24	1352
Peanuts, All Types, Dry-roasted, with Salt 1 peanut (1g)	6	0	0	0	0	0.1	0	0	8
Peanuts, All Types, Dry-Roasted, Without Salt 1 oz (28.35g)	166	14	2	0	6	2.3	1	7	2
Peanuts, All Types, Oil-roasted, with Salt 1 cup, halves and whole (144g)	863	76	13	0	22	13.5	6	40	461
Peanuts, All Types, Oil-roasted, Without Salt 1 oz, shelled (28.35g)	165	14	2	0	5	2.0	1	7	2
Peanuts, All Types, Raw 1 oz (28.35g)	161	14	2	0	5	2.4	1	7	5
Peanuts, Spanish, Oil-roasted, with Salt 1 oz (28.35g)	164	14	2	0	5	2.5	--	8	123
Peanuts, Spanish, Oil-roasted, Without Salt 1 oz (28.35g)	164	14	2	0	5	2.5	--	8	2
Peanuts, Spanish, Raw 1 oz (28.35g)	162	14	2	0	4	2.7	--	7	6
Peanuts, Valencia, Oil-roasted, with Salt 1 oz (28.35g)	167	15	2	0	5	2.5	--	8	219
Peanuts, Valencia, Oil-roasted, Without Salt 1 oz (28.35g)	167	15	2	0	5	2.5	--	8	2

Food Serving size	Cal.	(g) Total Fat	(g) Sat. Fat	(mg) Chol.	(g) Carb.	(g) Fiber	(g) Sug.	(g) Prot.	(mg) Sod.
Peanuts, Valencia, Raw 1 oz (28.35g)	162	13	2	0	6	2.5	--	7	0
Peanuts, Virginia, Oil-roasted, with Salt 1 oz (28.35g)	164	14	2	0	6	2.5	--	7	123
Peanuts, Virginia, Oil-roasted, Without Salt 1 oz (28.35g)	164	14	2	0	6	2.5	--	7	2
Peanuts, Virginia, Raw 1 oz (28.35g)	160	14	2	0	5	2.4	1	7	3
Pecans 1 cup, halves (99g)	684	71	6	0	14	9.5	4	9	0
Pecans, Dry Roasted, with Salt 1 oz (28.35g)	201	21	2	0	4	2.7	1	3	109
Pecans, Dry Roasted, Without Salt 1 oz (28.35g)	201	21	2	0	4	2.7	1	3	0
Pecans, Oil Roasted, with Salt 1 oz (15 halves) (28.35g)	203	21	2	0	4	2.7	1	3	111
Pecans, Oil Roasted, Without Salt 1 oz (15 halves) (28.35g)	203	21	2	0	4	2.7	1	3	0
Pine Nuts, Pinyon, Dried 10 nuts (1g)	6	1	0	0	0	0.1	--	0	1
Pistachio Nuts, Dry Roasted, with Salt 1 oz (49 kernels) (28.35g)	160	13	2	0	8	2.8	2	6	121
Pistachio Nuts, Dry Roasted, Without Salt 1 oz (49 kernels) (28.35g)	161	13	2	0	8	2.8	2	6	2
Pistachio Nuts, Raw 1 oz (49 kernels) (28.35g)	159	13	2	0	8	2.9	2	6	0
Safflower Seed Kernels, Dried 1 oz (28.35g)	147	11	1	0	10	--	--	5	1
Safflower Seed Meal, Part Defatted 1 oz (28.35g)	97	1	0	0	14	--	--	10	1
Seeds, Flaxseed 1 tbsp, whole (10.3g)	55	4	0	0	3	2.8	0	2	3
Sesame Butter, Paste 1 tbsp (16g)	94	8	1	0	4	0.9	--	3	2

Food Serving size	Cal.	(g) Total Fat	(g) Sat. Fat	(mg) Chol.	(g) Carb.	(g) Fiber	(g) Sug.	(g) Prot.	(mg) Sod.
Sesame Butter, Tahini, from Raw and Stone Ground Kernels									
1 oz (28.35g)	162	14	2	0	7	2.6	--	5	21
Sesame Butter, Tahini, from Roasted Kernels (Most Common Type)									
1 oz (28.35g)	169	15	2	0	6	2.6	0	5	33
Sesame Butter, Tahini, from Unroasted Kernels									
1 oz (28.35g)	172	16	2	0	5	2.6	--	5	0
Sesame Butter, Tahini, Kernels Unspecified									
1 tbsp (15g)	89	8	1	0	3	0.7	--	3	5
Sesame Seed Kernels, Dried (Decort)									
1 tbsp (8g)	50	5	1	0	1	0.9	0	2	4
Sesame Seed Kernels, Toasted, with Salt (Decort)									
1 oz (28.35g)	161	14	2	0	7	4.8	0	5	167
Sesame Seed Kernels, Toasted, Without Salt (Decort)									
1 oz (28.35g)	161	14	2	0	7	4.8	0	5	11
Sesame Seeds, Whole, Dried									
1 tbsp (9g)	52	4	1	0	2	1.1	0	2	1
Sesame Seeds, Whole, Roasted and Toasted									
1 oz (28.35g)	160	14	2	0	7	4.0	--	5	3
Sunflower Seed Butter, with Salt									
1 oz (28.35g)	175	16	1	0	7	1.6	3	5	94
Sunflower Seed Butter, Without Salt									
1 oz (28.35g)	175	16	1	0	7	1.6	3	5	1
Sunflower Seed Flour, Part Defatted									
1 tbsp (4g)	13	0	0	0	1	0.2	--	2	0
Sunflower Seed Kernels, Dried									
1 cup (140g)	818	72	6	0	28	12.0	4	29	13
Sunflower Seed Kernels, Dry Roasted, with Salt									
1 oz (28.35g)	165	14	1	0	7	2.6	1	5	116
Sunflower Seed Kernels, Dry Roasted, Without Salt									
1 oz (28.35g)	165	14	1	0	7	3.1	1	5	1
Sunflower Seed Kernels, Oil Roasted, with Salt									
1 oz (28.35g)	168	15	2	0	6	3.0	1	6	116
Sunflower Seed Kernels, Oil Roasted, Without Salt									
1 oz (28.35g)	168	15	2	0	6	3.0	1	6	1

Food Serving size	Cal.	(g) Total Fat	(g) Sat. Fat	(mg) Chol.	(g) Carb.	(g) Fiber	(g) Sug.	(g) Prot.	(mg) Sod.
Sunflower Seed Kernels, Toasted, with Salt									
1 oz (28.35g)	175	16	2	0	6	3.3	--	5	174
Sunflower Seed Kernels, Toasted, Without Salt									
1 oz (28.35g)	175	16	2	0	6	3.3	--	5	1
Walnuts, Black, Dried									
1 tbsp (7.8g)	48	5	0	0	1	0.5	0	2	0
Walnuts, English									
1 cup, ground (80g)	523	52	5	0	11	5.4	2	12	2
Watermelon Seed Kernels, Dried									
1 oz (28.35g)	158	13	3	0	4	--	--	8	28

Seafood (Fish, Shellfish, Misc. Seafood)

Food Serving size	Cal.	(g) Total Fat	(g) Sat. Fat	(mg) Chol.	(g) Carb.	(g) Fiber	(g) Sug.	(g) Prot.	(mg) Sod.
Abalone, Mixed Species, Cooked, Fried									
3 oz (85g)	161	6	1	80	9	0.0	--	17	502
Anchovy, European, Canned in Oil, Drained Solid									
1 anchovy (4g)	8	0	0	3	0	0.0	0	1	147
Bass, Fresh Water, Mixed Species, Cooked, Dry Heat									
3 oz (85g)	124	4	1	74	0	0.0	--	21	77
Bass, Striped, Cooked, Dry Heat									
3 oz (85g)	105	3	1	88	0	0.0	--	19	75
Bluefish, Cooked, Dry Heat									
3 oz (85g)	135	5	1	65	0	0.0	--	22	65
Burbot, Cooked, Dry Heat									
3 oz (85g)	98	1	0	65	0	0.0	--	21	105
Butterfish, Cooked, Dry Heat									
3 oz (85g)	159	9	--	71	0	0.0	--	19	97
Carp, Cooked, Dry Heat									
3 oz (85g)	138	6	1	71	0	0.0	--	19	54
Catfish, Channel, Cooked, Breaded and Fried									
3 oz (85g)	195	11	3	60	7	0.6	--	15	238
Catfish, Channel, Farmed, Cooked, Dry Heat									
3 oz (85g)	122	6	1	56	0	0.0	0	16	101
Catfish, Channel, Wild, Cooked, Dry Heat									
3 oz (85g)	89	2	1	61	0	0.0	--	16	43

Food Serving size	Cal.	(g) Total Fat	(g) Sat. Fat	(mg) Chol.	(g) Carb.	(g) Fiber	(g) Sug.	(g) Prot.	(mg) Sod.
Caviar, Black and Red, Granular 1 oz (28.35g)	75	5	1	167	1	0.0	0	7	425
Cisco, Smoked 3 oz (85g)	150	10	1	27	0	0.0	0	14	409
Clam, Mixed Species, Canned, Drained Solid 3 oz (85g)	121	1	0	43	5	0.0	0	21	95
Clam, Mixed Species, Canned, Liquid 3 oz (85g)	2	0	0	3	0	0.0	0	0	183
Clam, Mixed Species, Cooked, Breaded and Fried 20 small (188g)	380	21	5	115	19	--	--	27	684
Clam, Mixed Species, Cooked, Moist Heat 20 small (190g)	281	4	0	127	10	0.0	--	49	213
Cod, Atlantic, Canned, Solids and Liquid 3 oz (85g)	89	1	0	47	0	0.0	0	19	185
Cod, Atlantic, Cooked, Dry Heat 3 oz (85g)	89	1	0	47	0	0.0	0	19	66
Cod, Atlantic, Dried and Salted 1 piece (5-1/2" x 1-1/2" x 1/2") (80g)	232	2	0	122	0	0.0	0	50	5622
Cod, Pacific, Cooked, Dry Heat 3 oz (85g)	72	0	0	48	0	0.0	0	16	316
Crab, Alaska King, Cooked, Moist Heat 3 oz (85g)	82	1	0	45	0	0.0	--	16	911
Crab, Alaska King, Imitation, Made from Surimi 3 oz (85g)	81	0	0	17	13	0.4	5	6	715
Crab, Blue, Canned 1 oz (28.35g)	24	0	0	27	0	0.0	0	5	112
Crab, Blue, Cooked, Moist Heat 1 cup (not packed) (135g)	112	1	0	131	0	0.0	0	24	533
Crab, Blue, Crab Cakes 1 cake (60g)	93	5	1	90	0	0.0	--	12	198
Crab, Dungeness, Cooked, Moist Heat 1 crab (127g)	140	2	0	97	1	0.0	--	28	480
Crab, Queen, Cooked, Moist Heat 3 oz (85g)	98	1	0	60	0	0.0	--	20	587

Food Serving size	Cal.	(g) Total Fat	(g) Sat. Fat	(mg) Chol.	(g) Carb.	(g) Fiber	(g) Sug.	(g) Prot.	(mg) Sod.
Crayfish, Mixed Species, Farmed, Cooked, Moist Heat									
3 oz (85g)	74	1	0	116	0	0.0	--	15	82
Crayfish, Mixed Species, Wild, Cooked, Moist Heat									
3 oz (85g)	70	1	0	113	0	0.0	0	14	80
Croaker, Atlantic, Cooked, Breaded and Fried									
3 oz (85g)	188	11	3	71	6	0.3	--	15	296
Cusk, Cooked, Dry Heat									
3 oz (85g)	95	1	--	45	0	0.0	--	21	34
Cuttlefish, Mixed Species, Cooked, Moist Heat									
3 oz (85g)	134	1	0	190	1	0.0	--	28	632
Dolphinfish, Cooked, Dry Heat									
3 oz (85g)	93	1	0	80	0	0.0	--	20	96
Drum, Fresh Water, Cooked, Dry Heat									
3 oz (85g)	130	5	1	70	0	0.0	--	19	82
Eel, Mixed Species, Cooked, Dry Heat									
1 oz, with bone (yield after bone removed) (22g)	52	3	1	35	0	0.0	--	5	14
Fish Broth									
1 fl oz (30.5g)	5	0	0	0	0	0.0	0	1	97
Fish Sticks, Meatless									
1 stick (28g)	81	5	1	0	3	1.7	0	6	137
Flatfish (Flounder and Sole Species), Cooked, Dry Heat									
3 oz (85g)	73	2	0	48	0	0.0	0	13	309
Gefilte Fish, Commercial, Sweet Recipe									
1 piece (42g)	35	1	0	13	3	0.0	--	4	220
Grouper, Mixed Species, Cooked, Dry Heat									
3 oz (85g)	100	1	0	40	0	0.0	--	21	45
Haddock, Cooked, Dry Heat									
3 oz (85g)	77	0	0	56	0	0.0	0	17	222
Haddock, Smoked									
1 cubic inch, boneless (17g)	20	0	0	13	0	0.0	0	4	130
Halibut, Atlantic and Pacific, Cooked, Dry Heat									
3 oz (85g)	94	1	0	51	0	0.0	0	19	70
Halibut, Greenland, Cooked, Dry Heat									
3 oz (85g)	203	15	3	50	0	0.0	--	16	88

Food Serving size	Cal.	(g) Total Fat	(g) Sat. Fat	(mg) Chol.	(g) Carb.	(g) Fiber	(g) Sug.	(g) Prot.	(mg) Sod.
Herring, Atlantic, Cooked, Dry Heat									
3 oz (85g)	173	10	2	65	0	0.0	0	20	98
Herring, Atlantic, Kippered									
1 cubic inch, boneless (17g)	37	2	0	14	0	0.0	0	4	156
Herring, Atlantic, Pickled									
1 oz, boneless (28.35g)	74	5	1	4	3	0.0	2	4	247
Herring, Pacific, Cooked, Dry Heat									
3 oz (85g)	213	15	4	84	0	0.0	--	18	81
Jellyfish, Dried, Salted									
1 cup (58g)	21	1	0	3	0	0.0	--	3	5620
Ling, Cooked, Dry Heat									
3 oz (85g)	94	1	--	43	0	0.0	--	21	147
Lingcod, Cooked, Dry Heat									
3 oz (85g)	93	1	0	57	0	0.0	--	19	65
Lobster, Northern, Cooked, Moist Heat									
3 oz (85g)	76	1	0	124	0	0.0	0	16	413
Mackerel, Atlantic, Cooked, Dry Heat									
3 oz (85g)	223	15	4	64	0	0.0	--	20	71
Mackerel, Jack, Canned, Drained Solid									
1 oz, boneless (28.35g)	44	2	1	22	0	0.0	0	7	107
Mackerel, King, Cooked, Dry Heat									
3 oz (85g)	114	2	0	58	0	0.0	--	22	173
Mackerel, Pacific and Jack, Mixed Species, Cooked, Dry Heat									
1 cubic inch, boneless (17g)	34	2	0	10	0	0.0	0	4	19
Mackerel, Salted									
1 cup, cooked (136g)	415	34	10	129	0	0.0	0	25	6052
Mackerel, Spanish, Cooked, Dry Heat									
3 oz (85g)	134	5	2	62	0	0.0	--	20	56
Milkfish, Cooked, Dry Heat									
3 oz (85g)	162	7	--	57	0	0.0	--	22	78
Monkfish, Cooked, Dry Heat									
3 oz (85g)	82	2	--	27	0	0.0	--	16	20
Mullet, Striped, Cooked, Dry Heat									
3 oz (85g)	128	4	1	54	0	0.0	--	21	60

Food Serving size	Cal.	(g) Total Fat	(g) Sat. Fat	(mg) Chol.	(g) Carb.	(g) Fiber	(g) Sug.	(g) Prot.	(mg) Sod.
Octopus, Common, Cooked, Moist Heat 3 oz (85g)	139	2	0	82	4	0.0	0	25	391
Oyster, Eastern, Canned 1 cup, undrained (248g)	169	6	2	136	10	0.0	0	18	278
Oyster, Eastern, Cooked, Breaded and Fried 6 medium (88g)	175	11	3	62	10	--	--	8	367
Oyster, Eastern, Farmed, Cooked, Dry Heat 6 medium (59g)	47	1	0	22	4	0.0	--	4	96
Oyster, Eastern, Farmed, Raw 6 medium (84g)	50	1	0	21	5	0.0	--	4	150
Oyster, Eastern, Wild, Cooked, Dry Heat 6 medium (59g)	47	2	0	37	2	0.0	1	5	78
Oyster, Eastern, Wild, Cooked, Moist Heat 6 medium (42g)	43	1	0	33	2	0.0	1	5	70
Oyster, Pacific, Cooked, Moist Heat 3 oz (85g)	139	4	1	85	8	0.0	0	16	180
Oyster, Pacific, Raw 3 oz (85g)	69	2	0	43	4	0.0	--	8	90
Perch, Mixed Species, Cooked, Dry Heat 3 oz (85g)	99	1	0	98	0	0.0	--	21	67
Pike, Northern, Cooked, Dry Heat 3 oz (85g)	96	1	0	43	0	0.0	--	21	42
Pike, Walleye, Cooked, Dry Heat 3 oz (85g)	101	1	0	94	0	0.0	--	21	55
Pollock, Atlantic, Cooked, Dry Heat 3 oz (85g)	100	1	0	77	0	0.0	--	21	94
Pollock, Walleye, Cooked, Dry Heat 3 oz (85g)	94	1	0	73	0	0.0	0	20	88
Pompano, Florida, Cooked, Dry Heat 3 oz (85g)	179	10	4	54	0	0.0	--	20	65
Pout, Ocean, Cooked, Dry Heat 3 oz (85g)	87	1	0	57	0	0.0	--	18	66
Rockfish, Pacific, Mixed Species, Cooked, Dry Heat 3 oz (85g)	93	1	0	52	0	0.0	0	19	76

Food Serving size	Cal.	(g) Total Fat	(g) Sat. Fat	(mg) Chol.	(g) Carb.	(g) Fiber	(g) Sug.	(g) Prot.	(mg) Sod.
Roe, Mixed Species, Cooked, Dry Heat									
3 oz (85g)	173	7	2	407	2	0.0	--	24	99
Sablefish, Cooked, Dry Heat									
3 oz (85g)	213	17	3	54	0	0.0	--	15	61
Sablefish, Smoked									
3 oz (85g)	218	17	4	54	0	0.0	--	15	626
Salmon, Atlantic, Farmed, Cooked, Dry Heat									
3 oz (85g)	175	10	2	54	0	0.0	--	19	52
Salmon, Atlantic, Wild, Cooked, Dry Heat									
3 oz (85g)	155	7	1	60	0	0.0	--	22	48
Salmon, Chinook, Cooked, Dry Heat									
3 oz (85g)	196	11	3	72	0	0.0	--	22	51
Salmon, Chinook, Smoked									
1 oz, boneless (28.35g)	33	1	0	7	0	0.0	0	5	222
Salmon, Chinook, Smoked (Lox), Regular									
3 oz (85g)	99	4	1	20	0	0.0	--	16	1700
Salmon, Chum, Canned, Without Salt, Drained Solid with Bone									
3 oz (85g)	120	5	1	33	0	0.0	--	18	64
Salmon, Chum, Cooked, Dry Heat									
3 oz (85g)	131	4	1	81	0	0.0	--	22	54
Salmon, Chum, Drained Solid with Bone									
3 oz (85g)	120	5	1	33	0	0.0	0	18	414
Salmon, Coho, Farmed, Cooked, Dry Heat									
3 oz (85g)	151	7	2	54	0	0.0	--	21	44
Salmon, Coho, Wild, Cooked, Dry Heat									
3 oz (85g)	118	4	1	47	0	0.0	0	20	49
Salmon, Coho, Wild, Cooked, Moist Heat									
3 oz (85g)	156	6	1	48	0	0.0	--	23	45
Salmon, Pink, Canned, Solids with Bone and Liquid									
3 oz (85g)	118	5	1	47	0	0.0	0	17	471
Salmon, Pink, Canned, Without Salt, Solids with Bone and Liquid									
3 oz (85g)	118	5	1	47	0	0.0	--	17	64
Salmon, Pink, Cooked, Dry Heat									
.5 fillet (124g)	190	7	1	68	0	0.0	0	30	112

Food Serving size	Cal.	(g) Total Fat	(g) Sat. Fat	(mg) Chol.	(g) Carb.	(g) Fiber	(g) Sug.	(g) Prot.	(mg) Sod.
Salmon, Sockeye, Canned, Drained Solid with Bone									
3 oz (85g)	141	6	1	37	0	0.0	0	20	306
Salmon, Sockeye, Canned, Without Salt, Drained Solid with Bone									
3 oz (85g)	130	6	1	37	0	0.0	--	17	64
Salmon, Sockeye, Cooked, Dry Heat									
3 oz (85g)	144	6	1	54	0	0.0	0	22	114
Sardine, Atlantic, Canned in Oil, Drained Solid with Bone									
1 oz (28.35g)	59	3	0	40	0	0.0	0	7	143
Sardine, Pacific, Canned in Tomato Sauce, Drained Solid with Bone									
1 can (370g)	685	39	10	226	2	0.4	2	77	1532
Scallop, Mixed Species, Cooked, Breaded and Fried									
2 large (31g)	67	3	1	17	3	--	--	6	144
Scallop, Mixed Species, Imitation, Made from Surimi									
3 oz (85g)	84	0	0	19	9	0.0	--	11	676
Scup, Cooked, Dry Heat									
3 oz (85g)	115	3	--	57	0	0.0	--	21	46
Sea Bass, Mixed Species, Cooked, Dry Heat									
3 oz (85g)	105	2	1	45	0	0.0	--	20	74
Sea Trout, Mixed Species, Cooked, Dry Heat									
3 oz (85g)	113	4	1	90	0	0.0	--	18	63
Seaweed, Kelp, Raw									
2 tbsp (1/8 cup) (10g)	4	0	0	0	1	0.1	0	0	23
Shad, American, Cooked, Dry Heat									
3 oz (85g)	214	15	--	82	0	0.0	--	18	55
Shark, Mixed Species, Cooked, Batter-dipped and Fried									
3 oz (85g)	194	12	3	50	5	0.0	--	16	104
Shrimp, Mixed Species, Canned									
1 oz (28.35g)	28	0	0	71	0	0.0	0	6	220
Shrimp, Mixed Species, Cooked, Breaded and Fried									
4 large (30g)	73	4	1	41	3	0.1	0	6	103
Shrimp, Mixed Species, Cooked, Moist Heat									
4 large (22g)	26	0	0	46	0	0.0	0	5	208
Shrimp, Mixed Species, Imitation, Made from Surimi									
3 oz (85g)	86	1	0	31	8	0.0	--	11	599

Food Serving size	Cal.	(g) Total Fat	(g) Sat. Fat	(mg) Chol.	(g) Carb.	(g) Fiber	(g) Sug.	(g) Prot.	(mg) Sod.
Smelt, Rainbow, Cooked, Dry Heat 3 oz (85g)	105	3	0	77	0	0.0	--	19	65
Snapper, Mixed Species, Cooked, Dry Heat 3 oz (85g)	109	1	0	40	0	0.0	--	22	48
Spiny Lobster, Mixed Species, Cooked, Moist Heat 3 oz (85g)	122	2	0	77	3	0.0	--	22	193
Spot, Cooked, Dry Heat 3 oz (85g)	134	5	2	65	0	0.0	--	20	31
Squid, Mixed Species, Cooked, Fried 3 oz (85g)	149	6	2	221	7	0.0	--	15	260
Sturgeon, Mixed Species, Cooked, Dry Heat 1 oz, boneless (28.35g)	38	1	0	22	0	0.0	0	6	20
Sturgeon, Mixed Species, Smoked 3 oz (85g)	147	4	1	68	0	0.0	0	27	628
Sucker, White, Cooked, Dry Heat 3 oz (85g)	101	3	0	45	0	0.0	--	18	43
Sunfish, Pumpkin Seed, Cooked, Dry Heat 3 oz (85g)	97	1	0	73	0	0.0	--	21	88
Surimi 3 oz (85g)	84	1	0	26	6	0.0	0	13	122
Swordfish, Cooked, Dry Heat 3 oz (85g)	146	7	2	66	0	0.0	0	20	82
Tilefish, Cooked, Dry Heat 3 oz (85g)	125	4	1	54	0	0.0	--	21	50
Trout, Mixed Species, Cooked, Dry Heat 3 oz (85g)	162	7	1	63	0	0.0	--	23	57
Trout, Rainbow, Farmed, Cooked, Dry Heat 3 oz (85g)	143	6	1	60	0	0.0	0	20	52
Trout, Rainbow, Wild, Cooked, Dry Heat 3 oz (85g)	128	5	1	59	0	0.0	--	19	48
Tuna Salad 3 oz (85g)	159	8	1	11	8	0.0	--	14	342
Tuna, Fresh, Bluefin, Cooked, Dry Heat 3 oz (85g)	156	5	1	42	0	0.0	--	25	43

Food Serving size	Cal.	(g) Total Fat	(g) Sat. Fat	(mg) Chol.	(g) Carb.	(g) Fiber	(g) Sug.	(g) Prot.	(mg) Sod.
Tuna, Light, Canned in Oil, Drained Solid									
1 oz (28.35g)	56	2	0	5	0	0.0	0	8	100
Tuna, Light, Canned in Oil, Without Salt, Drained Solid									
3 oz (85g)	168	7	1	15	0	0.0	--	25	43
Tuna, Light, Canned in Water, Drained Solid									
1 oz (28.35g)	33	0	0	9	0	0.0	0	7	96
Tuna, Light, Canned in Water, Without Salt, Drained Solid									
3 oz (85g)	99	1	0	26	0	0.0	0	22	43
Tuna, Skipjack, Fresh, Cooked, Dry Heat									
3 oz (85g)	112	1	0	51	0	0.0	--	24	40
Tuna, White, Canned in Oil, Drained Solid									
3 oz (85g)	158	7	1	26	0	0.0	0	23	337
Tuna, White, Canned in Oil, Without Salt, Drained Solid									
3 oz (85g)	158	7	1	26	0	0.0	--	23	43
Tuna, White, Canned in Water, Drained Solid									
3 oz (85g)	109	3	1	36	0	0.0	0	20	320
Tuna, White, Canned in Water, Without Salt, Drained Solid									
3 oz (85g)	109	3	1	36	0	0.0	--	20	43
Tuna, Yellowfin, Fresh, Cooked, Dry Heat									
3 oz (85g)	111	1	0	40	0	0.0	0	25	46
Turbot, European, Cooked, Dry Heat									
3 oz (85g)	104	3	--	53	0	0.0	--	17	163
Whitefish, Mixed Species, Cooked, Dry Heat									
3 oz (85g)	146	6	1	65	0	0.0	--	21	55
Whitefish, Mixed Species, Smoked									
1 oz, boneless (28.35g)	31	0	0	9	0	0.0	0	7	289
Whiting, Mixed Species, Cooked, Dry Heat									
3 oz (85g)	99	1	0	71	0	0.0	0	20	112
Wolffish, Atlantic, Cooked, Dry Heat									
3 oz (85g)	105	3	0	50	0	0.0	--	19	93
Yellowtail, Mixed Species, Cooked, Dry Heat									
3 oz (85g)	159	6	--	60	0	0.0	--	25	43

Food Serving size	Cal.	(g) Total Fat	(g) Sat. Fat	(mg) Chol.	(g) Carb.	(g) Fiber	(g) Sug.	(g) Prot.	(mg) Sod.
Eggs									
Egg Substitute, Liquid or Frozen, Fat Free .25 cup (60g)	29	0	0	0	1	0.0	1	6	119
Egg Substitute, Powder .7 oz (20g)	89	3	1	114	4	0.0	4	11	160
Egg, White, Dried, Flakes, Glucose Reduced .5 lb (227g)	797	0	0	0	9	0.0	9	175	2624
Egg, White, Dried, Powder, Glucose Reduced 1 tbsp (7g)	26	0	0	0	0	0.0	0	6	87
Egg, White, Raw, Fresh 1 large (33g)	17	0	0	0	0	0.0	0	4	55
Egg, Whole, Cooked, Fried 1 large (46g)	90	7	2	184	0	0.0	0	6	95
Egg, Whole, Cooked, Hard-boiled 1 tbsp (8.5g)	13	1	0	32	0	0.0	0	1	11
Egg, Whole, Cooked, Omelet 1 large (61g)	94	7	2	191	0	0.0	0	6	95
Egg, Whole, Cooked, Poached 1 large (50g)	69	5	2	185	0	0.0	0	6	149
Egg, Whole, Cooked, Scrambled 1 tbsp (13.7g)	20	2	0	38	0	0.0	0	1	20
Egg, Whole, Dried 1 tbsp (5g)	30	2	1	75	0	0.0	0	2	26
Egg, Whole, Dried, Stabilized, Glucose Reduced 1 tbsp (5g)	31	2	1	101	0	0.0	--	2	27
Egg, Whole, Raw, Fresh 1 extra large (56g)	80	5	2	208	0	0.0	0	7	80
Egg, Yolk, Dried 1 tbsp (4g)	27	2	1	82	0	0.0	0	1	5
Egg, Yolk, Frozen, Salted .5 lb (227g)	622	52	16	2168	4	0.0	--	32	8581
Egg, Yolk, Raw, Fresh 1 large (17g)	55	5	2	184	1	0.0	0	3	8

Food Serving size	Cal.	(g) Total Fat	(g) Sat. Fat	(mg) Chol.	(g) Carb.	(g) Fiber	(g) Sug.	(g) Prot.	(mg) Sod.
Egg, Yolk, Raw, Frozen .5 lb (227g)	688	58	18	2145	3	0.0	1	35	152
Egg, Yolk, Raw, Frozen, Sugared .5 lb (227g)	697	52	16	2177	25	0.0	--	31	152

Soy Products

Food Serving size	Cal.	(g) Total Fat	(g) Sat. Fat	(mg) Chol.	(g) Carb.	(g) Fiber	(g) Sug.	(g) Prot.	(mg) Sod.
Soy Protein Concentrate, Crude Protein Basis (N x 6.25), Acid Wash 1 oz (28.35g)	93	0	0	0	7	1.6	--	18	255
Soy Protein Concentrate, Produced by Alcohol Extraction 1 oz (28.35g)	94	0	0	0	9	1.6	6	16	1
Soy Protein Concentrated, Produced by Acid Wash 1 oz (28.35g)	94	0	0	0	9	1.6	6	16	255
Soy Protein Isolate 1 oz (28.35g)	96	1	0	0	2	1.6	0	23	285
Soy Protein Isolate, Potassium 1 oz (28.35g)	92	0	0	0	3	1.6	0	23	14
Soy Protein Isolate, Potassium, Crude Protein Basis 1 oz (28.35g)	91	0	0	0	1	0.6	0	25	14
Soy Protein Isolate, Protein Technologies International, Proplus 1 oz (28.35g)	108	1	0	0	0	--	--	24	11
Soy Protein Isolate, Protein Technologies International, Supro 1 oz (28.35g)	110	1	0	0	0	--	--	25	337
Soybean, Curd, Cheese 1 cup (225g)	340	18	3	0	16	0.0	--	28	45
Soybeans, Green, Cooked, Boiled, Drained, with Salt 1 cup (180g)	254	12	1	0	20	7.6	--	22	450
Soybeans, Green, Cooked, Boiled, Drained, Without Salt 1 cup (180g)	254	12	1	0	20	7.6	--	22	25
Soybeans, Green, Raw 1 cup (256g)	376	17	2	0	28	10.8	--	33	38
Soybeans, Mature Seeds, Cooked, Boiled, with Salt 1 cup (172g)	298	15	2	0	17	10.3	5	29	408
Soybeans, Mature Seeds, Dry Roasted 1 cup (172g)	776	37	5	0	56	13.9	--	68	3

Food Serving size	Cal.	(g) Total Fat	(g) Sat. Fat	(mg) Chol.	(g) Carb.	(g) Fiber	(g) Sug.	(g) Prot.	(mg) Sod.
Soybeans, Mature Seeds, Raw									
1 cup (186g)	830	37	5	0	56	17.3	14	68	4
Soybeans, Mature Seeds, Roasted, No Salt Added									
1 cup (172g)	810	44	6	0	58	30.4	--	61	7
Soybeans, Mature Seeds, Roasted, Salted									
1 cup (172g)	810	44	6	0	58	30.4	7	61	280
Soybeans, Mature Seeds, Sprouted, Cooked, Raw									
10 sprouts (10g)	12	1	0	0	.1	0.1	--	1	1
Soybeans, Mature Seeds, Sprouted, Cooked, Steamed									
1 cup (94g)	76	4	1	0	6	0.8	0	8	9
Soybeans, Mature Seeds, Sprouted, Cooked, Steamed, with Salt									
1 cup (94g)	76	4	1	0	6	0.8	0	8	231
Soybeans, Mature, Cooked, Boiled, Without Salt									
1 tbsp (10.7g)	19	1	0	0	1	0.6	0	2	0
Tempeh									
1 cup (166g)	320	18	4	0	16	--	--	31	15

Tofu Products

Food Serving size	Cal.	(g) Total Fat	(g) Sat. Fat	(mg) Chol.	(g) Carb.	(g) Fiber	(g) Sug.	(g) Prot.	(mg) Sod.
Mori-nu, Tofu, Silken, Firm									
1 slice (84g)	52	2	0	0	2	0.1	1	6	30
Mori-nu, Tofu, Silken, Lite Extra Firm									
1 slice (84g)	32	1	0	0	1	0.0	0	6	82
Mori-nu, Tofu, Silken, Lite Firm									
1 slice (84g)	31	1	0	0	1	0.0	0	5	71
Mori-nu, Tofu, Silken, Soft									
1 slice (84g)	46	2	0	0	2	0.1	1	4	4
Mori-nu, Yofu, Silken, Extra Firm									
1 slice (84g)	46	2	0	0	2	0.1	1	6	53
Tofu, Dried-frozen (Koyadofu)									
1 piece (17g)	82	5	1	0	2	1.2	--	8	1
Tofu, Dried-frozen (Koyadofu), Prepared with Calcium Sulfate									
1 piece (17g)	80	5	1	0	2	0.2	--	8	1
Tofu, Extra Firm, Prepared with Nigari									
.2 block (91g)	83	5	0	0	2	0.4	0	9	7

Food Serving size	Cal.	(g) Total Fat	(g) Sat. Fat	(mg) Chol.	(g) Carb.	(g) Fiber	(g) Sug.	(g) Prot.	(mg) Sod.
Tofu, Firm, Prepared with Calcium Sulfate and Magnesium Chloride (Nigari) .25 block (81g)	57	3	1	0	1	0.7	0	7	10
Tofu, Fried 1 piece (13g)	35	3	0	0	1	0.5	0	2	2
Tofu, Fried, Prepared with Calcium Sulfate 1 piece (13g)	35	3	0	0	1	0.5	--	2	2
Tofu, Hard, Prepared with Nigari .25 block (122g)	178	12	2	0	5	0.7	--	15	2
Tofu, Okara 1 cup (122g)	94	2	0	0	15	--	--	4	11
Tofu, Raw, Firm, Prepared with Calcium Sulfate .25 block (81g)	117	7	1	0	3	1.9	--	13	11
Tofu, Raw, Regular, Prepared with Calcium Sulfate .25 block (116g)	88	6	1	0	2	0.3	--	9	8
Tofu, Salted and Fermented (Fuyu) 1 block (11g)	13	1	0	0	1	--	--	1	316
Tofu, Salted and Fermented (Fuyu), Prepared with Calcium Sulfate 1 block (11g)	13	1	0	0	1	--	--	1	316
Tofu, Soft, Prepared with Calcium Sulfate and Magnesium Chloride (Nigari) 1 cubic inch (18g)	11	1	0	0	0	0.0	0	1	1
VitaSoy USA, Light Vanilla Soy Milk 1 serving (243g)	73	2	0	0	10	0.2	7	4	119
VitaSoy USA, Nasoya Lite Firm Tofu 1 serving (79g)	43	1	0	0	1	0.5	0	7	27
VitaSoy USA, Organic Classic Original Soy Milk 1 serving (243g)	114	4	1	0	11	1.0	5	8	160
VitaSoy USA, Organic Creamy Original Soy Milk 1 serving (243g)	107	4	0	0	11	1.0	5	7	160
VitaSoy USA, Organic Nasoya Extra Firm Tofu 1 serving (79g)	77	4	1	0	2	1.0	0	8	3
VitaSoy USA, Organic Nasoya Firm Tofu 1 serving (79g)	66	3	0	0	2	0.6	0	7	3
VitaSoy USA, Organic Nasoya Super Firm Cubed Tofu .2 pkg (79g)	96	5	1	0	3	1.7	0	10	5

Fats and Oils

Why Eat Fats and Oils?

Fats and oils are not a food group, but they do provide essential nutrients. Most of the fats you eat should be polyunsaturated (PUFA) or monounsaturated (MUFA) fats. Some fatty acids are necessary for health; these are called "essential fatty acids." The MUFAs and PUFAs found in fish, nuts, and vegetable oils do not raise LDL ("bad") cholesterol levels in the blood. In addition to the essential fatty acids they contain, oils are the major source of vitamin E, a potent antioxidant.

Daily Goal

6 teaspoons for an adult on a 2000-calorie diet
One-teaspoon equivalents:
    1 tablespoon oil = 2.5 teaspoons
    1 tablespoon mayonnaise = 2.5 teaspoons
    2 tablespoons Italian dressing = 2 teaspoons
    4 large olives = ½ teaspoon
    1 oz nuts = 3 teaspoons
    2 tablespoons peanut butter = 4 teaspoons

Shopping Tips

- Choose fats and oils high in monounsaturated and polyunsaturated fatty acids, such as fish, nuts, seeds, and vegetable oils.
- Limit solid fats, such as butter, stick margarine, shortening, and animal fats.
- Choose fats high in omega-3, such as olive oil, soy oil, walnuts, and flaxseeds.

Shopping List Essentials

Olive oil
Canola oil
Soybean oil
Tub margarine
Nuts
Avocadoes

Red Flags

While consuming some oil is needed for health, oils still contain calories. In fact, oils and solid fats both contain about 120 calories per tablespoon. Therefore, the amount of oil consumed needs to be limited to balance total calorie intake.

Food Serving size	Cal.	(g) Total Fat	(g) Sat. Fat	(mg) Chol.	(g) Carb.	(g) Fiber	(g) Sug.	(g) Prot.	(mg) Sod.
Olives									
Olives, Pickled, Canned or Bottled, Green .1 olive (2.7g)	4	0	0	0	0	0.1	0	0	42
Olives, Ripe, Canned (Jumbo - Super Colossal) 1 super colossal (15g)	12	1	0	0	1	0.4	0	0	110
Olives, Ripe, Canned (Small - Extra Large) 1 large (4.4g)	5	0	0	0	0	0.1	0	0	32
Butter/Margarine									
Butter Oil, Anhydrous 1 tbsp (12.8g)	112	13	8	33	0	0.0	0	0	0
Butter Replacement, Without Fat, Powder 1 cup (80g)	298	1	0	2	71	0.0	2	2	960
Butter, Whipped, with Salt 1 tbsp (9.4g)	67	8	5	21	0	0.0	0	0	78
Butter, with Salt 1 tbsp (14.2g)	102	12	7	31	0	0.0	0	0	101
Butter, Without Salt 1 tbsp (14.2g)	102	12	7	31	0	0.0	0	0	2
Margarine Spread, Approximately 48% Fat, Tub 1 tbsp (14g)	59	7	1	0	0	0.0	--	0	90
Margarine, 80% Fat, Stick, Including Regular and Hydrogenated Corn and Soybean Oils 1 tbsp (14g)	100	11	2	0	0	0.0	--	0	92
Margarine, 80% Fat, Tub, Canola Harvest Soft Spread 1 tbsp (1 NLEA serving) (14g)	102	11	2	--	0	--	--	0	100
Margarine, Industrial, Non-diary, Cottonseed, Soy Oil (Part Hydrogenated) 1 tbsp (14g)	100	11	3	0	0	0.0	0	0	123
Margarine, Industrial, Soy and Part Hydrogenated Soy Oil, Baking, Sauces, Candy 1 cup (227g)	1621	182	37	0	2	0.0	0	0	2011
Margarine, Margarine-like Vegetable Oil Spread, 67-70% Fat, Tub 1 tbsp (1 NLEA serving) (14g)	85	10	2	--	0	--	--	0	75
Margarine, Regular, 80% Fat, Composite, Stick, with Salt 1 cup (227g)	1628	183	34	0	2	0.0	0	0	1705

Food Serving size	Cal.	(g) Total Fat	(g) Sat. Fat	(mg) Chol.	(g) Carb.	(g) Fiber	(g) Sug.	(g) Prot.	(mg) Sod.
Margarine, Regular, 80% Fat, Composite, Stick, with Salt, with Added Vitamin D									
1 cup (227g)	1628	183	34	0	2	0.0	0	0	1705
Margarine, Regular, 80% Fat, Composite, Stick, Without Salt									
1 cup (227g)	1628	183	34	0	2	0.0	0	0	5
Margarine, Regular, 80% Fat, Composite, Stick, Without Salt, with added Vitamin D									
1 cup (229g)	1642	185	35	0	2	0.0	0	0	5
Margarine, Regular, 80% Fat, Composite, Tub, with Salt									
1 cup (227g)	1619	182	32	0	2	0.0	0	0	1491
Margarine, Regular, 80% Fat, Composite, Tub, with Salt, with Added Vitamin D									
1 tbsp (14g)	100	11	2	0	0	0.0	0	0	92
Margarine, Regular, 80% Fat, Composite, Tub, Without Salt									
1 cup (227g)	1619	182	32	0	2	0.0	0	0	64
Margarine, Regular, Hard, Soybean (Hydrogenated)									
1 stick (113g)	812	91	19	0	1	0.0	0	1	1066
Margarine, Vegetable Oil Spread, 70% Fat, Soybean and Part Hydrogenated Soybean, Stick									
1 tbsp (1 NLEA serving) (14g)	88	10	2	0	0	--	--	0	98
Margarine-like Shortening, Industrial, Soy (Part Hydrogenated), Cottonseed and Soy									
1 tbsp (14g)	88	10	3	0	0	0.0	0	0	121
Margarine-like Spread with Yogurt, 70% Fat, Stick, with Salt									
1 tbsp (14g)	88	10	2	0	0	0.0	0	0	83
Margarine-like Spread with Yogurt, Approximately 40% Fat, Tub, with Salt									
1 tbsp (14g)	46	5	1	0	0	0.0	0	0	88
Margarine-like Spread, Benecol Light Spread									
1 tbsp (1 NLEA serving) (14g)	50	5	1	--	1	--	--	0	94
Margarine-like Spread, Smart Balance Light Buttery Spread									
1 tbsp (14g)	47	5	1	--	0	--	--	0	81
Margarine-like Spread, Smart Balance Omega Plus Spread									
1 tbsp (14g)	85	10	3	3	0	0.0	0	0	102
Margarine-like Spread, Smart Balance Regular Buttery Spread									
1 tbsp (14g)	82	9	2	0	0	0.0	0	0	90
Margarine-like Spread, Smart Beat, Smart Squeeze									
1 tbsp (14g)	7	0	0	0	1	0.0	0	0	116

Food Serving size	Cal.	(g) Total Fat	(g) Sat. Fat	(mg) Chol.	(g) Carb.	(g) Fiber	(g) Sug.	(g) Prot.	(mg) Sod.
Margarine-like Spread, Smart Beat, Super Light Without Saturated Fat									
1 tbsp (14g)	22	2	0	0	0	0.0	0	0	106
Margarine-like, Butter-margarine Blend, 80% Fat, Stick, Without Salt									
1 tbsp (14g)	101	11	4	12	0	0.0	--	0	4
Margarine-like, Margarine-butter Blend, Soybean Oil and Butter									
1 cup (227g)	1621	182	32	27	2	0.0	0	1	1437
Margarine-like, Vegetable Oil Spread, 20% Fat, Without Salt									
1 cup (205g)	359	40	6	0	1	0.0	0	0	0
Margarine-like, Vegetable Oil Spread, Fat Free, Liquid, with Salt									
1 tbsp (15g)	6	0	0	0	0	0.0	0	0	125
Margarine-like, Vegetable Oil Spread, Stick or Tub, Sweetened									
1 tbsp (14g)	75	7	1	0	2	0.0	--	0	76
Margarine-like, Vegetable Oil, Spread, 20% Fat, with Salt									
1 cup (240g)	420	47	7	0	1	0.0	0	0	1759
Margarine-like, Vegetable Oil, Spread, 60 % Fat, Stick, with Salt									
1 cup (229g)	1230	138	25	0	2	0.0	0	0	1798
Margarine-like, Vegetable Oil, Spread, 60% Fat, Stick/tub/bottle, with Salt									
1 cup (229g)	1205	135	23	2	0	0.0	0	1	1603
Margarine-like, Vegetable Oil, Spread, 60% Fat, Tub, with Salt									
1 cup (229g)	1221	137	28	2	2	0.0	0	0	1408
Margarine-like, Vegetable Oil, Spread, Fat Free, Tub									
1 cup (233g)	103	7	5	0	10	0.0	0	0	1351
Margarine-like, Vegetable Oil-butter Spread, Reduced Calorie, Tub with Salt									
1 tbsp (14g)	63	7	2	10	0	0.0	0	0	85
Margarine-like, Vegetable Oil-butter Spread, Tub, with Salt									
1 tbsp (14g)	51	6	1	0	0	0.0	0	0	110
Oil, Cocoa Butter									
1 cup (218g)	1927	218	130	0	0	0.0	0	0	0
Oil, Pam Cooking Spray, Original									
1 spray, about 1/3 second (1 NLEA serving) (0.3g)	2	0	0	0	0	0.0	0	0	0

Salad Dressings

Creamy Dressing, Made with Sour Cream and/or Buttermilk and Oil, **Reduced Calorie**									
1 cup (245g)	392	34	5	0	17	0.0	9	4	2744

Food Serving size	Cal.	(g) Total Fat	(g) Sat. Fat	(mg) Chol.	(g) Carb.	(g) Fiber	(g) Sug.	(g) Prot.	(mg) Sod.
Creamy Dressing, Made with Sour Cream and/or Buttermilk and Oil, Reduced Calorie, Fat Free									
1 cup (264g)	282	7	1	0	53	0.0	--	4	2368
Creamy Dressing, with Sour Cream and/or Buttermilk and Oil, Reduced Calorie, Cholesterol Free									
1 cup (234g)	328	19	3	0	37	0.0	--	2	2181
Mayonnaise Dressing, No Cholesterol									
1 cup (239g)	1644	186	26	0	1	0.0	90	0	1162
Mayonnaise, Low Sodium, Low Calorie or Diet									
1 cup (224g)	517	43	7	54	36	0.0	7	1	246
Mayonnaise, Made from Tofu									
1 cup (240g)	773	76	7	0	7	2.6	--	14	1855
Mayonnaise, Reduced Calorie or Diet, Cholesterol Free									
1 cup (231g)	769	77	11	0	15	0.0	--	2	1693
Oil, Almond									
1 cup (218g)	1927	218	18	0	0	0.0	0	0	0
Oil, Apricot Kernel									
1 cup (218g)	1927	218	14	0	0	0.0	0	0	0
Oil, Avocado									
1 cup (218g)	1927	218	25	--	0	0.0	--	0	0
Oil, Babassu									
1 cup (218g)	1927	218	177	0	0	0.0	0	0	0
Oil, Canola									
1 cup (218g)	1927	218	16	0	0	0.0	0	0	0
Oil, Coconut									
1 cup (218g)	1879	218	189	0	0	0.0	0	0	0
Oil, Cooking and Salad, Enova, 80% Diglycerides									
1 cup (214g)	1892	214	10	--	0	--	--	0	0
Oil, Corn or Canola									
1 cup (224g)	1980	224	18	0	0	0.0	14	0	0
Oil, Corn, Industrial and Retail, All Purpose Salad or Cooking									
1 cup (218g)	1927	218	28	0	0	0.0	0	0	0
Oil, Corn, Peanut, and Olive									
1 teaspoon (4.5g)	40	5	1	0	0	0.0	3	0	0
Oil, Cottonseed, Salad or Cooking									
1 cup (218g)	1927	218	56	0	0	0.0	0	0	0

Food Serving size	Cal.	(g) Total Fat	(g) Sat. Fat	(mg) Chol.	(g) Carb.	(g) Fiber	(g) Sug.	(g) Prot.	(mg) Sod.
Oil, Cupu Assu 1 cup (218g)	1927	218	116	0	0	0.0	0	0	0
Oil, Fish Oil, Cod Liver 1 tbsp (13.6g)	123	14	3	78	0	0.0	--	0	0
Oil, Fish Oil, Herring 1 tbsp (13.6g)	123	14	3	104	0	0.0	--	0	0
Oil, Fish Oil, Menhaden 1 tbsp (13.6g)	123	14	4	71	0	0.0	--	0	0
Oil, Fish Oil, Menhaden, Fully Hydrogenated 1 tbsp (12.5g)	113	13	12	63	0	0.0	--	0	0
Oil, Fish Oil, Salmon 1 tbsp (13.6g)	123	14	3	66	0	0.0	--	0	0
Oil, Fish Oil, Sardine 1 tbsp (13.6g)	123	14	4	97	0	0.0	--	0	0
Oil, Flaxseed 1 cup (218g)	1927	218	20	0	0	0.0	--	0	0
Oil, Grape Seed 1 cup (218g)	1927	218	21	0	0	0.0	0	0	0
Oil, Hazelnut 1 cup (218g)	1927	218	16	0	0	0.0	0	0	0
Oil, Industrial, Canola (Part Hydrogenated) Oil for Deep Fat Frying 1 tbsp (13.6g)	120	14	1	0	0	0.0	0	0	0
Oil, Industrial, Canola for Salads, Woks and Light Frying 1 teaspoon (4.5g)	40	5	0	0	0	0.0	0	0	0
Oil, Industrial, Canola with Antifoaming Agent 1 cup (218g)	1927	218	17	0	0	0.0	0	0	0
Oil, Industrial, Canola, Hi Oleic 1 cup (218g)	1962	218	15	0	0	0.0	0	0	0
Oil, Industrial, Coconut 1 cup (218g)	1927	218	187	0	0	0.0	0	0	0
Oil, Industrial, Coconut (Hydrogenated), for Toppings and Whiteners 1 cup (218g)	1918	217	204	0	0	0.0	0	0	15
Oil, Industrial, Coconut, Confection Fat, Ice Cream Coatings 1 cup (218g)	1927	218	189	0	0	0.0	0	0	11

Food Serving size	Cal.	(g) Total Fat	(g) Sat. Fat	(mg) Chol.	(g) Carb.	(g) Fiber	(g) Sug.	(g) Prot.	(mg) Sod.
Oil, Industrial, Mid Oleic, Sunflower									
1 tsp (4.5g)	40	5	0	0	0	0.0	0	0	0
Oil, Industrial, Palm and Palm Kernel, Filling Fat (Non-hydrogenated)									
1 cup (218g)	1918	217	156	0	0	0.0	0	0	13
Oil, Industrial, Palm Kernel (Hydrogenated) for Whipped Toppings									
1 cup (218g)	1927	218	194	0	0	0.0	0	0	13
Oil, Industrial, Palm Kernel (Hydrogenated), Confection Fat									
1 cup (218g)	1927	218	204	0	0	0.0	0	0	13
Oil, Industrial, Palm Kernel (Hydrogenated), Confection Fat									
1 cup (218g)	1927	218	202	0	0	0.0	0	0	13
Oil, Industrial, Palm Kernel (Hydrogenated), Filling Fat									
1 cup (218g)	1927	218	192	0	0	0.0	0	0	13
Oil, Industrial, Palm Kernel, Confection Fat									
1 cup (218g)	1927	218	191	0	0	0.0	0	0	13
Oil, Industrial, Soy (Part Hydrogenated) and Cottonseed, Tortilla Shortening									
1 cup (218g)	1927	218	56	0	0	0.0	0	0	0
Oil, Industrial, Soy (Part Hydrogenated) and Soy, Pourable Frying									
1 cup (218g)	1927	218	33	0	0	0.0	0	0	0
Oil, Industrial, Soy (Part Hydrogenated) for Non-diary Butter Flavor									
1 cup (218g)	1927	218	39	0	0	0.0	0	0	0
Oil, Industrial, Soy (Part Hydrogenated), All Purpose									
1 cup (218g)	1927	218	54	0	0	0.0	0	0	0
Oil, Industrial, Soy (Part Hydrogenated), for Popcorn and Flavoring Vegetables									
1 cup (218g)	1927	218	39	0	0	0.0	0	0	0
Oil, Industrial, Soy (Part Hydrogenated), Palm, Icings and Fillings									
1 cup (218g)	1927	218	62	0	0	0.0	0	0	0
Oil, Industrial, Soy, Fully Hydrogenated									
1 cup (218g)	1927	218	205	0	0	0.0	0	0	0
Oil, Industrial, Soy, Refined, for Woks and Light Frying									
1 cup (218g)	1927	218	33	0	0	0.0	0	0	0
Oil, Industrial, Soy, Ultra Lo Linolenic									
1 cup (218g)	1927	218	32	0	0	0.0	0	0	0
Oil, Mustard									
1 cup (218g)	1927	218	25	--	0	0.0	--	0	0

Food Serving size	Cal.	(g) Total Fat	(g) Sat. Fat	(mg) Chol.	(g) Carb.	(g) Fiber	(g) Sug.	(g) Prot.	(mg) Sod.
Oil, Nutmeg, Butter 1 cup (218g)	1927	218	196	0	0	0.0	0	0	0
Oil, Oat 1 cup (218g)	1927	218	43	0	0	0.0	0	0	0
Oil, Palm 1 cup (216g)	1909	216	106	0	0	0.0	0	0	0
Oil, Peanut, Salad or Cooking 1 cup (216g)	1909	216	37	0	0	0.0	0	0	0
Oil, Poppy Seed 1 cup (218g)	1927	218	29	0	0	0.0	0	0	0
Oil, Rice Bran 1 cup (218g)	1927	218	43	0	0	0.0	0	0	0
Oil, Safflower, Salad or Cooking, Hi Oleic 1 cup (218g)	1927	218	16	0	0	0.0	0	0	0
Oil, Safflower, Salad or Cooking, Linoleic (Over 70%) 1 cup (218g)	1927	218	14	0	0	0.0	0	0	0
Oil, Salad or Cooking 1 cup (216g)	1909	216	30	0	0	0.0	0	0	4
Oil, Sesame, Salad or Cooking 1 cup (218g)	1927	218	31	0	0	0.0	0	0	0
Oil, Sheanut 1 cup (218g)	1927	218	102	0	0	0.0	0	0	0
Oil, Soybean Lecithin 1 cup (218g)	1663	218	33	0	0	0.0	0	0	0
Oil, Soybean, Salad or Cooking 1 cup (218g)	1927	218	34	0	0	0.0	0	0	0
Oil, Soybean, Salad or Cooking (Partially Hydrogenated and Cottonseed) 1 cup (218g)	1927	218	39	0	0	0.0	0	0	0
Oil, Soybean, Salad or Cooking (Partially Hydrogenated) 1 cup (218g)	1927	218	32	0	0	0.0	0	0	0
Oil, Sunflower, Hi Oleic (70% and Over) 1 cup (218g)	1927	218	21	0	0	0.0	0	0	0
Oil, Sunflower, Linoleic (Approximately 65%) 1 cup (218g)	1927	218	22	0	0	0.0	0	0	0

Food Serving size	Cal.	(g) Total Fat	(g) Sat. Fat	(mg) Chol.	(g) Carb.	(g) Fiber	(g) Sug.	(g) Prot.	(mg) Sod.
Oil, Sunflower, Linoleic (Less than 60%)									
1 cup (218g)	1927	218	22	0	0	0.0	0	0	0
Oil, Sunflower, Linoleic (Partially Hydrogenated)									
1 cup (218g)	1927	218	28	0	0	0.0	0	0	0
Oil, Tea Seed									
1 cup (218g)	1927	218	46	0	0	0.0	0	0	0
Oil, Tomato Seed									
1 cup (218g)	1927	218	43	0	0	0.0	0	0	0
Oil, Ucuhuba Butter									
1 cup (218g)	1927	218	186	0	0	0.0	0	0	0
Oil, Vegetable, Natreon Canola, Hi Stability, Non Trans, Hi Oleic (70%)									
1 tbsp (14g)	124	14	1	0	0	0.0	0	0	0
Oil, Walnut									
1 cup (218g)	1927	218	20	0	0	0.0	0	0	0
Oil, Wheat Germ									
1 cup (218g)	1927	218	41	0	0	0.0	0	0	0
Salad Dressing, Bacon and Tomato									
1 cup (240g)	782	84	13	10	5	0.5	4	4	2172
Salad Dressing, Blue or Roquefort Cheese Dressing, Commercial, Regular									
1 cup (245g)	1166	125	20	76	11	1.0	9	3	2550
Salad Dressing, Blue or Roquefort Cheese Dressing, Fat Free									
1 cup (265g)	305	3	1	5	68	4.8	--	4	2157
Salad Dressing, Blue or Roquefort Cheese Dressing, Reduced Calorie									
1 cup (249g)	214	7	2	25	33	0.0	--	5	2338
Salad Dressing, Blue or Roquefort Cheese, Low Calorie									
1 cup (245g)	243	18	6	2	7	0.0	0	12	2301
Salad Dressing, Buttermilk, Lite									
1 serving (2 tbsp) (30g)	61	4	0	5	6	0.3	6	0	336
Salad Dressing, Caesar Dressing, Regular									
1 cup (235g)	1274	136	21	92	8	1.2	1	5	2841
Salad Dressing, Caesar, Low Calorie									
1 cup (240g)	264	11	2	5	45	0.2	0	1	2755
Salad Dressing, Cole Slaw									
1 cup (250g)	975	84	12	65	60	0.3	0	2	1775

Food Serving size	Cal.	(g) Total Fat	(g) Sat. Fat	(mg) Chol.	(g) Carb.	(g) Fiber	(g) Sug.	(g) Prot.	(mg) Sod.
Salad Dressing, Cole Slaw Dressing, Reduced Fat 1 cup (269g)	885	54	8	67	108	1.1	--	0	4304
Salad Dressing, French Dressing, Commercial, Regular 1 cup (250g)	1143	112	14	0	39	0.0	40	2	2090
Salad Dressing, French Dressing, Commercial, Regular, Without Salt 1 tbsp (15g)	69	7	1	0	2	0.0	2	0	0
Salad Dressing, French Dressing, Fat Free 1 cup (256g)	338	1	0	0	82	5.6	42	1	2184
Salad Dressing, French Dressing, Reduced Calorie 1 cup (260g)	520	34	5	0	70	0.0	--	1	2179
Salad Dressing, French Dressing, Reduced Fat 1 cup (260g)	577	30	2	0	81	3.9	44	2	2179
Salad Dressing, French Dressing, Reduced Fat, Without Salt 1 cup (260g)	606	35	3	0	76	2.9	74	2	78
Salad Dressing, French, Cottonseed, Oil, Home Recipe 1 cup (220g)	1388	154	40	0	7	0.0	--	0	1448
Salad Dressing, French, Home Recipe 1 cup (220g)	1388	154	28	0	7	0.0	--	0	1448
Salad Dressing, Green Goddess, Regular 1 cup (245g)	1046	106	15	98	18	0.2	0	5	2124
Salad Dressing, Home Recipe, Cooked 1 cup (255g)	400	24	7	145	38	0.0	23	11	1872
Salad Dressing, Home Recipe, Vinegar and Oil 1 cup (250g)	1123	125	23	0	6	0.0	6	0	3
Salad Dressing, Honey Mustard Dressing, Reduced Calorie 2 tbsp (1 serving) (30g)	62	3	0	0	9	0.2	5	0	270
Salad Dressing, Italian Dressing, Commercial, Regular 1 cup (235g)	684	67	11	0	25	0.0	20	1	2392
Salad Dressing, Italian Dressing, Commercial, Regular, Without Salt 1 cup (235g)	686	67	11	157	25	0.0	20	1	71
Salad Dressing, Italian Dressing, Fat Free 1 cup (231g)	109	2	1	5	20	1.4	20	2	2608
Salad Dressing, Italian Dressing, Reduced Calorie 1 cup (216g)	432	43	6	0	14	0.4	--	1	2320

Food Serving size	Cal.	(g) Total Fat	(g) Sat. Fat	(mg) Chol.	(g) Carb.	(g) Fiber	(g) Sug.	(g) Prot.	(mg) Sod.
Salad Dressing, Italian Dressing, Reduced Fat									
1 cup (240g)	180	15	1	14	11	0.0	11	1	2578
Salad Dressing, Italian Dressing, Reduced Fat, Without Salt									
1 cup (240g)	182	15	1	14	11	0.0	11	1	72
Salad Dressing, Kraft, Mayonnaise, Fat Free Mayonnaise									
1 tbsp (16g)	11	0	0	2	2	0.3	1	0	120
Salad Dressing, Kraft, Mayonnaise, Light Mayonnaise									
1 tbsp (15g)	50	5	1	5	1	0.0	1	0	120
Salad Dressing, Kraft, Miracle Whip Free Non-fat Dressing									
1 tbsp (16g)	13	0	0	1	2	0.3	2	0	126
Salad Dressing, Kraft, Miracle Whip Light Dressing									
1 tbsp (16g)	37	3	0	4	2	0.0	2	0	131
Salad Dressing, Mayonnaise and Mayonnaise-type, Low Calorie									
1 cup (232g)	610	44	7	60	55	0.0	0	2	1942
Salad Dressing, Mayonnaise Dressing, Diet, No Cholesterol									
1 cup (242g)	944	81	12	0	58	0.0	57	2	1721
Salad Dressing, Mayonnaise, Imitation, Milk Cream									
1 cup (240g)	233	12	7	103	27	0.0	--	5	1210
Salad Dressing, Mayonnaise, Imitation, Soybean									
1 tbsp (15g)	35	3	0	4	2	0.0	1	0	75
Salad Dressing, Mayonnaise, Imitation, Soybean Without Cholesterol									
1 cup (225g)	1085	107	17	0	36	0.0	14	0	794
Salad Dressing, Mayonnaise, Light									
1 tbsp (15g)	49	5	1	5	1	0.0	1	0	101
Salad Dressing, Mayonnaise, Light, Smart Balance, Omega Plus Light									
1 tbsp (1 NLEA serving) (14g)	47	5	0	5	1	0.0	1	0	119
Salad Dressing, Mayonnaise, Soybean and Safflower Oil, with Salt									
1 cup (220g)	1577	175	19	130	6	0.0	1	2	1250
Salad Dressing, Mayonnaise, Soybean Oil, with Salt									
1 cup (220g)	1580	175	26	84	7	0.0	2	2	1250
Salad Dressing, Mayonnaise, Soybean Oil, Without Salt									
1 cup (220g)	1577	175	26	130	6	0.0	--	2	66
Salad Dressing, Mayonnaise-like, Fat Free									
1 cup (256g)	215	7	2	23	40	4.9	--	1	2017

Food Serving size	Cal.	(g) Total Fat	(g) Sat. Fat	(mg) Chol.	(g) Carb.	(g) Fiber	(g) Sug.	(g) Prot.	(mg) Sod.
Salad Dressing, Mayonnaise-type, Regular with Salt 1 cup (235g)	917	78	12	61	56	0.0	15	2	1671
Salad Dressing, Peppercorn Dressing, Commercial, Regular 1 fl oz (26g)	147	16	3	13	1	0.0	--	0	287
Salad Dressing, Ranch Dressing, Commercial, Regular 1 tbsp (15g)	73	8	1	5	1	0.1	0	0	164
Salad Dressing, Ranch Dressing, Fat Free 1 tbsp (14g)	17	0	--	1	4	0.0	1	0	126
Salad Dressing, Ranch Dressing, Reduced Fat 1 serving (2 tbsp) (30g)	59	4	0	5	6	0.3	1	0	336
Salad Dressing, Russian Dressing 1 cup (245g)	870	64	6	0	78	1.7	43	2	2776
Salad Dressing, Russian Dressing, Low Calorie 1 cup (260g)	367	10	2	16	72	0.8	57	1	2257
Salad Dressing, Sesame Seed Dressing, Regular 1 cup (245g)	1085	111	15	0	21	2.5	20	8	2450
Salad Dressing, Spray-style Dressing, Assorted Flavors 1 serving (approximately 10 sprays) (8g)	13	1	0	0	1	0.0	1	0	88
Salad Dressing, Sweet and Sour 1 cup (250g)	38	0	0	0	9	0.0	0	0	520
Salad Dressing, Thousand Island Dressing, Commercial, Regular 1 cup (250g)	925	88	13	65	37	2.0	38	3	2158
Salad Dressing, Thousand Island Dressing, Fat Free 1 cup (256g)	338	4	1	13	75	8.4	43	1	2017
Salad Dressing, Thousand Island Dressing, Reduced Fat 1 cup (245g)	478	28	2	27	59	2.9	42	2	2340
Vinegar, Balsamic 1 tbsp (16g)	14	0	0	--	3	--	2	0	4
Vinegar, Cider 1 tbsp (14.9g)	3	0	0	0	0	0.0	0	0	1
Vinegar, Distilled 1 tbsp (14.9g)	3	0	0	0	0	0.0	0	0	0
Vinegar, Red Wine 1 tbsp (14.9g)	3	0	0	--	0	0.0	0	0	1

Snacks and Sweets

Why Eat Snacks?

Snacks are important to keep you energized throughout the day, especially when the time between meals is longer than 4 hours. This is the amount of time it takes for the food you eat to be digested, metabolized, and assimilated into your body cells, where it is used for energy and other maintenance tasks. After about 4 hours, your body will start sending hunger messages and may start slowing down, so a snack between meals can help you stay alert and not hungry. The important thing is to make nutritious snack choices that don't contain empty calories.

Daily Goal

Plan two healthy snacks each day.
Avoid "empty calories" in added sugar and solid fats.

Shopping Tips

- Keep raw nuts and seeds handy.
- Prepare cut-up fruits and vegetables and store in the refrigerator.
- Air-popped corn is a whole grain snack.
- Whole grain cereal makes a great snack.

Shopping List Essentials

Raw nuts
Raw seeds
Popcorn
Dried fruit
Fruits
Vegetables

Red Flags

Avoid "empty calories" in added sugar and solid fats. "Empty calorie" foods and beverages provide calories but few or no nutrients. Solid fats can be butter or shortening used in baking or fried foods, or they can be other fats added in processing that result in trans fats. Check ingredients lists for the term "partially hydrogenated fats." This term means the presence of "trans fats"—even when the Nutrition Facts say "0 grams trans fat."

Food Serving size	Cal.	(g) Total Fat	(g) Sat. Fat	(mg) Chol.	(g) Carb.	(g) Fiber	(g) Sug.	(g) Prot.	(mg) Sod.
Candies (Including Brand-name Bars)									
Candies, 5th Avenue Candy Bar 1 bar, snack size (16g)	77	4	1	1	10	0.5	8	1	36
Candies, Almond Joy Bites 18 pieces (40g)	225	14	8	4	23	1.7	21	2	16
Candies, Almond Joy, Candy Bar 1 bar, snack size (19g)	91	5	3	1	11	1.0	9	1	27
Candies, Butterscotch 3 pieces (16g)	63	1	0	1	14	0.0	13	0	63
Candies, Caramello Candy Bar 1 bar, 1.6 oz (45g)	208	10	6	12	29	0.5	26	3	55
Candies, Caramels 1 piece (10.1g)	39	1	0	1	8	0.0	7	0	25
Candies, Caramels, Chocolate-flavor Roll 1 piece (6.6g)	26	0	0	0	6	0.0	4	0	3
Candies, Carob, Unsweetened 1 bar (3 oz) (87g)	470	27	25	1	49	3.3	30	7	93
Candies, Chocolate Covered, Caramel with Nuts 1 piece (14g)	66	3	1	0	8	0.6	0	1	3
Candies, Confectioner's Coating, Butterscotch 1 oz (28.35g)	153	8	7	0	19	0.0	19	1	25
Candies, Dark Chocolate Coated Coffee Beans 1 serving, 28 pieces (40g)	216	12	6	5	24	3.0	17	3	10
Candies, Divinity, Prepared from Recipe 1 piece (11g)	40	0	0	0	10	0.0	9	0	4
Candies, Fudge, Chocolate Marshmallow, Prepared from Recipe 1 recipe, yield (60 pieces) (1229g)	5567	215	131	307	877	20.9	787	28	1045
Candies, Fudge, Chocolate, Prepared from Recipe 1 piece (17g)	70	2	1	2	13	0.3	12	0	8
Candies, Fudge, Peanut Butter, Prepared from Recipe 1 piece (16g)	62	1	0	0	12	0.1	12	1	19
Candies, Hard 1 piece (6g)	24	0	0	0	6	0.0	4	0	2

Food Serving size	Cal.	(g) Total Fat	(g) Sat. Fat	(mg) Chol.	(g) Carb.	(g) Fiber	(g) Sug.	(g) Prot.	(mg) Sod.
Candies, Hard, Dietetic or Low Calorie (Sorbitol)									
1 piece (3g)	12	0	0	0	3	0.0	0	0	0
Candies, Heath Bites									
15 pieces (39g)	207	12	6	7	25	0.8	23	2	96
Candies, Hershey, Kit Kat Big Kat Bar									
1 bar, king size 2.8 oz (79g)	411	22	14	7	50	1.5	43	5	51
Candies, Hershey, Reesesticks Crispy Wafers, Peanut Butter, Milk Chocolate									
1 serving, 1.5 oz (42g)	219	13	6	3	23	1.4	17	4	111
Candies, Hershey's Golden Almond Solitaires									
13 pieces (41g)	234	15	6	5	19	1.8	15	5	21
Candies, Hershey's Milk Chocolate with Almond Bites									
17 pieces (39g)	215	14	7	7	20	1.4	17	4	29
Candies, Hershey's Pot of Gold Almond Bar									
1 bar, 2.8 oz (78g)	450	30	13	10	36	3.0	30	10	50
Candies, Kit Kat Wafer Bar									
1 bar, miniature (.35 oz) (10g)	52	3	2	1	6	0.1	5	1	5
Candies, Krackel Chocolate Bar									
1 bar, 2 oz (56g)	287	15	9	6	36	1.2	29	4	110
Candies, Mars Snack US, Cocoavia Blueberry and Almond Chocolate Bar									
1 serving, 0.78 oz bar (22g)	116	6	3	0	13	2.0	9	1	2
Candies, Mars Snack US, Pop'ables 3 Musketeers Bite Size									
1 serving, 15 pieces (41g)	182	6	4	3	31	0.5	27	1	71
Candies, Mars Snack US, Starburst Fruit Chews, Fruit and Cream									
1 serving, fun size (8 chews) (40g)	163	3	3	0	33	0.0	23	0	1
Candies, Mars Snackfood US, 3 Musketeers Bar									
1 serving, 2 fun size bars (28g)	122	4	2	1	22	0.4	19	1	54
Candies, Mars Snackfood US, Cocoavia Chocolate Bar									
1 serving, 0.78 oz bar (22g)	119	6	3	0	14	1.9	9	1	2
Candies, Mars Snackfood US, Cocoavia Chocolate Covered Almonds									
1 serving, 1oz pack (28g)	160	10	3	0	14	2.9	8	3	3
Candies, Mars Snackfood US, Cocoavia Crispy Chocolate Bar									
1 serving, 0.7 oz bar (20g)	103	5	3	0	12	1.6	7	2	8
Candies, Mars Snackfood US, Dove Dark Chocolate									
1 serving, 7 pieces (42g)	218	14	8	3	25	3.2	19	2	2

Food Serving size	Cal.	(g) Total Fat	(g) Sat. Fat	(mg) Chol.	(g) Carb.	(g) Fiber	(g) Sug.	(g) Prot.	(mg) Sod.
Candies, Mars Snackfood US, Dove Milk Chocolate									
1 serving, 5 pieces (40g)	218	13	8	7	24	1.0	22	2	25
Candies, Mars Snackfood US, M&M's Crispy Chocolate Candies									
1 serving, 1.6 oz bag (47g)	223	9	5	6	34	0.9	28	2	64
Candies, Mars Snackfood US, M&M's Milk Chocolate Candies									
1 box (1.48 oz) (42g)	207	9	5	6	30	1.2	27	2	26
Candies, Mars Snackfood US, M&M's Minis Milk Chocolate Candies									
1 serving, 0.50 oz box (15g)	75	4	2	2	10	0.4	9	1	10
Candies, Mars Snackfood US, M&M's Peanut Chocolate Candies									
1 package, fun size (18g)	93	5	2	1	11	0.7	9	2	9
Candies, Mars Snackfood US, Mars Almond Bar									
1 bar (1.76 oz) (50g)	234	12	4	9	31	1.0	26	4	85
Candies, Mars Snackfood US, Milky Way Bar									
1 bar, fun size (17g)	78	3	2	2	12	0.2	10	1	28
Candies, Mars Snackfood US, Milky Way Caramel, Dark Chocolate Covered									
1 serving, 5 pieces (44g)	202	9	6	7	30	1.2	24	2	108
Candies, Mars Snackfood US, Milky Way Caramel, Milk Chocolate Covered									
1 serving, 5 pieces (44g)	204	8	6	9	30	0.3	26	2	120
Candies, Mars Snackfood US, Pop Milky Way Bite Size									
1 serving, 13 pieces (39g)	181	7	3	4	28	0.4	24	1	57
Candies, Mars Snackfood US, Pop Snickers Bite Size Candies									
1 serving, 13 pieces (39g)	187	9	4	5	24	0.9	20	3	87
Candies, Mars Snackfood US, Skittles Original Bite Size Candies									
1 cup (205g)	830	9	8	0	186	0.0	155	0	31
Candies, Mars Snackfood US, Skittles Sours Original									
1 serving, 1.80 oz bag (51g)	205	2	2	0	46	0.0	37	0	7
Candies, Mars Snackfood US, Skittles Tropical Bite Size Candies									
1 serving, fun size bag (20g)	81	1	--	0	18	0.0	15	0	3
Candies, Mars Snackfood US, Skittles Wild Berry Bite Size									
1 serving, fun size bag (20g)	80	1	1	0	18	0.0	15	0	3
Candies, Mars Snackfood US, Snickers Almond Bar									
1 serving, 1.76 oz bar (50g)	236	11	4	7	32	1.3	27	3	78
Candies, Mars Snackfood US, Snickers Bar									
1 bar, fun size (15g)	74	4	1	2	9	0.3	8	1	36

Food Serving size	Cal.	(g) Total Fat	(g) Sat. Fat	(mg) Chol.	(g) Carb.	(g) Fiber	(g) Sug.	(g) Prot.	(mg) Sod.
Candies, Mars Snackfood US, Snickers Cruncher									
1 bar, fun size (15g)	73	4	2	1	9	0.3	7	1	28
Candies, Mars Snackfood US, Snickers Munch Bar									
1 serving, 1.42 oz bar (40g)	214	14	4	10	17	1.9	12	6	143
Candies, Mars Snackfood US, Starburst Fruit Chews, Original Fruit									
1 serving, 2.07 oz pack (59g)	241	5	5	0	49	0.0	34	0	1
Candies, Mars Snackfood US, Starburst Fruit Chews, Tropical									
1 serving, 2.07 oz pack (59g)	241	5	5	0	49	0.0	34	0	1
Candies, Mars Snackfood US, Starburst Sour Fruit Chews									
1 serving, 2.07 oz pack (59g)	236	5	4	0	47	0.0	33	0	53
Candies, Mars Snackfood US, Twix Caramel Cookie Bars									
1 package (2.06 oz, 2 bars) (58g)	291	14	11	4	38	0.6	28	3	115
Candies, Mars Snackfood US, Twix Peanut Butter Cookie Bars									
1 package (2.06 oz, 2 bars) (58g)	311	19	9	3	31	1.8	21	5	131
Candies, Mars, M&M's Almond Chocolate Candies									
1 serving, about 1/4 cup (42g)	219	12	4	3	25	2.4	--	3	19
Candies, Mars, M&M's Peanut Butter Chocolate Candies									
1 cup (203g)	1074	60	38	14	115	8.1	--	21	432
Candies, Mars, Milky Way Midnight Bar									
1 bar, fun size (19g)	84	3	2	2	14	0.6	--	1	32
Candies, Marshmallows									
10 miniatures (7g)	22	0	0	0	6	0.0	4	0	6
Candies, Milk Chocolate									
1 bar, miniature (7g)	37	2	1	2	4	0.2	4	1	6
Candies, Milk Chocolate Coated Peanuts									
10 pieces (40g)	208	13	6	4	20	1.9	15	5	16
Candies, Milk Chocolate Coated Raisins									
10 pieces (10g)	39	1	1	0	7	0.3	6	0	4
Candies, Milk Chocolate, with Almonds									
1 bar (1.55 oz) (44g)	231	15	8	8	23	2.7	19	4	33
Candies, Milk Chocolate, with Rice Cereal									
1 bar (1.45 oz) (45g)	230	13	7	10	27	1.5	23	3	39

Food Serving size	Cal.	(g) Total Fat	(g) Sat. Fat	(mg) Chol.	(g) Carb.	(g) Fiber	(g) Sug.	(g) Prot.	(mg) Sod.
Candies, Mounds Candy Bar 1 package, 1.9 oz (53g)	258	14	11	1	31	2.0	24	2	77
Candies, Mr. Goodbar Chocolate Bar 1 bar, 2.6 oz (73g)	393	24	10	7	40	2.8	34	7	30
Candies, Nestle, 100 Grand Bar 1 bar, miniature (21g)	98	4	2	3	15	0.2	11	1	43
Candies, Nestle, After Eight Mints 1 piece (8.4g)	36	1	1	0	7	0.2	6	0	0
Candies, Nestle, Baby Ruth Bar 1 serving, fun size bar 0.65 oz (18g)	83	4	2	0	12	0.4	10	1	41
Candies, Nestle, Bit-O'-Honey Candy Chews 1 serving, 6 pieces (40g)	150	3	2	0	32	0.1	19	1	118
Candies, Nestle, Butterfinger Bar 1 serving, 1 fun size bar 0.65 oz (18g)	83	3	2	0	13	0.4	8	1	41
Candies, Nestle, Chunky Bar 1 serving, 1.4 oz bar (40g)	190	11	5	4	24	1.0	21	3	15
Candies, Nestle, Crunch Bar and Dessert Topping 1 bar, 0.5 oz (14.2g)	71	4	2	2	10	0.3	8	1	21
Candies, Nestle, Goobers Chocolate Covered Peanuts 1 serving, 0.25 cup (41g)	210	14	5	5	22	4.0	18	4	15
Candies, Nestle, Oh Henry! Bar 1 serving, fun size bar (26g)	120	6	2	2	17	0.5	12	2	50
Candies, Nestle, Raisinets Chocolate Covered Raisins 1 serving, fun size (48g)	203	8	5	5	34	1.1	28	2	16
Candies, Nougat, with Almonds 1 piece (14g)	56	0	0	0	13	0.5	0	0	5
Candies, Peanut Bar 1 bar, 1.4 oz (40g)	209	13	2	0	19	1.6	17	6	62
Candies, Praline, Prepared from Recipe 1 recipe, yield (907g)	4399	235	20	0	540	31.7	506	30	435
Candies, Reese's Bites 16 pieces (39g)	203	12	7	3	22	1.2	19	4	70

Food Serving size	Cal.	(g) Total Fat	(g) Sat. Fat	(mg) Chol.	(g) Carb.	(g) Fiber	(g) Sug.	(g) Prot.	(mg) Sod.
Candies, Reese's Fast Break, Candy Bar 1 serving, 1 bar (56g)	277	13	5	5	36	2.0	30	5	180
Candies, Reese's Nutrageous Candy Bar 2 bars (34g)	176	11	3	1	18	1.3	14	4	48
Candies, Reese's Peanut Butter Cups 1 package, 1.6 oz 2 cups (45g)	232	14	5	3	25	1.6	21	5	161
Candies, Reese's Pieces Candy 10 pieces (8g)	40	2	1	0	5	0.2	4	1	16
Candies, Reese's, Fast Break, Milk Chocolate Peanut Butter and Soft Nuggets 2 oz, bar (56g)	265	13	5	2	34	1.6	30	5	185
Candies, Rolo Caramels in Milk Chocolate 7 pieces (42g)	199	9	6	5	29	0.4	27	2	79
Candies, Semisweet Chocolate 1 cup, large chips (182g)	874	55	32	0	116	10.7	99	8	20
Candies, Semisweet Chocolate, Made with Butter 1 cup, large chips (182g)	868	54	32	33	115	10.7	--	8	20
Candies, Sesame Crunch 1 piece (1.8g)	9	1	0	0	1	0.1	1	0	3
Candies, Skor Toffee Bar 1 bar, 1.4 oz (39g)	209	13	7	21	24	0.5	23	1	124
Candies, Special Dark Chocolate Bar 1 bar, 2.6 oz (73g)	406	24	--	4	44	4.7	35	4	4
Candies, Sugar-coated Almonds 1 piece (3.5g)	17	1	0	0	2	0.1	2	0	0
Candies, Sweet Chocolate 1 bar, 1.45 oz (41g)	208	14	8	0	25	2.3	21	2	7
Candies, Sweet Chocolate Coated Fondant 1 patty, small (11g)	40	1	1	0	9	0.2	8	0	3
Candies, Symphony, Milk Chocolate Bar 1 bar, 2.4 oz (68g)	361	21	12	16	39	1.2	37	6	69
Candies, Taffy, Prepared from Recipe 1 piece (15g)	60	0	0	1	14	0.0	10	0	8
Candies, Toffee, Prepared from Recipe 1 piece (12g)	67	4	2	12	8	0.0	8	0	16
Candies, Tootsie Roll, Chocolate Flavor Roll 1 piece (6.6g)	26	0	0	0	6	0.0	4	0	3

Food Serving size	Cal.	(g) Total Fat	(g) Sat. Fat	(mg) Chol.	(g) Carb.	(g) Fiber	(g) Sug.	(g) Prot.	(mg) Sod.
Candies, Truffles, Prepared from Recipe 1 recipe, yield, recipe makes 49 1" x 1" pieces (612g)									
	3121	207	113	324	275	15.3	234	38	416
Candies, Twizzlers Cherry Bites 18 pieces (40g)	135	1	0	0	32	0.0	--	1	104
Candies, Twizzlers Nibs Cherry Bits 27 pieces (40g)	139	1	0	0	32	0.2	21	1	78
Candies, Twizzlers Strawberry Twists Candy 4 pieces, from 5 oz package (38g)	133	1	0	0	30	0.0	15	1	109
Candies, Whatchamacallit Candy Bar 1 bar, 1.7 oz (48g)	237	11	8	6	30	0.9	23	4	144
Candies, White Chocolate 1 bar, 3 oz (85g)	458	27	17	18	50	0.2	50	5	77
Candies, York Bites 15 pieces (39g)	154	3	2	0	32	0.8	29	1	18
Candies, York Peppermint Pattie 1 patty, 1.5 oz (43g)	165	3	2	0	35	0.9	27	1	12
Heinz, Weight Watchers, Chocolate Éclair, Frozen 1 eclair, frozen (59g)	142	4	1	28	24	1.2	10	3	177
McKee Baking, Little Debbie Nut Bar, Wafer with Peanut Butter, Chocolate Covered 1 serving (57g)	312	19	4	--	31	--	19	5	127
Snacks, Farley Candy, Farley Fruit Snacks, with Vitamins A, C and E 1 pouch (26g)	89	0	--	--	21	--	--	1	9
Snacks, General Mills, Betty Crocker Fruit Roll Ups, Berry Flavored with Vitamin C 2 rolls (28g)	104	1	0	--	24	--	11	0	89
Snacks, M&M Mars, Kudos Whole Grain Bar, M&M's Milk Chocolate 1 bar (24g)	100	3	2	1	18	0.6	0	1	82
Snacks, M&M Mars, Kudos Whole Grain Bar, Peanut Butter 1 bar (28g)	130	6	3	1	18	0.7	0	2	75
Snacks, M&M Mars, Kudos Whole Grain Bars, Chocolate Chip 1 bar (28g)	118	4	1	38	20	0.7	11	1	69
Snacks, Sunkist, Sunkist Fruit Roll, Strawberry with Vitamins A, C, and E 1 roll (21g)	72	0	--	--	17	1.6	--	0	23

Food Serving size	Cal.	(g) Total Fat	(g) Sat. Fat	(mg) Chol.	(g) Carb.	(g) Fiber	(g) Sug.	(g) Prot.	(mg) Sod.
Jellies, Jams, and Preserves									
Candies, Gumdrops, Dietetic or Low Calorie (Sorbitol)									
1 piece (5g)	8	0	0	0	4	0.9	0	0	0
Candies, Gumdrops, Starch Jelly Pieces									
10 gumdrops (36g)	143	0	0	0	36	0.0	21	0	16
Candies, Jelly Beans									
10 large, 1 oz (28g)	105	0	0	0	26	0.1	20	0	14
Cranberry-Orange Relish, Canned									
1 cup (275g)	490	0	0	0	127	0.0	--	1	88
Desserts, Flan, Caramel Custard, Prepared from Recipe									
1 recipe, yield (1531g)	2220	62	28	1378	349	0.0	354	69	811
Gelatin Dessert, Dry Mix									
1 portion, amount to make 1/2 cup (21g)	80	0	0	0	19	0.0	18	2	98
Gelatin Dessert, Dry Mix, Prepared with Water									
.5 cup (135g)	84	0	0	0	19	0.0	18	2	101
Gelatin Dessert, Dry Mix, Reduced Calorie with Aspartame									
1 serving (6.4g)	13	0	0	0	5	0.0	0	1	55
Gelatin Dessert, Dry Mix, Reduced Calorie with Aspartame, Added Phosphorus, Potassium, Sodium, Vitamin C									
1 package, 0.35 oz (10g)	35	0	0	0	3	0.0	--	6	275
Gelatin Dessert, Dry Mix, Reduced Calorie with Aspartame, No Added Sodium									
1 package, 0.35 oz (10g)	35	0	0	0	3	0.0	--	6	16
Gelatin Dessert, Dry Mix, Reduced Calorie with Aspartame, Prepared with Water									
1 package, yield (2 cups) (469g)	94	0	0	0	20	0.0	0	4	225
Gelatin Dessert, Dry Mix, with Added Vitamin C, Sodium-citrate and Salt									
1 portion, amount to make 1/2 cup (21g)	80	0	0	0	19	0.0	--	2	103
Gelatins, Dry Powder, Unsweetened									
1 package, 1 oz (28g)	94	0	0	0	0	0.0	0	24	55
Jams and Preserves									
1 packet, 0.5 oz (14g)	39	0	0	0	10	0.2	7	0	4
Jams and Preserves, Apricot									
1 packet, 0.5 oz (14g)	34	0	0	0	9	0.0	6	0	6

Food Serving size	Cal.	(g) Total Fat	(g) Sat. Fat	(mg) Chol.	(g) Carb.	(g) Fiber	(g) Sug.	(g) Prot.	(mg) Sod.
Jams and Preserves, Dietetic (with Sodium Saccharin), Any Flavor									
1 tbsp (14g)	18	0	0	0	8	0.4	1	0	0
Jellies									
1 packet, 0.5 oz (14g)	37	0	0	0	10	0.1	7	0	4
Jellies, Red Sugar, Home Preserved									
1 tbsp (19g)	34	0	0	0	9	0.2	2	0	0
Marmalade, Orange									
1 tbsp (20g)	49	0	0	0	13	0.1	12	0	11
Pectin, Unsweetened, Dry Mix									
1 package, 1.75 oz (50g)	163	0	0	0	45	4.3	--	0	100
Pie Fillings, Apple, Canned									
.125 can (74g)	74	0	0	0	19	0.7	10	0	35
Pie Fillings, Blueberry, Canned									
1 cup (262g)	474	1	0	0	116	6.8	124	1	31
Pie Fillings, Cherry, Canned									
.125 can (74g)	85	0	0	0	21	0.4	--	0	13
Pie Fillings, Cherry, Low Calorie									
1 cup (264g)	140	0	0	0	32	3.2	0	2	32

Misc. Candies (Gums, etc.)

Food Serving size	Cal.	(g) Total Fat	(g) Sat. Fat	(mg) Chol.	(g) Carb.	(g) Fiber	(g) Sug.	(g) Prot.	(mg) Sod.
Chewing Gum									
10 Chiclets (16g)	58	0	0	0	15	0.4	11	0	0
Chewing Gum, Sugarless									
1 piece (2g)	5	0	0	0	2	0.0	0	0	0
Snacks, Beef Sticks, Smoked									
1 stick (20g)	110	10	4	27	1	--	--	4	306

Chips and Pretzels

Food Serving size	Cal.	(g) Total Fat	(g) Sat. Fat	(mg) Chol.	(g) Carb.	(g) Fiber	(g) Sug.	(g) Prot.	(mg) Sod.
Banana Chips									
3 oz (85g)	441	29	25	0	50	6.5	30	2	5
Cheese Puffs and Twists, Corn Based, Baked, Low Fat									
1 oz (28.35g)	122	3	1	0	21	3.0	2	2	240
Corn-based, Extruded, Chips, Barbecue Flavor									
1 bag, 7 oz (198g)	1036	65	9	0	111	10.3	--	14	1511

Food Serving size	Cal.	(g) Total Fat	(g) Sat. Fat	(mg) Chol.	(g) Carb.	(g) Fiber	(g) Sug.	(g) Prot.	(mg) Sod.
Corn-based, Extruded, Chips, Barbecue Flavor, with Enriched Masa Flour									
1 oz (28.35g)	148	9	1	0	16	--	--	2	216
Corn-based, Extruded, Chips, Plain									
1 bag, 7 oz (198g)	1026	56	7	0	125	10.5	2	12	1079
Corn-based, Extruded, Chips, Unsalted									
1 bag, single serving (28g)	156	9	1	0	16	1.2	3	2	4
Corn-based, Extruded, Cones, Nacho Flavor									
1 oz (28.35g)	152	9	8	1	16	0.3	--	2	270
Corn-based, Extruded, Onion Flavor									
2 oz (57g)	284	13	2	0	37	2.2	3	4	542
Corn-based, Extruded, Puffs or Twists, Cheese Flavor									
32 pieces (28g)	158	10	2	2	15	0.5	1	2	255
Corn-based, Extruded, Puffs or Twists, Cheese Flavor, Unenriched									
1 bag (8 oz) (227g)	1267	81	13	9	123	5.0	6	13	2034
Cornnuts, Barbecue-flavor									
2 oz (57g)	249	8	1	0	41	4.8	--	5	342
Cornnuts, Nacho-flavor									
2 oz (57g)	250	8	1	1	41	4.6	--	5	361
Cornnuts, Plain									
2 oz (57g)	254	9	1	0	41	3.9	0	5	362
Doo Dads Snack Mix, Original Flavor									
.5 cup (28g)	128	5	1	0	18	1.9	--	3	356
Fritolay, SunChips, Multigrain Snack, Original Flavor									
1 oz (28.35g)	139	6	1	--	19	1.9	0	2	93
Fritolay, SunChips, Multigrain, French Onion Flavor									
1 oz (28.35g)	141	6	1	1	19	2.2	0	2	132
Fritolay, SunChips, Multigrain, Harvest Cheddar									
1 oz (28.35g)	139	6	1	1	18	2.3	0	2	153
M&M Mars, Combo Snacks, Cheddar Cheese Pretzel									
10 pieces (30g)	139	5	3	0	20	--	--	3	466
Plaintain Chips, Salted									
1 oz (28.35g)	151	8	2	0	18	1.0	0	1	57
Popcorn, Air-popped									
1 oz (28.35g)	110	1	0	0	22	4.1	0	4	2

Food Serving size	Cal.	(g) Total Fat	(g) Sat. Fat	(mg) Chol.	(g) Carb.	(g) Fiber	(g) Sug.	(g) Prot.	(mg) Sod.
Popcorn, Air-popped, White Popcorn 1 oz (28.35g)	108	1	0	0	22	4.3	--	3	1
Popcorn, Cakes 2 cakes (20g)	77	1	0	0	16	0.6	0	2	58
Popcorn, Caramel-coated, with Peanuts 2 oz (57g)	228	4	1	0	46	2.2	26	4	168
Popcorn, Caramel-coated, Without Peanuts 1 oz (28.35g)	122	4	1	1	22	1.5	15	1	58
Popcorn, Cheese Flavor 1 oz (28.35g)	149	9	2	3	15	2.8	--	3	252
Popcorn, Microwave, 94% Fat Free 1 oz (28.35g)	114	2	0	0	22	3.9	0	3	178
Popcorn, Microwave, Low Fat 1 oz (28.35g)	120	3	0	0	20	4.0	0	4	251
Popcorn, Micowave, Low Fat and Low Sodium 1 oz (28.35g)	122	3	0	0	21	4.0	0	4	139
Popcorn, Microwave, Regular (Butter) Flavor, with Partially Hydrogenated Oil 1 oz (28.35g)	149	8	2	1	16	2.8	0	2	219
Popcorn, Oil-popped, Microwave 1 oz (28.35g)	165	12	2	0	13	2.3	0	2	300
Popcorn, Oil-popped, White Popcorn 1 oz (28.35g)	142	8	1	0	16	2.8	--	3	251
Popcorn, Sugar Syrup, Caramel, Fat Free 1 oz (28.35g)	108	0	0	0	26	0.7	18	1	81
Popcorn, Unpopped Kernels 1 oz (28.35g)	106	1	0	--	21	3.6	0	3	2
Popovers, Dry Mix, Unenriched 1 package (6 oz) (170g)	631	7	2	0	121	--	--	18	1540
Potato Chips, Barbecue Flavor 1 bag (7 oz) (198g)	972	64	16	0	105	8.7	--	15	1485
Potato Chips, Cheese Flavor 1 bag (6 oz) (170g)	843	46	15	7	98	8.8	--	14	1348
Potato Chips, Fat Free, Made with Olestra 1 oz (28.35g)	78	0	0	0	18	1.9	0	2	157

Food Serving size	Cal.	(g) Total Fat	(g) Sat. Fat	(mg) Chol.	(g) Carb.	(g) Fiber	(g) Sug.	(g) Prot.	(mg) Sod.
Potato Chips, Fat Free, Salted 1 bag (8 oz) (227g)	860	1	0	0	190	17.0	8	22	1460
Potato Chips, from Dried Potatoes, Fat Free, with Olestra 1 oz (28.35g)	72	0	0	0	16	2.1	0	1	122
Potato Chips, Light 1 bag (6 oz) (170g)	801	35	7	0	114	10.0	0	12	836
Potato Chips, Made from Dried Potatoes, Cheese Flavor 1 can (6.25 oz) (191g)	1052	71	18	8	97	6.5	--	13	1442
Potato Chips, Made from Dried Potatoes, Light 1 can (6 oz) (170g)	853	44	11	0	110	5.4	1	8	699
Potato Chips, Made from Dried Potatoes, Plain 1 can (7 oz) (198g)	1107	76	19	0	103	6.1	2	9	768
Potato Chips, Made from Dried Potatoes, Sour Cream and Onion Flavor 1 can (6.75 oz) (198g)	1083	73	19	6	102	2.4	--	13	1426
Potato Chips, Plain, Made with Partially Hydrogenated Soybean Oil, Salted 1 bag (8 oz) (227g)	1217	79	12	0	120	10.9	--	16	1348
Potato Chips, Plain, Made with Partially Hydrogenated Soybean Oil, Unsalted 1 bag (8 oz) (227g)	1217	79	12	0	120	10.9	--	16	18
Potato Chips, Plain, Salted 1 bag (8 oz) (227g)	1230	83	9	0	115	10.0	1	15	1192
Potato Chips, Plain, Unsalted 1 bag (8 oz) (227g)	1217	79	25	0	120	10.9	0	16	18
Potato Chips, Sour Cream and Onion Flavor 1 bag (7 oz) (198g)	1051	67	18	14	102	10.3	--	16	1238
Potato Chips, White, Restructured, Baked 10 chips (12g)	56	2	0	0	9	0.6	0	1	76
Potato Chips, Without Salt, Reduced Fat 1 oz (28.35g)	138	6	1	0	19	1.7	0	2	2
Pretzels, Hard, Confectioner's Coating, Chocolate Flavor 1 pretzel (11g)	50	2	1	0	8	--	--	1	63
Pretzels, Hard, Plain, Made with Enriched Flour, Unsalted 10 twists (60g)	229	2	0	0	48	1.7	1	5	173
Pretzels, Hard, Plain, Made with Unenriched Flour, Salted 10 twists (60g)	229	2	0	0	48	1.7	--	5	1029

Food Serving size	Cal.	(g) Total Fat	(g) Sat. Fat	(mg) Chol.	(g) Carb.	(g) Fiber	(g) Sug.	(g) Prot.	(mg) Sod.
Pretzels, Hard, Plain, Made with Unenriched Flour, Unsalted 10 twists (60g)	229	2	0	0	48	1.7	--	5	173
Pretzels, Hard, Plain, Salted 10 twists (60g)	228	2	0	0	48	1.8	2	6	814
Pretzels, Hard, Whole Wheat 2 oz (57g)	206	1	0	0	46	4.4	--	6	116
Pretzels, Soft 1 medium (115g)	389	4	1	3	80	2.0	0	9	926
Pretzels, Soft, Unsalted 1 medium (115g)	389	4	1	3	82	2.0	0	9	794
Soy Chips or Crisps, Salted 1 oz (28.35g)	109	2	0	0	15	1.0	0	8	239
Sweet Potato Chips 1 oz (28.35g)	141	7	1	0	18	1.0	0	1	10
Taro Chips 10 chips (23g)	115	6	1	0	16	1.7	1	1	79
Tortilla Chips, Light (Baked with Less Oil) 10 chips (16g)	74	2	0	0	12	0.9	7	1	137
Tortilla Chips, Low Fat, Baked, Without Fat 1 oz (28.35g)	118	2	0	0	23	1.5	0	3	119
Tortilla Chips, Low Fat, Made with Olestra, Nacho Cheese 1 oz (28.35g)	90	1	0	1	18	1.8	1	2	171
Tortilla Chips, Low Fat, Unsalted 1 oz (28.35g)	118	2	0	0	23	1.5	0	3	4
Tortilla Chips, Nacho Cheese 1 oz (28.35g)	146	7	1	--	18	1.3	1	2	174
Tortilla Chips, Nacho Flavor, Made with Enriched Masa Flour 1 oz (28.35g)	141	7	1	1	18	1.5	--	2	201
Tortilla Chips, Nacho Flavor, Reduced Fat 1 bag (6 oz) (170g)	757	26	5	5	122	8.2	--	15	1705
Tortilla Chips, Ranch Flavor 1 bag (7 oz) (198g)	992	49	7	--	124	7.9	6	14	1028
Tortilla Chips, Taco Flavor 1 bag (8 oz) (227g)	1090	55	11	11	143	12.0	--	18	1786

Food Serving size	Cal.	(g) Total Fat	(g) Sat. Fat	(mg) Chol.	(g) Carb.	(g) Fiber	(g) Sug.	(g) Prot.	(mg) Sod.
Tortilla Chips, Unsalted, White Corn									
1 bag, single serving (28g)	141	7	1	0	18	1.5	1	2	4
Tortillas, Ready-to-bake or Fry, Corn									
1 enchilada (19g)	41	1	0	0	8	1.2	0	1	9
Tortillas, Ready-to-bake or Fry, Corn, Without Salt									
1 tortilla, medium (approx 6" dia) (26g)	58	1	0	0	12	1.4	--	1	3
Tostada Shells, Corn									
3 pieces (mean serving weight, aggregated over brands) (37g)	175	9	3	--	24	2.1	--	2	243
Tostada with Guacamole									
2 pieces (261g)	360	23	10	39	32	--	--	12	799
Trail Mix, Regular									
1 oz (28.35g)	131	8	2	0	13	--	--	4	65
Trail Mix, Regular, Unsalted									
1 oz (28.35g)	131	8	2	0	13	--	--	4	3
Trail Mix, Regular, with Chocolate Chips, Salted Nuts and Seeds									
1 oz (28.35g)	137	9	2	1	13	--	--	4	34
Trail Mix, Regular, with Chocolate Chips, Unsalted Nuts and Seeds									
1 oz (28.35g)	137	9	2	1	13	--	--	4	8
Trail Mix, Tropical									
1 oz (28.35g)	115	5	2	0	19	--	--	2	3

Sugars, Syrups, and Toppings

Food Serving size	Cal.	(g) Total Fat	(g) Sat. Fat	(mg) Chol.	(g) Carb.	(g) Fiber	(g) Sug.	(g) Prot.	(mg) Sod.
Candies, Confectioner's Coating, Peanut Butter									
1 oz (28.35g)	150	8	4	0	13	1.4	11	5	71
Candies, Confectioner's Coating, Yogurt									
1 cup, chips (170g)	887	46	41	2	109	0.0	106	10	150
Chocolate Syrup									
1 cup (300g)	837	3	2	0	195	7.8	149	6	216
Chocolate-flavored Hazelnut Spread									
1 serving, 2 tbsp (37g)	200	11	11	0	23	2.0	20	2	15
Frostings, Chocolate, Creamy, Dry Mix									
1 package (388g)	1509	20	--	0	357	9.3	--	5	295

Food Serving size	Cal.	(g) Total Fat	(g) Sat. Fat	(mg) Chol.	(g) Carb.	(g) Fiber	(g) Sug.	(g) Prot.	(mg) Sod.
Frostings, Chocolate, Creamy, Ready-to-eat									
2 tbsp, creamy (41g)	163	7	2	0	26	0.4	24	0	75
Frostings, Coconut-nut, Ready-to-eat									
.083 package (38g)	165	9	3	0	20	1.0	15	1	74
Frostings, Cream Cheese Flavor, Ready-to-eat									
2 tbsp, whipped (24g)	100	4	1	0	16	0.0	15	0	46
Frostings, Glaze, Prepared from Recipe									
1 recipe, yield (327g)	1115	2	1	3	274	0.0	263	1	20
Frostings, Vanilla, Creamy, Dry Mix									
.083 package (34g)	139	2	--	0	32	0.0	--	0	4
Frostings, Vanilla, Creamy, Ready-to-eat									
.083 package (38g)	159	6	1	0	26	0.0	24	0	70
Frostings, White, Fluffy, Dry Mix									
.083 package (17g)	63	0	--	0	16	0.0	--	0	40
Frostings, White, Fluffy, Dry Mix, Prepared with Water									
.083 package (26g)	63	0	0	0	16	0.0	--	0	41
Honey									
1 tbsp (21g)	64	0	0	0	17	0.0	17	0	1
Ice Cream Cones, Cake or Wafer-type									
1 cone (4g)	17	0	0	0	3	0.1	0	0	10
Ice Cream Cones, Sugar, Rolled-type									
1 cone (10g)	40	0	0	0	8	0.2	3	1	25
Molasses									
1 serving, 1 tbsp (20g)	58	0	0	0	15	0.0	11	0	7
Sugar, Brown									
1 cup, unpacked (145g)	551	0	0	0	142	0.0	141	0	41
Sugar, Granulated									
1 tsp (4.2g)	16	0	0	0	4	0.0	4	0	0
Sugar, Maple									
1 oz (28.35g)	100	0	0	0	26	0.0	24	0	3
Sugar, Powdered									
1 cup, sifted (100g)	389	0	0	0	100	0.0	98	0	2
Sweeteners, Tabletop, Aspartame, Equal, Packets									
1 serving, 1 packet (1g)	4	0	0	0	1	0.0	1	0	0

Food Serving size	Cal.	(g) Total Fat	(g) Sat. Fat	(mg) Chol.	(g) Carb.	(g) Fiber	(g) Sug.	(g) Prot.	(mg) Sod.
Sweeteners, Tabletop, Fructose, Dry, Powder 1 tsp (4.2g)	15	0	0	0	4	0.0	2	0	1
Sweeteners, Tabletop, Saccharin 1 serving, 1 packet (0.8g)	3	0	0	0	1	0.0	0	0	3
Sweeteners, Tabletop, Sucralose, Splenda Packets 1 serving, 1 packet (1g)	3	0	0	0	1	0.0	1	0	0
Syrup, Chocolate, Fudge-type 2 tbsp (38g)	133	3	2	0	24	1.1	13	2	131
Syrup, Chocolate, Hershey's Genuine Chocolate Flavor Lite Syrup 2 tbsp (35g)	54	0	0	0	12	0.0	10	0	35
Syrup, Corn, Dark 1 tbsp (20g)	57	0	0	0	16	0.0	5	0	31
Syrup, Corn, High Fructose 1 tbsp (19g)	53	0	0	0	14	0.0	5	0	0
Syrup, Corn, Light 1 tbsp (22g)	62	0	0	0	17	0.0	6	0	14
Syrup, Dietetic 1 tbsp (15g)	6	0	0	0	7	0.5	1	0	3
Syrup, Grenadine 1 tsp (6.7g)	18	0	0	0	4	0.0	0	0	2
Syrup, Malt 1 tbsp (24g)	76	0	0	0	17	0.0	17	1	8
Syrup, Maple 1 tbsp (20g)	52	0	0	0	13	0.0	12	0	2
Syrup, Sorghum 1 tbsp (21g)	61	0	0	0	16	0.0	16	0	2
Syrup, Table Blends, Pancake 1 tbsp (20g)	47	0	0	0	12	0.0	4	0	16
Syrup, Table Blends, Pancake, Reduced Calorie 1 tbsp (15g)	25	0	0	0	7	0.0	5	0	27
Syrup, Table Blends, Cane and 15% Maple 1 tbsp (20g)	56	0	0	0	14	0.0	14	0	21
Syrup, Table Blends, Corn, Refiner and Sugar 1 tbsp (20g)	64	0	0	0	17	0.0	--	0	14

Food Serving size	Cal.	(g) Total Fat	(g) Sat. Fat	(mg) Chol.	(g) Carb.	(g) Fiber	(g) Sug.	(g) Prot.	(mg) Sod.
Syrup, Table Blends, Pancake, with 2% Maple									
1 tbsp (20g)	53	0	0	0	14	0.0	8	0	12
Syrup, Table Blends, Pancake, with 2% Maple, with Potassium									
1 tbsp (20g)	53	0	0	0	14	0.0	--	0	12
Syrup, Table Blends, Pancake, with Butter									
1 tbsp (20g)	59	0	0	1	15	0.0	--	0	20
Toppings, Butterscotch or Caramel									
2 tbsp (41g)	103	0	0	0	27	0.4	--	1	143
Toppings, Marshmallow Cream									
1 jar (198g)	638	1	0	0	156	0.2	93	2	158
Toppings, Nuts in Syrup									
2 tbsp (41g)	184	9	1	0	24	0.9	15	2	17
Toppings, Pineapple									
2 tbsp (42g)	106	0	0	0	28	0.2	9	0	18
Toppings, Strawberry									
2 tbsp (42g)	107	0	0	0	28	0.3	11	0	9
Vanilla Extract									
1 tbsp (13g)	37	0	0	0	2	0.0	2	0	1
Vanilla Extract, Imitation, Alcohol									
1 tsp (4.2g)	10	0	--	0	0	0.0	--	0	0
Vanilla Extract, Imitation, No Alcohol									
1 tsp (4.2g)	2	0	0	0	1	0.0	1	0	0

Beverages

Why Drink Beverages?

Beverages provide hydration and needed nutrients. Water is the body's principle component and makes up 60% of your body weight. Every system in your body depends on water. Even mild dehydration can drain your energy and make you tired. Beverages can also provide needed nutrients such as calcium in milk and vitamin C in orange juice.

Daily Goal

"8 by 8 rule"—drinking eight 8-ounce glasses of fluid a day is the general rule.
Women actually need about 9 cups of total beverages a day.
Men actually need about 13 cups of total beverages a day.
Women who are expecting or breast-feeding need about 10 to 13 cups of fluids a day.

Shopping Tips

- Plain water is best for hydration.
- Choose 100% juices rather than juice drinks.
- Drink skim or fat-free milk.
- Use sports drinks in moderation.

Shopping List Essentials

Bottled water
Milk, fat-free or skim
Juice drinks, 100% juice

Red Flags

Drinks can be high in calories and sugars. Make sure that juice drinks don't have added sugars. A soda that only has sugar calories is an example of an "empty calories" choice. You need water for hydration but try not to drink calories with your water.

Food Serving size	Cal.	(g) Total Fat	(g) Sat. Fat	(mg) Chol.	(g) Carb.	(g) Fiber	(g) Sug.	(g) Prot.	(mg) Sod.
Alcoholic Beverages/Wines									
Alcoholic Beverage, Daiquiri, Prepared from Recipe									
1 cocktail (2 fl oz) (60g)	112	0	0	0	4	0.1	3	0	3
Alcoholic Beverage, Distilled, All (Gin, Rum, Vodka, Whiskey) 80 Proof									
1 jigger, 1.5 fl oz (42g)	97	0	0	0	0	0.0	0	0	0
Alcoholic Beverage, Distilled, All (Gin, Rum, Vodka, Whiskey) 86 Proof									
1 jigger, 1.5 fl oz (42g)	105	0	0	0	0	0.0	0	0	0
Alcoholic Beverage, Distilled, All (Gin, Rum, Vodka, Whiskey) 90 Proof									
1 jigger, 1.5 fl oz (42g)	110	0	0	0	0	0.0	0	0	0
Alcoholic Beverage, Distilled, All (Gin, Rum, Vodka, Whiskey) 94 Proof									
1 jigger, 1.5 fl oz (42g)	116	0	0	0	0	0.0	--	0	0
Alcoholic Beverage, Distilled, All (Gin, Rum, Vodka, Whiskey) 100 Proof									
1 jigger, 1.5 fl oz (42g)	124	0	0	0	0	0.0	--	0	0
Alcoholic Beverage, Distilled, Gin, 90 Proof									
1 jigger, 1.5 fl oz (42g)	110	0	0	0	0	0.0	0	0	1
Alcoholic Beverage, Distilled, Rum, 80 Proof									
1 jigger, 1.5 fl oz (42g)	97	0	0	0	0	0.0	0	0	0
Alcoholic Beverage, Distilled, Vodka, 80 Proof									
1 jigger, 1.5 fl oz (42g)	97	0	0	0	0	0.0	0	0	0
Alcoholic Beverage, Distilled, Whiskey, 86 Proof									
1 jigger, 1.5 fl oz (42g)	105	0	0	0	0	0.0	0	0	0
Beer, Light									
1 can, or bottle (12 fl oz) (354g)	103	0	0	0	6	0.0	0	1	14
Beer, Light, Bud Light									
12 fl oz (354g)	110	0	--	0	7	0.0	--	1	11
Beer, Light, Budweiser Select									
12 fluid ounce (355g)	99	0	--	0	3	0.0	--	1	11
Beer, Light, Michelob Ultra									
12 fl oz (354g)	96	0	--	0	3	0.0	--	1	11
Beer, Regular, All									
1 fl oz (29.7g)	13	0	0	0	1	0.0	0	0	1
Beer, Regular, Budweiser									
12 fl oz (357g)	146	0	--	0	11	0.0	--	1	11

Food Serving size	Cal.	(g) Total Fat	(g) Sat. Fat	(mg) Chol.	(g) Carb.	(g) Fiber	(g) Sug.	(g) Prot.	(mg) Sod.
Créme de Menthe, 72 Proof 1 jigger 1.5 fl oz (50g)	186	0	0	0	21	0.0	21	0	3
Daiquiri, Canned 1 can (6.8 fl oz, 200 ml) (207g)	259	0	0	0	32	0.0	--	0	83
Liqueur, Coffee, 53 Proof 1 jigger, 1.5 fl oz (52g)	170	0	0	0	24	0.0	24	0	4
Liqueur, Coffee, 63 Proof 1 jigger, 1.5 fl oz (52g)	160	0	0	0	17	0.0	17	0	4
Liqueur, Coffee, with Cream, 34 Proof 1 jigger, 1.5 fl oz (47g)	154	7	5	27	10	0.0	9	1	43
Pina Colada, Canned 1 can (6.8 fl oz, 200 ml) (222g)	526	17	15	0	61	0.2	--	1	15823
Pina Colada, Prepared from Recipe 1 cocktail (4.5 fl oz) (141g)	245	3	2	0	32	0.4	31	1	8
Rice (Sake) 1 fl oz (29.1g)	39	0	0	0	1	0.0	--	0	1
Tequila Sunrise, Canned 1 can (6.8 fl oz, 200 ml) (211g)	232	0	0	0	24	0.0	--	1	120
Whiskey Sour Mix, Bottled 2 fl oz (65g)	57	0	0	0	14	0.0	14	0	66
Whiskey Sour Mix, Bottled, with Added Potassium and Sodium 1 fl oz (32.3g)	27	0	0	0	7	0.0	--	0	11
Whiskey Sour Mix, Powder 1 packet (17g)	65	0	0	0	17	0.0	17	0	47
Whiskey Sour, Canned 1 can (6.8 fl oz, 200 ml) (209g)	249	0	0	0	28	0.2	--	0	92
Whiskey Sour, Prepared from Bottled Mix 1 portion (2 oz mix + 1.5 oz whiskey) (106g)	162	0	0	0	14	0.0	14	0	65
Whiskey Sour, Prepared from Bottled Mix, with Added Potassium and Sodium 1 portion (2 oz mix + 1.5 oz whiskey) (106g)	158	0	0	0	14	0.0	--	0	21

Food Serving size	Cal.	(g) Total Fat	(g) Sat. Fat	(mg) Chol.	(g) Carb.	(g) Fiber	(g) Sug.	(g) Prot.	(mg) Sod.
Whiskey Sour, Prepared with Water, Whiskey and Powder Mix 1 packet, prepared (103g)	169	0	0	0	16	0.0	16	0	48
Wine, Cooking 1 fl oz (29g)	15	0	0	0	2	0.0	0	0	182
Wine, Dessert, Dry 1 glass (3.5 fl oz) (103g)	157	0	0	0	12	0.0	1	0	9
Wine, Dessert, Sweet 1 glass (3.5 fl oz) (103g)	165	0	0	0	14	0.0	8	0	9
Wine, Light 1 serving, 5 fl oz (148g)	73	0	0	0	2	0.0	3	0	10
Wine, Non-alcoholic 1 fl oz (29g)	2	0	0	0	0	0.0	0	0	2
Wine, Table, All 1 fl oz (29.5g)	24	0	0	0	1	0.0	0	0	1
Wine, Table, Red 1 serving, 5 fl oz (147g)	125	0	0	0	4	0.0	1	0	6
Wine, Table, Red, Barbera 1 serving, 5 fl oz (147g)	125	0	--	--	4	--	--	0	--
Wine, Table, Red, Burgundy 1 serving, 5 fl oz (148g)	127	0	--	--	5	--	--	0	--
Wine, Table, Red, Cabernet Franc 1 serving, 5 fl oz (147g)	122	0	--	--	4	--	--	0	--
Wine, Table, Red, Cabernet Sauvignon 1 serving, 5 fl oz (147g)	122	0	--	--	4	--	--	0	--
Wine, Table, Red, Carignane 1 serving, 5 fl oz (147g)	109	0	--	--	4	--	--	0	--
Wine, Table, Red, Claret 1 serving, 5 fl oz (147g)	122	0	--	--	4	--	--	0	--
Wine, Table, Red, Gamay 1 serving, 5 fl oz (147g)	115	0	--	--	3	--	--	0	--
Wine, Table, Red, Lemberger 1 serving, 5 fl oz (147g)	118	0	--	--	4	--	--	0	--
Wine, Table, Red, Merlot 1 serving, 5 fl oz (147g)	122	0	--	--	4	0.0	1	0	6

Food Serving size	Cal.	(g) Total Fat	(g) Sat. Fat	(mg) Chol.	(g) Carb.	(g) Fiber	(g) Sug.	(g) Prot.	(mg) Sod.
Wine, Table, Red, Mouvedre 1 serving, 5 fl oz (147g)	129	0	--	--	4	--	--	0	--
Wine, Table, Red, Petite Sirah 1 serving, 5 fl oz (147g)	125	0	--	--	4	--	--	0	--
Wine, Table, Red, Pinot Noir 1 serving, 5 fl oz (147g)	121	0	--	--	3	--	--	0	--
Wine, Table, Red, Sangiovese 1 serving, 5 fl oz (147g)	126	0	--	--	4	--	--	0	--
Wine, Table, Red, Syrah 1 serving, 5 fl oz (147g)	122	0	--	--	4	--	--	0	--
Wine, Table, Red, Zinfandel 1 serving, 5 fl oz (147g)	129	0	--	--	4	--	--	0	--
Wine, Table, White 1 serving, 5 fl oz (147g)	121	0	0	0	4	0.0	1	0	7
Wine, Table, White, Chenin Blanc 1 serving, 5 fl oz (148g)	118	0	--	--	5	--	--	0	--
Wine, Table, White, Fume Blanc 1 serving, 5 fl oz (147g)	121	0	--	--	3	--	--	0	--
Wine, Table, White, Gewurztraminer 1 serving, 5 fl oz (147g)	119	0	--	--	4	--	--	0	--
Wine, Table, White, Late Harvest 1 serving, 5 fl oz (154g)	172	0	--	--	21	--	--	0	--
Wine, Table, White, Muller Thurgau 1 serving, 5 fl oz (148g)	112	0	--	--	5	--	--	0	--
Wine, Table, White, Muscat 1 serving, 5 fl oz (150g)	123	0	--	--	8	--	--	0	--
Wine, Table, White, Pinot Blanc 1 serving, 5 fl oz (147g)	119	0	--	--	3	--	--	0	--
Wine, Table, White, Pinot Gris (Grigio) 1 serving, 5 fl oz (147g)	122	0	--	--	3	--	--	0	--
Wine, Table, White, Riesling 1 serving, 5 fl oz (148g)	118	0	--	--	6	--	--	0	--

Food Serving size	Cal.	(g) Total Fat	(g) Sat. Fat	(mg) Chol.	(g) Carb.	(g) Fiber	(g) Sug.	(g) Prot.	(mg) Sod.
Wine, Table, White, Sauvignon Blanc 1 serving, 5 fl oz (147g)	119	0	--	--	3	--	--	0	--
Wine, Table, White, Semillon 1 serving, 5 fl oz (148g)	121	0	--	--	5	--	--	0	--

Non-alcoholic

Food Serving size	Cal.	(g) Total Fat	(g) Sat. Fat	(mg) Chol.	(g) Carb.	(g) Fiber	(g) Sug.	(g) Prot.	(mg) Sod.
Bean Beverage 1 fl oz (28.8g)	10	0	0	0	2	0.0	0	1	1
Beverage, Fruit Juice Drink, Reduced Sugar, with Vitamin E Added 1 ml (1.1g)	0	0	0	0	0	0.0	0	0	0
Beverage, Instant Breakfast Powder, Chocolate Sugar-free, Not Reconstituted 1 envelope (20g)	72	1	0	9	8	0.4	--	7	143
Beverage, Instant Breakfast Powder, Chocolate, Not Reconstituted 1 envelope (37g)	132	1	0	4	24	0.1	0	7	142
Beverage, Milkshake Mix, Dry, Not Chocolate 1 envelope (21g)	69	1	0	3	11	0.3	0	5	164
Beverage, Vegetables and Fruit Juice Blend, with Added Vitamins A, C, E 1 serving, 8 oz (246g)	113	0	0	0	27	0.0	26	1	71
Chocolate Syrup, Prepared with Whole Milk 1 cup (8 fl oz) (282g)	254	8	5	25	36	0.8	32	9	133
Chocolate-flavor Beverage Mix for Milk, Powder, with Added Nutrients 1 serving (22g)	88	0	1	0	20	1.0	18	1	30
Chocolate-flavor Beverage Mix for Milk, Powder, Without Added Nutrients 1 portion (2-3 heaping tsp) (22g)	89	1	0	0	20	1.1	18	1	46
Chocolate-flavor Beverage Mix with Added Nutrients, Prepared with Whole Milk 1 serving (266g)	237	8	5	27	32	1.1	31	9	133
Chocolate-flavor Beverage Mix, Powder, Prepared with Whole Milk 1 cup (8 fl oz) (266g)	226	9	5	24	32	1.1	--	9	154
Chocolate-flavor Drink, Whey and Milk-based 1 fl oz (30.5g)	15	0	0	0	3	0.2	1	0	28
Clam and Tomato Juice, Canned 1 can (5.5 oz) (166g)	80	0	0	0	18	0.7	5	1	601
Cocktail Mix, Non-alcoholic, Concentrated, Frozen 1 fl oz (36g)	103	0	0	0	26	0.0	3	0	0

Food Serving size	Cal.	(g) Total Fat	(g) Sat. Fat	(mg) Chol.	(g) Carb.	(g) Fiber	(g) Sug.	(g) Prot.	(mg) Sod.
Coconut milk, canned (Liquid Expressed from Grated Meat and Water)									
1 tbsp (15g)	30	3	3	0	0	--	--	0	2
Coconut Milk, Frozen (Liquid Expressed from Grated Meat and Water)									
1 tbsp (15g)	30	3	3	0	1	--	--	0	2
Coconut Milk, Raw (Liquid Expressed from Grated Meat and Water)									
1 tbsp (15g)	35	4	3	0	1	0.3	1	0	2
Coconut Water (Liquid from Coconuts)									
1 tbsp (15g)	3	0	0	0	1	0.2	0	0	16
Corn Beverage									
1 fl oz (30.2g)	12	0	0	0	3	0.1	--	0	42
Eggnog									
1 fl oz (31.8g)	28	1	1	19	3	0.0	3	1	17
Eggnog-flavor Mix, Powder, Prepared with Whole Milk									
1 cup (8 fl oz) (272g)	258	8	5	30	39	0.0	34	8	150
Fruit Punch Drink, Frozen Concentrate, Prepared with Water									
1 fl oz (30.9g)	14	0	0	0	4	0.0	0	0	2
Fruit Punch Drink, with Added Nutrients, Canned									
1 fl oz (31g)	15	0	0	0	4	0.1	3	0	12
Fruit Punch Juice Drink, Frozen Concentrate									
1 can (12 fl oz) (423g)	740	3	0	0	182	0.8	--	1	42
Fruit Punch Juice Drink, Frozen Concentrate, Prepared with Water									
1 fl oz (29.3g)	12	0	0	0	3	0.0	0	0	1
Fruit Punch-flavor Drink, Powder, Without Added Sodium, Prepared with Water									
1 fl oz (32.8g)	12	0	0	0	3	0.0	3	0	2
Fruit-flavored Drink Mix, Powder, Unsweetened									
2 tsp, rounded (25g)	57	0	0	0	23	0.0	0	0	682
Fruit-flavored Drink, Dry Powder Mix, Low Calorie, with Aspartame									
1 tsp (8g)	17	0	0	0	7	0.0	0	0	32
Fruit-flavored Drink, Powder, with Hi Vitamin C with Other Added Vitamins, Low Calorie									
1 tsp (2g)	5	0	0	0	2	0.0	0	0	0
Grape Drink, Canned									
1 fl oz (31.3g)	19	0	0	0	5	0.0	4	0	5

Food Serving size	Cal.	(g) Total Fat	(g) Sat. Fat	(mg) Chol.	(g) Carb.	(g) Fiber	(g) Sug.	(g) Prot.	(mg) Sod.
Horchata, Dry Mix, Unprepared, Variety of Brands, All with Morro Seeds									
1 cup (118g)	487	9	2	0	93	4.7	46	9	4
Malt Beverage									
1 fl oz (29.6g)	11	0	0	0	2	0.0	2	0	4
Malted Drink Mix, Chocolate, Powder									
1 serving (3 heaping tsp or 1 envelope) (21g)	86	1	1	0	18	1.0	14	1	40
Malted Drink Mix, Chocolate, Powder, Prepared with Whole Milk									
1 cup (8 fl oz) (265g)	225	9	5	27	30	1.3	18	9	159
Malted Drink Mix, Chocolate, with Added Nutrients, Powder									
1 serving (4 tbsp or 1 envelope) (21g)	82	1	0	0	18	1.0	15	1	125
Malted Drink Mix, Chocolate, with Added Nutrients, Powder, Prepared with Whole Milk									
1 cup (8 fl oz) (265g)	231	9	5	27	30	1.1	28	9	231
Malted Drink Mix, Natural, Powder									
1 serving (3 heaping tsp or 1 envelope) (21g)	90	2	1	5	15	0.0	10	3	85
Malted Drink Mix, Natural, Powder, Prepared with Whole Milk									
1 cup (8 fl oz) (265g)	233	10	5	32	27	0.3	25	10	209
Malted Drink Mix, Natural, with Added Nutrients, Powder									
1 serving (4 tbsp or 1 envelope) (21g)	78	0	0	0	18	0.4	13	2	54
Malted Drink Mix, Natural, with Added Nutrients, Powder, Prepared with Whole Milk									
1 cup (8 fl oz) (265g)	228	9	5	29	28	0.0	22	10	191
Meal Supplement Drink, Nestle, Supligen, Canned, Peanut Flavor									
1 cup (158g)	160	5	1	--	23	--	--	6	85
Water, Tap, Drinking									
1 cup, 8 fl oz (237g)	0	0	0	0	0	0.0	0	0	9
Water, Tap, Municipal									
1 cup, 8 fl oz (237g)	0	0	0	0	0	0.0	0	0	7
Water, Tap, Well									
1 cup, 8 fl oz (237g)	0	0	--	--	0	0.0	--	0	12

Food Serving size	Cal.	(g) Total Fat	(g) Sat. Fat	(mg) Chol.	(g) Carb.	(g) Fiber	(g) Sug.	(g) Prot.	(mg) Sod.
Bottled Waters									
Water, Bottled, Generic 1 cup (237g)	0	0	0	0	0	0.0	0	0	5
Water, Bottled, Non-carbonated, Calistoga 1 bottle, 16.9 fl oz (500g)	0	0	--	--	0	--	--	0	0
Water, Bottled, Non-carbonated, Crystal Geyser 1 bottle, 8 fl oz in packages of 8 (237g)	0	0	--	--	0	--	--	0	2
Water, Bottled, Non-carbonated, Dannon 1 bottle, 11.2 fl oz in package of 12 (331g)	0	0	--	--	0	--	--	0	0
Water, Bottled, Non-carbonated, Dannon Fluoride to Go 1 bottle, 8.5 fl oz in packages of 8 (251g)	0	0	--	--	0	--	--	0	3
Water, Bottled, Non-carbonated, Dasani 1 bottle, 16.9 fl oz in packages of 6 and 24 (500g)	0	0	--	--	0	--	--	0	0
Water, Bottled, Non-carbonated, Evian 1 bottle, 11.2 fl oz in package of 6 (331g)	0	0	--	--	0	--	--	0	0
Water, Bottled, Non-carbonated, Naya 1 fl oz (29.6g)	0	0	--	--	0	--	--	0	0
Water, Bottled, Non-carbonated, Pepsi, Aquafina 1 bottle, 16.9 fl oz in packages of 6, 12 or 24 (500g)	0	0	--	--	0	--	--	0	0
Water, Bottled, Perrier 1 bottle, 6.5 fl oz (192g)	0	0	0	0	0	0.0	--	0	2
Water, Bottled, Poland Spring 1 bottle, 16.9 fl oz in packages of 6 and 24 (500g)	0	0	0	0	0	0.0	--	0	5
Water, Non-carbonated, Fruit Flavors, Sweetened, with Low Calorie Sweetener 1 fl oz (29.6g)	0	0	0	0	0	0.0	0	0	1
Water, with Added Vitamins and Minerals, Sweetened, Fruit Flavors 1 serving (237g)	52	0	0	0	13	0.0	13	0	0
Water, with Corn Syrup and/or Sugar and Low Calorie Sweetener, Fruit Flavor 1 pouch (200g)	36	0	0	0	9	0.0	9	0	16

Food Serving size	Cal.	(g) Total Fat	(g) Sat. Fat	(mg) Chol.	(g) Carb.	(g) Fiber	(g) Sug.	(g) Prot.	(mg) Sod.
Coffees, Teas, and Cocoas									
Cocoa Mix, Nestle, Hot Cocoa Mix, Rich Chocolate with Marshmallows									
1 serving, 1 envelope (20g)	80	3	3	0	15	0.7	13	1	160
Cocoa Mix, Nestle, Rich Chocolate Hot Cocoa Mix									
1 serving, 1 envelope (20g)	80	3	2	0	15	0.8	12	1	170
Cocoa Mix, Powder									
1 serving (3 heaping tsp or 1 envelope) (28g)	111	1	1	0	23	1.0	18	2	141
Cocoa Mix, Powder, Prepared with Water									
1 fl oz (34.3g)	19	0	0	0	4	0.2	3	0	25
Cocoa Mix, Swiss Miss, No Sugar Added, Powder									
1 envelope (.53 oz) (15g)	57	0	0	0	11	1.1	6	2	131
Cocoa Mix, with Aspartame, Low Calorie, Powder, with Added Calcium, No Added Sodium or Vitamin A									
1 packet (0.675 oz) (19g)	68	1	0	2	11	0.2	11	5	124
Cocoa Mix, with Aspartame, Powder, Prepared with Water									
1 fl oz (32.1g)	9	0	0	0	2	0.2	1	0	23
Cocoa, Dry Powder, Hi-fat or Breakfast, Plain									
1 tbsp (5.4g)	26	1	1	0	3	1.6	0	1	1
Cocoa, Dry Powder, Unsweetened									
1 tbsp (5.4g)	12	1	0	0	3	1.8	0	1	1
Cocoa, Dry Powder, Unsweetened, Hershey's European Style Cocoa									
1 tbsp (5g)	20	1	0	0	3	1.0	0	1	0
Cocoa, Dry Powder, Unsweetened, Processed with Alkali									
1 tbsp (5.4g)	12	1	0	0	3	1.6	0	1	1
Coffee and Cocoa (Mocha) Powder, with Whitener and Low Calorie Sweetener									
1 tsp, dry (6.4g)	16	1	1	0	5	0.3	0	1	32
Coffee and Cocoa (Mocha) Powder, with Whitener and Low Calorie Sweetener, Decaffeinated									
1 tsp, dry (6.4g)	16	1	1	0	5	0.3	2	1	32
Coffee Substitute, Cereal Grain Beverage, Powder									
1 tsp (1 serving) (3g)	11	0	0	0	2	0.7	0	0	2
Coffee Substitute, Cereal Grain Beverage, Powder, Prepared with Whole Milk									
6 fl oz (185g)	120	6	4	24	10	0.2	--	6	91

Food Serving size	Cal.	(g) Total Fat	(g) Sat. Fat	(mg) Chol.	(g) Carb.	(g) Fiber	(g) Sug.	(g) Prot.	(mg) Sod.
Coffee Substitute, Cereal Grain Beverage, Prepared with Water									
1 fl oz (30.1g)	2	0	0	0	0	0.1	0	0	2
Coffee Substitute, Roasted Grain Beverage, Natural Touch Kaffree Roma, Powder									
1 tsp, rounded (1 serving) (2g)	7	0	--	0	2	0.0	0	0	3
Coffee, Brewed from Grounds, Prepared with Tap Water									
1 fl oz (29.6g)	0	0	0	0	0	0.0	0	0	1
Coffee, Brewed from Grounds, Prepared with Tap Water, Decaffeinated									
1 fl oz (29.6g)	0	0	0	0	0	0.0	0	0	1
Coffee, Brewed, Espresso, Restaurant Prepared									
1 fluid ounce (30g)	1	0	0	0	0	0.0	0	0	4
Coffee, Brewed, Espresso, Restaurant Prepared, Decaffeinated									
1 fluid ounce (30g)	0	0	0	0	0	0.0	0	0	4
Coffee, Dry, Powder, with Whitener, Reduced Calorie									
1 tsp, dry (1.7g)	9	0	0	0	1	0.0	--	0	14
Coffee, Instant, Decaffeinated, Powder									
1 tsp, rounded (1.8g)	4	0	0	0	1	0.0	0	0	0
Coffee, Instant, Decaffeinated, Powder, Prepared with Water									
1 fl oz (29.9g)	1	0	0	0	0	0.0	0	0	1
Coffee, Instant, Regular, Powder									
1 packet (2g)	5	0	0	0	1	0.0	0	0	1
Coffee, Instant, Regular, Powder, Half the Caffeine									
1 packet (2g)	7	0	0	0	1	0.0	0	0	1
Coffee, Instant, Regular, Prepared with Water									
1 fl oz (29.8g)	1	0	0	0	0	0.0	0	0	1
Coffee, Instant, with Chicory, Powder									
1 tsp, rounded (1.8g)	6	0	0	0	1	0.0	--	0	5
Coffee, Instant, with Chicory, Prepared with Water									
1 fl oz (29.9g)	1	0	0	0	0	0.0	0	0	2
Coffee, Instant, with Sugar, Cappuccino-flavor Powder									
4 teaspoon (1 serving) (13g)	53	1	0	0	11	0.2	9	0	23
Coffee, Instant, with Sugar, French-flavor, Powder									
4 teaspoon (1 serving) (13g)	63	3	1	0	9	0.0	5	1	72
Coffee, Instant, with Sugar, Mocha-flavor, Powder									
1 serving, 2 tbsp (13g)	60	2	1	0	10	0.2	8	1	41

Food Serving size	Cal.	(g) Total Fat	(g) Sat. Fat	(mg) Chol.	(g) Carb.	(g) Fiber	(g) Sug.	(g) Prot.	(mg) Sod.
Tea, Brewed, Prepared with Distilled Water 6 fl oz (178g)	2	0	0	0	1	0.0	--	0	0
Tea, Brewed, Prepared with Tap Water 1 fl oz (29.6g)	0	0	0	0	0	0.0	0	0	1
Tea, Brewed, Prepared with Tap Water, Decaffeinated 6 fl oz (178g)	2	0	0	0	1	0.0	0	0	5
Tea, Herb, Chamomile, Brewed 6 fl oz (178g)	2	0	0	0	0	0.0	0	0	2
Tea, Herb, Other than Chamomile, Brewed 6 fl oz (178g)	2	0	0	0	0	0.0	0	0	2
Tea, Instant, Sweetened with Sodium Saccharin, Lemon-flavored, Powder 4 tbsp (1/4 cup) (14.4g)	49	0	0	0	12	0.0	0	0	59
Tea, Instant, Sweetened with Sodium Saccharin, Lemon-flavored, Powder, Decaffeinated 2 tsp (1.6g)	5	0	0	0	1	0.0	0	0	7
Tea, Instant, Sweetened with Sodium Saccharin, Lemon-flavored, Prepared 1 fl oz (29.8g)	1	0	0	0	0	0.0	0	0	2
Tea, Instant, Sweetened with Sugar, Lemon-flavored, with Vitamin C, Powder 1 serving, (3 heaping tsp) (23g)	89	0	0	0	22	0.0	--	0	1
Tea, Instant, Sweetened with Sugar, Lemon-flavored, Without Vitamin C, Powder 1 serving (3 heaping tsp) (23g)	92	0	0	0	23	0.2	22	0	1
Tea, Instant, Sweetened with Sugar, Lemon-flavored, Without Vitamin C, Powder, Decaffeinated 1 serving (3 heaping tsp) (23g)	89	0	0	0	23	0.0	22	0	1
Tea, Instant, Sweetened with Sugar, Lemon-flavored, Without Vitamin C, Powder, Prepared 1 cup (8 fl oz) (259g)	91	0	0	0	22	0.3	22	0	5
Tea, Instant, Unsweetened, Lemon-flavored, Powder 2 tbsp, rounded (11.3g)	39	0	0	0	9	0.6	1	1	6
Tea, Instant, Unsweetened, Powder 1 serving, 1 tsp (0.7g)	2	0	0	0	0	0.1	0	0	1
Tea, Instant, Unsweetened, Powder, Decaffeinated 1 serving, 2 tsp (0.7g)	2	0	0	0	0	0.1	0	0	1
Tea, Instant, Unsweetened, Powder, Prepared 1 fl oz (29.7g)	0	0	0	0	0	0.0	0	0	1

Food Serving size	Cal.	(g) Total Fat	(g) Sat. Fat	(mg) Chol.	(g) Carb.	(g) Fiber	(g) Sug.	(g) Prot.	(mg) Sod.
Tea, Ready-to-drink, Arizona Iced Tea, with Lemon Flavor									
1 serving, 8 fl oz (227g)	89	0	0	0	22	0.0	22	0	9
Tea, Ready-to-drink, Lipton Brisk Iced Tea, with Lemon Flavor									
1 serving, 8 fl oz (245g)	86	0	0	0	22	0.0	21	0	51
Tea, Ready-to-drink, Nestle, Cool Nestea Iced tea, with Lemon Flavor									
1 serving, 8 fl oz (245g)	88	0	--	--	22	0.0	22	0	51

Energy and Sports Drinks

Food Serving size	Cal.	(g) Total Fat	(g) Sat. Fat	(mg) Chol.	(g) Carb.	(g) Fiber	(g) Sug.	(g) Prot.	(mg) Sod.
Drink Mix, Quaker Oats, Gatorade, Orange Flavor, Powder									
1 scoop, powder (23g)	89	0	0	0	22	0.0	19	0	14
Energy Drink, Amp									
1 serving (240g)	110	0	0	0	29	0.0	29	1	65
Energy Drink, Amp, Sugar-free									
1 serving, 8 fl oz (240g)	5	0	0	0	2	0.0	0	0	74
Energy Drink, Full Throttle									
1 serving, 8 fluid oz (240g)	110	0	0	0	29	0.0	29	1	84
Energy Drink, Monster									
1 serving (240g)	101	0	0	0	27	0.0	27	0	180
Energy Drink, Red Bull, Sugar Free, with Added Caffeine, Niacin, Panto, Vitamin B6 and B12									
1 serving, 8.3 fl oz can (250g)	13	0	0	0	2	0.0	0	1	98
Energy Drink, Red Bull, with Added Caffeine, Niacin, Panto, Vitamin B6 and B12									
1 can, 12 fl oz (369g)	166	0	0	0	40	0.0	37	1	140
Energy Drink, Rockstar									
1 serving (240g)	139	0	0	0	30	0.0	30	0	41
Energy Drink, Rockstar, Sugar-free									
8 fl oz (1 serving) (240g)	10	0	0	0	2	0.0	0	1	125
Energy Drink, Vault Zero, Sugar-free, Citrus Flavor									
12 fl oz (360g)	4	0	0	0	3	0.0	0	1	50
Energy Drink, Vault, Citrus Flavor									
1 oz (31g)	15	0	0	0	4	0.0	4	0	4
Ensure Plus, Liquid Nutrition									
1 fl oz (31.5g)	44	1	0	1	6	0.0	--	2	30
Fluid Replacement, Electrolyte Solin (Including Pedialyte)									
1 fl oz (31.2g)	3	0	0	0	1	0.0	0	0	32

Food Serving size	Cal.	(g) Total Fat	(g) Sat. Fat	(mg) Chol.	(g) Carb.	(g) Fiber	(g) Sug.	(g) Prot.	(mg) Sod.
Protein Supplement, Milk-based, Muscle Milk, Powder									
1 tbsp (11g)	45	2	0	2	2	0.8	1	5	36
Quaker Oats, Propel Fitness Water, Fruit-flavored, Non-carbonated									
1 bottle, 16.9 fl oz in packages of 6 (501g)	25	0	0	0	6	0.0	6	0	65
Rice Drink, Unsweetened, with Added Calcium, Vitamins A and D									
8 fl oz (approximate weight, 1 serving) (240g)	113	2	0	0	22	0.7	13	1	94
Sports Drink, Coca-Cola, Powerade, Lemon-lime Flavor, Ready-to-drink									
8 fl oz (244g)	78	0	0	0	19	0.0	15	0	54
Sports Drink, Fruit-flavored, Low Calorie, Ready-to-drink									
1 fl oz (30g)	3	0	0	0	1	0.0	0	0	11
Sports Drink, Pepsico, Gatorade, Fruit-flavored, Ready-to-drink									
8 fl oz (244g)	63	0	0	0	16	0.0	13	0	95

Soft Drinks and Sodas and Drink Mixes

Food Serving size	Cal.	(g) Total Fat	(g) Sat. Fat	(mg) Chol.	(g) Carb.	(g) Fiber	(g) Sug.	(g) Prot.	(mg) Sod.
Carbonated Beverage, Chocolate-flavored Soda									
1 can, or bottle (16 fl oz) (492g)	207	0	0	0	53	0.0	53	0	433
Carbonated Beverage, Club Soda									
1 can, or bottle (16 fl oz) (474g)	0	0	0	0	0	0.0	0	0	100
Carbonated Beverage, Cola, Contains Caffeine									
1 can, 12 fl oz (368g)	136	0	0	0	35	0.0	33	0	15
Carbonated Beverage, Cola, with Higher Caffeine									
1 can, 12 fl oz (368g)	151	0	0	0	39	0.0	39	0	15
Carbonated Beverage, Cola, Without Caffeine									
1 can, 12 fl oz (368g)	151	0	0	0	39	0.0	39	0	15
Carbonated Beverage, Cream Soda									
1 can, or bottle (16 fl oz) (494g)	252	0	0	0	66	0.0	66	0	59
Carbonated Beverage, Dr Pepper-type, Contains Caffeine									
1 can, or bottle (16 fl oz) (491g)	201	0	0	0	51	0.0	--	0	49
Carbonated Beverage, Ginger Ale									
1 can, or bottle (16 fl oz) (488g)	166	0	0	0	43	0.0	42	0	34

Food Serving size	Cal.	(g) Total Fat	(g) Sat. Fat	(mg) Chol.	(g) Carb.	(g) Fiber	(g) Sug.	(g) Prot.	(mg) Sod.
Carbonated Beverage, Grape Soda 1 can, or bottle (12 fl oz) (372g)	160	0	0	0	42	0.0	--	0	56
Carbonated Beverage, Lemon-lime Soda, Contains Caffeine 1 can, 12 fl oz (369g)	151	0	0	0	38	0.0	38	0	37
Carbonated Beverage, Local, Other than Cola or Dr Pepper, with Saccharin, Without Caffeine 1 can (12 fl oz) (355g)	0	0	0	0	0	0.0	--	0	57
Carbonated Beverage, Low Calorie, Cola or Dr Pepper, with Aspartame, Caffeine 1 can, 12 fl oz (355g)	7	0	0	0	1	0.0	0	0	28
Carbonated Beverage, Low Calorie, Cola or Dr Pepper, with Sodium Saccharin, Contains Caffeine 1 bottle (16 fl oz) (474g)	0	0	0	0	0	0.0	0	0	76
Carbonated Beverage, Low Calorie, Cola or Dr Pepper-type, with Aspartame, Without Caffeine 1 bottle 16 fl oz (473g)	5	0	0	0	1	0.0	0	1	19
Carbonated Beverage, Low calorie, Not Cola or Dr Pepper-type, with Aspartame, Contains Caffeine 1 can (12 fl oz) (355g)	0	0	0	0	0	0.0	0	0	21
Carbonated Beverage, Low Calorie, Other than Cola or Dr Pepper, Without Caffeine 1 can (12 fl oz) (355g)	0	0	0	0	0	0.0	0	0	21
Carbonated Beverage, Orange 1 can, or bottle (16 fl oz) (496g)	238	0	0	0	61	0.0	--	0	60
Carbonated Beverage, Reduced Sugar, Cola, Contains Caffeine and Sweeteners 1 can (8 fl oz) (355g)	71	0	0	0	18	0.0	18	0	14
Carbonated Beverage, Root Beer 1 can, or bottle (16 fl oz) (493g)	202	0	0	0	52	0.0	52	0	64
Carbonated Beverage, Sprite, Lemon-lime, Without Caffeine 1 can, 12 fl oz (369g)	148	0	0	0	37	0.0	33	0	33
Carbonated Beverage, Tonic Water 1 bottle (11 fl oz) (336g)	114	0	0	0	30	0.0	30	0	40
Carob-flavor Beverage Mix, Powder 1 tbsp (12g)	45	0	0	0	11	1.0	--	0	12

Food Serving size	Cal.	(g) Total Fat	(g) Sat. Fat	(mg) Chol.	(g) Carb.	(g) Fiber	(g) Sug.	(g) Prot.	(mg) Sod.
Carob-flavor Beverage Mix, Powder, Prepared with Whole Milk									
1 cup (8 fl oz) (256g)	192	8	5	26	22	1.0	--	8	118
Lemonade, Powder									
1 cup (218g)	824	2	0	0	212	0.9	206	0	111
Lemonade, Powder, Prepared with Water									
1 fl oz (33g)	5	0	0	0	1	0.0	1	0	2
Lemonade-flavor Drink, Powder									
1 serving (18g)	68	0	0	0	18	0.0	17	0	23
Lemonade-flavor Drink, Powder, Prepared with Water									
1 fl oz (31.8g)	9	0	0	0	2	0.0	2	0	4
Shake, Fast Food, Chocolate									
1 small, 12 fl oz (282g)	358	10	7	37	58	5.4	52	10	274
Shake, Fast Food, Strawberry									
1 small, 12 fl oz (282g)	319	8	5	31	53	1.1	--	10	234
Shake, Fast Food, Vanilla									
1 fl oz (20.8g)	31	1	1	5	4	0.2	3	1	17
Strawberry-flavored Beverage Mix, Powder									
1 serving (2-3 heaping tsp) (22g)	86	0	0	0	22	0.0	21	0	8
Strawberry-flavored Beverage Mix, Powder, Prepared with Whole Milk									
1 cup (8 fl oz) (266g)	234	8	5	32	33	0.0	--	8	128

Mixed Dishes

Why Eat Mixed Dishes?

Mixed dishes are convenient and enjoyable to eat but they don't fit neatly into one food group. For example, a cheese pizza counts in several groups: the crust in the grains group, the tomato sauce in the vegetable group, and the cheese in the milk group. Frozen and shelf-stable, partially prepared foods are convenient and can be healthy.

Daily Goal

Compare each mixed food selection to MyPlate.
A prepared entrée should have:

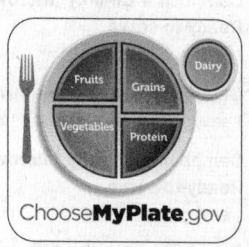

    300 to 500 calories
    10g or more protein
    30% or less fat calories (10 to 28 grams total fat)
    10% or less saturated fat (1 to 2 grams)
    480 mg or less sodium

Shopping Tips

- Most prepared entrées don't include a serving of dairy. If the calcium level is below 10% Daily Value, plan to add milk.
- Fresh fruits and vegetables are usually lacking in prepared meals. Plan a side salad or vegetable.
- Purchase fruit for a sweet ending to the meal.
- Choose mixed dishes with sauces in separate packets so that you can decide how much to use.
- Look for low-sodium soups.

Shopping List Essentials

    Healthy frozen dinners and prepackaged entrées
    Low-sodium soups
    Whole grain-based entrées: brown rice, quinoa, whole grain pasta
    Vegetables
    Fruits

Red Flags

Some mixed foods can contain a lot of fat or sugar, which adds empty calories. Mixed dishes are also usually high in sodium. Look for those that claim "Healthy." These have limits on fat, saturated fat, and sodium and must contain a good source of at least one positive nutrient. See the guidelines for "Healthy" on page vii.

Food Serving size	Cal.	(g) Total Fat	(g) Sat. Fat	(mg) Chol.	(g) Carb.	(g) Fiber	(g) Sug.	(g) Prot.	(mg) Sod.
Soups (Including Soup-related Products)									
Beef Stew, Canned Entrée									
1 cup (1 serving) (196g)	194	11	4	25	15	1.8	5	9	760
Campbell's Bowls, 98% Fat Free, New England Clam Chowder									
1 cup (245g)	110	2	1	10	17	1.0	1	6	480
Campbell's Brown Sugar and Bacon Flavor Baked Beans									
1 serving (130g)	160	2	1	5	30	8.1	13	5	471
Campbell's Chunky Microwavable Bowls, Beef with Country Vegetables, Ready-to-serve									
1 serving, 1 cup (245g)	149	3	1	20	21	4.9	3	10	899
Campbell's Chunky Microwavable Bowls, Chicken Dumplings Soup									
1 serving, 1 cup (245g)	191	9	2	25	18	2.9	2	8	889
Campbell's Chunky Microwavable Bowls, Classic Chicken Noodle, Ready-to-serve									
1 serving, 1 cup (245g)	110	3	1	25	14	2.0	3	6	789
Campbell's Chunky Microwavable Bowls, Grilled Chicken and Sausage Gumbo, Ready-to-serve									
1 serving, 1 cup (245g)	140	4	2	15	18	1.0	5	7	779
Campbell's Chunky Microwavable Bowls, Grilled Chicken with Vegetables and Pasta, Ready-to-serve									
1 serving, 1 cup (245g)	110	2	0	15	14	2.9	2	7	850
Campbell's Chunky Microwavable Bowls, New England Clam Chowder, Ready-to-serve									
1 serving, 1 cup (245g)	201	12	2	10	17	2.9	1	6	870
Campbell's Chunky Microwavable Bowls, Old Fashioned Vegetable Beef, Ready-to-serve									
1 serving, 1 cup (245g)	100	1	0	10	14	2.9	4	7	880
Campbell's Chunky Microwavable Bowls, Sirloin Burger with Country Vegetables, Ready-to-serve									
1 serving, 1 cup (245g)	140	4	1	15	18	2.9	4	8	801
Campbell's Chunky Soups, Baked Potato Cheddar Bacon Bits Soup									
1 cup (245g)	191	9	3	10	23	2.0	3	5	789
Campbell's Chunky Soups, Baked Potato with Steak and Cheese Soup									
1 cup (245g)	201	10	2	15	21	2.9	3	8	840

Food Serving size	Cal.	(g) Total Fat	(g) Sat. Fat	(mg) Chol.	(g) Carb.	(g) Fiber	(g) Sug.	(g) Prot.	(mg) Sod.
Campbell's Chunky Soups, Barbecue Seasoned Burger Soup									
1 serving (245g)	206	6	2	15	28	4.9	10	10	899
Campbell's Chunky Soups, Barbecue Seasoned Pork Soup									
1 serving (245g)	167	4	1	15	22	4.9	5	12	921
Campbell's Chunky Soups, Beef Rib Roast Potatoe Herbs Soup									
1 cup (245g)	108	1	1	10	17	2.0	6	7	889
Campbell's Chunky Soups, Beef Stew - Fully Loaded									
1 cup (245g)	169	5	2	20	20	2.9	0	10	811
Campbell's Chunky Soups, Beef Stroganoff									
1 serving (245g)	250	14	4	39	18	3.9	0	12	811
Campbell's Chunky Soups, Beef with Country Vegetable Soup									
1 cup (245g)	130	3	1	15	18	2.9	4	8	921
Campbell's Chunky Soups, Beef with White and Wild Rice Soup									
1 cup (245g)	140	1	0	10	24	2.0	5	8	889
Campbell's Chunky Soups, Chicken and Dumplings Soup									
1 cup (245g)	181	8	2	29	19	2.9	12	8	889
Campbell's Chunky Soups, Chicken Broccoli Cheese and Potato Soup									
1 cup (245g)	211	11	4	20	20	2.9	6	7	880
Campbell's Chunky Soups, Chicken Corn Chowder									
1 cup (245g)	201	10	3	15	20	2.0	3	7	860
Campbell's Chunky Soups, Chicken Mushroom Chowder									
1 serving (245g)	191	9	1	25	19	2.9	4	8	850
Campbell's Chunky Soups, Classic Chicken Noodle Soup									
1 cup (245g)	120	3	1	25	14	2.0	2	8	789
Campbell's Chunky Soups, Fajita Chicken with Rice and Beans Soup									
1 cup (245g)	130	1	0	15	23	2.0	7	7	850
Campbell's Chunky Soups, Firehouse – Hot Spicy Beef Bean Chili									
1 cup (245g)	233	8	4	25	25	5.9	7	15	870
Campbell's Chunky Soups, Grilled Chicken Sausage Gumbo Soup									
1 cup (245g)	140	3	1	20	21	2.0	4	7	850
Campbell's Chunky Soups, Grilled Chicken Vegetable and Pasta Soup									
1 cup (245g)	100	2	0	15	14	2.0	2	6	880
Campbell's Chunky Soups, Grilled Sirloin Steak and Hearty Vegetables Soup									
1 cup (245g)	130	2	1	10	19	3.9	15	8	889

Food Serving size	Cal.	(g) Total Fat	(g) Sat. Fat	(mg) Chol.	(g) Carb.	(g) Fiber	(g) Sug.	(g) Prot.	(mg) Sod.
Campbell's Chunky Soups, Healthy Request									
1 cup (245g)	130	3	1	10	20	2.0	0	5	409
Campbell's Chunky Soups, Healthy Request, Beef Barley Soup									
1 serving (245g)	140	2	1	15	21	4.9	0	9	480
Campbell's Chunky Soups, Healthy Request, Chicken Noodle Soup									
1 cup (245g)	120	2	1	10	17	2.0	3	8	409
Campbell's Chunky Soups, Healthy Request, Microwavable Bowls, Chicken Noodle Soup									
1 serving (245g)	120	2	1	15	17	1.0	0	7	409
Campbell's Chunky Soups, Healthy Request, Microwavable Bowls, Grilled, Chicken Sausage Gumbo Soup									
1 cup (245g)	130	3	1	10	18	2.0	0	7	409
Campbell's Chunky Soups, Healthy Request, Vegetable Soup									
1 cup (245g)	120	1	0	0	24	3.9	8	4	409
Campbell's Chunky Soups, Hearty Bean 'n' Ham Soup									
1 cup (245g)	181	2	0	10	30	8.1	5	11	779
Campbell's Chunky Soups, Hearty Beef Barley Soup									
1 cup (245g)	159	2	0	10	26	3.9	5	9	789
Campbell's Chunky Soups, Hearty Chicken with Vegetable Soup									
1 serving (245g)	110	2	0	15	17	2.9	3	6	711
Campbell's Chunky Soups, Hearty Vegetable with Pasta Soup									
1 cup (245g)	125	2	0	5	23	2.9	9	4	931
Campbell's Chunky Soups, Herb Roasted Chicken with Potatoes and Garlic Soup									
1 serving (245g)	113	1	1	15	17	2.9	4	8	870
Campbell's Chunky Soups, Honey Roasted Ham with Potatoes Soup									
1 serving (245g)	135	2	1	15	20	2.9	7	8	811
Campbell's Chunky Soups, Italian Sausage and Peppers Soup									
1 serving (245g)	152	5	1	20	20	2.9	8	7	801
Campbell's Chunky Soups, Manhattan Clam Chowder									
1 cup (245g)	127	4	1	5	19	2.9	4	5	831
Campbell's Chunky Soups, New England Clam Chowder									
1 cup (245g)	230	13	2	10	20	2.9	1	7	889
Campbell's Chunky Soups, Old Fashioned Potato Ham Chowder									
1 cup (245g)	191	11	4	20	17	2.9	1	6	801

Food Serving size	Cal.	(g) Total Fat	(g) Sat. Fat	(mg) Chol.	(g) Carb.	(g) Fiber	(g) Sug.	(g) Prot.	(mg) Sod.
Campbell's Chunky Soups, Old Fashioned Vegetable Beef Soup									
1 cup (245g)	120	2	1	15	17	2.9	4	8	889
Campbell's Chunky Soups, Pepper Steak Soup									
1 serving (245g)	118	1	0	15	18	2.9	4	8	801
Campbell's Chunky Soups, Pork Roast with Carrots and Potatoe Soup									
1 serving (245g)	123	3	1	15	16	2.9	3	8	889
Campbell's Chunky Soups, Rigatoni and Meat									
1 cup (245g)	211	7	3	20	25	2.9	0	11	801
Campbell's Chunky Soups, Roadhouse – Beef Bean Chili									
1 cup (245g)	233	8	4	25	25	5.9	7	15	880
Campbell's Chunky Soups, Salisbury Steak, Mushroom and Onion Soup									
1 serving (245g)	140	5	2	15	19	2.0	6	7	801
Campbell's Chunky Soups, Savory Chicken White Wild Rice Soup									
1 cup (245g)	110	2	0	10	18	2.0	1	7	811
Campbell's Chunky Soups, Savory Pot Roast Soup									
1 cup (245g)	120	1	0	10	20	2.0	4	7	789
Campbell's Chunky Soups, Savory Vegetable Soup									
1 cup (245g)	108	1	0	0	22	3.9	6	3	769
Campbell's Chunky Soups, Sizzlin' Steak – Grilled Steak with Chili Beans									
1 cup (245g)	198	3	1	15	27	7.1	9	16	870
Campbell's Chunky Soups, Slow Roasted Beef with Mushroom Soup									
1 cup (245g)	118	1	1	15	18	2.9	5	8	831
Campbell's Chunky Soups, Smoked Chicken with Roasted Corn Chowder									
1 serving (245g)	206	10	2	15	19	4.9	3	10	889
Campbell's Chunky Soups, Split Pea 'n' Ham Soup									
1 cup (245g)	191	2	1	10	30	4.9	5	12	779
Campbell's Chunky Soups, Steak 'n' Potato Soup									
1 cup (245g)	120	2	0	15	18	2.9	1	8	921
Campbell's Chunky Soups, Tantalizin' Turkey – Turkey Chili Beans Soup									
1 serving (245g)	191	2	1	15	27	8.1	9	15	880
Campbell's Chunky Soups, Turkey Pot Pie									
1 cup (245g)	201	8	1	34	21	3.9	0	11	801
Campbell's Healthy Request, Chicken Noodle Soup, Condensed									
1 serving, 1/2 cup (126g)	60	2	1	10	8	1.0	1	3	410

Food Serving size	Cal.	(g) Total Fat	(g) Sat. Fat	(mg) Chol.	(g) Carb.	(g) Fiber	(g) Sug.	(g) Prot.	(mg) Sod.
Campbell's Healthy Request, Chicken with Rice Soup, Condensed									
.5 cup (126g)	71	1	1	5	9	1.0	1	2	410
Campbell's Healthy Request, Cream of Celery Soup, Condensed									
1 serving, 1/2 cup (124g)	69	2	0	5	12	1.0	2	1	410
Campbell's Healthy Request, Cream of Chicken Soup, Condensed									
1 serving, 1/2 cup (124g)	81	3	1	5	12	1.0	7	2	410
Campbell's Healthy Request, Cream of Mushroom Soup, Condensed									
1 serving, 1/2 cup (124g)	69	2	0	5	10	1.0	2	2	410
Campbell's Healthy Request, Homestyle Chicken Noodle Soup, Condensed									
1 serving, 1/2 cup (126g)	60	1	1	10	10	1.0	1	3	410
Campbell's Healthy Request, Minestrone Soup, Condensed									
1 serving, 1/2 cup (120g)	76	0	0	0	14	2.9	4	3	390
Campbell's Healthy Request, Tomato Juice									
1 serving (243g)	51	0	0	0	11	1.9	0	2	481
Campbell's Healthy Request, Tomato Soup, Condensed									
1 serving, 1/2 cup (124g)	91	2	0	0	17	1.0	10	2	410
Campbell's Healthy Request, Vegetable Soup, Condensed									
1 serving, 1/2 cup (126g)	100	1	0	0	20	3.0	5	4	410
Campbell's Low Sodium Soups, Chicken Broth									
1 serving, 1 container (298g)	30	1	1	6	1	0.0	1	3	140
Campbell's Low Sodium Soups, Chicken with Noodle Soup									
1 serving, 1 container (305g)	159	5	2	31	17	2.1	4	12	140
Campbell's Low Sodium Soups, Cream of Mushroom Soup									
1 serving, 1 container (298g)	161	8	3	15	19	0.0	6	3	60
Campbell's Organic Tomato Juice									
1 serving (243g)	51	0	0	0	10	1.9	0	2	680
Campbell's Pace, Diced Green Chilies, Green Chilies									
1 serving (30g)	8	0	0	0	2	1.0	0	0	100
Campbell's Pace, Dry Taco Seasoning Mix									
2 tbsp (1 serving) (5.3g)	10	0	0	0	3	1.0	1	0	428
Campbell's Pace, Jalapenos Nacho Sliced Peppers									
1 serving (30g)	4	0	0	0	1	1.0	0	0	300
Campbell's Pace, Pico de Gallo									
2 tbsp (32g)	10	0	0	0	3	--	0	0	150

Food Serving size	Cal.	(g) Total Fat	(g) Sat. Fat	(mg) Chol.	(g) Carb.	(g) Fiber	(g) Sug.	(g) Prot.	(mg) Sod.
Campbell's Pace, Salsa Refried Beans 1 serving (120g)	72	0	0	0	14	4.0	4	4	590
Campbell's Pace, Salsa Verde 2 tbsp (32g)	15	0	0	0	2	0.0	0	0	230
Campbell's Pace, Spicy Jalapeno Refried Beans 1 serving (120g)	76	0	0	0	14	5.0	4	5	590
Campbell's Pace, Tequila Lime Salsa 2 tbsp (32g)	15	0	0	0	3	0.0	0	0	190
Campbell's Pace, Traditional Refried Beans 1 serving (120g)	80	0	0	0	13	5.0	3	5	690
Campbell's Pace, Triple Pepper Salsa 2 tbsp (32g)	15	0	0	0	3	1.0	0	1	190
Campbell's Pork and Beans 1 serving (130g)	140	1	1	5	25	7.0	8	6	439
Campbell's Red and White - Microwavable Bowls, Tomato Soup 1 serving (245g)	108	0	0	0	24	2.9	18	3	789
Campbell's Red and White - Microwavable Bowls, Vegetable Beef Soup 1 serving (245g)	83	0	0	10	15	2.9	2	5	880
Campbell's Red and White - Microwavable Bowls, Chicken Rice Soup 1 serving (245g)	74	1	0	5	14	1.0	1	2	801
Campbell's Red and White - Microwavable Bowls, Creamy Tomato Soup 1 serving (245g)	157	5	1	5	25	2.9	16	3	750
Campbell's Red and White, 25% Less Sodium, Chicken Noodle Soup, Condensed 1 serving, 1/2 cup (126g)	60	2	1	15	8	1.0	1	3	660
Campbell's Red and White, 25% Less Sodium, Cream of Mushroom Soup, Condensed 1 serving, 1/2 cup (124g)	110	8	1	5	8	2.0	1	2	650
Campbell's Red and White, 25% Less Sodium, Tomato Soup, Condensed 1 serving, 1/2 cup (124g)	91	0	0	--	20	1.0	12	2	480
Campbell's Red and White, 98% Fat Free, Broccoli Cheese Soup, Condensed 1 serving, 1/2 cup (124g)	69	2	1	5	12	1.0	3	2	480
Campbell's Red and White, 98% Fat Free, Cream of Broccoli Soup, Condensed 1 serving, 1/2 cup (124g)	69	2	0	5	10	2.0	1	2	701

Food Serving size	Cal.	(g) Total Fat	(g) Sat. Fat	(mg) Chol.	(g) Carb.	(g) Fiber	(g) Sug.	(g) Prot.	(mg) Sod.
Campbell's Red and White, 98% Fat Free, Cream of Celery Soup, Condensed									
1 serving, 1/2 cup (124g)	69	3	1	5	9	2.0	1	1	480
Campbell's Red and White, 98% Fat Free, Cream of Chicken Soup, Condensed									
1 serving, 1/2 cup (124g)	69	3	1	5	10	1.0	1	2	480
Campbell's Red and White, 98% Fat Free, Cream of Mushroom Soup, Condensed									
1 serving, 1/2 cup (124g)	60	3	0	5	9	1.0	0	1	480
Campbell's Red and White, Batman Fun Shapes Soup, Condensed									
1 serving, 1/2 cup (126g)	71	2	1	5	10	1.0	1	3	580
Campbell's Red and White, Bean with Bacon Soup, Condensed									
1 serving, 1/2 cup (128g)	160	3	2	5	25	8.1	4	8	860
Campbell's Red and White, Beef Broth, Condensed									
1 serving, 1/2 cup (124g)	15	0	0	0	1	0.0	1	3	861
Campbell's Red and White, Beef Consommé, Condensed									
1 serving, 1/2 cup (124g)	20	0	0	0	1	0.0	1	4	810
Campbell's Red and White, Beef Noodle Soup, Condensed									
1 serving, 1/2 cup (126g)	71	2	1	10	8	1.0	1	4	820
Campbell's Red and White, Beef with Vegetable and Barley Soup, Condensed									
1 serving, 1/2 cup (126g)	89	1	1	10	15	3.0	2	5	890
Campbell's Red and White, Beefy Mushroom Soup, Condensed									
1 serving, 1/2 cup (126g)	50	2	1	5	6	0.0	1	3	890
Campbell's Red and White, Broccoli Cheese Soup, Condensed									
1 serving, 1/2 cup (124g)	100	5	2	5	12	0.0	3	2	820
Campbell's Red and White, Cheddar Cheese Soup, Condensed									
1 serving, 1/2 cup (124g)	100	5	2	5	11	1.0	2	2	650
Campbell's Red and White, Chicken Alphabet Soup, Condensed									
1 serving, 1/2 cup (126g)	71	1	1	5	12	1.0	1	3	480
Campbell's Red and White, Chicken and Dumplings Soup, Condensed									
1 serving, 1/2 cup (126g)	71	2	1	10	10	1.0	1	3	760
Campbell's Red and White, Chicken and Stars Soup, Condensed									
1 serving, 1/2 cup (126g)	71	2	1	5	11	1.0	1	3	480
Campbell's Red and White, Chicken Barley with Mushroom Soup, Condensed									
1 serving (126g)	89	1	1	5	16	3.0	0	4	719
Campbell's Red and White, Chicken Broth, Condensed									
1 serving, 1/2 cup (124g)	20	1	0	5	1	0.0	1	1	770

Food Serving size	Cal.	(g) Total Fat	(g) Sat. Fat	(mg) Chol.	(g) Carb.	(g) Fiber	(g) Sug.	(g) Prot.	(mg) Sod.
Campbell's Red and White, Chicken Gumbo Soup, Condensed									
1 serving, 1/2 cup (126g)	60	1	1	5	10	1.0	2	2	869
Campbell's Red and White, Chicken NOODLEO'S Soup, Condensed									
1 serving, 1/2 cup (126g)	89	2	1	20	15	1.0	2	3	480
Campbell's Red and White, Chicken Noodle Soup, Condensed									
1 serving, 1/2 cup (126g)	60	2	1	15	8	1.0	1	3	890
Campbell's Red and White, Chicken Vegetable Soup, Condensed									
1 serving, 1/2 cup (126g)	79	1	1	5	15	2.0	3	3	890
Campbell's Red and White, Chicken with Rice Soup, Condensed									
1 serving, 1/2 cup (126g)	71	1	1	5	13	1.0	1	2	610
Campbell's Red and White, Chicken Won Ton Soup, Condensed									
1 serving, 1/2 cup (126g)	50	1	1	5	8	0.0	1	3	869
Campbell's Red and White, Cream of Asparagus Soup, Condensed									
1 serving, 1/2 cup (124g)	110	7	2	5	9	3.0	2	2	830
Campbell's Red and White, Cream of Broccoli Soup, Condensed									
1 serving, 1/2 cup (124g)	91	5	2	5	12	1.0	3	2	750
Campbell's Red and White, Cream of Celery Soup, Condensed									
1 serving, 1/2 cup (124g)	91	6	1	5	9	3.0	1	1	640
Campbell's Red and White, Cream of Chicken Soup, Condensed									
1 serving, 1/2 cup (124g)	120	8	2	10	10	2.0	1	2	870
Campbell's Red and White, Cream of Chicken with Herbs Soup, Condensed									
1 serving, 1/2 cup (124g)	81	4	2	10	9	0.0	1	2	800
Campbell's Red and White, Cream of Mushroom Soup, Condensed									
1 serving, 1/2 cup (124g)	100	6	2	5	9	2.0	1	1	870
Campbell's Red and White, Cream of Mushroom with Roasted Garlic Soup, Condensed									
1 serving, 1/2 cup (124g)	69	3	1	5	10	2.0	1	2	480
Campbell's Red and White, Cream of Onion Soup, Condensed									
1 serving, 1/2 cup (124g)	100	6	2	5	10	3.0	4	1	800
Campbell's Red and White, Cream of Potato Soup, Condensed									
1 serving, 1/2 cup (124g)	91	2	1	5	15	2.0	1	2	600
Campbell's Red and White, Cream of Shrimp Soup, Condensed									
1 serving, 1/2 cup (124g)	100	6	2	20	8	0.0	0	3	861
Campbell's Red and White, Creamy Chicken Noodle Soup, Condensed									
1 serving, 1/2 cup (124g)	120	7	2	15	11	4.0	1	4	870

Food Serving size	Cal.	(g) Total Fat	(g) Sat. Fat	(mg) Chol.	(g) Carb.	(g) Fiber	(g) Sug.	(g) Prot.	(mg) Sod.
Campbell's Red and White, Creamy Chicken Verde Soup, Condensed									
1 serving, 1/2 cup (124g)	110	7	2	10	10	3.0	1	2	780
Campbell's Red and White, Curly Noodle Soup, Condensed									
1 serving, 1/2 cup (126g)	79	2	1	15	11	1.0	1	4	480
Campbell's Red and White, Danny Phantom Shaped Pasta									
1 serving, 1/2 cup (126g)	71	2	1	5	10	1.0	1	4	559
Campbell's Red and White, Dora the Explorer Soup, Condensed									
1 serving, 1/2 cup (126g)	79	2	1	5	13	1.0	3	3	480
Campbell's Red and White, Double Noodle in Chicken Broth Soup, Condensed									
1 serving, 1/ 2 cup (126g)	110	2	1	10	20	1.0	1	3	480
Campbell's Red and White, Fiesta Nacho Cheese Soup, Condensed									
1 serving, 1/2 cup (124g)	120	8	3	10	10	1.0	2	3	790
Campbell's Red and White, French Onion Soup, Condensed									
1 serving, 1/2 cup (126g)	45	1	1	5	6	1.0	4	2	650
Campbell's Red and White, Golden Mushroom Soup, Condensed									
1 serving, 1/2 cup (124g)	81	3	1	0	10	1.0	1	2	650
Campbell's Red and White, Goldfish Pasta with Chicken Soup									
1 serving, 1/2 cup (126g)	79	2	1	5	12	1.0	1	3	480
Campbell's Red and White, Goldfish Pasta with Meatballs									
1 serving, 1/2 cup (126g)	89	3	1	10	11	1.0	1	4	4
Campbell's Red and White, Green Pea Soup, Condensed									
1 serving, 1/2 cup (128g)	180	3	1	0	28	4.0	6	9	870
Campbell's Red and White, Hearty Vegetable with Pasta Soup, Condensed									
1 serving, 1/2 cup (126g)	89	1	0	0	19	2.0	8	3	890
Campbell's Red and White, Home Style Chicken Noodle Soup, Condensed									
1 serving, 1/2 cup (126g)	71	2	1	10	10	1.0	1	4	650
Campbell's Red and White, Italian Style Wedding Soup, Condensed									
1 serving (126g)	89	2	1	10	12	3.0	0	4	810
Campbell's Red and White, Lentil Soup, Condensed									
1 serving (126g)	140	1	1	0	24	5.0	0	8	800
Campbell's Red and White, Manhattan Clam Chowder, Condensed									
1 serving, 1/2 cup (126g)	60	1	1	0	12	2.0	2	2	879
Campbell's Red and White, Mega Noodle in Chicken Broth, Condensed									
1 serving, 1/2 cup (126g)	89	2	1	15	15	1.0	1	3	480

Food Serving size	Cal.	(g) Total Fat	(g) Sat. Fat	(mg) Chol.	(g) Carb.	(g) Fiber	(g) Sug.	(g) Prot.	(mg) Sod.
Campbell's Red and White, Microwavable Bowls, Chicken Noodle Soup									
1 serving (245g)	74	2	0	15	10	1.0	0	4	870
Campbell's Red and White, Minestrone Soup, Condensed									
1 serving, 1/2 cup (126g)	89	1	1	5	17	3.0	3	4	650
Campbell's Red and White, New England Clam Chowder, Condensed									
1 serving, 1/2 cup (126g)	89	2	1	5	13	1.0	1	4	650
Campbell's Red and White, Old Fashioned Tomato Rice Soup, Condensed									
1 serving, 1/2 cup (126g)	110	2	1	0	23	1.0	10	1	770
Campbell's Red and White, Oyster Stew, Condensed									
1 serving, 1/2 cup (126g)	79	6	3	20	3	0.0	0	3	910
Campbell's Red and White, Pepper Pot Soup, Condensed									
1 serving, 1/2 cup (126g)	89	4	1	25	9	1.0	1	5	980
Campbell's Red and White, Scotch Broth, Condensed									
1 serving, 1/2 cup (124g)	60	1	0	5	10	2.0	1	3	861
Campbell's Red and White, Shrek Shaped Pasta with Chicken in Chicken Broth									
1 serving (126g)	79	2	1	5	12	1.0	0	3	480
Campbell's Red and White, Souper Shapes									
1 serving (126g)	79	2	1	5	11	1.0	0	4	480
Campbell's Red and White, Southwest Style Pepper Jack Special, Condensed									
1 serving, 1/2 cup (124g)	110	6	2	5	13	4.0	3	2	880
Campbell's Red and White, Southwestern-Style Chicken Vegetable Soup, Condensed									
1 serving, 1/2 cup (126g)	110	1	1	5	21	4.0	3	5	830
Campbell's Red and White, Split Pea with Ham and Bacon Soup, Condensed									
1 serving, 1/2 cup (128g)	180	2	1	5	30	4.0	4	10	850
Campbell's Red and White, Tomato Bisque, Condensed									
1 serving, 1/2 cup (126g)	130	4	1	5	23	1.0	15	2	879
Campbell's Red and White, Tomato Soup, Condensed									
1 serving, 1/2 cup (124g)	91	0	0	0	20	1.0	12	2	480
Campbell's Red and White, Vegetable Beef Soup, Condensed									
1 serving, 1/2 cup (126g)	89	1	1	5	15	3.0	2	5	890
Campbell's Red and White, Vegetable Soup, Condensed									
1 serving, 1/2 cup (126g)	100	1	1	5	21	3.0	7	4	650
Campbell's Red and White, Vegetarian Vegetable Soup, Condensed									
1 serving, 1/2 cup (126g)	89	1	0	0	18	2.0	6	3	480

Food Serving size	Cal.	(g) Total Fat	(g) Sat. Fat	(mg) Chol.	(g) Carb.	(g) Fiber	(g) Sug.	(g) Prot.	(mg) Sod.
Campbell's Select Gold Label Soups, Blended Red Pepper Black Bean Soup									
1 serving (245g)	120	1	1	5	23	3.9	10	3	821
Campbell's Select Gold Label Soups, Creamy Portobello Mushroom Soup									
1 serving (245g)	103	4	3	10	14	2.0	2	3	789
Campbell's Select Gold Label Soups, Golden Butternut Squash Soup									
1 serving (245g)	91	1	1	5	18	2.9	8	2	811
Campbell's Select Gold Label Soups, Italian Tomato and Basil Soup									
1 serving (245g)	91	0	0	0	19	2.9	0	3	769
Campbell's Select Gold Label Soups, Southwestern Corn Chowder									
1 serving (245g)	149	3	0	0	26	2.0	0	3	620
Campbell's Select Microwavable Bowls, Chicken with Egg Noodles Soup									
1 cup (245g)	120	4	1	25	12	1.0	2	8	480
Campbell's Select Microwavable Bowls, Healthy Request, Italian Style Wedding Soup									
1 cup (245g)	120	3	1	10	18	2.0	--	6	409
Campbell's Select Microwavable Bowls, Healthy Request, Mexican Style Tortilla									
1 cup (245g)	130	2	0	10	20	2.0	--	8	409
Campbell's Select Microwavable Bowls, Italian Sausage Pasta and Pepperoni Soup									
1 serving (245g)	130	6	2	15	15	2.0	5	7	870
Campbell's Select Microwavable Bowls, Italian Style Wedding Soup									
1 cup (245g)	130	4	2	15	16	2.0	3	7	480
Campbell's Select Microwavable Bowls, Mexican Style Chicken Tortilla Soup									
1 cup (245g)	127	2	1	20	19	2.0	3	8	480
Campbell's Select Microwavable Bowls, Minestrone Soup									
1 cup (245g)	96	1	0	5	19	2.9	5	4	480
Campbell's Select Microwavable Bowls, Savory Chicken and Long Grain Rice Soup									
1 cup (245g)	110	1	0	15	15	1.0	3	6	480
Campbell's Select Soup, 98% Fat Free, New England Clam Chowder									
1 cup (245g)	110	2	1	10	17	1.0	1	6	480
Campbell's Select Soup, Beef with Roasted Barley Soup									
1 cup (245g)	132	1	0	10	21	2.0	4	9	480

Food Serving size	Cal.	(g) Total Fat	(g) Sat. Fat	(mg) Chol.	(g) Carb.	(g) Fiber	(g) Sug.	(g) Prot.	(mg) Sod.
Campbell's Select Soup, Chicken and Pasta with Roasted Garlic Soup									
1 serving (245g)	113	1	0	15	18	2.0	2	8	821
Campbell's Select Soup, Chicken Vegetable Medley Soup									
1 cup (245g)	120	1	0	20	19	1.0	4	7	480
Campbell's Select Soup, Creamy Chicken Alfredo Soup									
1 cup (245g)	221	13	4	20	15	1.0	1	10	480
Campbell's Select Soup, Harvest Tomato with Basil Soup									
1 cup (245g)	100	0	0	0	22	2.0	--	3	480
Campbell's Select Soup, Healthy Request									
1 serving (245g)	100	2	1	15	13	2.0	--	7	480
Campbell's Select Soup, Healthy Request, Mexican Style Chicken Tortilla									
1 cup (245g)	140	2	1	15	22	2.0	2	8	409
Campbell's Select Soup, Italian Sausage with Pasta Pepperoni Soup									
1 cup (245g)	159	7	2	15	18	2.0	3	7	480
Campbell's Select Soup, Italian Style Wedding Soup									
1 cup (245g)	130	5	3	15	13	1.0	3	7	480
Campbell's Select Soup, Mediterranean Meatball Bowtie Pasta Soup									
1 cup (245g)	120	4	1	20	15	2.0	3	7	480
Campbell's Select Soup, Mexican Style Chicken Tortilla Soup									
1 cup (245g)	110	2	1	10	15	2.0	3	7	480
Campbell's Select Soup, Minestrone Soup									
1 cup (245g)	100	0	0	0	20	2.9	5	5	480
Campbell's Select Soup, New England Clam Chowder									
1 cup (245g)	179	10	2	10	17	1.0	1	6	480
Campbell's Select Soup, Potato Broccoli Cheese Soup									
1 cup (245g)	149	9	1	5	15	2.9	3	3	480
Campbell's Select Soup, Roasted Chicken with Long Grain Wild Rice Soup									
1 cup (245g)	110	0	0	15	20	1.0	2	6	480
Campbell's Select Soup, Roasted Chicken with Rotini and Penne Pasta Soup									
1 cup (245g)	91	1	0	10	13	1.0	2	8	480
Campbell's Select Soup, Savory White Bean with Roasted Ham Soup									
1 cup (245g)	169	1	0	5	30	7.1	4	9	480
Campbell's Select Soup, Slow Roasted Beef and Vegetable Soup									
1 cup (245g)	100	0	0	10	16	2.0	4	7	480

Food Serving size	Cal.	(g) Total Fat	(g) Sat. Fat	(mg) Chol.	(g) Carb.	(g) Fiber	(g) Sug.	(g) Prot.	(mg) Sod.
Campbell's Select Soup, Split Pea with Roasted Ham Soup									
1 cup (245g)	149	1	0	5	29	4.9	5	9	480
Campbell's Select Soup, Tomato Garden Soup									
1 cup (245g)	100	0	0	5	21	2.0	10	3	480
Campbell's Select Soup, Vegetable Medley Soup									
1 cup (245g)	81	0	0	0	16	2.9	6	3	480
Campbell's Select Soup, Zesty Azteca Meatball									
1 cup (245g)	130	5	2	15	18	1.0	--	5	480
Campbell's Soup at Hand, 25% Less Sodium, Chicken with Mini Noodles Soup									
1 container (305g)	79	2	1	9	11	2.1	--	4	729
Campbell's Soup at Hand, 25% Less Sodium, Classic Tomato									
1 container (305g)	119	0	0	0	27	2.1	0	3	659
Campbell's Soup at Hand, Blended Vegetable Medley Soup									
1 container (305g)	101	1	1	6	19	4.0	9	3	891
Campbell's Soup at Hand, Chicken and Stars Soup									
1 container (305g)	64	1	1	6	10	2.1	1	3	891
Campbell's Soup at Hand, Chicken with Mini Noodles Soup									
1 container (305g)	79	2	1	9	11	2.1	2	4	979
Campbell's Soup at Hand, Cream of Broccoli Soup									
1 container (305g)	143	7	2	6	17	7.0	3	3	891
Campbell's Soup at Hand, Creamy Chicken Soup									
1 container (305g)	131	9	2	6	13	4.0	1	4	891
Campbell's Soup at Hand, Creamy Tomato Soup									
1 container (305g)	189	4	1	6	34	4.0	23	4	939
Campbell's Soup at Hand, Italian Style Wedding Soup									
1 container (305g)	73	3	1	9	10	0.9	3	3	860
Campbell's Soup at Hand, New England Clam Chowder									
1 container (305g)	122	6	1	6	13	4.0	0	4	891
Campbell's Soup at Hand, Vegetable Beef Soup									
1 container (305g)	61	1	1	6	10	0.9	5	3	930
Campbell's Soup at Hand, Velvety Potato Soup									
1 container (305g)	156	7	1	6	21	4.0	5	2	869

Food Serving size	Cal.	(g) Total Fat	(g) Sat. Fat	(mg) Chol.	(g) Carb.	(g) Fiber	(g) Sug.	(g) Prot.	(mg) Sod.
Campbell's SpaghettiOs A to Z 1 cup (1 serving) (252g)	169	1	0	5	35	3.0	55	6	600
Campbell's SpaghettiOs A to Z with Meatballs 1 cup (1 serving) (252g)	239	7	2	20	32	4.0	0	11	600
Campbell's SpaghettiOs in Meat Sauce 1 cup (1 serving) (252g)	174	2	1	10	31	3.0	0	8	890
Campbell's SpaghettiOs Original 1 cup (1 serving) (252g)	169	1	0	5	35	3.0	187	6	600
Campbell's SpaghettiOs Original, Easy Open 1 can (1 serving) (213g)	149	1	1	4	31	3.0	2	5	479
Campbell's SpaghettiOs Plus Calcium 1 cup (1 serving) (252g)	169	1	0	5	35	3.0	90	6	600
Campbell's SpaghettiOs with Meatballs 1 cup (1 serving) (252g)	239	7	2	20	32	4.0	7	11	600
Campbell's SpaghettiOs with Meatballs, Easy Open 1 can (1 serving) (206g)	179	5	2	21	24	3.1	19	9	490
Campbell's SpaghettiOs with Sliced Franks 1 cup (1 serving) (252g)	219	6	2	20	32	4.0	56	9	600
Campbell's SpaghettiOs, Mini Beef Ravioli in Meat Sauce 1 serving (259g)	256	5	2	10	43	4.9	89	11	1059
Campbell's SpaghettiOs, Raviolios Beef Ravioli in Meat Sauce 1 cup (1 serving) (252g)	267	8	4	20	38	4.0	55	11	1091
Campbell's SpaghettiOs, Spaghetti in Tomato and Cheese Sauce 1 cup (1 serving) (252g)	202	2	0	5	40	3.0	9	7	950
Campbell's Supper Bakes Meal Kits, Herb Chicken with Rice .167 box (NLEA serving) (94g)	185	1	1	5	40	1.0	0	4	780
Campbell's Supper Bakes Meal Kits, Lemon Chicken with Herb Rice 1 serving (NLEA serving) (94g)	197	1	1	5	43	2.0	16	4	780
Campbell's Supper Bakes Meal Kits, Savory Pork Chops with Herb Stuffing .167 box (85g)	154	1	1	5	31	2.0	29	5	784
Campbell's Swanson Broth, Certified Organic Vegetable Broth 1 serving (235g)	12	0	0	0	3	0.0	2	0	550
Campbell's Swanson Broth, Vegetable Broth 1 serving (235g)	12	0	0°	0	3	0.0	2	0	940

Food Serving size	Cal.	(g) Total Fat	(g) Sat. Fat	(mg) Chol.	(g) Carb.	(g) Fiber	(g) Sug.	(g) Prot.	(mg) Sod.
Campbell's Swanson, Chicken a la King									
1 can (1 serving) (298g)	212	12	3	21	12	2.1	33	14	1371
Campbell's Swanson, Chicken and Dumplings									
1 cup (1 serving) (247g)	230	10	5	35	24	2.0	20	11	990
Campbell's Tomato Juice									
1 serving (243g)	51	0	0	0	10	1.9	0	2	680
Campbell's Tomato Juice, Low Sodium									
1 serving (243g)	51	0	0	0	10	1.9	0	2	141
Campbell's V8 60% Vegetable Juice, V8 V-lite									
1 serving (243g)	34	0	0	0	7	1.0	0	1	360
Campbell's V8 Splash Juice Drinks, Berry Blend									
1 serving, 8 oz (243g)	70	0	--	--	18	--	18	0	51
Campbell's V8 Splash Juice Drinks, Diet Berry Blend									
1 serving, 8 oz (243g)	10	0	--	--	3	--	1	0	34
Campbell's V8 Splash Juice Drinks, Diet Fruit Medley									
1 serving, 8 oz (238g)	10	0	--	--	3	--	2	0	31
Campbell's V8 Splash Juice Drinks, Diet Strawberry Kiwi									
1 serving (238g)	10	0	--	--	3	--	2	0	31
Campbell's V8 Splash Juice Drinks, Diet Tropical Blend									
1 serving, 8 oz (238g)	10	0	--	--	3	--	1	0	36
Campbell's V8 Splash Juice Drinks, Fruit Medley									
1 serving, 8 oz (243g)	80	0	--	--	19	--	19	0	51
Campbell's V8 Splash Juice Drinks, Guava Passion Fruit									
1 serving, 8 oz (243g)	80	0	--	--	19	--	19	0	34
Campbell's V8 Splash Juice Drinks, Mango Peach									
1 serving, 8 oz (243g)	80	0	--	--	20	--	20	0	39
Campbell's V8 Splash Juice Drinks, Orange Pineapple									
1 serving, 8 oz (243g)	70	0	--	--	18	--	18	0	51
Campbell's V8 Splash Juice Drinks, Orchard Blend									
1 serving, 8 oz (243g)	80	0	--	--	19	--	19	0	51
Campbell's V8 Splash Juice Drinks, Strawberry Banana									
1 serving, 8 oz (243g)	70	0	--	--	18	--	18	0	51
Campbell's V8 Splash Juice Drinks, Strawberry Kiwi									
1 serving, 8 oz (243g)	70	0	--	--	18	--	18	0	51

Food Serving size	Cal.	(g) Total Fat	(g) Sat. Fat	(mg) Chol.	(g) Carb.	(g) Fiber	(g) Sug.	(g) Prot.	(mg) Sod.
Campbell's V8 Splash Juice Drinks, Tropical Blend									
1 serving, 8 oz (243g)	70	0	--	--	18	--	18	0	51
Campbell's V8 Splash Smoothies, Peach Mango									
1 serving, 8 oz (245g)	91	0	0	0	19	0.0	18	3	71
Campbell's V8 Splash Smoothies, Strawberry Banana									
1 serving, 8 oz (245g)	91	0	0	0	20	0.0	18	3	71
Campbell's V8 Splash Smoothies, Tropical Colada									
1 serving, 8 oz (246g)	101	0	0	0	21	1.0	18	3	49
Campbell's V8 Vegetable Juice, Calcium Enriched V8									
1 serving (243g)	51	0	0	0	11	1.9	0	2	481
Campbell's V8 Vegetable Juice, Essential Antioxidants V8									
1 serving (243g)	51	0	0	0	11	1.9	0	2	481
Campbell's V8 Vegetable Juice, Hi Fiber V8									
1 serving (243g)	61	0	0	0	13	5.1	0	2	481
Campbell's V8 Vegetable Juice, Low Sodium Spicy Hot									
1 serving (243g)	51	0	0	--	11	1.9	0	2	141
Campbell's V8 Vegetable Juice, Low Sodium V8									
1 serving (243g)	51	0	0	0	10	1.9	0	2	141
Campbell's V8 Vegetable Juice, Organic V8									
1 serving (243g)	49	0	0	0	11	1.9	0	1	481
Campbell's V8 Vegetable Juice, Spicy Hot V8									
1 serving (243g)	51	0	0	0	10	1.9	0	2	481
Campbell's V8 V-Fusion Juices, Acai Berry									
1 serving, 8 oz (246g)	111	0	0	0	27	0.0	26	0	69
Campbell's V8 V-Fusion Juices, Peach Mango									
1 serving, 8 oz (246g)	121	0	--	--	28	0.0	26	1	69
Campbell's V8 V-Fusion Juices, Strawberry Banana									
1 serving, 8 oz (246g)	121	0	--	--	29	0.0	25	1	69
Campbell's V8 V-Fusion Juices, Tropical									
1 serving, 8 oz (246g)	121	0	--	--	28	0.0	25	1	81
Chili Con Carne with Beans, Canned Entrée									
1 cup (246g)	298	13	4	32	28	9.6	6	17	1043

Food Serving size	Cal.	(g) Total Fat	(g) Sat. Fat	(mg) Chol.	(g) Carb.	(g) Fiber	(g) Sug.	(g) Prot.	(mg) Sod.
Chili with Beans, Canned 1 tbsp (16g)	18	1	0	3	2	0.7	0	1	84
Oriental Mix, Rice-based 2 oz (57g)	288	15	2	0	29	7.5	2	10	235
Soup, Bean with Bacon, Condensed, Single Brand 1 serving (135g)	158	3	1	4	24	6.2	--	9	994
Soup, Bean with Bacon, Dry, Mix, Prepared with Water 1 cup (8 fl oz) (265g)	106	2	1	3	16	9.0	1	5	928
Soup, Beans with Frankfurters, Canned, Condensed 1 can (11.25 oz) (319g)	453	17	5	29	53	14.7	--	24	2651
Soup, Beans with Frankfurters, Canned, Prepared with Equal Volume of Water 1 can (11.25 oz), prepared (607g)	455	17	5	30	53	--	--	24	2653
Soup, Beans with Ham, Canned, Chunky, Ready-to-serve 1 can (19.25 oz) (546g)	519	19	7	49	61	25.1	--	28	2184
Soup, Beans with Pork, Canned, Condensed .5 cup (130g)	168	6	1	3	22	7.7	4	8	922
Soup, Beans with Pork, Canned, Prepared with Equal Volume of Water 1 fl oz (33.3g)	21	1	0	0	3	1.0	0	1	116
Soup, Beef and Mushroom, Low Sodium, Chunk Style 1 cup (251g)	173	6	4	15	24	0.5	2	11	63
Soup, Beef Broth Bouillon and Consommé, Canned, Condensed 1 can (10.5 oz) (310g)	40	0	0	0	3	0.0	0	8	2024
Soup, Beef Broth or Bouillon, Canned, Ready-to-serve 1 can, 14.5 oz (435g)	30	1	0	0	0	0.0	0	5	1618
Soup, Beef Broth or Bouillon, Powder, Dry 1 packet (6g)	14	1	0	1	1	0.0	1	1	1019
Soup, Beef Broth or Bouillon, Powder, Prepared with Water 1 fl oz (30g)	1	0	0	0	0	0.0	0	0	78
Soup, Beef Broth, Bouillon, Consommé, Prepared with Equal Volume of Water 1 can (10.5 oz), prepared (586g)	70	0	0	0	4	0.0	--	13	1547
Soup, Beef Broth, Cubed, Dry 1 cube (3.6g)	6	0	0	0	1	0.0	1	1	864

Food Serving size	Cal.	(g) Total Fat	(g) Sat. Fat	(mg) Chol.	(g) Carb.	(g) Fiber	(g) Sug.	(g) Prot.	(mg) Sod.
Soup, Beef Broth, Cubed, Prepared with Water									
1 fl oz (30g)	1	0	0	0	0	0.0	0	0	78
Soup, Beef Mushroom, Canned, Condensed									
1 can (10.75 oz) (305g)	186	7	4	15	16	0.6	--	14	2162
Soup, Beef Mushroom, Canned, Prepared with Equal Volume of Water									
1 can (10.75 oz), prepared (593g)	178	7	4	18	15	0.6	--	14	2289
Soup, Beef Noodle, Canned, Condensed									
1 can (10.75 oz) (305g)	204	8	3	12	22	1.8	6	12	1992
Soup, Beef Noodle, Canned, Prepared with Equal Volume of Water									
1 can (10.75 oz), prepared (593g)	202	7	3	12	21	1.8	6	11	2259
Soup, Beef Noodle, Dry, Mix									
1 packet (9.2g)	30	1	0	1	4	0.2	0	2	774
Soup, Beef Stroganoff, Canned, Chunky Style, Ready-to-serve									
1 cup (240g)	235	11	6	50	22	1.4	4	12	1044
Soup, Beef with Vegetables and Barley, Canned, Condensed, Single Brand									
1 serving (127g)	77	2	1	8	10	--	--	5	898
Soup, Black Bean, Canned, Condensed									
1 can (11 oz), undiluted (312g)	284	4	1	0	48	21.2	8	15	3026
Soup, Black Bean, Canned, Prepared with Equal Volume of Water									
1 can (11 oz), prepared (600g)	276	4	1	0	46	20.4	7	15	2922
Soup, Bouillon Cubes and Granules, Low Sodium, Dry									
1 cube (3.6g)	16	1	0	0	2	0.0	1	1	38
Soup, Broccoli Cheese, Canned, Condensed, Commercial									
1 serving, 1/2 cup (121g)	105	6	2	5	9	2.2	3	3	800
Soup, Cheese, Canned, Condensed									
1 can (11 oz), undiluted (312g)	378	25	16	72	26	2.5	2	13	2162
Soup, Cheese, Canned, Prepared with Equal Volume of Milk									
1 can (11 oz), prepared (609g)	560	35	22	116	39	2.4	--	23	2473

Food Serving size	Cal.	(g) Total Fat	(g) Sat. Fat	(mg) Chol.	(g) Carb.	(g) Fiber	(g) Sug.	(g) Prot.	(mg) Sod.
Soup, Cheese, Canned, Prepared with Equal Volume of Water 1 can (11 oz), prepared (600g)	378	25	16	72	26	2.4	--	13	2328
Soup, Chicken Broth Cubes, Dry 1 cube (4.8g)	10	0	0	1	1	0.0	0	1	1152
Soup, Chicken Broth Cubes, Dry, Prepared with Water 1 cube (6 fl oz prepared) (182g)	9	0	0	0	1	--	--	1	593
Soup, Chicken Broth or Bouillon, Dry 1 tsp (2g)	5	0	0	0	0	0.0	0	0	478
Soup, Chicken Broth or Bouillon, Dry, Prepared with Water 1 fl oz (30.1g)	1	0	0	0	0	0.0	0	0	121
Soup, Chicken Broth, Canned, Condensed 1 can (10.75 oz) (305g)	95	3	1	3	2	0.0	.1	13	1894
Soup, Chicken Broth, Canned, Less/Reduced Sodium 1 cup (240g)	17	0	0	0	1	0.0	1	3	554
Soup, Chicken Broth, Canned, Prepared with Equal Volume of Water 1 can (10.75 oz), prepared (593g)	95	3	1	0	2	0.0	2	12	1815
Soup, Chicken Broth, Low Sodium, Canned 1 cup (240g)	38	1	0	0	3	0.0	0	5	72
Soup, Chicken Corn Chowder, Chunky, Ready-to-serve, Single Brand 1 serving (240g)	238	15	4	26	18	2.2	--	7	718
Soup, Chicken Gumbo, Canned, Condensed 1 can (10.75 oz) (305g)	137	3	1	9	20	4.9	6	6	2114
Soup, Chicken Gumbo, Canned, Prepared with Equal Volume of Water 1 can (10.75 oz), prepared (593g)	136	3	1	12	20	4.7	6	6	2319
Soup, Chicken Mushroom Chowder, Chunky, Ready-to-serve, Single Brand 1 serving (240g)	192	11	3	14	17	3.4	--	7	814
Soup, Chicken Mushroom, Canned, Condensed 1 can (10.75 oz) (305g)	332	22	6	24	23	0.6	4	11	2016
Soup, Chicken Mushroom, Canned, Prepared with Equal Volume of Water 1 can (10.75 oz), prepared (593g)	320	22	6	24	23	0.6	--	11	1939
Soup, Chicken Noodle, Canned, Condensed 1 can (10.7oz) (303g)	158	6	2	33	18	0.9	2	8	2139

Food Serving size	Cal.	(g) Total Fat	(g) Sat. Fat	(mg) Chol.	(g) Carb.	(g) Fiber	(g) Sug.	(g) Prot.	(mg) Sod.
Soup, Chicken Noodle, Canned, Prepared with Equal Volume of Water 1 serving, 1 cup (248g)	62	2	1	12	7	0.5	1	3	866
Soup, Chicken Noodle, Dry, Mix 1 packet (6 fl oz) (11.1g)	42	1	0	8	7	0.4	0	2	404
Soup, Chicken Noodle, Dry, Mix, Prepared with Water 1 cup (245g)	56	1	0	10	9	0.2	1	2	561
Soup, Chicken Noodle, Low Sodium, Canned, Prepared with Equal Volume of Water 1 fl oz (31g)	8	0	0	2	1	0.1	0	0	54
Soup, Chicken Rice, Canned, Chunky, Ready-to-serve 1 can, 19 oz (539g)	286	7	2	27	29	2.2	3	28	1994
Soup, Chicken Rice, Dry, Mix, Prepared with Water 1 fl oz (30g)	7	0	0	0	1	0.1	0	0	116
Soup, Chicken Vegetable, Canned, Condensed 1 can (10.7 oz) (303g)	185	7	2	21	21	2.1	4	9	2221
Soup, Chicken Vegetable, Canned, Prepared with Equal Volume of Water 1 cup (8 fl oz) (248g)	77	3	1	10	9	1.0	1	4	972
Soup, Chicken Vegetable, Chunky, Canned, Ready-to-serve 1 can (19 oz) (539g)	372	11	3	38	42	--	--	28	1870
Soup, Chicken Vegetable, Chunky, Reduced Fat, Ready-to-serve, Single Brand 1 serving (240g)	96	1	0	10	15	--	--	6	461
Soup, Chicken with Dumplings, Canned, Condensed 1 can (10.5 oz) (298g)	235	13	3	80	15	1.2	1	14	1842
Soup, Chicken with Dumplings, Canned, Prepared with Equal Volume of Water 1 can (10.5 oz), prepared (586g)	234	13	3	82	15	1.2	2	14	1787
Soup, Chicken with Rice, Canned, Condensed 1 can (10.5 oz) (298g)	146	5	1	15	17	1.5	0	9	1442
Soup, Chicken with Rice, Canned, Prepared with Equal Volume of Water 1 serving, 1 cup (243g)	58	2	0	7	7	0.7	0	4	578
Soup, Chicken with Star-shaped Pasta, Canned, Condensed, Single Brand 1 serving (125g)	63	2	0	5	9	--	--	3	915
Soup, Chicken, Canned, Chunky, Ready-to-serve 1 cup (245g)	174	6	2	29	17	1.5	2	12	867

Food Serving size	Cal.	(g) Total Fat	(g) Sat. Fat	(mg) Chol.	(g) Carb.	(g) Fiber	(g) Sug.	(g) Prot.	(mg) Sod.
Soup, Chili Beef, Canned, Condensed									
1 can (11.25 oz) (319g)	373	8	4	32	60	8.0	16	16	2514
Soup, Chili Beef, Canned, Prepared with Equal Volume of Water									
1 fl oz (32.6g)	19	0	0	2	3	0.4	1	1	126
Soup, Chunky Beef with Country Vegetables, Ready-to-serve									
1 serving (243g)	151	3	1	24	21	--	--	10	892
Soup, Chunky Beef, Canned, Ready-to-serve									
1 can (19 oz) (539g)	356	6	3	32	54	3.2	4	21	1822
Soup, Chunky Chicken Noodle, Canned, Ready-to-serve									
1 can (18.6 oz) (527g)	195	5	2	26	21	2.1	4	17	1808
Soup, Chunky Vegetable, Canned, Ready-to-serve									
1 can (19 oz) (539g)	275	8	1	0	43	2.7	10	8	1935
Soup, Clam Chowder, Manhattan Style, Canned, Chunky, Ready-to-serve									
1 can (19 oz) (539g)	302	8	5	32	42	6.5	9	16	2248
Soup, Clam Chowder, Manhattan, Canned, Condensed									
1 can (10.75 oz) (305g)	186	5	1	6	30	3.7	8	5	1394
Soup, Clam Chowder, Manhattan, Canned, Prepared with Equal Volume of Water									
1 fl oz (31.1g)	9	0	0	0	1	0.2	0	0	70
Soup, Clam Chowder, New England, Canned, Condensed									
1 can (10.7 oz) (303g)	218	6	3	18	31	2.1	1	10	1563
Soup, Clam Chowder, New England, Canned, Prepared with Equal Volume of Low Fat (2%) Milk									
1 fl oz (31.5g)	19	1	0	2	2	0.1	1	1	86
Soup, Clam Chowder, New England, Canned, Prepared with Equal Volume of Water									
1 fl oz (31g)	11	0	0	1	2	0.1	0	0	79
Soup, Consomm with Gelatin, Dry, Mix, Prepared with Water									
1 fl oz (31.1g)	2	0	0	0	0	0.0	0	0	412
Soup, Crab, Canned, Ready-to-serve									
1 can (13 oz) (369g)	114	2	1	15	16	1.1	--	8	1867
Soup, Cream of Asparagus, Canned, Condensed									
1 can (10.75 oz) (305g)	210	10	3	12	26	1.2	2	6	2016
Soup, Cream of Asparagus, Canned, Prepared with Equal Volume of Milk									
1 can (10.75 oz), prepared (602g)	391	20	8	54	40	1.8	--	15	2528

Food Serving size	Cal.	(g) Total Fat	(g) Sat. Fat	(mg) Chol.	(g) Carb.	(g) Fiber	(g) Sug.	(g) Prot.	(mg) Sod.
Soup, Cream of Asparagus, Canned, Prepared with Equal Volume of Water 1 can (10.75 oz), prepared (593g)									
	208	10	3	12	26	1.2	--	6	2384
Soup, Cream of Celery, Canned, Condensed 1 can (10.75 oz) (305g)	220	14	3	34	21	1.8	4	4	1574
Soup, Cream of Celery, Canned, Prepared with Equal Volume of Milk 1 can (10.75 oz), prepared (602g)									
	397	24	10	78	35	1.8	--	14	1637
Soup, Cream of Celery, Canned, prepared with Equal Volume of Water 1 can (10.75 oz), prepared (593g)									
	219	14	3	36	21	1.8	--	4	1506
Soup, Cream of Chicken, Canned, Condensed 1 can (10.75 oz) (305g)	275	18	5	24	22	0.0	2	7	2141
Soup, Cream of Chicken, Canned, Condensed, Single Brand 1 serving (126g)	125	8	2	9	10	--	--	3	993
Soup, Cream of Chicken, Canned, Prepared with Equal Volume of Milk 1 fl oz (31g)	24	1	1	3	2	0.0	--	1	112
Soup, Cream of Chicken, Canned, Prepared with Equal Volume of Water 1 fl oz (30.5g)	15	1	0	1	1	0.0	--	0	106
Soup, Cream of Chicken, Dry, Mix, Prepared with Water 1 fl oz (32.6g)	13	1	0	0	2	0.0	1	0	148
Soup, Cream of Mushroom, Canned, Condensed, Reduced Sodium 1 cup (251g)	131	4	1	8	20	1.5	5	3	961
Soup, Cream of Mushroom, Canned, Condensed 1 can (10.7 oz) (303g)	258	18	4	0	20	0.0	4	5	2127
Soup, Cream of Mushroom, Canned, Prepared with Equal Volume of Low Fat (2%) Milk 1 fl oz (31.5g)	21	1	0	1	2	0.0	1	1	106
Soup, Cream of Mushroom, Canned, Prepared with Equal Volume of Water 1 fl oz (31g)	13	1	0	0	1	0.0	0	0	99
Soup, Cream of Mushroom, Low Sodium, Ready-to-serve, Canned 1 can (10.75 oz) (305g)	162	11	3	3	14	0.6	5	3	61
Soup, Cream of Onion, Canned, Condensed 1 can (10.75 oz) (305g)	268	13	4	37	32	1.2	11	7	1943

Food Serving size	Cal.	(g) Total Fat	(g) Sat. Fat	(mg) Chol.	(g) Carb.	(g) Fiber	(g) Sug.	(g) Prot.	(mg) Sod.
Soup, Cream of Onion, Canned, Prepared with Equal Volume of Milk 1 can (10.75 oz), prepared (602g)	452	23	10	78	45	1.8	--	16	2438
Soup, Cream of Onion, Canned, Prepared with Equal Volume of Water 1 can (10.75 oz), prepared (593g)	261	13	4	36	31	2.4	--	7	2253
Soup, Cream of Potato, Canned, Condensed 1 can (10.75 oz) (305g)	180	6	3	15	28	1.2	5	4	1476
Soup, Cream of Potato, Canned, Prepared with Equal Volume of Milk 1 can (10.75 oz), prepared (602g)	361	16	9	54	42	1.2	--	14	1385
Soup, Cream of Potato, Canned, Prepared with Equal Volume of Water 1 can (10.75 oz), prepared (593g)	178	6	3	12	28	1.2	--	4	1411
Soup, Cream of Shrimp, Canned, Condensed 1 can (10.75 oz) (305g)	220	13	8	40	20	0.6	--	7	2089
Soup, Cream of Shrimp, Canned, Prepared with Equal Volume of Low Fat (2%) Milk 1 fl oz (31.6g)	19	1	1	3	2	0.0	1	1	112
Soup, Cream of Shrimp, Canned, Prepared with Equal Volume of Water 1 can (10.75 oz), prepared (593g)	213	12	8	42	19	0.6	1	7	2319
Soup, Cream of Vegetable, Dry, Powder 1 packet (18g)	80	4	1	0	9	0.5	3	1	892
Soup, Egg Drop, Chinese Restaurant 1 cup (241g)	65	1	0	55	10	1.0	0	3	892
Soup, Escarole, Canned, Ready-to-serve 1 can (19.5 oz) (553g)	61	4	1	6	4	--	--	3	8616
Soup, Gazpacho, Canned, Ready-to-serve 1 can (13 oz) (369g)	70	0	0	0	7	0.7	2	11	1118
Soup, Healthy Choice Chicken Noodle Soup, Condensed 1 serving, 1 cup (243g)	100	2	1	12	13	1.9	1	9	474
Soup, Healthy Choice, Chicken and Rice Soup, Condensed 1 serving, 1 cup (240g)	89	1	0	17	14	1.9	1	6	434
Soup, Healthy Choice, Garden Vegetable Soup, Condensed 1 serving, 1 cup (246g)	125	1	0	2	25	4.7	5	5	480

Food Serving size	Cal.	(g) Total Fat	(g) Sat. Fat	(mg) Chol.	(g) Carb.	(g) Fiber	(g) Sug.	(g) Prot.	(mg) Sod.
Soup, Hot and Sour, Chinese Restaurant 1 cup (233g)	91	3	1	49	10	1.2	0	6	876
Soup, Lentil with Ham, Canned, Ready-to-serve 1 can (20 oz) (567g)	318	6	3	17	46	--	--	21	3016
Soup, Minestrone, Canned, Chunk, Ready-to-serve 1 can (19 oz) (539g)	286	6	3	11	47	12.9	12	11	1552
Soup, Minestrone, Canned, Condensed 1 can (10.5 oz) (298g)	203	6	1	3	27	2.4	4	10	1538
Soup, Minestrone, Canned, Prepared with Equal Volume of Water 1 can (10.5 oz), prepared (586g)	199	6	1	6	27	2.3	--	10	1488
Soup, Mushroom Barley, Canned, Condensed 1 can (10.75 oz) (305g)	186	5	1	0	29	--	--	5	1748
Soup, Mushroom Barley, Canned, Prepared with Equal Volume of Water 1 can (10.75 oz), prepared (593g)	178	6	1	0	28	1.8	--	5	2164
Soup, Mushroom with Beef Stock, Canned, Condensed 1 can (10.75 oz) (305g)	207	10	4	18	23	0.3	7	8	2358
Soup, Mushroom with Beef Stock, Canned, Prepared with Equal Volume of Water 1 can (10.75 oz), prepared (593g)	208	10	4	18	23	1.8	--	8	2354
Soup, Mushroom, Dry, Mix, Prepared with Water 1 packet (6 fl oz prepared) (194g)	64	4	1	0	9	0.4	0	1	782
Soup, Onion Dry, Mix 1 packet (39g)	114	0	0	0	25	2.6	2	3	3132
Soup, Onion, Canned, Condensed 1 can (10.5 oz) (298g)	137	4	1	0	20	2.1	8	9	2181
Soup, Onion, Canned, Prepared with Equal Volume of Water 1 fl oz (30.4g)	7	0	0	0	1	0.1	0	0	129
Soup, Onion, Dry, Mix, Prepared with Water 1 fl oz (28.7g)	3	0	0	0	1	0.1	0	0	99
Soup, Oxtail, Dry, Mix, Prepared with Water 1 cup (244g)	68	2	1	0	9	0.2	2	3	1159
Soup, Oyster Stew, Canned, Condensed 1 can (10.5 oz) (298g)	143	9	6	33	10	0.0	--	5	2205

Food Serving size	Cal.	(g) Total Fat	(g) Sat. Fat	(mg) Chol.	(g) Carb.	(g) Fiber	(g) Sug.	(g) Prot.	(mg) Sod.
Soup, Oyster Stew, Canned, Prepared with Equal Volume of Milk 1 can (10.5 oz), prepared (595g)	327	19	12	77	24	0.0	--	15	2529
Soup, Oyster Stew, Canned, Prepared with Equal Volume of Water 1 can (10.5 oz), prepared (586g)	141	9	6	35	10	--	--	5	2385
Soup, Pea, Green, Canned, Condensed 1 can (11.2 oz) (319g)	399	7	3	0	64	12.4	21	21	2169
Soup, Pea, Green, Canned, Prepared with Equal Volume of Milk 1 can (11.25 oz), prepared (616g)	579	17	10	43	78	6.8	--	31	2168
Soup, Pea, Green, Canned, Prepared with Equal Volume of Water 1 fl oz (32.4g)	20	0	0	0	3	0.6	1	1	109
Soup, Pea, Low Sodium, Prepared with Equal Volume of Water 1 fl oz (32.4g)	20	0	0	0	3	0.6	1	1	3
Soup, Pepper Pot, Canned, Condensed 1 can (10.5 oz) (298g)	250	11	5	24	23	1.2	--	15	2318
Soup, Pepper Pot, Canned, Prepared with Equal Volume of Water 1 fl oz (30.4g)	12	1	0	1	1	0.1	0	1	117
Soup, Potato Ham Chowder, Chunky, Ready-to-serve, Single Brand 1 serving (240g)	192	12	4	22	13	1.4	--	6	874
Soup, Ramen Noodle, Any Flavor, Dry 1 package (85g)	371	13	6	0	54	2.0	1	9	1731
Soup, Ramen Noodle, Beef Flavor, Dry 1 package (85g)	371	13	7	--	54	1.9	2	9	1702
Soup, Ramen Noodle, Chicken Flavor, Dry 1 package (85g)	371	13	6	--	54	2.0	1	9	1760
Soup, Ramen Noodle, Dry, Any Flavor, Reduced Fat, Reduced Sodium 1.41 oz, dry (half noodle block) (40g)	140	1	0	0	28	1.1	0	4	480
Soup, Scotch Broth, Canned, Condensed 1 can (10.5 oz) (298g)	197	6	3	12	23	3.0	--	12	2134
Soup, Scotch Broth, Canned, Prepared with Equal Volume of Water 1 can (10.5 oz), prepared (586g)	193	6	3	12	23	2.9	2	12	2432

Food Serving size	Cal.	(g) Total Fat	(g) Sat. Fat	(mg) Chol.	(g) Carb.	(g) Fiber	(g) Sug.	(g) Prot.	(mg) Sod.
Soup, Shark Fin, Restaurant-prepared 1 cup (216g)	99	4	1	4	8	0.0	--	7	1082
Soup, Sirloin Burger with Vegetables, Ready-to-serve, Single Brand 1 serving (240g)	185	9	3	26	16	5.5	--	10	866
Soup, Split Pea with Ham, Canned, Chunky, Ready-to-serve 1 can (19 oz) (539g)	415	9	4	16	60	9.2	10	25	1622
Soup, Split Pea with Ham, Canned, Condensed 1 can (11.5 oz) (326g)	460	11	4	20	68	5.5	--	25	2054
Soup, Split Pea with Ham, Canned, Prepared with Equal Volume of Water 1 can (11.5 oz), prepared (614g)	461	11	4	18	68	5.5	--	25	2444
Soup, Split Pea with Ham, Chunky, Reduced Fat, Reduced Sodium, Ready-to-serve, Single Brand 1 serving (243g)	185	3	1	15	27	--	--	13	833
Soup, Split Pea, Canned, Reduced Sodium, Prepared with Water or Ready-to-serve 1 cup (253g)	180	2	1	5	30	4.8	13	10	420
Soup, Split Pea, with Ham and Bacon, Canned, Condensed, Single Brand 1 serving (135g)	189	3	1	4	29	4.1	--	12	984
Soup, Stock, Beef, Home-prepared 1 cup (240g)	31	0	0	0	3	0.0	1	5	475
Soup, Stock, Chicken, Home-prepared 1 cup (240g)	86	3	1	7	8	0.0	4	6	343
Soup, Stock, Fish, Home-prepared 1 cup (233g)	40	2	0	2	0	0.0	0	5	363
Soup, Stockpot, Canned, Condensed 1 can (11 oz), undiluted (312g)	243	9	2	9	28	--	--	12	2546
Soup, Stockpot, Canned, Prepared with Equal Volume of Water 1 can (11 oz), prepared (600g)	240	9	2	12	28	--	--	12	2544
Soup, Swanson Chicken Broth, 99% Fat Free 1 serving, 1 cup 8 oz (227g)	9	0	0	0	0	0.0	0	1	928
Soup, Tomato Beef with Noodle, Canned, Condensed 1 can (10.75 oz) (305g)	342	10	4	9	51	3.7	--	11	2230
Soup, Tomato Beef with Noodle, Canned, Prepared with Equal Volume of Water 1 can (10.75 oz), prepared (593g)	332	10	4	12	50	3.6	4	11	2176

Food Serving size	Cal.	(g) Total Fat	(g) Sat. Fat	(mg) Chol.	(g) Carb.	(g) Fiber	(g) Sug.	(g) Prot.	(mg) Sod.
Soup, Tomato Bisque, Canned, Condensed 1 can (11 oz), undiluted (312g)	300	6	1	12	58	2.5	--	5	2137
Soup, Tomato Bisque, Canned, Prepared with Equal Volume of Milk 1 can (11 oz), prepared (609g)	481	16	8	55	71	1.2	--	15	2692
Soup, Tomato Bisque, Canned, Prepared with Equal Volume of Water 1 can (11 oz), prepared (600g)	300	6	1	12	58	1.2	--	6	2544
Soup, Tomato Rice, Canned, Condensed 1 can (11 oz), undiluted (312g)	290	7	1	3	53	4.1	18	5	1981
Soup, Tomato Rice, Canned, Prepared with Equal Volume of Water 1 can (11 oz), prepared (600g)	282	6	1	6	51	4.2	18	5	1914
Soup, Tomato Vegetable, Dry, Mix 1 packet (39g)	127	2	1	1	23	1.2	1	5	2622
Soup, Tomato Vegetable, Dry, Mix, Prepared with Water 1 cup, 8 fl oz (245g)	54	1	0	0	10	0.7	2	2	323
Soup, Tomato, Canned, Condensed 1 can (10.7 oz) (303g)	182	2	0	0	41	3.6	25	5	1173
Soup, Tomato, Canned, Condensed, Reduced Sodium 1 serving, 1/2 cup (121g)	79	1	0	0	16	1.5	10	2	27
Soup, Tomato, Canned, Prepared with Equal Volume of Low Fat (2%) Milk 1 fl oz (31.5g)	17	0	0	1	3	0.2	2	1	66
Soup, Tomato, Canned, Prepared with Equal Volume of Water, Commercial 1 fl oz (31g)	9	0	0	0	2	0.2	1	0	59
Soup, Tomato, Dry, Mix, Prepared with Water 1 cup, 8 fl oz (265g)	101	2	1	5	19	1.1	10	2	943
Soup, Tomato, Low Sodium, with Water 1 fl oz (31g)	9	0	0	0	2	0.2	1	0	7
Soup, Turkey Noodle, Canned, Condensed 1 can (10.75 oz) (305g)	168	5	1	12	21	1.8	1	9	1983
Soup, Turkey Noodle, Canned, Prepared with Equal Volume of Water 1 fl oz (30.5g)	9	0	0	1	1	0.1	--	0	102

Food Serving size	Cal.	(g) Total Fat	(g) Sat. Fat	(mg) Chol.	(g) Carb.	(g) Fiber	(g) Sug.	(g) Prot.	(mg) Sod.
Soup, Turkey Vegetable, Canned, Condensed									
1 can (10.5 oz) (298g)	179	7	2	3	21	1.5	3	8	2202
Soup, Turkey Vegetable, Canned, Prepared with Equal Volume of Water									
1 fl oz (30.1g)	9	0	0	0	1	0.1	--	0	113
Soup, Turkey, Chunky, Canned, Ready-to-serve									
1 can (18.75 oz) (532g)	303	10	3	21	32	--	--	23	2080
Soup, Vegetable Beef, Canned, Condensed									
1 can (10.75 oz) (305g)	192	5	2	12	25	4.9	3	14	2153
Soup, Vegetable Beef, Canned, Condensed, Single Brand									
1 serving (136g)	72	1	0	7	10	--	--	5	755
Soup, Vegetable Beef, Canned, Prepared with Equal Volume of Water									
1 can (10.75 oz), prepared (593g)	184	5	2	12	24	4.7	3	13	2070
Soup, Vegetable Beef, Dry, Mix, Prepared with Water									
1 cup, 8 fl oz (253g)	53	1	1	0	8	0.8	1	3	789
Soup, Vegetable Beef, Microwavable, Ready-to-serve, Single Brand									
1 serving (292g)	128	2	1	9	10	4.4	--	18	1098
Soup, Vegetable Chicken, Canned, Prepared with Water, Low sodium									
1 cup (241g)	166	5	1	17	21	1.0	3	12	84
Soup, Vegetable Soup, Low Sodium, Condensed, Prepared with Equal Volume of Water									
1 cup (253g)	83	1	0	0	15	2.8	5	3	491
Soup, Vegetable with Beef Broth, Canned, Condensed									
1 can (10.5 oz) (298g)	197	5	1	3	32	3.9	5	7	1535
Soup, Vegetables with Beef Broth, Canned, Prepared with Equal Volume of Water									
1 can (10.5 oz), prepared (586g)	193	5	1	6	31	4.1	5	7	1483
Soup, Vegetarian Vegetable, Canned, Condensed									
1 can (10.5 oz) (298g)	176	5	1	0	29	1.5	9	5	2003
Soup, Vegetarian Vegetable, Canned, Prepared with Equal Volume of Water									
1 can (10.5 oz), prepared (586g)	164	5	1	0	29	1.8	9	5	1981

Food Serving size	Cal.	(g) Total Fat	(g) Sat. Fat	(mg) Chol.	(g) Carb.	(g) Fiber	(g) Sug.	(g) Prot.	(mg) Sod.
Sauces and Gravies									
Campbell's Au Jus Gravy .25 cup (59g)	5	0	0	0	0	--	--	1	230
Campbell's Beef Gravy .25 cup (59g)	25	1	0	5	3	0.0	1	1	270
Campbell's Brown Gravy, with Onions .25 cup (59g)	25	1	0	0	4	0.0	2	0	330
Campbell's, Chicken Gravy .25 cup (59g)	40	3	1	5	3	0.0	1	0	260
Campbell's, Country Style Cream Gravy .25 cup (59g)	45	3	1	5	3	0.0	1	1	190
Campbell's, Country Style Sausage Gravy .25 cup (59g)	70	6	1	10	3	0.0	1	2	270
Campbell's, Fat Free Beef Gravy .25 cup (59g)	15	0	0	0	3	0.0	--	1	300
Campbell's, Fat Free Chicken Gravy .25 cup (59g)	15	0	0	5	3	--	--	1	310
Campbell's, Fat Free Turkey Gravy .25 cup (60g)	20	0	0	5	4	--	--	1	290
Campbell's, Franco-American, Fat Free Slow Roasted Beef Gravy .25 cup (59g)	20	0	0	5	3	--	--	1	300
Campbell's, Franco-American, Fat Free Slow Roasted Chicken Gravy .25 cup (59g)	20	0	0	5	4	--	--	1	250
Campbell's, Franco-American, Slow Roasted Beef Gravy .25 cup (59g)	25	1	0	5	3	0.0	0	1	310
Campbell's, Franco-American, Slow Roasted Chicken Gravy .25 cup (59g)	20	1	0	5	3	--	--	1	240
Campbell's, Franco-American, Slow Roasted Turkey Gravy .25 cup (59g)	25	1	0	5	4	--	--	1	320
Campbell's, Golden Pork Gravy .25 cup (59g)	45	3	1	5	3	0.0	1	1	310
Campbell's, Microwavable Beef Gravy .25 cup (59g)	25	1	0	0	3	0.0	1	1	280
Campbell's, Microwavable Chicken Gravy .25 cup (60g)	40	3	1	5	3	0.0	1	0	260

Food Serving size	Cal.	(g) Total Fat	(g) Sat. Fat	(mg) Chol.	(g) Carb.	(g) Fiber	(g) Sug.	(g) Prot.	(mg) Sod.
Campbell's, Microwavable Turkey Gravy .25 cup (60g)	25	1	0	0	3	0.0	1	1	270
Campbell's, Mushroom Gravy .25 cup (59g)	20	1	0	5	3	--	1	0	280
Campbell's, Pace, Chipotle Chunky Salsa 2 tbsp (32g)	8	0	0	0	2	1.0	2	0	230
Campbell's, Pace, Cilantro Chunky Salsa 2 tbsp (32g)	8	0	0	0	2	1.0	2	0	270
Campbell's, Pace, Enchilada Sauce 1 serving (60g)	24	0	0	0	5	1.0	4	1	520
Campbell's, Pace, Green Taco Sauce 2 tbsp (16g)	4	0	0	0	1	--	1	0	100
Campbell's, Pace, Lime and Garlic Chunky Salsa 2 tbsp (32g)	12	0	0	0	3	1.0	2	0	210
Campbell's, Pace, Organic Picante Sauce 2 tbsp (32g)	8	0	0	0	2	1.0	2	0	220
Campbell's, Pace, Picante Sauce 2 tbsp (32g)	8	0	--	0	2	1.0	2	0	250
Campbell's, Pace, Red Taco Sauce 1 serving (16g)	8	0	0	0	2	0.0	1	0	130
Campbell's, Pace, Thick and Chunky Salsa 2 tbsp (32g)	8	0	0	0	2	1.0	2	0	230
Campbell's, Prego Pasta, Chunky Garden Combo Italian Sauce, Ready-to-serve 1 serving, 1/2 cup (130g)	70	1	0	0	13	3.0	10	2	471
Campbell's, Prego Pasta, Chunky Garden Tomato, Onion and Garlic Italian Sauce, Ready-to-serve 1 serving, 1/2 cup (130g)	94	3	0	0	14	3.1	10	2	489
Campbell's, Prego Pasta, Heart Smart - Traditional Sauce .5 cup (130g)	70	1	0	0	13	3.0	0	2	360
Campbell's, Prego Sauce, Chunky Garden Mushroom and Green Pepper with Italian Sausage, Ready-to-serve 1 serving, 1/2 cup (130g)	90	3	0	0	13	3.0	10	2	471
Campbell's, Prego Sauce, Chunky Garden Mushroom with Italian Sausage, Ready-to-serve 1 serving, 1/2 cup (130g)	90	3	1	0	13	3.0	10	2	460

Food Serving size	Cal.	(g) Total Fat	(g) Sat. Fat	(mg) Chol.	(g) Carb.	(g) Fiber	(g) Sug.	(g) Prot.	(mg) Sod.
Campbell's, Prego Sauce, Diced Onion and Garlic with Italian Sausage, Ready-to-serve									
1 serving, 1/2 cup (130g)	120	4	2	0	18	3.0	12	2	480
Campbell's, Prego Sauce, Flavored with Italian Sausage, Ready-to-serve									
1 serving, 1/2 cup (130g)	81	2	1	5	13	3.0	10	2	480
Campbell's, Prego Sauce, Fresh Mushroom with Italian Sausage, Ready-to-serve									
1 serving, 1/2 cup (130g)	70	1	1	0	13	3.0	11	2	480
Campbell's, Prego Sauce, Garlic and Italian Sausage, Ready-to-serve									
1 serving, 1/2 cup (125g)	90	3	1	5	13	3.0	10	3	480
Campbell's, Prego Sauce, Garlic Supreme with Italian Sausage, Ready-to-serve									
1 serving, 1/2 cup (130g)	111	4	2	0	17	3.0	13	2	530
Campbell's, Prego Sauce, Heart Smart, Ricotta, Parmesan with Italian Sausage, Ready-to-serve									
1 serving, 1/2 cup (125g)	90	3	1	5	13	3.0	10	3	360
Campbell's, Prego Sauce, Heart Smart, Roasted Red Peppers and Garlic with Italian Sausage, Ready-to-serve									
1 serving, 1/2 cup (125g)	70	2	0	0	13	3.0	9	2	360
Campbell's, Prego Sauce, Mini Meatballs and Italian Sausage, Ready-to-serve									
1 serving, 1/2 cup (130g)	100	3	1	5	13	3.0	10	4	480
Campbell's, Prego Sauce, Mushroom and Garlic with Italian Sausage, Ready-to-serve									
1 serving, 1/2 cup (130g)	81	2	0	0	13	3.0	10	2	471
Campbell's, Prego Sauce, Mushroom and Parmesan Italian Sausage, Ready-to-serve									
1 serving, 1/2 cup (125g)	130	4	2	5	22	3.0	13	3	480
Campbell's, Prego Sauce, Organic Mushroom with Italian Sausage, Ready-to-serve									
1 serving, 1/2 cup (125g)	90	3	1	0	13	4.0	9	2	470
Campbell's, Prego Sauce, Organic Tomato and Basil with Italian Sausage, Ready-to-serve									
1 serving, 1/2 cup (125g)	90	3	0	0	13	4.0	9	2	470
Campbell's, Prego Sauce, Roasted Garlic and Herb Italian Sausage, Ready-to-serve									
1 serving, 1/2 cup (130g)	90	3	0	0	13	3.0	9	2	460

Food Serving size	Cal.	(g) Total Fat	(g) Sat. Fat	(mg) Chol.	(g) Carb.	(g) Fiber	(g) Sug.	(g) Prot.	(mg) Sod.
Campbell's, Prego Sauce, Roasted Garlic with Parmesan Italian Sausage, Ready-to-serve									
1 serving, 1/2 cup (130g)	100	1	1	5	13	3.0	10	3	480
Campbell's, Prego Sauce, Tomato, Basil and Garlic with Italian Sausage, Ready-to-serve									
1 serving, 1/2 cup (125g)	80	3	0	0	12	3.0	9	2	420
Campbell's, Prego Sauce, Traditional Italian, Ready-to-serve									
1 serving, 1/2 cup (130g)	70	1	0	0	13	3.0	10	2	480
Campbell's, Prego Sauce, Zesty Mushroom with Italian Sausage, Ready-to-serve									
1 serving, 1/2 cup (130g)	111	3	1	0	18	3.0	12	2	530
Campbell's, Turkey Gravy									
.25 cup (59g)	25	1	0	0	3	0.0	1	1	270
Gravy, Au Jus, Canned									
1 can (298g)	48	1	0	0	7	0.0	--	4	149
Gravy, Au Jus, Dry									
1 tsp (3g)	9	0	0	0	1	--	--	0	348
Gravy, Beef, Canned, Ready-to-serve									
1 can (291g)	154	7	3	9	14	1.2	1	11	1630
Gravy, Brown Instant, Dry									
1 serving (6.7g)	25	1	0	1	4	0.2	1	1	339
Gravy, Brown, Dry									
1 tbsp (6g)	22	1	0	0	4	0.1	--	1	291
Gravy, Chicken, Canned, Ready-to-serve									
1 can (298g)	235	17	4	6	16	1.2	2	6	1264
Gravy, Chicken, Dry									
1 serving (8g)	30	1	0	2	5	--	--	1	332
Gravy, Heinz Home Style Savory Beef Gravy									
1 serving, 1/4 cup 2 oz (57g)	22	1	0	1	4	0.4	0	1	335
Gravy, Instant Beef, Dry									
1 pkg (16 oz) (454g)	1675	43	22	50	277	19.5	109	44	236
Gravy, Instant Turkey, Dry									
1 pkg (16 oz) (454g)	1857	67	22	109	261	17.3	35	53	185
Gravy, Meat or Poultry, Low Sodium, Prepared									
1 cup (236g)	125	6	2	7	15	0.7	0	9	42

Food Serving size	Cal.	(g) Total Fat	(g) Sat. Fat	(mg) Chol.	(g) Carb.	(g) Fiber	(g) Sug.	(g) Prot.	(mg) Sod.
Gravy, Mushroom, Canned 1 can (298g)	149	8	1	0	16	1.2	--	4	1699
Gravy, Mushroom, Dry, Powder 1 cup (8 fl oz) (21g)	69	1	0	1	14	1.0	1	2	1382
Gravy, Onion, Dry, Mix 1 cup (8 fl oz) (24g)	77	1	0	0	16	1.4	--	2	1005
Gravy, Pork, Dry, Powder 1 serving (6.7g)	25	1	0	1	4	0.2	2	1	359
Gravy, Turkey, Canned, Ready-to-serve 1 tbsp (14.9g)	8	0	0	0	1	0.1	0	0	86
Gravy, Turkey, Dry 1 serving (7g)	26	1	0	1	5	--	--	1	307
Guava Sauce, Cooked 1 cup (238g)	86	0	0	0	23	8.6	14	1	10
Kraft, Stove Top Stuffing Mix, Chicken Flavor 1 NLEA serving (makes 1/2 cup prepared) (28g)	107	1	0	1	20	0.7	3	4	429
Roast Beef Spread 1 serving, .25 cup (57g)	127	9	4	40	2	0.1	0	9	413
Sandwich Spread, Meatless 1 tbsp (15g)	22	1	0	0	1	0.5	0	1	95
Sandwich Spread, Pork, Beef 1 oz (28.35g)	67	5	2	11	3	0.1	0	2	287
Sandwich Spread, with Chopped Pickle, Regular, Unspecified Oils 1 cup (245g)	953	83	12	186	55	1.0	37	2	2450
Sauce, Barbecue 1 packet (9.3g)	14	0	0	0	3	0.1	2	0	79
Sauce, Barbecue, Low Sodium 1 cup (250g)	375	1	0	0	91	1.5	65	0	333
Sauce, Cheese, Dry, Powder 1 packet (35g)	157	9	4	18	12	0.4	9	8	1299
Sauce, Cheese, Ready-to-serve .25 cup (63g)	110	8	4	18	4	0.3	0	4	522
Sauce, Chili, Peppers, Hot, Immature Greens, Canned 1 tbsp (15g)	3	0	0	0	1	0.3	0	0	4

Food Serving size	Cal.	(g) Total Fat	(g) Sat. Fat	(mg) Chol.	(g) Carb.	(g) Fiber	(g) Sug.	(g) Prot.	(mg) Sod.
Sauce, Fish, Ready-to-serve 1 tbsp (18g)	6	0	0	0	1	0.0	1	1	1413
Sauce, Hoisin, Ready-to-serve 1 tbsp (16g)	35	1	0	0	7	0.4	4	1	258
Sauce, Homemade, White, Medium .5 cup (125g)	184	13	4	9	11	0.3	5	5	443
Sauce, Homemade, White, Thick .5 cup (125g)	233	17	4	8	15	0.4	5	5	466
Sauce, Homemade, White, Thin .5 cup (125g)	131	8	3	10	9	0.1	6	5	410
Sauce, Mole Poblano, Dry Mix, Single Brand 1 cup, sauce (265g)	1513	110	--	--	111	26.8	--	20	3085
Sauce, Oyster, Ready-to-serve 1 tbsp (18g)	9	0	0	0	2	0.1	0	0	492
Sauce, Pasta, Spaghetti, Marinara, Ready-to-serve 1 cup (257g)	224	7	2	5	35	6.7	23	5	1054
Sauce, Pasta, Spaghetti, Marinara, Ready-to-serve, Low Sodium 1 cup (257g)	224	7	2	5	35	6.7	23	5	77
Sauce, Peppers, Hot, Chili, Mature Red, Canned 1 tbsp (15g)	3	0	0	0	1	0.1	0	0	4
Sauce, Pizza, Canned, Ready-to-serve .25 cup (63g)	34	1	0	2	5	1.3	1	1	117
Sauce, Plum, Ready-to-serve 1 tbsp (19g)	35	0	0	0	8	0.1	--	0	102
Sauce, Ready-to-serve, Pepper or Hot .25 tsp (1.2g)	0	0	0	0	0	0.0	0	0	32
Sauce, Ready-to-serve, Pepper, Tabasco .25 tsp (1.2g)	0	0	0	0	0	0.0	0	0	8
Sauce, Salsa, Ready-to-serve 1 tbsp (16g)	4	0	0	0	1	0.3	0	0	96
Sauce, Sofrito, Prepared from Recipe .5 cup (103g)	244	19	--	--	6	1.8	--	13	1179
Sauce, Teriyaki, Ready-to-serve 1 tbsp (18g)	16	0	0	0	3	0.0	3	1	690

Food Serving size	Cal.	(g) Total Fat	(g) Sat. Fat	(mg) Chol.	(g) Carb.	(g) Fiber	(g) Sug.	(g) Prot.	(mg) Sod.
Sauce, Tomato Chili Sauce, Bottled, No Salt, Low Sodium 1 tbsp (17g)	18	0	0	0	5	0.1	2	0	3
Sauce, Tomato Chili Sauce, Bottled, with Salt 1 packet (6g)	6	0	0	0	1	0.4	1	0	80
Sauce, Worcestershire 1 tbsp (17g)	13	0	0	0	3	0.0	2	0	167
Soy Sauce, Made from Hydrolyzed Vegetable Protein 1 tsp (6g)	2	0	0	0	0	0.0	0	0	341
Soy Sauce, Made from Soy and Wheat (Shoyu) 1 tbsp (16g)	8	0	0	0	1	0.1	0	1	902
Soy Sauce, Made from Soy and Wheat (Shoyu), Low Sodium 1 tbsp (16g)	8	0	0	0	1	0.1	0	1	533
Soy Sauce, Made from Soy (Tamari) 1 tsp (6g)	4	0	0	0	0	0.0	0	1	335
Tomato Products, Canned, Paste, with Salt 1 can (6 oz) (170g)	139	1	0	0	32	7.0	21	7	1343
Tomato Products, Canned, Paste, Without Salt Added 1 tbsp (16g)	13	0	0	0	3	0.7	2	1	16
Tomato Products, Canned, Puree, with Salt 1 can (29 oz) (401 x 411) (822g)	312	2	0	0	74	15.6	40	14	3280
Tomato Products, Canned, Puree, Without Salt 1 can (29 oz) (401 x 411) (822g)	312	2	0	0	74	15.6	40	14	230
Tomato Products, Canned, Sauce 1 cup (245g)	59	0	0	0	13	3.7	10	3	1284
Tomato Products, Canned, Sauce, Spanish Style 1 can, 15 oz (303 x 406) (425g)	140	1	0	0	31	6.0	--	6	2006
Tomato Products, Canned, Sauce, with Herbs and Cheese 1 can, 15 oz (303 x 406) (425g)	251	8	3	13	44	9.4	--	9	2308
Tomato Products, Canned, Sauce, with Mushrooms 1 cup (245g)	86	0	0	0	21	3.7	14	4	1107
Tomato Products, Canned, Sauce, with Onions 1 cup (245g)	103	0	0	0	24	4.4	--	4	1350

Food Serving size	Cal.	(g) Total Fat	(g) Sat. Fat	(mg) Chol.	(g) Carb.	(g) Fiber	(g) Sug.	(g) Prot.	(mg) Sod.
Tomato Products, Canned, Sauce, with Onions, Green Peppers and Celery 1 can, 15 oz (303 x 406) (411g)	169	3	1	0	36	5.8	30	4	2244
Tomato Products, Canned, Sauce, with Tomato Tidbits 1 can, 15 oz (303 x 406) (425g)	136	2	0	0	30	6.0	--	6	64
Tomato Sauce, No Salt 1 cup (245g)	103	0	0	0	21	3.7	1	3	27
Worthington Saucettes, Canned, Unprepared 1 link (38g)	83	6	--	1	2	1.1	0	6	202

Frozen Dinners/Meals

Food Serving size	Cal.	(g) Total Fat	(g) Sat. Fat	(mg) Chol.	(g) Carb.	(g) Fiber	(g) Sug.	(g) Prot.	(mg) Sod.
Beef Pot Pie, Frozen Entrée, Prepared 1 pie, cooked (average weight) (268g)	590	31	11	56	59	2.1	10	19	978
Chicken Pot Pie, Frozen Entrée, Prepared 1 pie (average weight of prepared pie) (234g)	501	25	8	56	54	2.8	7	14	889
DiGiorno Pizza, Cheese Topping, Cheese Stuffed Crust, Frozen, Baked 1 pie, 12" diameter (688g)	1920	80	39	193	205	13.1	--	93	5545
DiGiorno Pizza, Cheese Topping, Rising Crust, Frozen, Baked 1 pie, 12" diameter (729g)	1866	63	26	109	232	17.5	25	93	5074
DiGiorno Pizza, Cheese Topping, Thin Crispy Crust, Frozen, Baked 1 pie, 23 oz (643g)	1588	64	30	135	170	19.3	21	83	3254
DiGiorno Pizza, Pepperoni Topping, Cheese Stuffed Crust, Frozen, Baked 1 pie, 12" diameter (732g)	2042	86	37	176	216	15.4	20	102	5512
DiGiorno Pizza, Pepperoni Topping, Rising Crust, Frozen, Baked 1 pie, 12" diameter (759g)	2011	77	29	137	236	17.5	28	95	5639
DiGiorno Pizza, Pepperoni Topping, Thin Crispy Crust, Frozen, Baked 1 pie, 22.1 oz (548g)	1551	70	27	153	157	15.3	18	72	3633
DiGiorno Pizza, Supreme Topping, Rising Crust, Frozen, Baked 1 pie, 12" diameter (876g)	2234	94	35	166	245	20.1	32	103	6237
DiGiorno Pizza, Supreme Topping, Thin Crispy Crust, Frozen, Baked 1 pie, 24.8 oz (595g)	1517	64	26	119	167	16.7	21	68	3302
Egg Rolls, Chicken, Refrigerated, Heated 1 oz (28.35g)	56	1	0	4	8	0.7	7	3	159

Food Serving size	Cal.	(g) Total Fat	(g) Sat. Fat	(mg) Chol.	(g) Carb.	(g) Fiber	(g) Sug.	(g) Prot.	(mg) Sod.
Egg Rolls, Pork, Refrigerated, Heated 1 oz (28.35g)	63	2	0	4	8	0.6	6	3	149
Egg Rolls, Vegetable, Refrigerated, Heated 1 oz (28.35g)	56	1	0	0	9	0.8	7	2	159
Entrees, Crab Cake 1 cake (60g)	160	10	2	82	5	0.2	--	11	491
Entrees, Fish Fillet, Battered or Breaded and Fried 1 fillet (91g)	211	11	3	31	15	0.5	--	13	484
Fish Portions and Sticks, Frozen, Preheated 1 stick (4" x 1" x 1/2") (28g)	70	4	1	8	6	0.4	1	3	118
French Toast, Frozen, Ready-to-heat 1 piece (59g)	126	4	1	48	19	0.6	--	4	292
Hot Pockets Ham 'n Cheese Stuffed Sandwich, Frozen 1 serving (1 hot pocket) (127g)	306	12	5	29	39	1.9	4	12	640
Hot Pockets, Croissant Pockets Chicken, Broccoli and Cheddar Stuffed Sandwich, Frozen 1 serving (1 hot pocket) (127g)	298	11	3	37	39	1.4	5	11	439
Hot Pockets, Meatballs and Mozzarella Stuffed Sandwich, Frozen 1 hot pocket (analytical weight) (131g)	331	14	5	26	40	2.9	32	12	811
Kellogg, Kellogg's Eggo, Banana Bread Waffles 1 serving (78g)	212	7	1	0	32	2.0	5	5	280
Kellogg, Kellogg's Eggo, Buttermilk Pancake 3 pancakes (NLEA serving) (116g)	270	8	2	13	44	1.3	10	7	589
Kellogg's Eggo Golden Oat Waffles 1 serving (70g)	139	2	0	1	26	2.5	2	5	270
Kellogg's Eggo Low Fat Blueberry Nutri-Grain Waffles 1 serving (70g)	146	2	0	0	30	2.5	6	4	414
Kellogg's Eggo Low Fat Homestyle Waffles 1 serving (70g)	165	2	1	18	31	0.7	2	5	309
Lasagna with Meat and Sauce, Frozen Entrée 1 serving (297g)	377	14	7	45	38	3.6	11	25	832
Lasagna with Meat and Sauce, Low Fat, Frozen Entrée 1 oz (28.35g)	29	1	0	2	4	0.4	1	2	51

Food Serving size	Cal.	(g) Total Fat	(g) Sat. Fat	(mg) Chol.	(g) Carb.	(g) Fiber	(g) Sug.	(g) Prot.	(mg) Sod.
Lasagna, Cheese, Frozen, Prepared									
1 oz (28.35g)	37	2	1	4	4	0.5	1	2	81
Lasagna, Vegetable, Frozen, Baked									
1 cup (226g)	314	14	5	32	32	4.3	44	16	796
Lean Pockets, Ham 'n Cheddar									
1 each (analytical measurement) (129g)	297	8	3	26	42	2.2	27	13	637
Morningstar Farms Asian Veggie Patties, Frozen, Unprepared									
1 patty (67g)	104	4	1	0	10	2.0	3	7	486
Morningstar Farms BBQ Riblets, Frozen, Unprepared									
1 piece, with sauce (142g)	223	4	0	0	35	6.8	24	19	815
Morningstar Farms Breakfast Pattie, Made with Organic Soy, Frozen, Unprepared									
1 patty (38g)	78	3	0	1	4	1.6	1	8	240
Morningstar Farms California Turkey Burger, Frozen, Unprepared									
1 patty (64g)	91	5	1	0	7	5.0	1	9	390
Morningstar Farms Chik Patties, Frozen, Unprepared									
1 patty (71g)	140	5	1	0	16	2.1	1	8	593
Morningstar Farms Chik'n Grill Veggie Patties, Frozen, Unprepared									
1 patty (67g)	79	3	0	0	7	3.8	0	9	348
Morningstar Farms Chik'n Nuggets, Frozen, Unprepared									
4 pieces (86g)	190	9	1	0	19	4.2	2	12	604
Morningstar Farms Garden Veggie Patties, Frozen, Unprepared									
1 patty (67g)	118	4	1	1	9	3.0	2	12	352
Morningstar Farms Grillers Original, Frozen, Unprepared									
1 patty (64g)	136	6	1	2	5	2.8	1	15	270
Morningstar Farms Grillers Prime, Frozen, Unprepared									
1 patty (71g)	169	9	1	1	4	1.8	0	17	356
Morningstar Farms Grillers Quarter Pound Veggie Burger, Frozen, Unprepared									
1 patty (114g)	252	12	2	1	10	2.9	1	26	489
Morningstar Farms Hot and Spicy Veggie Sausage Patties, Frozen, Unprepared									
1 patty (38g)	71	3	0	0	3	0.9	0	8	209
Morningstar Farms Italian Herb Chik Patties, Frozen, Unprepared									
1 patty (71g)	168	5	1	0	22	2.4	1	10	484
Morningstar Farms Lasagna with Veggie Sausage, Frozen, Unprepared									
1 serving (284g)	304	7	3	11	41	6.5	5	20	591

Food Serving size	Cal.	(g) Total Fat	(g) Sat. Fat	(mg) Chol.	(g) Carb.	(g) Fiber	(g) Sug.	(g) Prot.	(mg) Sod.
Morningstar Farms Maple Flavor Veggie Sausage Patties, Frozen, Unprepared 1 patty (38g)	84	3	0	0	5	0.8	2	10	249
Morningstar Farms Meal Starters Chik'n Strips, Frozen, Unprepared 12 strips (85g)	139	3	1	0	6	1.2	1	23	507
Morningstar Farms Meatfree Buffalo Wings, Frozen, Unprepared 5 pieces (85g)	196	8	1	0	20	3.1	2	12	644
Morningstar Farms Mushroom Lover's Burger, Frozen, Unprepared 1 patty (64g)	108	6	1	0	8	0.8	1	7	221
Morningstar Farms Original Chik'n Tenders, Frozen, Unprepared 2 pieces (81g)	189	7	1	0	20	2.9	0	12	578
Morningstar Farms Sausage Style Recipe Crumbles, Frozen, Unprepared 1 cup (55g)	89	3	0	0	5	2.5	1	11	417
Morningstar Farms Tomato and Basil Pizza Burger, Frozen, Unprepared 1 patty (67g)	121	6	1	7	7	2.5	2	10	261
Morningstar Farms Veggie Breakfast Bacon Strips, Frozen, Unprepared 2 strips (16g)	55	4	1	0	2	0.8	0	2	234
Morningstar Farms Veggie Breakfast Sausage Links, Frozen, Unprepared 2 links (45g)	72	3	0	1	3	1.8	0	9	302
Morningstar Farms Veggie Italian Style Sausage, Frozen, Unprepared 1 link (64g)	120	6	1	--	7	1.3	1	11	351
Morningstar Farms Veggie Sweet and Sour Chick'n, Frozen, Unprepared 1 serving (284g)	346	7	1	0	58	3.7	12	14	545
Morningstar Farms, Grillers Burger Style Recipe Crumbles, Frozen, Unprepared .667 cup (1 serving) (55g)	77	2	0	0	5	2.6	2	10	235
Morningstar Farms, Grillers Vegan, Frozen, Unprepared 1 patty (71g)	94	2	0	0	6	3.7	2	12	280
Morningstar Farms, Spicy Black Bean Burger, Frozen, Unprepared 1 patty (67g)	115	4	1	1	13	4.6	2	11	348
Morningstar Farms, Veggie Breakfast Sausage Patties, Frozen, Unprepared 1 patty (38g)	80	3	0	1	3	1.6	1	10	255
Onion Rings, Breaded, Partially Fried, Frozen, Unprepared 1 pkg (9 oz) (255g)	658	36	12	0	78	4.6	--	8	627
Pizza Pepperoni Topping, Regular Crust, Frozen, Cooked 1 pizza (428g)	1267	65	21	64	122	9.4	14	48	2645

Food Serving size	Cal.	(g) Total Fat	(g) Sat. Fat	(mg) Chol.	(g) Carb.	(g) Fiber	(g) Sug.	(g) Prot.	(mg) Sod.
Pizza, Cheese Topping, Regular Crust, Frozen, Cooked 1 pkg, 15.1 oz pizza (452g)	1211	56	19	63	131	9.9	17	47	2020
Pizza, Cheese Topping, Rising Crust, Frozen, Cooked 1 pkg, 19.7 oz pizza (595g)	1547	52	23	95	196	14.9	21	74	3308
Pizza, Meat and Vegetable Topping, Regular Crust, Frozen, Cooked 1 pkg, 22.85 oz pizza (644g)	1777	93	33	103	162	14.2	33	73	3574
Pizza, Meat and Vegetable Topping, Rising Crust, Frozen, Cooked 1 pkg, 30.7 oz pizza (891g)	2415	105	41	169	256	20.5	43	113	5702
Supper Bakes Meal Kit, Creamy Stroganoff Sauce with Pasta 1 serving (125g)	184	4	2	10	31	1.0	11	6	650
Supper Bakes Meal Kit, Garlic Chicken with Pasta .167 box (NLEA serving) (103g)	227	1	1	5	44	2.1	25	10	763
Supper Bakes Meal Kit, Southwestern-style Chicken with Rice 1 serving (81g)	153	1	0	5	32	2.0	20	4	600
Supper Bakes Meal, Cheesy Chicken with Pasta (Chicken Not Included) .167 box (NLEA serving size) (85g)	168	4	1	5	27	1.0	0	6	840
Supper Bakes Meal, Chicken with Stuffing (Chicken Not Included) 1 box (505g)	960	18	6	30	174	12.1	48	30	4439
Turkey Pot Pie, Frozen Entrée 1 serving (397g)	699	35	11	64	70	4.4	15	26	1390
Turkey Roast, Boneless, Frozen, Seasoned, Light and Dark Meat, Roasted 1 box (net weight, 1.72 lb) (782g)	1212	45	15	414	24	0.0	0	167	5318
Turkey, Stuffing, Mashed Potatoes with Gravy, Assorted Vegetables, Frozen, Microwave 1 package (422g)	540	16	4	59	69	5.5	107	29	1772
Waffles, Buttermilk, Frozen, Ready-to-heat 1 waffle, round (38g)	104	4	1	6	16	0.8	2	3	236
Waffles, Buttermilk, Frozen, Ready-to-heat, Microwaved 1 waffle (35g)	101	3	1	6	15	0.8	2	2	232

Food Serving size	Cal.	(g) Total Fat	(g) Sat. Fat	(mg) Chol.	(g) Carb.	(g) Fiber	(g) Sug.	(g) Prot.	(mg) Sod.
Waffles, Buttermilk, Frozen, Ready-to-heat, Toasted 1 waffle, round (4" dia) (33g)	102	3	1	4	16	0.9	1	2	234
Waffles, Chocolate Chip, Frozen, Ready-to-heat 2 waffles, round (70g)	195	7	2	15	29	1.0	9	4	380
Waffles, Plain, Frozen, Ready-to-heat 1 waffle, square (4" square) (include frozen) (35g)	100	3	1	5	15	0.8	2	2	223
Waffles, Plain, Frozen, Ready-to-heat, Microwave 1 waffle, round (4"dia) (32g)	95	3	1	5	15	0.8	2	2	218
Waffles, Plain, Frozen, Ready-to-heat, Toasted 1 waffle, round (4" dia) (33g)	103	3	1	5	16	0.8	2	2	241
Waffles, Plain, Prepared from Recipe 1 waffle, round (7" dia) (75g)	218	11	2	52	25	--	--	6	383
Worthington Chic-ketts, Frozen, Unprepared 2 slices (3/8" thick) (55g)	110	5	1	0	3	0.7	0	13	353
Worthington Chili, Canned, Unprepared 1 cup (230g)	290	10	2	0	25	7.8	3	24	1042
Worthington Dinner Roasted, Frozen, Unprepared 1 slice, 3/4" (85g)	181	11	2	1	6	2.6	1	14	570
Worthington Fri Chik Original, Canned, Unprepared 2 pieces (90g)	144	9	1	1	3	1.4	0	12	361
Worthington Fripats, Frozen, Unprepared 1 patty (64g)	134	6	1	1	5	1.8	1	15	331
Worthington Leanies, Frozen, Unprepared 1 link (40g)	100	7	1	1	2	1.5	0	8	431
Worthington Low Fat Fri Chik, Canned, Unprepared 2 pieces (85g)	87	2	0	1	4	0.9	0	12	354
Worthington Low Fat Veja-Links, Canned, Unprepared 1 link (31g)	38	1	0	1	1	0.4	0	5	190
Worthington Meatless Chicken Roll, Frozen, Unprepared 1 slice, 3/8" (55g)	85	4	1	1	2	1.3	0	9	249
Worthington Meatless Corned Beef Roll, Frozen, Unprepared 2 slices, 3/8" (55g)	135	8	1	1	5	0.0	1	10	417
Worthington Multi-grain Cutlets, Canned, Unprepared 2 slices (92g)	99	1	0	0	6	2.9	1	17	288

Food Serving size	Cal.	(g) Total Fat	(g) Sat. Fat	(mg) Chol.	(g) Carb.	(g) Fiber	(g) Sug.	(g) Prot.	(mg) Sod.
Worthington Prime Stakes, Canned, Unprepared									
1 piece (92g)	124	7	1	1	7	1.3	0	9	442
Worthington Prosage Links, Frozen, Unprepared									
2 links (45g)	64	2	0	1	2	1.3	0	9	369
Worthington Prosage Roll, Frozen, Unprepared									
1 slice, 5/8" (55g)	144	10	2	1	3	1.9	0	11	367
Worthington Smoked Turkey Roll, Frozen, Unprepared									
1 slice, 3/8" (55g)	138	9	1	0	4	0.6	1	10	472
Worthington Stakelets, Frozen, Unprepared									
1 piece (71g)	150	7	1	1	7	2.0	1	14	462
Worthington Stripples, Frozen, Unprepared									
2 strips (16g)	55	4	1	0	2	0.8	0	2	234
Worthington Super Links, Canned, Unprepared									
1 link (48g)	105	7	1	0	3	0.9	0	7	340
Worthington Vegetable Steaks, Canned, Unprepared									
2 slices (72g)	81	1	--	0	4	1.6	0	15	300
Worthington Vegetarian Burger, Canned, Unprepared									
.25 cup (55g)	68	2	0	0	3	1.5	0	10	248
Worthington Wham (Roll), Frozen, Unprepared									
1 slice, 3/8" (55g)	108	6	1	0	3	0.0	2	10	394

Meal Replacement Bars

Food Serving size	Cal.	(g) Total Fat	(g) Sat. Fat	(mg) Chol.	(g) Carb.	(g) Fiber	(g) Sug.	(g) Prot.	(mg) Sod.
Formulated Bar, Luna Bar, Nutz Over Chocolate									
1 bar (48g)	193	6	3	0	25	2.1	0	10	185
Formulated Bar, Mars Snackfood US, Cocoavia, Chocolate Almond									
1 bar (22g)	76	3	1	0	11	1.1	0	2	57
Formulated Bar, Mars Snackfood US, Cocoavia, Chocolate Blueberry									
1 bar (22g)	72	2	1	0	13	1.0	0	1	57
Formulated Bar, Mars Snackfood US, Snickers Marathon Chewy Chocolate Peanut Bar									
1 bar (55g)	218	7	3	2	26	1.4	0	13	254
Formulated Bar, Mars Snackfood US, Snickers Marathon Double Chocolate Nut Bar									
1 bar (55g)	189	5	3	2	29	5.8	0	12	183

Food Serving size	Cal.	(g) Total Fat	(g) Sat. Fat	(mg) Chol.	(g) Carb.	(g) Fiber	(g) Sug.	(g) Prot.	(mg) Sod.
Formulated Bar, Mars Snackfood US, Snickers Marathon Energy Bar, All Flavors									
1 bar (44g)	170	5	2	2	22	2.9	0	10	169
Formulated Bar, Mars Snackfood US, Snickers Marathon Multi-grain Crunch									
1 bar (55g)	232	7	3	2	31	1.5	0	10	230
Formulated Bar, Mars Snackfood US, Snickers Marathon, Honey Nut Oat Bar									
1 bar (55g)	208	4	2	--	30	6.1	0	12	175
Formulated Bar, Power Bar, Chocolate									
1 bar (68g)	247	2	1	0	47	3.9	0	10	99
Formulated Bar, Slim-Fast Optima Meal Bar, Milk Chocolate Peanut									
1 bar (55g)	212	5	3	4	33	2.8	0	9	139
Formulated, Wheat-based, All Flavors Except Macadamia, Without Salt									
1 oz (28.35g)	183	18	3	0	6	1.5	--	4	26
Formulated, Wheat-based, Flavor, Macadamia Flavor, Without Salt									
1 oz (28.35g)	175	16	2	0	8	1.5	--	3	13
Formulated, Wheat-based, Unflavored, with Salt									
1 oz (28.35g)	176	16	2	0	7	1.5	--	4	143

Baby Foods/Beverages

Feeding Infants, Toddlers, and Children

Good nutrition is a must to support the rapid growth and development your baby will undergo in the first two years of life. Providing the right foods during this critical time will support good health and encourage enjoyment of new tastes and textures as they grow, as well as build the beginning of healthy eating habits. Use this information to help raise healthy and happy children.

What Is a Healthy Diet for Your Baby, Toddler, and Child?

The chart on the next page gives the daily estimated calories and recommended servings of each of the major food groups for infants and children from birth to age 8 (see page 362). Calorie estimates are based on a moderately active child. Food portions are assumed to be nutrient-dense.

Why Are Nutrition Facts for Children Different?

Because young children have unique nutritional needs for their growing bodies, yet require fewer calories than the 2000 that the regular Nutrition Facts labels are based on, the Nutrition Facts for children's foods and beverages are different. First, foods specifically for children less than 4 years do not provide % Daily Values for the macronutrients, carbohydrates and fat, as well as sodium, fiber, cholesterol, saturated fat, and trans fat. Since protein is an important nutrient for growing children, a % Daily Value is provided, along with % Daily Values for vitamins A and C, calcium and iron. Unfortunately, the % Daily Values are based on a 2000-calorie diet and are not specific to the needs of children. Also, food labels for children less than 2 years of age do not present information on calories from fat, nor do they include amounts for saturated fat, polyunsaturated fat, monounsaturated fat, and cholesterol. Because fat is essential to growth, it should not be restricted during these early years. In addition, serving sizes for infant foods are based on average amounts that infants under two years usually eat. (See page 363.)

	0 to 6 months	6 months to 1 year	1 to 2 years	2 to 3 years	4 to 8 years
Calories	Variable	Variable	Variable	1000 to 1400	1400 to 1600
Milk/Dairy	18 to 45 oz (breast milk or formula)	24 to 32 oz (breast milk or formula)	24 to 32 oz (breast milk or formula) or 2 cups whole milk	2 to 2.5 cups whole milk	2.5 to 3 cups (can switch to low-fat milk)
Lean Meat/Beans	None	Begin to offer well cooked, soft, finely cut or pureed meats or cheese.	1 to 2 oz soft, finely cut meats or other protein foods	2 to 3 oz lean meat, poultry, or seafood; 1 egg; 1 T peanut butter	3 to 4 oz lean meat, poultry, or seafood; 1 egg; 1 T peanut butter
Fruits	None	2 to 4 oz 100% juice; begin to offer plain cooked, mashed or strained baby food.	2 to 4 oz 100% juice or 1 cup fruit	1 cup 100% juice or 1 cup fruit	1.5 cups 100% juice or 1 cup fruit
Vegetables	None	Begin to offer plain cooked, mashed, or strained baby food.	1 cup raw or cooked	1 cup raw or cooked	1.5 cups raw or cooked
Grains	None	2 to 6 T iron-fortified baby cereal or other soft breads, cereals, etc.	2 oz (1 oz = 1 slice whole grain bread; ½ cup cooked cereal, rice, or pasta, 1 cup dry cereal)	3 oz (1 oz = 1 slice whole grain bread; ½ cup cooked cereal, rice, or pasta, 1 cup dry cereal)	4 to 5 oz (1 oz = 1 slice whole grain bread; ½ cup cooked cereal, rice, or pasta, 1 cup dry cereal)
Oils (g)	None	NA	NA	15 to 17 g	17 to 22 g

Adapted from 2010 US Dietary Guidelines, Appendix 7; Start Healthy Feeding Guidelines, the American Dietetic Association; and Feeding Recommendations (American Academy of Pediatrics).

Nutrition Facts

Serving Size 1 jar (140g)

Amount Per Serving	
Calories 110	
Total Fat	0g
Trans Fat	0g
Sodium	10mg
Total Carbohydrate	27g
Dietary Fiber	4g
Sugars	0g
Protein	0g

% Daily Value

Protein 0%	•	Vitamin A 6%
Vitamin C 45%	•	Calcium 2%
Iron 2%		

Nutrition Facts

Serving Size 1 jar (140g)

Amount Per Serving	
Calories 110	Calories from Fat 0
Total Fat	0g
Saturated Fat	0g
Trans Fat	0g
Cholesterol	0mg
Sodium	10mg
Total Carbohydrate	27g
Dietary Fiber	4g
Sugars	0g
Protein	0g

% Daily Value

Protein 0%	•	Vitamin A 6%
Vitamin C 45%	•	Calcium 2%
Iron 2%		

How Do the Food Label Reference Values (Daily Values) Compare to the Nutritional Recommendations for Children (DRIs)?

Nutrient Recommendations by Age (DRIs)

Nutrient	Daily Value	2 to 3 years	4 to 8 years
Protein (grams)	50	13	19
Iron (mg)	18	7	10
Calcium (mg)	1000	700	1000
Vitamin A (IU)	5000	1000	1333
Vitamin C (mg)	60	15	25

Sources: 2010 Dietary Guidelines and IOM Dietary Reference Intakes 2006 and 2010.

Tips for Raising Healthy Children

1. **Offer a variety of healthy foods.** When children eat a variety of foods, they get the nutrients they need from every food group. They will be more likely to try new foods and to like more foods. This will make it easier to plan family meals.

2. **Start with small portions.** Offer children small, easy-to-eat amounts to make eating easy and more enjoyable. Use smaller bowls, plates, and utensils for your child to eat with. Don't insist that children finish all the food on their plate. Let your child know it is okay to only eat as much as he or she wants. We are born with an internal mechanism that signals when we are full—don't mess with it.

3. **Follow a meal and snack schedule.** Regularly scheduled meal and snack times help your child learn structure for eating. Your child is more likely to eat healthy meals and try new foods if snacks are not offered too close to mealtime.

4. **Make mealtime an enjoyable family time.** Family meals allow your child to focus on the task of eating and give you a chance to model good behaviors. You may not be able to eat together all the time, but try to plan a family meal at least once a day. It takes a little work to bring everyone together for meals, but it's worth it. Involve your child in conversation. Ask questions like:

   - What made you feel really happy today?
   - What did you have to eat at lunch today?
   - What's your favorite veggie? Why?
   - Tell me one thing you learned today?
   - Wha't made you laugh today?

5. **Make food fun for picky eaters.** Picky eating is temporary, so don't get discouraged. Get your child involved in planning, shopping for, and preparing the food. Let them create snacks, salads, or desserts. Be creative with the food—try fun and interesting food shapes.

6. **Set a good example.** Your child picks up all of your attitudes and behaviors—including your eating habits. Children love to copy what their parents do. They are likely to mimic your table manners, your likes and dislikes, your willingness to try new foods, and your physical activities.

Food Serving size	Cal.	(g) Total Fat	(g) Sat. Fat	(mg) Chol.	(g) Carb.	(g) Fiber	(g) Sug.	(g) Prot.	(mg) Sod.
Baby Foods/Baby Formulas									
Baby Face, Juice, Fruit Punch, with Calcium 1 fl oz (31.2g)	16	0	0	0	4	0.1	3	0	1
Baby Food, Apple Yogurt Dessert, Strained 1 jar, NFS (113g)	108	2	1	7	22	0.6	--	1	23
Baby Food, Apple-Banana Juice 1 bottle, Earth's Best (4.2 fl oz) (131g)	67	0	0	0	16	0.3	14	0	5
Baby Food, Apple-Cranberry Juice 1 fl oz (31.2g)	14	0	0	0	4	0.0	2	0	2
Baby Food, Apples, Diced, Toddler 1 oz (28.35g)	14	0	0	0	3	0.3	3	0	2
Baby Food, Apples, with Ham, Strained 1 jar, NFS (113g)	70	1	0	9	12	2.0	9	3	10
Baby Food, Baked Product, Finger Snacks Cereal 1 cookie (1.7g)	7	0	0	0	1	0.0	0	0	6
Baby Food, Banana Apple Dessert, Strained 1 jar, NFS (113g)	77	0	0	0	18	1.1	10	0	8
Baby Food, Banana Juice, with Low Fat Yogurt 1 bottle, NFS (126g)	112	1	1	4	22	0.5	--	3	47
Baby Food, Banana, No Tapioca, Strained 1 jar, NFS (113g)	103	0	0	0	24	1.8	0	1	2
Baby Food, Carrots and Beef, Strained 1 jar, NFS (113g)	67	3	1	9	6	2.9	2	4	78
Baby Food, Carrots, Toddler 1 oz (28.35g)	7	0	0	0	1	0.7	1	0	14
Baby Food, Cereal, Barley, Dry .5 oz (15g)	55	1	0	0	11	1.2	0	2	2
Baby Food, Cereal, Barley, Prepared with Whole Milk 1 oz (28.35g)	24	1	0	3	3	0.2	1	1	12
Baby Food, Cereal, Brown Rice, Dry, Instant 1 tbsp (3.7g)	15	0	0	0	3	0.2	0	0	0
Baby Food, Cereal, Egg Yolks and Bacon, Junior 1 jar (170g)	134	9	3	160	11	1.5	--	4	82

Food Serving size	Cal.	(g) Total Fat	(g) Sat. Fat	(mg) Chol.	(g) Carb.	(g) Fiber	(g) Sug.	(g) Prot.	(mg) Sod.
Baby Food, Cereal, Hi Protein, Prepared with Whole Milk									
1 oz (28.35g)	31	1	--	--	3	--	--	2	14
Baby Food, Cereal, Hi Protein, with Apples and Orange, Prepared with Whole Milk									
1 oz (28.35g)	32	1	--	--	4	--	--	2	16
Baby Food, Cereal, High Protein, with Apples and Orange, Dry									
.5 oz (14.2g)	53	1	0	0	8	1.0	--	4	15
Baby Food, Cereal, Mixed, Dry									
.5 oz (15g)	57	1	0	0	11	1.1	0	2	0
Baby Food, Cereal, Mixed, Prepared with Whole Milk									
1 oz (28.35g)	27	1	0	3	3	0.2	1	1	12
Baby Food, Cereal, Mixed, with Applesauce and Bananas, Junior									
1 jar (170g)	141	1	0	0	31	2.0	13	2	5
Baby Food, Cereal, Mixed, with Applesauce and Bananas, Strained									
1 jar (113g)	93	1	0	0	20	1.4	9	1	3
Baby Food, Cereal, Mixed, with Bananas, Dry									
.5 oz (15g)	59	1	0	0	12	1.2	1	2	0
Baby Food, Cereal, Mixed, with Bananas, Prepared with Whole Milk									
1 oz (28.35g)	24	1	1	3	3	0.1	2	1	14
Baby Food, Cereal, Mixed, with Honey, Prepared with Whole Milk									
1 oz (28.35g)	33	1	--	--	5	--	--	1	14
Baby Food, Cereal, Oatmeal, Dry									
.5 oz (15g)	60	1	0	0	10	1.4	1	2	1
Baby Food, Cereal, Oatmeal, Prepared with Whole Milk									
1 oz (28.35g)	33	1	1	3	4	0.3	--	1	13
Baby Food, Cereal, Oatmeal, with Applesauce and Bananas, Junior									
1 jar (170g)	128	1	0	0	27	1.4	16	2	5
Baby Food, Cereal, Oatmeal, with Applesauce and Bananas, Strained									
1 jar (113g)	84	1	0	0	17	0.9	12	1	3
Baby Food, Cereal, Oatmeal, with Bananas, Dry									
.5 oz (15g)	59	1	0	0	11	0.8	2	2	1
Baby Food, Cereal, Oatmeal, with Bananas, Prepared with Whole Milk									
1 oz (28.35g)	24	1	1	3	3	0.1	2	1	14
Baby Food, Cereal, Oatmeal, with Honey, Dry									
.5 oz (14.2g)	56	1	--	--	10	--	--	2	7

Food Serving size	Cal.	(g) Total Fat	(g) Sat. Fat	(mg) Chol.	(g) Carb.	(g) Fiber	(g) Sug.	(g) Prot.	(mg) Sod.
Baby Food, Cereal, Oatmeal, with Honey, Prepared with Whole Milk									
1 oz (28.35g)	33	1	--	--	4	--	--	1	14
Baby Food, Cereal, Rice, Dry									
.5 oz (15g)	59	1	0	0	12	0.1	0	1	1
Baby Food, Cereal, Rice, Prepared with Whole Milk									
1 oz (28.35g)	24	1	1	3	3	0.0	1	1	12
Baby Food, Cereal, Rice, with Applesauce and Bananas, Strained									
1 oz (28.35g)	23	0	0	0	5	0.3	1	0	1
Baby Food, Cereal, Rice, with Bananas, Dry									
.5 oz (15g)	61	1	0	0	12	0.2	3	1	0
Baby Food, Cereal, Rice, with Bananas, Prepared with Whole Milk									
1 oz (28.35g)	24	1	1	3	3	0.0	2	1	13
Baby Food, Cereal, Rice, with Honey, Prepared with Whole Milk									
1 oz (28.35g)	33	1	--	--	5	--	--	1	14
Baby Food, Cereal, Rice, with Mixed Fruit, Junior									
1 oz (28.35g)	23	0	0	0	5	0.2	3	0	3
Baby Food, Cereal, Whole Wheat, with Apples, Dry									
.5 oz (15g)	60	1	0	0	12	1.8	3	2	4
Baby Food, Cereal, with Egg Yolks, Junior									
1 jar (170g)	88	3	1	107	12	1.5	--	3	56
Baby Food, Cereal, with Egg Yolks, Strained									
1 jar (113g)	58	2	1	71	8	1.0	--	2	37
Baby Food, Cereal, with Eggs, Strained									
1 jar (113g)	66	2	1	58	9	--	--	2	43
Baby Food, Cherry Cobbler, Junior									
1 oz (28.35g)	22	0	0	0	5	0.1	3	0	0
Baby Food, Cookie, Fruit									
1 cookie (8g)	35	1	0	0	6	0.3	2	1	1
Baby Food, Cookies									
1 cookie (6.5g)	28	1	0	1	4	0.0	2	1	23
Baby Food, Cookies, Arrowroot									
1 cookie (5g)	22	1	0	0	4	0.0	--	0	16
Baby Food, Corn and Sweet Potatoes, Strained									
1 oz (28.35g)	19	0	0	0	4	0.5	1	0	4

Food Serving size	Cal.	(g) Total Fat	(g) Sat. Fat	(mg) Chol.	(g) Carb.	(g) Fiber	(g) Sug.	(g) Prot.	(mg) Sod.
Baby Food, Crackers, Vegetable									
1 cracker (0.7g)	3	0	0	0	0	0.0	0	0	4
Baby Food, Dessert, Banana Pudding, Strained									
1 jar, NFS (113g)	77	1	0	33	16	0.9	0	1	61
Baby Food, Dessert, Banana Yogurt, Strained									
1 jar, NFS (113g)	89	1	0	1	20	0.6	3	1	16
Baby Food, Dessert, Blueberry Yogurt, Strained									
1 jar, NFS (113g)	87	1	1	5	19	0.5	13	1	16
Baby Food, Dessert, Cherry Vanilla Pudding, Junior									
1 jar (170g)	117	0	0	17	31	0.5	29	0	0
Baby Food, Dessert, Cherry Vanilla Pudding, Strained									
1 jar (113g)	77	0	0	11	20	0.3	10	0	0
Baby Food, Dessert, Custard Pudding, Vanilla, Junior									
1 tbsp (14g)	12	0	0	5	2	0.0	2	0	4
Baby Food, Dessert, Custard Pudding, Vanilla, Strained									
1 tbsp (14g)	12	0	0	1	2	0.0	2	0	0
Baby Food, Dessert, Dutch Apple, Junior									
1 jar (170g)	134	0	0	0	33	2.4	30	0	5
Baby Food, Dessert, Dutch Apple, Strained									
1 jar (113g)	85	0	0	0	22	1.6	20	0	0
Baby Food, Dessert, Fruit Dessert, Without Vitamin C, Junior									
1 oz (28.35g)	18	0	0	0	5	0.2	3	0	0
Baby Food, Dessert, Fruit Dessert, Without Vitamin C, Strained									
1 oz (28.35g)	17	0	0	0	5	0.2	4	0	0
Baby Food, Dessert, Fruit Pudding, Orange, Strained									
1 jar (113g)	90	1	1	3	20	0.7	--	1	23
Baby Food, Dessert, Fruit Pudding, Pineapple, Strained									
1 oz (28.35g)	23	0	0	0	6	0.2	3	0	0
Baby Food, Dessert, Peach Cobbler, Junior									
1 oz (28.35g)	19	0	0	0	5	0.2	3	0	0
Baby Food, Dessert, Peach Cobbler, Strained									
1 oz (28.35g)	18	0	0	0	5	0.2	3	0	2
Baby Food, Dessert, Peach Yogurt									
1 jar, NFS (113g)	86	0	0	5	20	0.5	10	1	16

Food Serving size	Cal.	(g) Total Fat	(g) Sat. Fat	(mg) Chol.	(g) Carb.	(g) Fiber	(g) Sug.	(g) Prot.	(mg) Sod.
Baby Food, Dessert, Tropical Fruit, Junior									
1 jar (113g)	68	0	--	--	19	--	--	0	8
Baby Food, Dinner, Apples and Chicken, Strained									
1 jar (113g)	73	2	0	6	12	2.0	9	2	14
Baby Food, Dinner, Beef and Rice, Toddler									
1 jar (170g)	139	5	--	--	15	--	0	9	54
Baby Food, Dinner, Beef Lasagna, Toddler									
1 jar (170g)	131	4	--	--	17	--	0	7	70
Baby Food, Dinner, Beef Noodle, Junior									
1 oz (28.35g)	16	1	0	2	2	0.3	0	1	7
Baby Food, Dinner, Beef Noodle, Strained									
1 oz (28.35g)	18	1	0	2	2	0.4	0	1	4
Baby Food, Dinner, Beef Stew, Toddler									
1 jar (170g)	87	2	1	22	9	1.9	2	9	180
Baby Food, Dinner, Beef with Vegetables									
1 jar, Beech-Nut Stage 2 (4 oz) (113g)	108	8	3	14	7	2.0	2	2	43
Baby Food, Dinner, Broccoli and Chicken, Junior									
1 container (162g)	100	4	1	21	10	2.3	2	6	28
Baby Food, Dinner, Chicken and Noodle, with Vegetables, Toddler									
1 jar, NFS (170g)	112	3	1	48	15	1.0	0	6	400
Baby Food, Dinner, Chicken and Rice									
1 jar, Gerber (4 oz) (113g)	58	1	0	11	10	1.2	1	2	28
Baby Food, Dinner, Chicken Noodle, Junior									
1 oz (28.35g)	16	0	0	3	2	0.3	0	1	10
Baby Food, Dinner, Chicken Noodle, Strained									
1 oz (28.35g)	19	1	0	5	3	0.6	1	1	11
Baby Food, Dinner, Chicken Soup, Strained									
1 tbsp (16g)	8	0	0	1	1	0.2	0	0	3
Baby Food, Dinner, Chicken Stew, Toddler									
1 oz (28.35g)	22	1	0	8	2	0.2	0	1	7
Baby Food, Dinner, Macaroni and Cheese, Junior									
1 jar (170g)	104	3	2	10	14	0.5	2	4	452
Baby Food, Dinner, Macaroni and Cheese, Strained									
1 jar (113g)	76	2	1	8	10	0.8	1	4	134

Food Serving size	Cal.	(g) Total Fat	(g) Sat. Fat	(mg) Chol.	(g) Carb.	(g) Fiber	(g) Sug.	(g) Prot.	(mg) Sod.
Baby Food, Dinner, Macaroni and Tomato and Beef, Junior									
1 oz (28.35g)	17	0	0	1	3	0.3	1	1	10
Baby Food, Dinner, Macaroni and Tomato and Beef, Strained									
1 oz (28.35g)	17	0	0	2	3	0.3	1	1	11
Baby Food, Dinner, Macaroni, Beef and Tomato, Sauce, Toddler									
1 tbsp (16g)	13	0	0	1	2	0.2	--	1	6
Baby Food, Dinner, Mixed Vegetables, Junior									
1 jar (170g)	56	0	--	--	14	--	--	2	65
Baby Food, Dinner, Mixed Vegetables, Strained									
1 jar (113g)	46	0	--	--	11	--	--	1	43
Baby Food, Dinner, Pasta, with Vegetables									
1 jar, Gerber (4 oz) (113g)	68	2	1	6	9	1.7	1	2	12
Baby Food, Dinner, Potatoes, with Cheese and Ham, Toddler									
1 oz (28.35g)	22	1	0	2	3	0.3	0	1	58
Baby Food, Dinner, Spaghetti and Tomato and Meat, Junior									
1 oz (28.35g)	19	0	0	1	3	0.3	1	1	9
Baby Food, Dinner, Spaghetti and Tomato and Meat, Toddler									
1 jar (170g)	128	2	--	--	18	--	--	9	406
Baby Food, Dinner, Sweet Potatoes and Chicken, Strained									
1 jar, Beech-Nut Stage 2 (4 oz) (113g)	84	2	1	12	12	1.5	6	3	25
Baby Food, Dinner, Turkey and Rice, Junior									
1 oz (28.35g)	16	0	0	1	3	0.3	0	1	7
Baby Food, Dinner, Turkey and Rice, Strained									
1 oz (28.35g)	15	0	0	1	2	0.3	0	1	5
Baby Food, Dinner, Turkey, Rice, and Vegetables, Toddler									
1 jar, Beech nut (170g)	102	3	1	12	13	1.4	1	6	469
Baby Food, Dinner, Vegetables and Bacon, Strained									
1 tbsp (16g)	11	0	0	1	1	0.3	0	0	8
Baby Food, Dinner, Vegetables and Beef, Junior									
1 tbsp (16g)	12	1	0	1	1	0.2	0	0	5
Baby Food, Dinner, Vegetables and Beef, Strained									
1 tbsp (16g)	12	1	0	1	1	0.2	0	0	5
Baby Food, Dinner, Vegetables and Chicken, Junior									
1 tbsp (16g)	8	0	0	1	1	0.2	0	0	5

Food Serving size	Cal.	(g) Total Fat	(g) Sat. Fat	(mg) Chol.	(g) Carb.	(g) Fiber	(g) Sug.	(g) Prot.	(mg) Sod.
Baby Food, Dinner, Vegetables and Chicken, Strained									
1 tbsp (16g)	9	0	0	2	1	0.3	0	0	4
Baby Food, Dinner, Vegetables and Dumplings and Beef, Junior									
1 jar (170g)	82	1	--	--	14	--	0	4	88
Baby Food, Dinner, Vegetables and Dumplings and Beef, Strained									
1 jar (113g)	54	1	--	--	9	--	0	2	55
Baby Food, Dinner, Vegetables and Ham, Junior									
1 tbsp (16g)	10	0	0	0	1	0.2	0	0	7
Baby Food, Dinner, Vegetables and Ham, Strained									
1 tbsp (16g)	9	0	0	1	1	0.3	0	0	3
Baby Food, Dinner, Vegetables and Lamb, Junior									
1 jar (170g)	87	3	1	9	12	1.9	2	4	22
Baby Food, Dinner, Vegetables and Lamb, Strained									
1 tbsp (16g)	8	0	0	1	1	0.2	0	0	3
Baby Food, Dinner, Vegetables and Noodles and Turkey, Junior									
1 jar (170g)	88	3	--	--	13	1.9	--	3	29
Baby Food, Dinner, Vegetables and Noodles and Turkey, Strained									
1 jar (113g)	50	1	--	--	8	1.2	--	1	24
Baby Food, Dinner, Vegetables and Turkey, Junior									
1 tbsp (16g)	8	0	0	1	1	0.1	0	0	7
Baby Food, Dinner, Vegetables and Turkey, Strained									
1 tbsp (16g)	8	0	0	1	1	0.2	0	0	3
Baby Food, Dinner, Vegetables and Turkey, Toddler									
1 jar (170g)	136	6	--	--	14	--	0	8	70
Baby Food, Dinner, Vegetables, Noodles and Chicken, Junior									
1 jar (170g)	109	4	--	--	15	1.9	--	3	44
Baby Food, Dinner, Vegetables, Noodles and Chicken, Strained									
1 jar (113g)	71	3	--	--	9	1.2	--	2	23
Baby Food, Fruit and Vegetable, Apple and Sweet Potato									
1 jar, Gerber (4 oz) (113g)	72	0	0	0	17	1.6	13	0	3
Baby Food, Fruit Dessert, Mango, with Tapioca									
1 oz (28.35g)	20	0	0	0	5	0.3	4	0	1
Baby Food, Fruit Supreme Dessert									
1 tbsp (15g)	11	0	0	0	3	0.3	2	0	0

Food Serving size	Cal.	(g) Total Fat	(g) Sat. Fat	(mg) Chol.	(g) Carb.	(g) Fiber	(g) Sug.	(g) Prot.	(mg) Sod.
Baby Food, Fruit, Apples and Blueberry, Junior 1 jar (170g)	105	0	0	0	28	3.1	15	0	2
Baby Food, Fruit, Apples and Blueberry, Strained 1 jar (113g)	69	0	0	0	18	2.0	16	0	1
Baby Food, Fruit, Applesauce and Apricots, Junior 1 oz (28.35g)	13	0	0	0	4	0.5	2	0	0
Baby Food, Fruit, Applesauce and Apricots, Strained 1 oz (28.35g)	12	0	0	0	3	0.5	3	0	0
Baby Food, Fruit, Applesauce and Cherries, Junior 1 jar (170g)	87	0	0	0	24	1.9	18	0	2
Baby Food, Fruit, Applesauce and Cherries, Strained 1 jar (113g)	58	0	0	0	16	1.2	12	0	1
Baby Food, Fruit, Applesauce and Pineapple, Junior 1 jar (170g)	66	0	0	0	18	2.6	--	0	3
Baby Food, Fruit, Applesauce and Pineapple, Strained 1 jar (113g)	42	0	0	0	11	1.7	--	0	2
Baby Food, Fruit, Applesauce and Raspberry, Junior 1 jar (170g)	99	0	0	0	26	3.6	22	0	0
Baby Food, Fruit, Applesauce and Raspberry, Strained 1 jar (113g)	66	0	0	0	18	2.4	15	0	0
Baby Food, Fruit, Applesauce, Junior 1 oz (28.35g)	10	0	0	0	3	0.5	2	0	0
Baby Food, Fruit, Applesauce, Strained 1 oz (28.35g)	12	0	0	0	3	0.5	3	0	0
Baby Food, Fruit, Applesauce, with Banana, Junior 1 jar, NFS (170g)	112	0	0	0	27	2.7	7	1	5
Baby Food, Fruit, Apricot, with Tapioca, Junior 1 oz (28.35g)	18	0	0	0	5	0.4	0	0	0
Baby Food, Fruit, Apricot, with Tapioca, Strained 1 oz (28.35g)	17	0	0	0	5	0.4	0	0	0
Baby Food, Fruit, Bananas and Pineapple, with Tapioca, Junior 1 oz (28.35g)	19	0	0	0	5	0.5	2	0	0
Baby Food, Fruit, Bananas and Pineapple, with Tapioca, Strained 1 oz (28.35g)	18	0	0	0	5	0.5	3	0	0

Food Serving size	Cal.	(g) Total Fat	(g) Sat. Fat	(mg) Chol.	(g) Carb.	(g) Fiber	(g) Sug.	(g) Prot.	(mg) Sod.
Baby Food, Fruit, Bananas, with Apples and Pears, Strained									
1 jar, NFS (113g)	94	0	0	0	22	1.6	14	1	2
Baby Food, Fruit, Banana, with Tapioca, Junior									
1 oz (28.35g)	19	0	0	0	5	0.5	2	0	0
Baby Food, Fruit, Bananas, with Tapioca, Strained									
1 oz (28.35g)	16	0	0	0	4	0.5	0	0	0
Baby Food, Fruit, Guava and Papaya, with Tapioca, Strained									
1 jar (113g)	71	0	--	--	19	--	--	0	5
Baby Food, Fruit, Papaya and Applesauce, with Tapioca, Strained									
1 jar (113g)	79	0	--	--	21	1.6	--	0	6
Baby Food, Fruit, Peaches, Junior									
1 oz (28.35g)	18	0	0	0	4	0.4	3	0	1
Baby Food, Fruit, Peaches, Strained									
1 oz (28.35g)	18	0	0	0	4	0.4	3	0	1
Baby Food, Fruit, Pears and Pineapple, Junior									
1 oz (28.35g)	12	0	0	0	3	0.7	2	0	0
Baby Food, Fruit, Pears and Pineapple, Strained									
1 oz (28.35g)	12	0	0	0	3	0.7	2	0	0
Baby Food, Fruit, Pears, Junior									
1 oz (28.35g)	12	0	0	0	3	1.0	2	0	0
Baby Food, Fruit, Pears, Strained									
1 oz (28.35g)	12	0	0	0	3	1.0	2	0	0
Baby Food, Fruit, Plums, with Tapioca, Without Vitamin C, Junior									
1 oz (28.35g)	21	0	0	0	6	0.3	4	0	0
Baby Food, Fruit, Plums, with Tapioca, Without Vitamin C, Strained									
1 oz (28.35g)	20	0	0	0	6	0.3	4	0	0
Baby Food, Fruit, Prunes, with Tapioca, Without Vitamin C, Junior									
1 jar (170g)	119	0	0	0	32	4.6	19	1	3
Baby Food, Fruit, Prunes, with Tapioca, Without Vitamin C, Strained									
1 oz (28.35g)	20	0	0	0	5	0.8	3	0	1
Baby Food, Fruit, Tutti Fruitti, Junior									
1 jar, NFS (170g)	117	1	0	26	27	0.7	1	1	29
Baby Food, Fruit, Tutti Frutti, Strained									
1 jar, NFS (113g)	75	0	0	17	17	0.7	0	0	28

Food Serving size	Cal.	(g) Total Fat	(g) Sat. Fat	(mg) Chol.	(g) Carb.	(g) Fiber	(g) Sug.	(g) Prot.	(mg) Sod.
Baby Food, Green Beans, Diced, Toddler 1 jar (128g)	37	0	0	0	7	1.7	1	2	47
Baby Food, Juice Treats, Fruit Medley, Toddler 1 packet (28g)	97	0	0	0	24	0.0	16	0	25
Baby Food, Juice, Apple 1 jar (127g)	60	0	0	0	15	0.1	14	0	10
Baby Food, Juice, Apple and Cherry 1 jar (127g)	52	0	0	0	13	0.1	11	0	0
Baby Food, Juice, Apple and Grape 1 jar (127g)	58	0	0	0	14	0.1	14	0	0
Baby Food, Juice, Apple and Peach 1 jar (127g)	55	0	0	0	13	0.1	12	0	0
Baby Food, Juice, Apple and Plum 1 jar (127g)	62	0	0	0	16	0.1	15	0	0
Baby Food, Juice, Apple and Prune 1 jar (127g)	91	0	0	0	23	0.1	13	0	10
Baby Food, Juice, Apple, with Calcium 1 serving (189g)	87	0	0	0	21	0.8	17	0	6
Baby Food, Juice, Apple-Cherry 1 bottle, Heinz Strained (4 fl oz) (125g)	59	0	0	0	14	0.4	--	0	5
Baby Food, Juice, Apple-Sweet Potato 1 fl oz (30.8g)	15	0	0	0	4	0.2	--	0	2
Baby Food, Juice, Mixed Fruit 1 jar (127g)	60	0	0	0	15	0.1	11	0	10
Baby Food, Juice, Orange 1 jar (127g)	57	0	0	0	13	0.1	10	1	0
Baby Food, Juice, Orange and Apple 1 jar (127g)	55	0	--	--	13	--	--	1	4
Baby Food, Juice, Orange and Apricot 1 jar (127g)	58	0	0	0	14	0.1	--	1	8
Baby Food, Juice, Orange and Banana 1 jar (127g)	64	0	--	--	15	--	--	1	4
Baby Food, Juice, Orange and Pineapple 1 jar (127g)	61	0	0	0	15	0.1	--	1	3

Food Serving size	Cal.	(g) Total Fat	(g) Sat. Fat	(mg) Chol.	(g) Carb.	(g) Fiber	(g) Sug.	(g) Prot.	(mg) Sod.
Baby Food, Juice, Orange, Apple and Banana									
1 jar (127g)	60	0	0	0	15	0.1	13	1	0
Baby Food, Juice, Orange-Carrot									
1 fl oz (30.8g)	13	0	0	0	3	0.1	--	0	3
Baby Food, Juice, Pear									
1 bottle, Earth's Best (4.2 fl oz) (131g)	62	0	0	0	16	0.1	10	0	10
Baby Food, Juice, Prune and Orange									
1 jar (127g)	89	0	--	--	21	--	--	1	3
Baby Food, Mashed Cheddar Potatoes and Broccoli, Toddler									
1 container (170g)	82	2	1	5	13	1.5	2	2	299
Baby Food, Meat, Beef, Strained									
1 oz (28.35g)	23	1	0	14	1	0.0	0	3	12
Baby Food, Meat, Beef, Strained									
1 tbsp (14.7g)	12	0	0	7	0	0.0	0	2	6
Baby Food, Meat, Beef, with Vegetables, Toddler									
1 jar, NFS (179g)	122	4	2	21	16	0.9	2	6	47
Baby Food, Meat, Chicken Sticks, Junior									
1 jar (71g)	133	10	3	55	1	0.1	1	10	290
Baby Food, Meat, Chicken, Junior									
1 oz (28.35g)	41	3	1	17	0	0.0	0	4	14
Baby Food, Meat, Chicken, Strained									
1 oz (28.35g)	37	2	1	17	0	0.0	0	4	14
Baby Food, Meat, Ham, Junior									
1 jar (71g)	69	3	1	21	3	0.0	0	8	31
Baby Food, Meat, Ham, Strained									
1 oz (28.35g)	27	1	0	7	1	0.0	0	3	12
Baby Food, Meat, Lamb, Junior									
1 jar (71g)	80	4	2	27	0	0.0	0	11	30
Baby Food, Meat, Lamb, Strained									
1 oz (28.35g)	25	1	0	10	0	0.0	0	4	12
Baby Food, Meat, Meat Sticks, Junior									
1 jar (71g)	131	10	4	50	1	0.1	1	10	300
Baby Food, Meat, Pork, Strained									
1 jar (71g)	88	5	2	34	0	0.0	0	10	30

Food Serving size	Cal.	(g) Total Fat	(g) Sat. Fat	(mg) Chol.	(g) Carb.	(g) Fiber	(g) Sug.	(g) Prot.	(mg) Sod.
Baby Food, Meat, Turkey Sticks, Junior 1 jar (71g)	133	10	3	46	1	0.4	1	10	312
Baby Food, Meat, Turkey, Junior 1 container (68g)	75	4	1	39	1	0.0	0	8	33
Baby Food, Meat, Turkey, Strained 1 oz (28.35g)	31	2	0	16	0	0.0	0	3	14
Baby Food, Meat, Veal, Strained 1 oz (28.35g)	23	1	0	9	0	0.0	0	4	11
Baby Food, Mixed Fruit Juice, with Low Fat Yogurt 1 bottle, NFS (126g)	96	1	1	4	18	0.5	--	3	45
Baby Food, Mixed Fruit Yogurt, Strained 1 jar, NFS (113g)	85	1	1	0	18	0.5	--	1	18
Baby Food, Oatmeal Cereal, with Fruit, Dry, Instant, Toddler 1 packet (.75 oz) (21g)	84	1	0	0	16	1.6	2	2	0
Baby Food, Peaches, Diced, Toddler 1 jar, Gerber (128g)	65	0	0	0	15	1.0	12	1	12
Baby Food, Pears, Diced, Toddler 1 jar, Gerber (128g)	73	0	0	0	17	1.5	11	0	8
Baby Food, Peas and Brown Rice 1 tbsp (14.4g)	9	0	0	0	2	0.4	0	0	1
Baby Food, Peas, Diced, Toddler 1 oz (28.35g)	18	0	0	0	3	1.1	1	1	14
Baby Food, Plums, Bananas and Rice, Strained 1 jar, Earth's Best (113g)	64	0	0	0	14	1.5	11	1	0
Baby Food, Potatoes, Toddler 1 tbsp (10g)	5	0	0	0	1	0.1	0	0	6
Baby Food, Pretzels 1 pretzel (6g)	24	0	0	0	5	0.1	0	1	16
Baby Food, Prunes, Without Vitamin C, Strained 1 jar, Gerber First Foods (2.5 oz) (71g)	71	0	0	0	17	1.9	15	1	1
Baby Food, Ravioli, Cheese-filled, with Tomato Sauce 1 piece (8g)	8	0	0	1	1	0.0	0	0	23
Baby Food, Rice and Apples, Dry 1 tbsp (2.5g)	10	0	0	0	2	0.1	--	0	0

Food Serving size	Cal.	(g) Total Fat	(g) Sat. Fat	(mg) Chol.	(g) Carb.	(g) Fiber	(g) Sug.	(g) Prot.	(mg) Sod.
Baby Food, Teething Biscuits									
1 biscuit (11g)	43	0	0	1	8	0.2	1	1	25
Baby Food, Vegetable and Brown Rice, Strained									
1 tbsp (14.4g)	10	0	0	0	2	0.2	--	0	2
Baby Food, Vegetable, Beets, Strained									
1 tbsp (14g)	5	0	0	0	1	0.3	1	0	12
Baby Food, Vegetable, Butternut Squash and Corn									
1 jar, Gerber (4 oz) (113g)	57	1	0	0	10	2.3	3	2	6
Baby Food, Vegetable, Carrots, Junior									
1 tbsp (14g)	4	0	0	0	1	0.2	0	0	7
Baby Food, Vegetable, Carrots, Strained									
1 tbsp (14g)	4	0	0	0	1	0.2	1	0	10
Baby Food, Vegetable, Corn, Creamed, Junior									
1 tbsp (15g)	10	0	0	0	2	0.3	0	0	8
Baby Food, Vegetable, Corn, Creamed, Strained									
1 tbsp (15g)	9	0	0	0	2	0.3	0	0	6
Baby Food, Vegetable, Garden Vegetables, Strained									
1 jar (113g)	36	0	0	0	8	1.7	3	3	35
Baby Food, Vegetable, Green Beans and Potatoes									
1 jar, Gerber (4 oz) (113g)	70	2	1	6	10	1.6	3	2	20
Baby Food, Vegetable, Green Beans, Junior									
1 tbsp (15g)	4	0	0	0	1	0.3	0	0	1
Baby Food, Vegetable, Green Beans, Strained									
1 tbsp (15g)	4	0	0	0	1	0.3	0	0	1
Baby Food, Vegetable, Mixed Vegetables, Junior									
1 tbsp (15g)	5	0	0	0	1	0.2	0	0	5
Baby Food, Vegetable, Mixed Vegetables, Strained									
1 jar (113g)	41	1	0	0	9	1.7	2	1	0
Baby Food, Vegetable, Peas, Strained									
1 oz (28.35g)	14	0	0	0	2	0.6	1	1	1
Baby Food, Vegetable, Spinach, Creamed, Strained									
1 tbsp (15g)	6	0	0	1	1	0.3	0	0	7
Baby Food, Vegetable, Squash, Junior									
1 oz (28.35g)	7	0	0	0	2	0.3	1	0	1

Food Serving size	Cal.	(g) Total Fat	(g) Sat. Fat	(mg) Chol.	(g) Carb.	(g) Fiber	(g) Sug.	(g) Prot.	(mg) Sod.
Baby Food, Vegetable, Squash, Strained 1 oz (28.35g)	8	0	0	0	2	0.3	1	0	1
Baby Food, Vegetable, Sweet Potatoes, Junior 1 tbsp (14g)	8	0	0	0	2	0.2	1	0	3
Baby Food, Vegetable, Sweet Potatoes, Strained 1 tbsp (14g)	8	0	0	0	2	0.2	1	0	3
Baby Food, Yogurt, Whole Milk, with Fruit, Multigrain Cereal and Added DHA 1 container (113g)	111	4	2	16	15	0.3	13	4	46
Child Formula, Abbott Nutrition, Pediasure, Ready-to-feed 1 fl oz (31g)	31	1	0	1	3	0.0	3	1	11
Child Formula, Abbott Nutrition, Pediasure, Ready-to-feed, with Iron 1 fl oz (31g)	31	1	0	1	3	0.2	2	1	11
Child Formula, Mead Johnson, Portagen, with Iron, Powder, Not Reconstituted 1 scoop (9.4g)	45	2	2	0	5	0.0	5	2	24
Child Formula, Mead Johnson, Portagen, with Iron, Prepared from Powder 1 fl oz (31g)	27	1	1	0	3	0.0	2	1	16
Infant Formula, Mead Johnson, Prosobee, with Iron, Ready-to-feed 1 fl oz (30.5g)	19	1	0	0	2	0.0	2	1	7
Infant Formula, Abbott Nutrition, Similac, Advance with Iron, Liquid, Concentrate 1 fl oz (31.4g)	40	2	1	1	4	0.0	4	1	10
Infant Formula, Abbott Nutrition, Similac, Advance with Iron, Powder 1 scoop (8.5g)	44	2	1	1	5	0.0	5	1	11
Infant Formula, Abbott Nutrition, Similac, Advance with Iron, Ready-to-feed 1 fl oz (30.4g)	20	1	0	1	2	0.0	2	0	5
Infant Formula, Abbott Nutrition, Similac, Ailment Advance, Ready-to-feed, with ARA and DHA 1 fl oz (30.5g)	20	1	1	0	2	0.0	1	1	9
Infant Formula, Abbott Nutrition, Similac, Alimentum, with Iron, Ready-to-feed 1 fl oz (30.5g)	20	1	1	0	2	0.0	1	1	9
Infant Formula, Abbott Nutrition, Similac, Isomil, Advance, with Iron, Liquid Concentrate 1 fl oz (31.4g)	40	2	1	0	4	0.0	4	1	18
Infant Formula, Abbott Nutrition, Similac, Isomil, Advance, with Iron, Powder 1 scoop (8.7g)	45	2	1	0	5	0.0	5	1	20

Food Serving size	Cal.	(g) Total Fat	(g) Sat. Fat	(mg) Chol.	(g) Carb.	(g) Fiber	(g) Sug.	(g) Prot.	(mg) Sod.
Infant Formula, Abbott Nutrition, Similac, Isomil, Advance, with Iron, Ready-to-feed									
1 fl oz (30.5g)	20	1	0	0	2	0.0	2	0	9
Infant Formula, Abbott Nutrition, Similac, Isomil, with Iron, Liquid Concentrate, Not Reconstituted									
1 fl oz (31.4g)	40	2	1	0	4	0.0	4	1	18
Infant Formula, Abbott Nutrition, Similac, Isomil, with Iron, Powder, Not Reconstituted									
1 scoop (8.7g)	45	2	1	0	5	0.0	5	1	20
Infant Formula, Abbott Nutrition, Similac, Isomil, with Iron, Ready-to-feed									
1 fl oz (30.5g)	20	1	0	0	2	0.0	2	0	9
Infant Formula, Abbott Nutrition, Similac, Low Iron, Liquid Concentrate									
1 fl oz (31.4g)	40	2	1	1	4	0.0	4	1	10
Infant Formula, Abbott Nutrition, Similac, Low Iron, Powder									
1 scoop (8.7g)	45	3	1	1	5	0.0	5	1	11
Infant Formula, Abbott Nutrition, Similac, Low Iron, Ready-to-feed									
1 fl oz (31g)	20	1	0	1	2	0.0	2	0	5
Infant Formula, Abbott Nutrition, Similac, Natural Care, Advance, Ready-to-feed, with ARA and DHA									
1 fl oz (30.5g)	24	1	1	1	3	0.0	3	1	10
Infant Formula, Abbott Nutrition, Similac, Neosure Advance, Powder, with ARA and DHA									
1 fl oz (30.5g)	159	9	3	4	16	0.0	16	4	52
Infant Formula, Abbott Nutrition, Similac, Neosure, Ready-to-feed, with ARA and DHA									
1 fl oz (30.5g)	21	1	1	1	2	0.0	2	1	7
Infant Formula, Abbott Nutrition, Similac, PM 60/40, Powder, Not Reconstituted									
1 scoop (8.7g)	46	2	1	1	5	0.0	5	1	11
Infant Formula, Abbott Nutrition, Similac, Sensitive (Lactose Free), Liquid Concentrate, with ARA and DHA									
1 fl oz (30.5g)	39	2	1	1	4	0.0	4	1	12
Infant Formula, Abbott Nutrition, Similac, Sensitive (Lactose Free), Powder, with ARA and DHA									
1 fl oz (30.5g)	159	9	6	5	17	0.0	17	3	48
Infant Formula, Abbott Nutrition, Similac, Sensitive (Lactose Free), Ready-to-feed, with ARA and DHA									
1 fl oz (30.5g)	21	1	1	1	2	0.0	2	0	6

Food Serving size	Cal.	(g) Total Fat	(g) Sat. Fat	(mg) Chol.	(g) Carb.	(g) Fiber	(g) Sug.	(g) Prot.	(mg) Sod.
Infant Formula, Abbott Nutrition, Similac, Special Care, Advance 24, with Iron, Ready-to-feed, with ARA and DHA									
1 fl oz (30.8g)	22	1	1	1	3	0.0	3	1	10
Infant Formula, Abbott Nutrition, Similac, with Iron, Liquid Concentrate									
1 fl oz (31.4g)	40	2	1	1	4	0.0	4	1	10
Infant Formula, Abbott Nutrition, Similac, with Iron, Powder									
1 scoop (8.5g)	44	2	1	1	5	0.0	5	1	11
Infant Formula, Abbott Nutrition, Similac, with Iron, Ready-to-feed									
1 fl oz (30.4g)	20	1	0	1	2	0.0	2	0	5
Infant Formula, Abbott, Alimentum Advance, Iron, Powder, Not Reconstituted, with DHA and ARA									
1 scoop (8.7g)	45	2	1	1	5	0.0	3	1	19
Infant Formula, Mead Johnson, Enfamil, AR Lipil, Powder, with ARA and DHA									
1 serving, 100 ml (106g)	540	28	12	18	59	0.0	59	13	216
Infant Formula, Mead Johnson, Enfamil, AR Lipil, Ready-to-feed, with ARA and DHA									
1 fl oz (30.5g)	21	1	0	0	2	0.0	2	1	8
Infant Formula, Mead Johnson, Enfamil, Enfacare Lipil, Ready-to-feed, with ARA and DHA									
1 fl oz (30.8g)	22	1	0	0	2	0.0	2	1	8
Infant Formula, Mead Johnson, Enfamil, Enfacare, Lipil, Powder, with ARA and DHA									
1 Serving, 100 ml (104g)	528	27	11	--	57	0.0	53	15	180
Infant Formula, Mead Johnson, Enfamil, Lactofree Lipil, with Iron, Liquid Concentrate, Not Reconstituted, with ARA and DHA									
1 fl oz (31.3g)	41	2	1	1	5	0.0	4	1	12
Infant Formula, Mead Johnson, Enfamil, Lactofree Lipil, with Iron, Powder, with ARA and DHA									
1 scoop (8.5g)	44	2	1	1	5	0.0	5	1	13
Infant Formula, Mead Johnson, Enfamil, Lactofree, Ready-to-feed									
1 fl oz (30.5g)	19	1	0	0	2	0.0	2	0	6
Infant Formula, Mead Johnson, Enfamil, Lactofree, with Iron, Liquid Concentrate, Not Reconstituted									
1 fl oz (30.4g)	40	2	1	1	4	0.0	4	1	12
Infant Formula, Mead Johnson, Enfamil, Lactofree, with Iron, Not Reconstituted									
1 scoop (8.5g)	44	2	1	1	5	0.0	5	1	13

Food Serving size	Cal.	(g) Total Fat	(g) Sat. Fat	(mg) Chol.	(g) Carb.	(g) Fiber	(g) Sug.	(g) Prot.	(mg) Sod.
Infant Formula, Mead Johnson, Enfamil, Lipil, Low Iron, Liquid Concentrate, with ARA and DHA									
1 fl oz (31.3g)	41	2	1	1	4	0.0	4	1	12
Infant Formula, Mead Johnson, Enfamil, Lipil, Low Iron, Powder, with ARA and DHA									
1 scoop (8.5g)	43	2	1	1	5	0.0	5	1	12
Infant Formula, Mead Johnson, Enfamil, Lipil, Low Iron, Ready to feed, with ARA and DHA									
1 fl oz (30.5g)	20	1	0	0	2	0.0	2	0	5
Infant Formula, Mead Johnson, Enfamil, Lipil, Ready-to-feed, with ARA and DHA									
1 fl oz (30.5g)	20	1	0	0	2	0.0	2	0	6
Infant Formula, Mead Johnson, Enfamil, Lipil, with Iron, Liquid Concentrate, with ARA and DHA									
1 fl oz (31.3g)	41	2	1	0	4	0.0	4	1	11
Infant Formula, Mead Johnson, Enfamil, Lipil, with Iron, Powder, with ARA and DHA									
1 scoop (8.5g)	43	2	1	1	5	0.0	5	1	12
Infant Formula, Mead Johnson, Enfamil, Lipil, with Iron, Ready-to-feed, with ARA and DHA									
1 fl oz (30.5g)	20	1	0	0	2	0.0	2	0	5
Infant Formula, Mead Johnson, Enfamil, Low Iron, Liquid Concentrate, Not Reconstituted									
1 fl oz (31.4g)	41	2	1	0	4	0.0	4	1	11
Infant Formula, Mead Johnson, Enfamil, Low Iron, Powder, Not Reconstituted									
1 scoop (8.3g)	42	2	1	1	5	0.0	5	1	12
Infant Formula, Mead Johnson, Enfamil, Low Iron, Ready-to-feed									
1 fl oz (30.5g)	19	1	0	0	2	0.0	2	0	5
Infant Formula, Mead Johnson, Enfamil, Nutramigen Lipil, with Iron, Powder, Not Reconstituted, with ARA and DHA									
1 scoop (9g)	44	2	1	0	5	0.0	5	1	21
Infant Formula, Mead Johnson, Enfamil, Nutramigen Lipil, with Iron, Ready-to-feed, with ARA and DHA									
1 fl oz (30.5g)	20	1	0	0	2	0.0	2	1	9
Infant Formula, Mead Johnson, Enfamil, Nutramigen, with Iron, Liquid Concentrate, Not Reconstituted									
1 fl oz (31.5g)	40	2	1	0	4	0.0	4	1	19

Food Serving size	Cal.	(g) Total Fat	(g) Sat. Fat	(mg) Chol.	(g) Carb.	(g) Fiber	(g) Sug.	(g) Prot.	(mg) Sod.
Infant Formula, Mead Johnson, Enfamil, Nutramigen, with Iron, Powder, Not Reconstituted 1 scoop (9.6g)	48	2	1	0	5	0.0	5	1	22
Infant Formula, Mead Johnson, Enfamil, Nutramigen, with Iron, Ready-to-feed 1 fl oz (30.8g)	20	1	0	0	2	0.0	2	1	10
Infant Formula, Mead Johnson, Enfamil, Prosobee, Iron, Powder, Not Reconstituted 1 scoop (8.8g)	45	2	1	0	5	0.0	5	1	16
Infant Formula, Mead Johnson, Enfamil, Prosobee, Lipil, Liquid Concentrate, Not Reconstituted, with ARA and DHA 1 fl oz (31.3g)	41	2	1	0	4	0.0	4	1	14
Infant Formula, Mead Johnson, Enfamil, Prosobee, Lipil, with Iron, Powder, Not Reconstituted, with ARA and DHA 1 scoop (8.8g)	45	2	1	0	5	0.0	5	1	15
Infant Formula, Mead Johnson, Enfamil, with Iron, Liquid Concentrate, Not Reconstituted 1 fl oz (31.4g)	40	2	1	0	4	0.0	4	1	11
Infant Formula, Mead Johnson, Enfamil, with Iron, Powder 1 scoop (8.3g)	43	2	1	1	5	0.0	5	1	12
Infant Formula, Mead Johnson, Enfamil, with Iron, Ready-to-feed 1 fl oz (30.5g)	19	1	0	0	2	0.0	2	0	5
Infant Formula, Mead Johnson, Next Step Prosobee, Powder 1 scoop (9.3g)	45	2	1	0	5	0.0	5	1	16
Infant Formula, Mead Johnson, Next Step Prosobee, Prepared from Powder 1 fl oz (30.5g)	20	1	0	0	2	0.0	2	1	7
Infant Formula, Mead Johnson, Next Step, Prosobee, Lipil, Powder, with ARA and DHA 3 scoop (28g)	134	6	2	0	16	0.0	16	4	48
Infant Formula, Mead Johnson, Next Step, Prosobee, Lipil, Ready-to-feed, with ARA and DHA 1 fl oz (30.5g)	20	1	0	0	2	0.0	2	1	7
Infant Formula, Mead Johnson, Nutramigen, Lipil, with Iron, Liquid Concentrate, Not Reconstituted, with ARA and DHA 1 fl oz (31.6g)	40	2	1	0	4	0.0	3	1	19
Infant Formula, Mead Johnson, Pregestimil, with Iron, Powder, Not Reconstituted 1 scoop (8.8g)	46	2	1	0	5	0.0	4	1	21

Food Serving size	Cal.	(g) Total Fat	(g) Sat. Fat	(mg) Chol.	(g) Carb.	(g) Fiber	(g) Sug.	(g) Prot.	(mg) Sod.
Infant Formula, Mead Johnson, Pregestimil, with Iron, Prepared from Powder									
1 fl oz (30.8g)	21	1	1	0	2	0.0	2	1	10
Infant Formula, Mead Johnson, Prosobee, Lipil, with Iron, Ready-to-feed, with ARA and DHA									
1 fl oz (30.5g)	20	1	0	0	2	0.0	2	1	7
Infant Formula, Mead Johnson, Prosobee, with Iron, Liquid, Concentrate, Not Reconstituted									
1 fl oz (30.8g)	40	2	1	0	4	0.0	4	1	14
Infant Formula, Nestle, Good Start 2 Essentials, with Iron, Liquid Concentrate									
1 fl oz (31.9g)	40	2	1	1	5	0.0	4	1	16
Infant Formula, Nestle, Good Start 2 Essentials, with Iron, Powder									
1 scoop (9.4g)	44	2	1	1	6	0.0	4	1	17
Infant Formula, Nestle, Good Start 2 Essentials, with Iron, Ready-to-feed									
1 fl oz (30.5g)	20	1	0	0	3	0.0	2	1	8
Infant Formula, Nestle, Good Start Essentials Soy, with Iron, Powder									
1 scoop (4.3g)	22	1	0	0	2	0.0	2	1	8
Infant Formula, Nestle, Good Start Essentials Soy, with Iron, Ready-to-feed									
1 fl oz (30.5g)	20	1	0	0	2	0.0	2	0	7
Infant Formula, Nestle, Good Start Essentials, Soy, with Iron, Liquid Concentrate									
1 fl oz (31.4g)	40	2	1	0	4	0.0	4	1	14
Infant Formula, Nestle, Good Start Supreme, Iron, DHA and ARA, Prepared from Liquid Concentrate									
1 fl oz (31.4g)	21	1	0	1	2	0.0	2	0	6
Infant Formula, Nestle, Good Start Supreme, with Iron, Liquid, Concentrate, Not Reconstituted									
1 fl oz (31.4g)	40	2	1	1	4	0.0	3	1	11
Infant Formula, Nestle, Good Start Supreme, with Iron, Powder									
1 scoop (8.7g)	44	2	1	3	5	0.0	3	1	12
Infant Formula, Nestle, Good Start Supreme, with Iron, Ready-to-feed									
1 fl oz (30.5g)	20	1	0	1	2	0.0	2	0	5
Infant Formula, Nestle, Good Start Supreme, with Iron, with DHA and ARA, Ready-to-feed									
1 fl oz (30.5g)	20	1	0	1	2	0.0	2	0	5
Infant Formula, PBM Products, Store Brand, Liquid Concentrate, Not Reconstituted									
1 fl oz (31.4g)	41	2	1	3	4	0.0	4	1	9

Food Serving size	Cal.	(g) Total Fat	(g) Sat. Fat	(mg) Chol.	(g) Carb.	(g) Fiber	(g) Sug.	(g) Prot.	(mg) Sod.
Infant Formula, PBM Products, Store Brand, Powder									
1 scoop (8.4g)	44	2	1	3	5	0.0	5	1	10
Infant Formula, PBM Products, Store Brand, Ready-to-feed									
1 fl oz (30.4g)	19	1	0	1	2	0.0	2	0	4
Infant Formula, PBM Products, Store Brand, Soy, Liquid Concentrate									
1 fl oz (31.4g)	40	2	1	0	4	0.0	4	1	11
Infant Formula, PBM Products, Store Brand, Soy, Powder									
1 scoop (8.7g)	44	2	1	0	5	0.0	5	1	13
Infant Formula, PBM Products, Store Brand, Soy, Ready-to-feed									
1 fl oz (30.4g)	19	1	0	0	2	0.0	2	1	5
Infant Formula, PBM Products, Ultra Bright Beginnings, Liquid Concentrate, Not Reconstituted									
1 fl oz (31.4g)	41	2	1	3	4	0.0	4	1	9
Infant Formula, PBM Products, Ultra Bright Beginnings, Powder									
1 scoop (8.4g)	44	2	1	3	5	0.0	5	1	10
Infant Formula, PBM Products, Ultra Bright Beginnings, Ready-to-feed									
1 fl oz (30.4g)	19	1	0	1	2	0.0	2	0	4
Infant Formula, PBM Products, Ultra Bright Beginnings, Soy, Liquid Concentrate									
1 fl oz (31.4g)	40	2	1	0	4	0.0	4	1	11
Infant Formula, PBM Products, Ultra Bright Beginnings, Soy, Ready-to-feed									
1 fl oz (30.4g)	19	1	0	0	2	0.0	2	1	5
Infant Formula, PBM, Ultra Bright Beginnings, Soy, Powder									
1 scoop (8.7g)	44	2	1	0	5	0.0	5	1	13
Zwieback									
1 piece (7g)	30	1	0	1	5	0.2	1	1	16

Restaurant Chains

Healthy Eating Out

Eating out can be a dietary danger zone, but the nutrition information in this book will help you plan ahead and make sensible choices. The goal is to enjoy your meal with control. The problem with eating out is that you lose control of portion sizes and preparation. Here are some tips for healthy eating in restaurants.

Plan Ahead

Set some reasonable guidelines for your meal.

- Set a calorie guideline and compare the nutrient information for different restaurants in this book.
- Decide on portion sizes of meat, bread, etc. Be sure to have a visual reference, such as the palm of your hand for a 3 to 4 oz. portion of meat, a die for 1 oz. of cheese, and what 4 oz. of wine looks like in a wine glass.
- Decide on which items you are going to include in your meal: only half the bun, wine but no dessert; only 10 French fries or chips, skip the bread or have bread without butter.

Know your restaurant and be familiar with the menu.

- Check out the restaurants included in this book. If your favorite restaurant is not included, there may be a similar one. A hamburger and French fries don't vary much from one restaurant to another.
- Highlight the healthiest options for each restaurant.
- Decide on dishes at home before you are tempted by the sight of the food or what others are ordering.

Never arrive at a restaurant hungry. Hungry people make bad ordering decisions. Don't skip meals thinking that this will give you more calories to eat. Eat an apple and drink a glass of water before you go out. This will help you control your hunger.

Ask Questions

If you feel awkward doing this at the table, call the restaurant ahead of time and ask to speak to the chef or a waiter.

How are items prepared? Can they alter the preparation?

- Baked rather than fried?
- Saute in broth rather than oil?
- Sauces on the side rather than on top?
- Plain bread rather than buttered?

Control Portion Sizes

- Order a main dish from the appetizer menu.
- Plan to take half the entrée home for a future meal. Ask your waiter to put half in a to-go box and just to serve you the other half.
- Stay away from buffets, especially an "all you can eat" buffet.

Savor your food. Try to never finish everything on your plate. Always leave a bite or two to prove to yourself that you are in control of your food rather than the food controlling how much you eat. You don't have to clean your plate!

Course-by-Course Suggestions

Beverages

- Drink plenty of water.
- Alcoholic beverages can stimulate your appetite. Plus, the calories (about 200 calories per ounce) in alcohol can add up fast. Best choice is a glass of wine sipped slowly.
- Stick to water, reduced-fat milk, tea, coffee, or diet soda.

Starters

- Soup can fill you up. A clear, broth-based soup with vegetables is good as an appetizer because a soup in general tends to decrease your appetite. Soup takes a long time to eat, is filling and low in calories, and is good for you.
- Salads are a great way to start a meal because they can take the edge off your appetite. Order a tossed green or spinach salad with the dressing served on the side. You decide how much salad dressing you will eat. Dipping your fork into the dressing and then spearing some veggies can cut down on the amount of dressing you eat. Avoid bacon bits, cheese, croutons, meats, and prepared salads like potato salad.

  - 1 tablespoon of grated cheese adds 28 calories and 2 grams of fat.
  - 1 tablespoon of bacon bits adds 30 calories and 1 gram of fat.
  - 1 tablespoon of salad dressing adds 60 to 90 calories and 6 to 9 grams of fat.

Entrees

- Choose a baked, broiled, grilled, poached, roasted, or steamed entrée. Ask that dishes be prepared without extra salt, butter, or oil. Meats and vegetables sautéed or stir-fried in a small amount of oil, broth, or water are usually lower in fat.
- Avoid entrees that are high in fat (check out the Red Flag Menu Terms below).
- Choose fish often. Some fish are higher in fat than others, but the type of fat is good for you. Ask that the fish be steamed, grilled, broiled, or poached.
- Choose white meat chicken over dark meat. Ask for the skin to be removed or remove it yourself. Order poultry steamed, poached, roasted, broiled, boiled, grilled, or baked.
- Allow yourself a red meat a few times a week. Be sure to choose lean cuts of meat like loin, flank, or tenderloin.
- Request sauces on the side so that you can determine if they contain fat and then decide how much you will eat. "Dry" is a good term to use when ordering.

Side Dishes

- Choose vegetables and ask for them to be steamed.
- Baked potatoes, boiled new potatoes, and rice also may be good options if they are prepared without added fats.
- Top your baked potato with salsa instead of butter or sour cream.
- Skip the French fries, potato chips, and onion rings, as well as vegetables slathered in cheese or cream sauces.

Dessert

- Leave a little time for your food to digest before ordering dessert. It takes about 20 minutes for your stomach to feel full and send this message to your brain.
- If you still want dessert, consider splitting the dessert with a friend. Half the dessert is half the calories.
- Healthy dessert choices include berries, melon, sorbet, or frozen yogurt.

Green Flag Menu Terms

Baked, broiled, boiled, poached, grilled, roasted, steamed, lean, dry, fat-free, low-fat, fresh, light, marinated, reduced, vinaigrette, high fiber, whole grain, multi-grain, vegetarian.

Red Flag Menu Terms

Fried, creamed or creamy, buttered or buttery, oil, breaded, Alfredo, battered or batter-dipped, gravy, smothered, fried, fricasseed, creamed, sautéed, stir-fried, stuffed, breaded, basted, au gratin, Alfredo, parmigiana, béarnaise or hollandaise, crispy, crunchy, giant, loaded, super-sized.

Food Serving size	Cal.	(g) Total Fat	(g) Sat. Fat	(mg) Chol.	(g) Carb.	(g) Fiber	(g) Sug.	(g) Prot.	(mg) Sod.

APPLEBEE'S

Chicken - Includes Sides

Chicken Fried Chicken									
	1230	59	12	NA	112	11	NA	61	3400
Chicken Parmesan									
	1410	63	20	NA	125	13	NA	85	3580
Chicken Tenders Basket									
	1020	60	11	NA	84	7	NA	36	2190
Chicken Tenders Platter									
	1320	78	14	NA	107	10	NA	49	2780
Crispy Orange Chicken									
	1520	53	10	NA	208	11	NA	64	2500
Fiesta Lime Chicken									
	1160	67	16	NA	94	7	NA	60	3190
Grilled Dijon Chicken and Portobellos									
	470	16	7	NA	30	5	NA	55	1820
Margherita Chicken									
	710	25	7	NA	67	7	NA	55	2300
Riblet and Chicken Tenders Basket									
	1250-1340	73	18	NA	92-115	6 to 7	NA	58	3040-3230
Riblet and Chicken Tenders Platter									
	1730-1870	101	26 to 27	NA	119-153	9 to 10	NA	88 to 89	4180-4800
Smothered Grilled Chicken									
	860	41	14	NA	61	10	NA	63	2950
Weight Watchers Chipotle Lime Chicken									
	490	12	2	NA	51	7	NA	49	4990

Desserts - As Served

Blue Ribbon Brownie									
	1310	63	32	NA	176	6	NA	16	740
Brownie Bite									
	360	17	9	NA	49	2	NA	4	200
Chocolate Chip Cookie Sundae									
	1540	74	46	NA	210	7	NA	18	910
Chocolate Mousse Shooter									
	450	31	19	NA	42	2	NA	3	260

Food Serving size	Cal.	(g) Total Fat	(g) Sat. Fat	(mg) Chol.	(g) Carb.	(g) Fiber	(g) Sug.	(g) Prot.	(mg) Sod.
Hot Fudge Sundae Shooter									
	350	18	13	NA	43	<1	NA	4	125
Maple Butter Blondie									
	1100	63	33	NA	115	2	NA	13	790
Sizzling Apple Pie									
	900	33	16	NA	145	4	NA	9	980
Strawberry Cheesecake Shooter									
	380	23	14	NA	37	1	NA	6	240
Triple Chocolate Meltdown									
	820	48	30	NA	97	4	NA	9	430

Drinks - As Served

Food Serving size	Cal.	(g) Total Fat	(g) Sat. Fat	(mg) Chol.	(g) Carb.	(g) Fiber	(g) Sug.	(g) Prot.	(mg) Sod.
Applebee's Limeades (20 oz)									
	230	0	0	NA	59	0	NA	0	15
Caffeine Free Diet Pepsi (20 oz)									
	0	0	0	NA	0	0	NA	0	25
Coffee (8 oz)									
	0	0	0	NA	0	0	NA	0	0
Decadent Shakes (20 oz)									
	890-940	44-50	25-27	NA	92-127	0-2	NA	15-16	330-490
Diet Mountain Dew (20 oz)									
	0	0	0	NA	0	0	NA	0	40
Diet Pepsi (20 oz)									
	0	0	0	NA	0	0	NA	0	25
Dr Pepper (20 oz)									
	100	0	0	NA	27	0	NA	0	35
Flavored Lemonades and Iced Teas (20 oz)									
	30-150	0	0	NA	7 to 40	0	NA	0	35-110
Frozen Lemonade (20 oz)									
	250-260	0	0	NA	63-65	0-<1	NA	0	0-5
Iced Tea (20 oz)									
	0	0	0	NA	<1	0	NA	0	30
Lipton Brisk Raspberry Iced Tea (20 oz)									
	80	0	0	NA	21	0	NA	0	25
Mountain Dew (20 oz)									
	110	0	0	NA	29	0	NA	0	35

Food Serving size	Cal.	(g) Total Fat	(g) Sat. Fat	(mg) Chol.	(g) Carb.	(g) Fiber	(g) Sug.	(g) Prot.	(mg) Sod.
Mug Root Beer (20 oz)									
	100	0	0	NA	26	0	NA	0	15
Pepsi (20 oz)									
	100	0	0	NA	28	0	NA	0	25
Sierra Mist (20 oz)									
	100	0	0	NA	27	0	NA	0	20
Tropicana Lemonade (20 oz)									
	100	0	0	NA	27	0	NA	0	105
Wild Cherry Pepsi (20 oz)									
	100	0	0	NA	28	0	NA	0	20

Extras - As Served

Food Serving size	Cal.	(g) Total Fat	(g) Sat. Fat	(mg) Chol.	(g) Carb.	(g) Fiber	(g) Sug.	(g) Prot.	(mg) Sod.
Applebee's House Salad (Without Dressing)									
	230	15	7	NA	12	2	NA	13	380
Baked Potato Soup (Bowl)									
	420	32	14	NA	27	2	NA	18	1240
Broccoli Cheddar Soup (Bowl)									
	340	26	16	NA	19	2	NA	13	1660
Cheesy Corn									
	350	20	10	NA	28	3	NA	15	620
Chicken Noodle Soup (Bowl)									
	160	4	1	NA	17	1	NA	13	1100
Chicken Tortilla Soup (Bowl)									
	180	8	2.5	NA	18	2	NA	9	1540
Chili (Bowl)									
	370	28	14	NA	16	5	NA	28	1020
Chili Cheese Fries, Side									
	550	33	11	NA	59	6	NA	17	1500
Clam Chowder (Bowl)									
	350	24	14	NA	22	1	NA	13	980
Crunchy Onion Rings, Side									
	530	28	5	NA	63	4	NA	7	1320
Dressing, Bleu Cheese									
	240	26	5	NA	<1<	0	NA	2	260
Dressing, Buttermilk Ranch									
	200	21	3.5	NA	1	0	NA	<1	310

Food Serving size	Cal.	(g) Total Fat	(g) Sat. Fat	(mg) Chol.	(g) Carb.	(g) Fiber	(g) Sug.	(g) Prot.	(mg) Sod.
Dressing, Dijon Honey Mustard									
	220	18	2.5	NA	13	0	NA	<1	470
Dressing, Mexi-Ranch									
	140	14	2.5	NA	2	0	NA	<1	490
French Onion Soup (Bowl)									
	260	14	9	NA	16	1	NA	15	1360
Fresh Fruit, Side									
	90	0	0	NA	24	3	NA	<1	0
Fries, Side									
	390	18	3.5	NA	53	4	NA	5	720
Garlic Mashed Potatoes									
	330	18	3.5	NA	38	4	NA	6	900
Loaded Baked Potato									
	500	35	20	NA	42	3	NA	12	500
Loaded Mashed Potatoes									
	550	42	17	NA	41	4	NA	18	1340
Red Beans and Rice									
	290	6	2.5	NA	48	5	NA	10	770
Seasonal Vegetables									
	35 to 50	0	0	NA	7 to 9	2 to 3	NA	1 to 3	260-340
Seasonal Vegetables, Side									
	35-50	0	0	NA	7 to 9	2 to 3	NA	1 to 3	260-340
Small Caesar Salad (with Dressing)									
	310	27	5	NA	12	3	NA	6	510
Small Caesar Salad (with Dressing) and Fried Shrimp									
	390	21	4	NA	35	2	NA	14	1270
Small Caesar Salad (with Dressing) and Grilled Shrimp									
	230	17	3	NA	2	0	NA	16	1070
Toasted Garlic Bread Basket									
	1120	78	23	NA	89	6	NA	19	1320
Tomato Basil Soup (Bowl)									
	250	14	7	NA	28	3	NA	5	1320

Kid's Menu - Without Sides or Drinks (unless otherwise indicated)

Food Serving size	Cal.	(g) Total Fat	(g) Sat. Fat	(mg) Chol.	(g) Carb.	(g) Fiber	(g) Sug.	(g) Prot.	(mg) Sod.
Fries, Side									
	390	18	3.5	NA	53	4	NA	5	720

Food Serving size	Cal.	(g) Total Fat	(g) Sat. Fat	(mg) Chol.	(g) Carb.	(g) Fiber	(g) Sug.	(g) Prot.	(mg) Sod.
Kids 4 oz Sirloin Steak									
	140	7	2.5	NA	0	0	NA	20	410
Kids Apple Juice (6.75 oz)									
	70	0	0	NA	17	0	NA	<1	5
Kids Applesauce Side									
	50	0	0	NA	27	1	NA	0	0
Kids Celery Side with Dressing									
	220	22	3.5	NA	5	2	NA	2	420
Kids Cheese Pizza									
	550	31	13	NA	44	3	NA	21	1280
Kids Chicken Tenders									
	240	14	3	NA	11	1	NA	18	600
Kids Chocolate Milk (1% 8 oz)									
	160-270	2.5-6	1.5-3	NA	27-45	0 - <1	NA	8 to 11	170-210
Kids Corn Dog									
	260	14	4	NA	28	<1	NA	6	440
Kids Fried Shrimp									
	230	14	2.5	NA	16	<1	NA	9	540
Kids Grape Juice (6.75 oz)									
	80	0	0	NA	20	0	NA	0	5
Kids Grilled Cheese [Hawaiian Bread]									
	610	36	15	NA	51	2	NA	19	1160
Kids Grilled Cheese [Sourdough Bread]									
	630	36	13	NA	54	2	NA	23	1440
Kids Grilled Chicken Sandwich									
	230	5	1.5	NA	23	<1	NA	24	560
Kids Hot Dog									
	330	18	7	NA	31	<1	NA	11	750
Kids Hot Fudge Sundae									
	350	18	13	NA	45	<1	NA	4	125
Kids Kraft Macaroni and Cheese									
	300	9	2.5	NA	45	2	NA	11	570
Kids Milk (1% or 2% 8 oz)									
	110-150	2.5-6	1.5-3	NA	13-15	0	NA	9 to 10	130-140
Kids Mini Cheeseburger - 1									
	430	30	9	NA	24	<1	NA	17	610

Food Serving size	Cal.	(g) Total Fat	(g) Sat. Fat	(mg) Chol.	(g) Carb.	(g) Fiber	(g) Sug.	(g) Prot.	(mg) Sod.
Kids Mini Cheeseburgers - 2									
	740	46	16	NA	47	1	NA	33	1110
Kids Mini Hamburger - 1									
	390	27	7	NA	23	<1	NA	15	490
Kids Mini Hamburgers - 2									
	660	40	12	NA	46	1	NA	29	870
Kids Orange-Tangerine Juice (6.75 oz)									
	70	0	0	NA	17	0	NA	1	0
Kids Oreo Cookie Milkshake									
	780	41	26	NA	97	1	NA	12	420
Kids Oreo Cookie Sundae									
	360	19	12	NA	43	<1	NA	4	170
Kids Pasta with Marina Sauce									
	360	7	2	NA	60	5	NA	14	1030
Kids Soda (12 oz)									
	0-70	0	0	NA	0-19	0	NA	0	10 to 65
Kids Steamed Broccoli Side									
	30	0	0	NA	4	3	NA	3	25
Kids Strawberry Sundae									
	260	14	9	NA	31	<1	NA	3	65
Kids Tropicana Fruit Punch (12 oz)									
	70	0	0	NA	19	0	NA	0	15
Kids Vanilla Sundae									
	230	14	9	NA	24	0	NA	3	65
Kids Vanilla Sundae with Hershey's Syrup									
	330	14	9	NA	49	0	NA	4	90

Menu Item

Food	Cal.	(g) Total Fat	(g) Sat. Fat	(mg) Chol.	(g) Carb.	(g) Fiber	(g) Sug.	(g) Prot.	(mg) Sod.
Appetizer Sampler									
	2320-2430	154-166	44-48	NA	156-182	14-15	NA	91-92	5490-6070
Boneless Wings, Classic Buffalo									
	1160	69	16	NA	66	8	NA	70	3730
Boneless Wings, Honey BBQ									
	1250	55	11	NA	116	8	NA	71	3060
Boneless Wings, Hot Buffalo									
	1170	69	16	NA	67	8	NA	71	3840

Food Serving size	Cal.	(g) Total Fat	(g) Sat. Fat	(mg) Chol.	(g) Carb.	(g) Fiber	(g) Sug.	(g) Prot.	(mg) Sod.
Boneless Wings, Southern BBQ									
	1110	55	11	NA	83	8	NA	70	2780
Boneless Wings, Sweet and Spicy Sauce									
	1150	55	11	NA	90	8	NA	71	3400
Cheese Quesadilla Grande									
	1120	87	36	NA	85	5	NA	44	3090
Cheeseburger Sliders									
	1270	81	25	NA	82	3	NA	51	2270
Cheeseburger Sliders with Applewood Smoked Bacon									
	1330	87	27	NA	82	3	NA	56	2510
Chicken Quesadilla Grande									
	1270	92	37	NA	89	5	NA	65	3790
Chili Cheese Nachos									
	1680	107	40	NA	134	17	NA	48	4270
Chips and Spicy Chipotle Lime Salsa									
	960	53	10	NA	106	11	NA	14	810
Classic Wings, Classic Buffalo									
	710	49	14	NA	8	2	NA	61	2000
Classic Wings, Honey BBQ									
	790	35	9	NA	59	3	NA	61	1340
Classic Wings, Hot Buffalo									
	720	49	14	NA	9	3	NA	61	2120
Classic Wings, Southern BBQ									
	660	35	9	NA	25	2	NA	61	1060
Classic Wings, Sweet and Spicy Sauce									
	690	35	9	NA	32	2	NA	62	1670
Crunchy Onion Rings									
	1290	56	10	NA	181	9	NA	16	3620
Grilled Chicken Wonton Tacos									
	590	24	4.5	NA	58	4	NA	36	2150
Mozzarella Sticks									
	940	48	21	NA	84	3	NA	43	2640
Pork Wonton Tacos									
	820	41	12	NA	68	4	NA	43	2240
Potato Skins									
	1090	103	50	NA	66	7	NA	64	1910

Food Serving size	Cal.	(g) Total Fat	(g) Sat. Fat	(mg) Chol.	(g) Carb.	(g) Fiber	(g) Sug.	(g) Prot.	(mg) Sod.
Potato Twisters									
	970	60	20	NA	81	8	NA	26	3520
Queso Blanco									
	1330	82	27	NA	114	12	NA	34	2400
Queso Blanco with Chili									
	1440	89	30	NA	118	14	NA	42	2680
Spicy Chili Cheese Nachos									
	1610	103	36	NA	125	16	NA	48	3240
Spinach and Artichoke Dip									
	1470-1580	96-107	23-30	NA	122-126	17	NA	34-36	2440-2560
Steak Quesadilla Towers									
	1110	73	32	NA	79	5	NA	59	3760
Trios Boneless Wings, Classic Buffalo									
	580	35	8	NA	33	4	NA	35	1880
Trios Boneless Wings, Honey BBQ									
	620	28	5	NA	58	4	NA	35	1530
Trios Boneless Wings, Hot Buffalo									
	590	35	8	NA	33	4	NA	35	1920
Trios Boneless Wings, Southern BBQ									
	550	28	5	NA	42	4	NA	35	1390
Trios Boneless Wings, Sweet and Spicy Sauce									
	570	28	5	NA	45	4	NA	36	1700
Trios Cheese Quesadilla Grande									
	510	44	16	NA	31	2	NA	20	1530
Trios Cheeseburger Sliders									
	880	59	18	NA	54	2	NA	34	1550
Trios Chicken Quesadilla Grande									
	580	46	16	NA	33	2	NA	30	1880
Trios Classic Wings, Classic Buffalo									
	360	24	7	NA	4	1	NA	30	1010
Trios Classic Wings, Honey BBQ									
	400	17	4.5	NA	29	1	NA	31	670
Trios Classic Wings, Hot Buffalo									
	360	25	7	NA	4	1	NA	30	1060
Trios Classic Wings, Southern BBQ									
	330	17	4.5	NA	13	1	NA	30	530

Food Serving size	Cal.	(g) Total Fat	(g) Sat. Fat	(mg) Chol.	(g) Carb.	(g) Fiber	(g) Sug.	(g) Prot.	(mg) Sod.
Trios Classic Wings, Sweet and Spicy Sauce									
	350	18	4.5	NA	16	<1	NA	31	840
Trios Grilled Chicken Wonton Tacos									
	430	18	3.5	NA	43	3	NA	25	1520
Trios Mozzarella Sticks									
	430	21	9	NA	39	2	NA	20	1270
Trios Pork Wonton Tacos									
	560	28	8	NA	48	3	NA	27	1460
Trios Spicy Queso Blanco									
	520	33	12	NA	40	4	NA	16	1090
Trios Spinach Artichoke Dip									
	560	39	10	NA	41	6	NA	14	890
Trios Steak Quesadilla Towers									
	560	38	14	NA	37	2	NA	28	1870
Trios Wings Bleu Cheese Dipping Sauce									
	240	26	5	NA	<1	0	NA	2	260
Trios Wings Ranch Dipping Sauce									
	200	21	3.5	NA	1	0	NA	<1	310
Veggie Patch Pizza									
	930	67	22	NA	50	5	NA	32	2210
Wings Bleu Cheese Dipping Sauce									
	240	26	5	NA	<1	0	NA	2	260
Wings Ranch Dipping Sauce									
	200	21	3.5	NA	1	0	NA	<1	310

Menu Items - Steak and Toppers - Without Sides (unless indicated)

Food Serving size	Cal.	(g) Total Fat	(g) Sat. Fat	(mg) Chol.	(g) Carb.	(g) Fiber	(g) Sug.	(g) Prot.	(mg) Sod.
12 oz New York Strip									
	590	39	18	NA	0	0	NA	60	550
12 oz Ribeye									
	670	47	21	NA	3	0	NA	57	950
7 oz House Sirloin									
	250	12	5	NA	0	0	NA	35	860
9 oz House Sirloin									
	310	13	5	NA	0	0	NA	48	970

Food Serving size	Cal.	(g) Total Fat	(g) Sat. Fat	(mg) Chol.	(g) Carb.	(g) Fiber	(g) Sug.	(g) Prot.	(mg) Sod.
Asiago Peppercorn Steak with Sides									
	380	14	6	NA	25	5	NA	44	1520
Baked Potato									
	430	28	17	NA	42	3	NA	7	300
Chicken Fried Steak (with Mashed Potatoes, Gravy and Vegetable)									
	1260	61	15	NA	118	10	NA	59	3840
Fried Red Potatoes									
	150	5	1	NA	22	3	NA	4	680
Garlic Mashed Potatoes									
	330	18	3.5	NA	38	4	NA	6	900
Seasonal Vegetables									
	35-50	0	0	NA	7 to 9	2 to 3	NA	1 to 3	260-340
Shrimp 'N Parmesan Sirloin									
	660	42	16	NA	4	0	NA	66	2140
Signature Sirloin with Garlic Herb Shrimp									
	500	21	8	NA	31	6	NA	51	2440
Steak and Fried Shrimp Combo									
	650	34	9	NA	37	2	NA	50	2220
Steak and Grilled Shrimp Combo									
	530	35	9	NA	2	0	NA	51	1950
Steak and Honey BBQ Chicken Combo									
	600	15	6	NA	37	<1	NA	78	2160
Steak and Riblets Combo									
	910-1040	49-50	20	NA	23-56	0-1	NA	93-94	2860-3470
Topper - Grilled Onions									
	45	2.5	0.5	NA	5	<1	NA	<1	280
Topper - Sauteed Garlic Mushrooms									
	130	12	4	NA	4	<1	NA	2	180
Topper - Shrimp 'N Parmesan									
	230	15	9	NA	4	0	NA	18	1060

Menu Items - Unbelievably Great Tasting and Under 550 Calories

Asiago Peppercorn Steak									
	380	14	6	NA	25	5	NA	44	1520
Grilled Dijon Chicken and Portobellos									
	470	16	7	NA	30	5	NA	55	1820

Food Serving size	Cal.	(g) Total Fat	(g) Sat. Fat	(mg) Chol.	(g) Carb.	(g) Fiber	(g) Sug.	(g) Prot.	(mg) Sod.
Grilled Shrimp and Island Rice									
	370	4.5	1	NA	56	5	NA	29	1990
Signature Sirloin with Garlic Herb Shrimp									
	500	21	8	NA	31	6	NA	51	2440
Teriyaki Chicken Pasta									
	450	8	2	NA	73	10	NA	34	2900
Teriyaki Shrimp Pasta									
	440	8	2	NA	74	10	NA	30	3410

Pasta - As Served

Food Serving size	Cal.	Total Fat	Sat. Fat	Chol.	Carb.	Fiber	Sug.	Prot.	Sod.
Cajun Shrimp Pasta									
	1170	69	26	NA	95	8	NA	43	3010
Chicken Broccoli Pasta Alfredo									
	1350	72	36	NA	111	9	NA	68	2410
Florentine Ravioli with Chicken									
	1300	82	40	NA	77	7	NA	67	3520
Provolone-Stuffed Meatballs with Fettuccine									
	1520	90	43	NA	116	10	NA	61	3700
Shrimp Fettuccine Alfredo									
	1430	81	40	NA	113	9	NA	64	3230
Teriyaki Chicken Pasta									
	450	8	2	NA	73	10	NA	34	2900
Teriyaki Shrimp Pasta									
	440	8	2	NA	74	10	NA	30	3410
Three-Cheese Chicken Penne									
	1460	75	36	NA	127	8	NA	71	2930

Pick 'N Pair and Lunch Combos

Food Serving size	Cal.	Total Fat	Sat. Fat	Chol.	Carb.	Fiber	Sug.	Prot.	Sod.
Applebee's Reuben									
	630	47	15	NA	25	4	NA	27	1830
Baked Potato Soup									
	360	28	13	NA	20	2	NA	16	1050
Black Bean Soup									
	190	9	5	NA	21	6	NA	9	900
Breadstick									
	290	19	6	NA	22	1	NA	5	330

Food Serving size	Cal.	(g) Total Fat	(g) Sat. Fat	(mg) Chol.	(g) Carb.	(g) Fiber	(g) Sug.	(g) Prot.	(mg) Sod.
Broccoli Cheddar Soup	280	23	14	NA	12	2	NA	11	1400
Caesar Salad	220	19	4	NA	8	2	NA	4	370
Chicken Caesar Salad	310	20	4.5	NA	8	2	NA	25	690
Chicken Fajita Rollup	560	41	16	NA	45	3	NA	32	2090
Chicken Noodle Soup	110	3	1	NA	11	<1	NA	11	900
Chicken Tortilla Soup	140	7	2	NA	12	1	NA	8	1290
Chili	310	26	13	NA	10	4	NA	25	860
Clam Chowder	290	20	12	NA	16	1	NA	11	800
Dressing, Bleu Cheese	160	17	3.5	NA	<1	0	NA	1	170
Dressing, Buttermilk Ranch	130	14	2.5	NA	<1	0	NA	0	210
Dressing, Dijon Honey Mustard	140	12	2	NA	9	0	NA	<1	320
Dressing, Mexi-Ranch	90	9	1.5	NA	2	0	NA	<1	320
French Dip Sliders	590	36	12	NA	50	1	NA	23	1630
French Onion Soup	260	14	9	NA	15	1	NA	15	1210
Fried Chicken Salad	380	27	6	NA	20	3	NA	18	790
Grilled Shrimp 'N Spinach Salad	260	15	3	NA	20	2	NA	13	940
House Salad	130	8	3	NA	9	2	NA	7	240
Oriental Chicken Salad	420	29	4.5	NA	25	3	NA	15	500

Food Serving size	Cal.	(g) Total Fat	(g) Sat. Fat	(mg) Chol.	(g) Carb.	(g) Fiber	(g) Sug.	(g) Prot.	(mg) Sod.
Oriental Grilled Chicken Salad									
	430	21	3	NA	36	2	NA	25	1400
Santa Fe Chicken Salad									
	530	37	10	NA	28	5	NA	28	1560
Spinach Salad									
	230	15	3	NA	19	2	NA	7	500
Three-Cheese Chicken Penne									
	940	49	22	NA	77	5	NA	50	1950
Tomato Basil Soup									
	220	13	6	NA	22	2	NA	4	1180
Wonton Tacos									
	430-560	18-28	3.5-8	NA	43-48	3	NA	25-27	1460-1520

Realburgers - Without Fries (unless otherwise indicated)

Food Serving size	Cal.	(g) Total Fat	(g) Sat. Fat	(mg) Chol.	(g) Carb.	(g) Fiber	(g) Sug.	(g) Prot.	(mg) Sod.
Bacon Cheddar Cheeseburger									
	970	60	22	NA	51	3	NA	57	1630
Cheeseburger									
	940	58	22	NA	52	3	NA	54	1660
Cowboy Burger									
	1180	70	25	NA	77	5	NA	61	2670
Fire Pit Bacon Burger									
	1100	73	24	NA	53	3	NA	57	1920
Hamburger									
	790	46	15	NA	50	3	NA	46	1180
Philly Burger									
	1130	67	26	NA	70	5	NA	61	2570
Quesadilla Burger									
	1240	103	43	NA	44	4	NA	78	3530
Southwest Jalapeño Burger									
	1140	72	25	NA	68	3	NA	54	2130
Steakhouse Burger with A.1. Steak Sauce									
	1250	84	26	NA	68	5	NA	55	2230
Veggie Burger									
	550	22	4.5	NA	60	7	NA	29	1560

Food Serving size	Cal.	(g) Total Fat	(g) Sat. Fat	(mg) Chol.	(g) Carb.	(g) Fiber	(g) Sug.	(g) Prot.	(mg) Sod.
Ribs - Includes Sides									
Applebee's Riblets Basket									
	1050-1180	55	19	NA	76-109	5 to 6	NA	62-63	2720-3340
Applebee's Riblets Platter									
	1590-1820	86-87	29	NA	107-162	7 to 9	NA	98-100	4170-5630
Double-Glazed Baby Back Ribs									
	1230-1460	71-74	23-24	NA	88-130	7	NA	60-69	2490-3620
Double-Glazed Baby Back Ribs - Half Rack									
	880-990	49-50	14	NA	78-99	7	NA	33-37	1700-2270
Salads - As Served									
Apple Walnut Chicken Salad, Half									
	630	43	12	NA	33	4	NA	33	1160
Apple Walnut Chicken Salad, Half (Without Dressing)									
	350	20	9	NA	15	3	NA	33	950
Apple Walnut Chicken Salad, Regular									
	1030	67	16	NA	54	5	NA	55	1700
Apple Walnut Chicken Salad, Regular (Without Dressing)									
	470	22	9	NA	18	5	NA	55	1280
Bruschetta Chicken Salad, Half									
	740	44	14	NA	45	5	NA	41	2080
Bruschetta Chicken Salad, Half (Without Dressing)									
	580	30	12	NA	40	5	NA	41	1780
Bruschetta Chicken Salad, Regular									
	1110	66	18	NA	67	8	NA	65	3100
Bruschetta Chicken Salad, Regular (Without Dressing)									
	790	36	13	NA	56	8	NA	65	2500
California Shrimp Salad, Half									
	500	42	8	NA	16	5	NA	23	1200
California Shrimp Salad, Half (Without Dressing)									
	330	23	4.5	NA	14	4	NA	22	740
California Shrimp Salad, Regular									
	740	61	11	NA	21	7	NA	33	2100
California Shrimp Salad, Regular (Without Dressing)									
	380	24	4.5	NA	16	5	NA	32	1160
Fried Chicken Salad, Half									
	520	42	12	NA	26	3	NA	27	1100

Food Serving size	Cal.	(g) Total Fat	(g) Sat. Fat	(mg) Chol.	(g) Carb.	(g) Fiber	(g) Sug.	(g) Prot.	(mg) Sod.
Fried Chicken Salad, Half (Without Dressing)	310	23	9	NA	12	3	NA	26	630
Fried Chicken Salad, Regular	970	79	22	NA	49	6	NA	48	2150
Fried Chicken Salad, Regular (Without Dressing)	540	42	17	NA	23	5	NA	46	1200
Grilled Chicken Caesar, Half	410	29	6	NA	12	3	NA	27	830
Grilled Chicken Caesar, Half (Without Dressing)	180	5	2	NA	10	3	NA	26	450
Grilled Chicken Caesar, Regular	820	57	11	NA	25	6	NA	53	1660
Grilled Chicken Caesar, Regular (Without Dressing)	370	10	4	NA	21	5	NA	52	910
Grilled Shrimp 'N Spinach Salad, Half	620	44	9	NA	33	6	NA	32	1690
Grilled Shrimp 'N Spinach Salad, Half (Without Dressing)	460	35	7	NA	12	5	NA	31	1280
Grilled Shrimp 'N Spinach Salad, Regular	1010	69	12	NA	63	11	NA	50	2650
Grilled Shrimp 'N Spinach Salad, Regular (Without Dressing)	680	51	9	NA	20	10	NA	48	1820
Grilled Steak Caesar, Half	460	34	8	NA	13	3	NA	26	910
Grilled Steak Caesar, Half (Without Dressing)	230	10	4	NA	11	3	NA	25	540
Grilled Steak Caesar, Regular	910	68	15	NA	25	6	NA	52	1820
Grilled Steak Caesar, Regular (Without Dressing)	460	21	8	NA	21	5	NA	50	1080
Oriental Chicken Salad, Half	670	49	7	NA	42	6	NA	19	600
Oriental Chicken Salad, Half (Without Dressing)	340	20	3	NA	25	5	NA	19	480
Oriental Chicken Salad, Regular	1340	98	15	NA	85	11	NA	37	1200

Food Serving size	Cal.	(g) Total Fat	(g) Sat. Fat	(mg) Chol.	(g) Carb.	(g) Fiber	(g) Sug.	(g) Prot.	(mg) Sod.
Oriental Chicken Salad, Regular (Without Dressing)									
	680	41	6	NA	50	11	NA	37	970
Oriental Grilled Chicken Salad, Half									
	680	40	6	NA	55	5	NA	28	1640
Oriental Grilled Chicken Salad, Half (Without Dressing)									
	340	9	1.5	NA	38	5	NA	27	1520
Oriental Grilled Chicken Salad, Regular									
	1290	79	12	NA	92	10	NA	54	2290
Oriental Grilled Chicken Salad, Regular (Without Dressing)									
	590	19	3	NA	58	9	NA	53	2060
Pecan-Crusted Chicken Salad, Half									
	820	48	11	NA	72	8	NA	27	1520
Pecan-Crusted Chicken Salad, Half (Without Dressing)									
	580	31	9	NA	53	8	NA	27	1220
Pecan-Crusted Chicken Salad, Regular									
	1350	80	17	NA	114	13	NA	46	2610
Pecan-Crusted Chicken Salad, Regular (Without Dressing)									
	880	46	12	NA	76	12	NA	46	2000
Santa Fe Chicken Salad, Half									
	940	73	21	NA	52	9	NA	37	2500
Santa Fe Chicken Salad, Half (Without Dressing)									
	760	55	18	NA	49	8	NA	36	1850
Santa Fe Chicken Salad, Regular									
	1240	93	25	NA	58	10	NA	60	3480
Santa Fe Chicken Salad, Regular (Without Dressing)									
	870	56	19	NA	52	10	NA	58	2190
Weight Watchers Paradise Chicken Salad									
	340	4	1	NA	35	6	NA	45	2060
Weight Watchers Steak and Potato Salad									
	380	12	4	NA	32	6	NA	35	1860

Sandwiches - Without Sides (unless otherwise indicated)

Food	Cal.	Total Fat	Sat. Fat	Chol.	Carb.	Fiber	Sug.	Prot.	Sod.
Applebee's Reuben									
	1140	81	28	NA	49	7	NA	54	3550
Bacon Cheese Chicken Grill									
	750	33	11	NA	50	3	NA	62	1830

Food Serving size	Cal.	(g) Total Fat	(g) Sat. Fat	(mg) Chol.	(g) Carb.	(g) Fiber	(g) Sug.	(g) Prot.	(mg) Sod.
Blackened Tilapia Sandwich									
	740	42	8	NA	54	4	NA	37	1790
California Turkey Club									
	980	55	18	NA	61	4	NA	59	3310
Chicken Fajita Rollup									
	850	65	28	NA	63	3	NA	59	3170
Classic Club House Grill									
	1150	67	22	NA	77	3	NA	58	3470
Cole Slaw									
	140	9	1.5	NA	15	2	NA	1	190
Hand-Battered Fish Sandwich									
	860	58	10	NA	63	4	NA	22	1190
Honey BBQ Chicken Sandwich									
	1000	42	17	NA	87	4	NA	70	2640
Oriental Chicken Rollup									
	1160	60	11	NA	121	6	NA	32	3160
Slow Simmered Tender Beef Sandwich									
	980	50	13	NA	101	8	NA	35	2140
Stuffed Meatball Sandwich									
	1090	58	28	NA	90	7	NA	52	3540
Zesty Ranch Chicken Sandwich									
	1150	72	21	NA	76	6	NA	46	2720

Seafood - As Served

Food Serving size	Cal.	(g) Total Fat	(g) Sat. Fat	(mg) Chol.	(g) Carb.	(g) Fiber	(g) Sug.	(g) Prot.	(mg) Sod.
Double Crunch Shrimp									
	1280	69	13	NA	133	10	NA	33	3270
Garlic Herb Salmon									
	690	29	8	NA	61	5	NA	46	1460
Grilled Shrimp and Island Rice									
	370	4.5	1	NA	56	5	NA	29	1990
Hand-Battered Fish and Chips									
	1570	106	18	NA	108	10	NA	46	1980
New England Fish and Chips									
	1930	138	24	NA	121	12	NA	51	3180
Orange Glazed Salmon									
	730	17	3.5	NA	98	6	NA	46	1840

Food Serving size	Cal.	(g) Total Fat	(g) Sat. Fat	(mg) Chol.	(g) Carb.	(g) Fiber	(g) Sug.	(g) Prot.	(mg) Sod.
Weight Watchers Cajun Lime Tilapia									
	350	5	1.5	NA	43	7	NA	36	1640
Weight Watchers Spicy Pineapple Glazed Shrimp and Spinach									
	310	5	1	NA	48	5	NA	22	1690

Sizzling Entrees - Includes Sides

Food Serving size	Cal.	(g) Total Fat	(g) Sat. Fat	(mg) Chol.	(g) Carb.	(g) Fiber	(g) Sug.	(g) Prot.	(mg) Sod.
Add Guacamole									
	70	6	1	NA	3	2	NA	<1	150
Bourbon Street Chicken and Shrimp									
	750	45	10	NA	31	4	NA	57	2560
Bourbon Street Steak									
	750	43	11	NA	35	5	NA	55	2450
Sizzling Asian Shrimp									
	850	33	7	NA	118	7	NA	30	3500
Sizzling Cajun Steak and Shrimp									
	850	41	13	NA	63	8	NA	58	3660
Sizzling Chicken with Spicy Queso Blanco									
	570	22	8	NA	40	6	NA	54	2530
Sizzling Skillet Fajitas - Chicken									
	1370	52	24	NA	149	11	NA	78	4860
Sizzling Skillet Fajitas - Combo									
	1390-1470	54-67	25-27	NA	150-151	11	NA	65-78	5140-5520
Sizzling Skillet Fajitas - Shrimp									
	1400	65	26	NA	151	11	NA	53	5250
Sizzling Skillet Fajitas - Steak									
	1410	55	25	NA	152	11	NA	78	5630
Sizzling Smokehouse Chicken Stack									
	1170	59	25	NA	78	6	NA	82	3030
Sizzling Steak and Cheese									
	1050	65	22	NA	49	6	NA	68	3090

Sliders - Without Sides (unless otherwise indicated)

Food Serving size	Cal.	(g) Total Fat	(g) Sat. Fat	(mg) Chol.	(g) Carb.	(g) Fiber	(g) Sug.	(g) Prot.	(mg) Sod.
BBQ Pulled Pork Sliders									
	1030	48	15	NA	90	3	NA	56	2040
Cheeseburger Sliders									
	1270	81	25	NA	82	3	NA	51	2270

Food Serving size	Cal.	(g) Total Fat	(g) Sat. Fat	(mg) Chol.	(g) Carb.	(g) Fiber	(g) Sug.	(g) Prot.	(mg) Sod.
Cheeseburger Sliders, Add Bacon									
	1330	87	27	NA	82	3	NA	56	2510
French Dip Sliders									
	840	49	17	NA	75	2	NA	39	2440

BLIMPIE

Breads/Wraps

Food Serving size	Cal.	(g) Total Fat	(g) Sat. Fat	(mg) Chol.	(g) Carb.	(g) Fiber	(g) Sug.	(g) Prot.	(mg) Sod.
Bread, Cheddar Jalapeno, 12"									
	540	11	4	15	91	3	8	20	1180
Bread, Cheddar Jalapeno, 6"									
	210	4.5	1.5	5	36	1	3	8	470
Bread, Ciabatta, Serving									
	230	2.5	0	0	43	2	2	8	590
Bread, Honey Oat 12"									
	520	15	3	0	82	10	11	20	810
Bread, Honey Oat 6"									
	260	8	1.5	0	41	5	5	10	400
Bread, Marble Rye 12"									
	480	5	1	0	93	5	4	18	1170
Bread, Marble Rye 6"									
	240	2.5	0.5	0	46	2	2	9	590
Bread, Pretzel									
	320	4	1	0	65	2	8	8	350
Bread, Wheat, 12"									
	430	8	2	0	76	10	5	20	810
Bread, Wheat, 6"									
	210	4	1	0	38	5	3	10	400
Bread, White, 12"									
	430	6	1	0	79	3	7	15	840
Bread, White, 6"									
	210	3	0.5	0	40	1	4	7	420
Bread, Zesty Parmesan, 12"									
	470	9	3.5	10	77	3	7	19	980
Bread, Zesty Parmesan, 6"									
	240	4.5	2	5	39	2	4	9	490

Food Serving size	Cal.	(g) Total Fat	(g) Sat. Fat	(mg) Chol.	(g) Carb.	(g) Fiber	(g) Sug.	(g) Prot.	(mg) Sod.
Wrap, Spinach Herb 12"									
	310	8	3	0	52	3	3	9	840
Wrap, Traditional 12"									
	310	8	2.5	0	52	5	1	9	670

Breakfast Items

Food Serving size	Cal.	(g) Total Fat	(g) Sat. Fat	(mg) Chol.	(g) Carb.	(g) Fiber	(g) Sug.	(g) Prot.	(mg) Sod.
Bagel									
	290	1	0	0	58	3	12	11	700
Bagel, Cream Cheese									
	390	11	6	30	59	3	12	13	780
Biscuit with Sausage Gravy									
	460	27	14	25	43	2	4	12	1320
Biscuit, Bacon, Egg and Cheese									
	520	30	18	190	38	1	4	22	1940
Biscuit, Egg, and Cheese									
	380	20	15	165	37	1	4	13	1380
Biscuit, Ham, Egg and Cheese									
	420	21	15	185	39	1	5	19	1660
Biscuit, Sausage, Egg and Cheese									
	530	34	20	195	37	1	4	19	1690
Bluffin, Bacon, Egg and Cheese									
	270	12	5	170	27	2	2	14	890
Bluffin, Egg and Cheese									
	240	10	5	165	27	2	2	12	770
Bluffin, Ham, Egg and Cheese									
	280	10	5	180	29	2	4	17	1050
Bluffin, Plain									
	130	1	0	0	25	2	2	5	240
Bluffin, Sausage, Egg and Cheese									
	390	24	10	195	27	2	2	18	1080
Burrito, Bacon, Egg and Cheese									
	580	28	12	335	57	5	2	26	2320
Burrito, Egg, and Cheese									
	500	23	10	325	57	5	2	21	2010
Burrito, Ham, Egg and Cheese									
	580	24	10	355	60	5	5	32	2560

Food Serving size	Cal.	(g) Total Fat	(g) Sat. Fat	(mg) Chol.	(g) Carb.	(g) Fiber	(g) Sug.	(g) Prot.	(mg) Sod.
Burrito, Sausage, Egg and Cheese									
	800	50	20	385	57	5	2	33	2620
Burrito, Turkey, Egg and Cheese									
	560	23	10	345	59	5	3	29	2530
Cinnamon Roll									
	450	20	9	30	60	2	17	9	730
Egg and Cheese on a Roll									
	200	9	4	160	22	1	2	10	650
Grilled Breakfast Sandwich, Bacon									
	480	23	10	335	44	1	4	25	1620
Grilled Breakfast Sandwich, Ham									
	480	19	9	355	47	1	7	30	1860
Grilled Breakfast Sandwich, Sausage									
	710	45	18	385	44	1	4	32	1920
Grilled Breakfast Sandwich, Turkey									
	460	18	8	345	46	1	5	28	1830

Cheese

Food Serving size	Cal.	Total Fat	Sat. Fat	Chol.	Carb.	Fiber	Sug.	Prot.	Sod.
American									
	100	9	5	25	1	NA	1	5	510
Cheddar Shredded, Serving									
	110	9	6	30	0	0	0	7	180
Parmesan Shredded, Serving									
	50	4	2	10	1	0	0	4	150
Pepper Jack, Serving									
	80	7	4	25	0	0	0	6	135
Provolone, Serving									
	80	6	4	15	0	NA	NA	5	190
Smoked Cheddar, Serving									
	80	6	4	20	1	NA	0	4	380
Swiss, Serving									
	80	6	4	20	0	0	0	6	45

Chips/Snacks

Food Serving size	Cal.	Total Fat	Sat. Fat	Chol.	Carb.	Fiber	Sug.	Prot.	Sod.
Baked BBQ									
	130	3.5	0	0	25	2	2	2	240

Food Serving size	Cal.	(g) Total Fat	(g) Sat. Fat	(mg) Chol.	(g) Carb.	(g) Fiber	(g) Sug.	(g) Prot.	(mg) Sod.
Cheddar Sour Cream	240	15	4.5	0	21	2	3	3	280
Cheetos Crunchy	160	10	2.5	0	15	1	1	2	290
Doritos Cooler Ranch	240	12	2.5	0	31	2	2	3	300
Doritos Nacho Cheese	240	12	2.5	0	30	2	3	3	330
Fritos	320	20	2	0	30	2	0	4	210
KC Master BBQ	240	15	4.5	0	22	1	3	3	300
Potato, Baked	120	1.5	0	0	26	2	2	2	170
Potato, Regular	220	15	4.5	0	22	1	0	3	270
Pretzels Classic Thin Style	220	2	0	0	47	2	2	4	NA
SunChips Multigrain Harvest Cheddar	210	9	1.5	0	28	3	3	3	280
SunChips Multigrain Original	210	9	1	0	29	4	3	3	140

Desserts, Snacks, and Sides

Food Serving size	Cal.	(g) Total Fat	(g) Sat. Fat	(mg) Chol.	(g) Carb.	(g) Fiber	(g) Sug.	(g) Prot.	(mg) Sod.
Brownie	230	10	4	22	28	1	21	3	115
Chocolate Chunk Cookie	200	10	4.5	15	25	0	16	2	150
Oatmeal Raisin Cookie	180	7	3	10	27	<1	16	2	150
Peanut Butter Cookie	210	13	5	10	21	<1	13	3	170
Sugar Cookie	320	16	6	35	42	0	23	3	240
White Chocolate Macadamia Nut Cookie	200	11	4.5	15	25	0	16	2	110

Food Serving size	Cal.	(g) Total Fat	(g) Sat. Fat	(mg) Chol.	(g) Carb.	(g) Fiber	(g) Sug.	(g) Prot.	(mg) Sod.
Dressings/Sauces									
Blimpie Special Sauce	40	4.5	0	0	0	NA	NA	0	0
Blue Cheese	230	24	4.5	25	2	NA	2	2	440
Buttermilk Ranch	230	24	3.5	10	2	NA	1	1	380
Creamy Caesar	210	21	3.5	10	2	NA	1	1	520
Creamy Italian	180	18	2.5	0	4	0	3	0	420
Dijon Honey Mustard	180	17	2.5	15	8	NA	7	1	240
Fat-Free Italian	25	0	NA	0	5	0	3	0	390
Light Buttermilk Ranch	70	4	0.5	0	8	NA	3	1	310
Light Italian	20	1	0	0	2	NA	2	0	770
Mayonnaise	200	22	3	20	0	0	0	0	200
Mustard, Honey	20	0.5	0	0	4	1	3	1	85
Mustard, Spicy Brown	15	0	0	0	0	NA	0	0	170
Mustard, Yellow Deli Style	15	0	0	NA	0	0	0	0	170
Oil, Blend	130	14	2	NA	0	0	0	0	0
Peppercorn	240	26	4.5	20	1	0	1	1	450
Red Wine Vinegar	5	0	0	0	1	0	0	0	0
Sauce, Red Hot Original	10	0	0	0	2	0	0	0	760

Food Serving size	Cal.	(g) Total Fat	(g) Sat. Fat	(mg) Chol.	(g) Carb.	(g) Fiber	(g) Sug.	(g) Prot.	(mg) Sod.
Thousand Island	210	20	3	15	6	0	6	0	350

Kid's Meals

Food Serving size	Cal.	(g) Total Fat	(g) Sat. Fat	(mg) Chol.	(g) Carb.	(g) Fiber	(g) Sug.	(g) Prot.	(mg) Sod.
3" Ham and American Cheese	260	8	4.5	15	32	2	6	14	900
3" Tuna	280	11	1.5	25	30	2	4	14	460
3" Turkey	190	2.5	0	10	31	2	5	10	600

Meats/Protein

Food Serving size	Cal.	(g) Total Fat	(g) Sat. Fat	(mg) Chol.	(g) Carb.	(g) Fiber	(g) Sug.	(g) Prot.	(mg) Sod.
Bacon	110	8	3	15	0	0	0	7	450
Cappacola	20	0.5	0	10	0	NA	0	3	160
Chicken (Grilled) Strips	110	3.5	1	50	0	0	0	19	300
Corned Beef	35	1	0	15	1	0	1	6	250
Ham	35	1	0	15	2	NA	2	5	280
Meatballs	220	16	6	45	8	2	2	11	1010
Pastrami	45	2.5	1	15	1	0	1	6	250
Pepperoni	70	6	2.5	15	1	NA	NA	3	230
Philly Steak and Onion	210	15	6	55	5	0	3	13	630
Prosciuttini	15	0	0	5	1	0	1	2	180
Roast Beef	30	1	0	15	0	0	0	6	150
Salami	35	3	1	10	0	0	0	2	135

Food Serving size	Cal.	(g) Total Fat	(g) Sat. Fat	(mg) Chol.	(g) Carb.	(g) Fiber	(g) Sug.	(g) Prot.	(mg) Sod.
Seafood Salad	90	4	0.5	20	10	1	2	4	410
Tuna	240	18	2.5	55	0	0	0	16	350
Turkey	30	0.3	0	12	1	NA	1	5	316

Salads

Food Serving size	Cal.	(g) Total Fat	(g) Sat. Fat	(mg) Chol.	(g) Carb.	(g) Fiber	(g) Sug.	(g) Prot.	(mg) Sod.
Antipasto	250	14	6	60	12	4	6	20	1630
Buffalo Chicken	220	14	6	60	12	4	5	20	1630
Chicken Caesar	190	8	4	65	6	3	3	25	460
Cole Slaw Salad, Side	160	9	1.5	5	20	2	17	1	240
Garden	30	0	0	0	6	3	3	2	15
Macaroni Salad, Side	330	22	5	15	28	2	8	5	790
Northwest Potato Salad, Side	260	17	4	25	22	3	3	3	390
Potato Salad, Side	230	12	2.5	10	28	3	8	3	490
Tuna	270	19	2.5	55	6	3	3	18	370
Ultimate Club	260	14	7	65	10	3	5	23	1070

Sandwiches (Lighter and Under 400 Calories)

Food Serving size	Cal.	(g) Total Fat	(g) Sat. Fat	(mg) Chol.	(g) Carb.	(g) Fiber	(g) Sug.	(g) Prot.	(mg) Sod.
6" Chicken Teriyaki, No Cheese	370	6	1.5	50	52	2	13	28	1090
6" Club, No Cheese/Sauce	310	4	1	25	49	3	9	18	1020
6" Ham, No Cheese/Sauce	310	4.5	1	30	49	3	10	19	980

Food Serving size	Cal.	(g) Total Fat	(g) Sat. Fat	(mg) Chol.	(g) Carb.	(g) Fiber	(g) Sug.	(g) Prot.	(mg) Sod.
6" Roast Beef, No Cheese/Sauce									
	330	5	1.5	45	46	3	7	25	870
6" Turkey, No Cheese/Sauce									
	320	3.5	0.5	30	49	3	8	21	1220
6" Veggie and Provolone, No Sauce									
	330	9	4	15	49	3	8	14	940
6" VegiMax, No Cheese/Sauce									
	390	8	1	0	55	5	7	23	950

Sandwiches/Wraps

Food Serving size	Cal.	(g) Total Fat	(g) Sat. Fat	(mg) Chol.	(g) Carb.	(g) Fiber	(g) Sug.	(g) Prot.	(mg) Sod.
Blimpie Best, 12"									
	900	35	12	105	99	6	19	49	2680
Blimpie Best, 12" Super Stacked									
	1100	44	15	185	104	6	24	71	4190
Blimpie Best, 6"									
	450	17	6	50	49	3	10	24	1330
Blimpie Best, 6" Super Stacked									
	550	22	8	90	52	3	12	36	2090
Blimpie Burger									
	460	24	10	70	42	1	4	21	1280
Blimpie Dog									
	510	29	12	55	45	1	7	17	1420
Blimpie Trio, 12" Super Stacked									
	1030	31	10	180	102	6	21	80	3530
Blimpie Trio, 6" Super Stacked									
	510	15	4.5	90	51	3	11	40	1760
BLT, 12"									
	870	44	10	55	86	5	11	30	1940
BLT, 12" Super Stacked									
	1270	82	18	110	84	4	10	43	2870
BLT, 6"									
	430	22	5	25	43	2	6	15	960
BLT, 6" Super Stacked									
	640	41	9	55	43	2	6	22	1440
Chicken Cheddar Bacon Ranch, 6"									
	600	29	10	85	48	3	8	36	1570

Food Serving size	Cal.	(g) Total Fat	(g) Sat. Fat	(mg) Chol.	(g) Carb.	(g) Fiber	(g) Sug.	(g) Prot.	(mg) Sod.
Chicken Cheddar Bacon Ranch, 12"	1190	58	19	175	95	6	15	72	3140
Chicken Teriyaki, 12"	860	25	11	130	94	3	19	65	2370
Chicken Teriyaki, 6"	450	12	5	65	52	2	13	33	1280
Chicken Teriyaki, 6" Wheat	450	14	6	65	50	5	12	35	1260
Ciabatta, Buffalo Chicken	540	23	7	65	49	3	5	31	1970
Ciabatta, French Dip	430	11	4.5	65	49	2	2	31	1820
Ciabatta, Grilled Chicken Caesar	580	20	5	65	62	3	4	34	1480
Ciabatta, Mediterranean	450	8	3	35	65	3	6	26	1720
Ciabatta, Roast Beef, Turkey and Cheddar	520	24	8	65	51	3	6	25	1780
Ciabatta, Sicilian	590	22	6	60	66	3	9	29	2170
Ciabatta, Spicy Chicken and Pepperoni	710	34	11	80	65	3	4	33	2070
Ciabatta, Tuscan	570	20	6	50	65	3	6	28	2030
Ciabatta, Ultimate Club	520	24	7	65	47	2	5	27	1600
Club, 12"	830	27	8	90	98	6	18	47	2110
Club, 6"	410	13	4	45	49	3	9	23	1050
Club, 6" Wheat	410	14	4.5	45	47	6	8	26	1040
Cuban, 12"	830	21	9	130	86	3	12	59	3260
Cuban, 6"	410	11	4.5	65	43	1	6	29	1630

Food Serving size	Cal.	(g) Total Fat	(g) Sat. Fat	(mg) Chol.	(g) Carb.	(g) Fiber	(g) Sug.	(g) Prot.	(mg) Sod.
French Dip, 12"	800	22	10	130	86	3	7	60	2550
French Dip, 6"	410	11	5	65	46	1	3	30	1650
Ham and Swiss, 12"	840	28	9	95	99	6	20	47	2040
Ham and Swiss, 6"	420	14	4.5	45	49	3	10	23	1020
Ham and Swiss, 6" Wheat	420	15	4.5	45	47	6	9	26	1000
Ham, Salami and Provolone, 12"	940	40	14	105	99	6	18	48	2550
Ham, Salami and Provolone, 6"	470	20	7	55	49	3	9	24	1270
Hot Pastrami, 12"	880	32	14	130	83	3	10	59	2780
Hot Pastrami, 12" Super Stacked	1150	47	20	220	86	3	13	93	4290
Hot Pastrami, 6"	430	16	7	65	42	1	5	30	1350
Hot Pastrami, 6" Super Stacked	570	23	10	110	43	1	7	46	2110
Meatball, 12"	1140	59	25	145	100	8	12	53	3790
Meatball, 6"	580	31	13	75	50	4	6	27	1960
Philly Steak and Onion, 12"	1200	70	23	155	92	3	14	50	2830
Philly Steak and Onion, 6"	600	35	11	80	46	1	7	25	1410
Pretzel, Ham and Swiss	520	15	4.5	45	75	4	14	24	940
Pretzel, Turkey Bacon	560	18	8	60	70	3	11	28	1800
Reuben, 12"	1060	40	12	145	105	6	13	67	3480

Food Serving size	Cal.	(g) Total Fat	(g) Sat. Fat	(mg) Chol.	(g) Carb.	(g) Fiber	(g) Sug.	(g) Prot.	(mg) Sod.
Reuben, 6"	530	20	6	70	52	3	7	34	1740
Roast Beef and Provolone, 12"	870	29	9	115	93	6	14	58	2010
Roast Beef and Provolone, 6"	430	14	5	55	46	3	7	28	980
Roast Beef and Provolone, 6" Wheat	430	16	5	60	44	6	6	32	1000
Special Vegetarian (Doritos Sub), 12"	1180	59	18	70	131	8	20	33	3540
Special Vegetarian (Doritos Sub), 6"	590	30	9	35	66	4	10	16	1170
Tuna, 12"	940	42	6	110	85	5	11	49	1550
Tuna, 6"	470	21	3	55	43	2	5	24	770
Turkey and Avocado, 12"	720	15	2	60	102	8	17	41	2690
Turkey and Avocado, 6"	360	7	1	30	51	4	8	21	1340
Turkey and Bacon, 12" Super Stacked	1250	57	21	180	96	5	17	79	5250
Turkey and Bacon, 6" Super Stacked	640	29	10	100	49	2	9	43	2830
Turkey and Cranberry, 12"	700	7	1.5	60	116	6	29	40	2440
Turkey and Cranberry, 6"	350	4	0.5	30	58	3	14	20	1220
Turkey and Provolone, 12"	840	27	8	85	99	6	17	49	2690
Turkey and Provolone, 6"	410	13	4	40	49	3	8	24	1310
Turkey and Provolone, 6" Wheat	420	14	5	45	47	6	8	27	1350
Veggie and Cheese, 12"	920	42	18	80	100	7	18	37	3290

Food Serving size	Cal.	(g) Total Fat	(g) Sat. Fat	(mg) Chol.	(g) Carb.	(g) Fiber	(g) Sug.	(g) Prot.	(mg) Sod.
Veggie and Cheese, 6"									
	460	21	9	40	50	3	9	19	1420
Veggie Supreme, 12"									
	1080	55	26	125	96	6	15	51	2330
Veggie Supreme, 6"									
	550	27	13	60	50	3	9	26	1500
VegieMax, 12"									
	1050	41	11	25	113	11	17	55	2550
VegieMax, 6"									
	520	20	6	15	56	5	8	28	1270
VegieMax, Wheat 6"									
	520	21	6	15	54	9	7	31	1250
Wrap, Chicken Caesar									
	560	24	8	60	56	4	5	30	1480
Wrap, Southwestern									
	530	22	6	55	61	4	10	23	1770

Soups

Food Serving size	Cal.	(g) Total Fat	(g) Sat. Fat	(mg) Chol.	(g) Carb.	(g) Fiber	(g) Sug.	(g) Prot.	(mg) Sod.
Bean with Ham									
	140	1	0	0	23	11	2	8	1070
Beef Steak and Noodle									
	120	4	1.5	30	14	0	4	8	780
Beef Stew									
	170	4	3.5	45	18	2	2	17	890
Captain's Corn Chowder									
	210	7	2.5	5	29	4	7	6	890
Chicken and Dumpling									
	170	7	3	50	19	3	4	11	970
Chicken Gumbo									
	90	2	0	10	13	2	4	6	1280
Chicken Noodle									
	130	4	1	30	18	2	5	7	1040
Chicken with White and Wild Rice									
	250	10	2.5	30	15	4	4	14	1030
Cream of Broccoli with Cheese									
	250	19	11	55	13	<1	2	7	1040

Food Serving size	Cal.	(g) Total Fat	(g) Sat. Fat	(mg) Chol.	(g) Carb.	(g) Fiber	(g) Sug.	(g) Prot.	(mg) Sod.
Cream of Potato	190	9	2.5	<5	24	3	3	5	860
French Onion	80	4	0.5	0	11	1	6	2	1020
Garden Vegetable	80	1	0	0	14	3	5	5	620
Grande Chili with Bean and Beef	310	9	4	20	31	9	9	20	1440
Harvest Vegetable	100	1	0	0	19	3	4	4	920
Italian Style Wedding	130	4	1.5	10	17	0	0	7	900
Minestrone	90	3	0	0	14	4	4	4	1150
New England Clam Chowder	170	3	2	25	28	2	5	7	1060
Pasta Fagioli with Sausage	150	5	1.5	20	22	4	2	7	910
Split Pea with Ham	130	2	0	5	21	6	1	8	1090
Tomato Basil with Raviolini	110	1	0	10	22	0	5	4	720
Vegetable Beef	80	2	0.5	5	13	2	3	4	1010
Yankee Pot Roast	80	2	0.5	10	12	2	2	5	750

Toppings

Food Serving size	Cal.	(g) Total Fat	(g) Sat. Fat	(mg) Chol.	(g) Carb.	(g) Fiber	(g) Sug.	(g) Prot.	(mg) Sod.
Guacamole	45	4	0.5	0	2	1	0	0	135
Lettuce, Serving	5	0	0	0	1	0	1	0	0
Olives, Serving	15	1.5	0	0	1	0	0	0	125
Onion, Serving	10	0	0	0	3	0	1	0	0

Food Serving size	Cal.	(g) Total Fat	(g) Sat. Fat	(mg) Chol.	(g) Carb.	(g) Fiber	(g) Sug.	(g) Prot.	(mg) Sod.
Peppers, Hot Ring, 12 Pieces									
	0	0	0	0	1	0	0	0	450
Peppers, Jalapeno, 18 Pieces									
	10	0	0	0	1	0	0	0	490
Peppers, Red Roasted, Serving									
	10	0	0	0	2	0	1	0	100
Peppers, Sweet Strips, 6 Pieces									
	20	0	0	0	5	0	5	0	115
Tomato, Serving									
	5	0	0	0	2	0	1	0	0

CARVEL

Blended Drinks (Small, 16 oz)

Food Serving size	Cal.	(g) Total Fat	(g) Sat. Fat	(mg) Chol.	(g) Carb.	(g) Fiber	(g) Sug.	(g) Prot.	(mg) Sod.
Arctic Blender - Cookie Dough									
	920	40	22	115	126	1	91	15	460
Arctic Blender - Fried Ice Cream									
	670	31	18	100	85	2	60	13	330
Arctic Blender - Peanut Butter									
	870	33	17	90	88	3	72	18	510
Carvelanche - Butterfinger									
	730	38	24	135	92	1	72	10	340
Carvelanche - Cake Mix									
	770	31	20	135	110	0	77	10	500
Carvelanche - Cookies and Cream									
	610	33	19	135	70	0	54	8	310
Carvelanche - M&M'S									
	760	39	18	135	88	0	75	11	230
Carvelanche - Reese's									
	750	39	28	135	85	0	74	14	320
Carvelatte - Caramel Macchiato									
	680	27	17	90	97	0	74	11	420
Carvelatte - Coffee									
	670	32	20	115	84	0	73	14	340
Carvelatte - Mocha									
	610	25	15	90	88	1	70	10	280

Food Serving size	Cal.	(g) Total Fat	(g) Sat. Fat	(mg) Chol.	(g) Carb.	(g) Fiber	(g) Sug.	(g) Prot.	(mg) Sod.
Float - Chocolate Ice Cream and Coke									
	360	14	8	35	54	1	49	6	150
Float - Chocolate Ice Cream and Soda Water									
	420	15	8	35	69	1	47	6	220
Float - Vanilla Ice Cream and Coke									
	380	17	11	85	53	0	48	4	150
Float - Vanilla Ice Cream and Soda Water									
	440	18	11	85	68	0	46	4	220
Iceberg - Barq's Root Beer									
	550	27	18	120	67	0	60	10	290
Iceberg - Coke									
	550	27	18	120	65	0	47	10	280
Iceberg - Fanta Orange									
	550	27	18	120	65	0	47	10	280
Thick Chocolate Shake									
	650	27	16	70	93	2	69	14	320
Thick Shake Float - Chocolate									
	790	34	20	90	109	3	83	17	390
Thick Shake Float - Strawberry									
	750	39	26	190	85	1	74	13	340
Thick Shake Float - Vanilla									
	810	39	26	190	102	0	92	13	350
Thick Strawberry Shake									
	600	31	20	150	70	1	61	11	280
Thick Vanilla Shake									
	660	31	20	150	86	0	79	11	280

Classic Sundaes (Small)

Food Serving size	Cal.	Total Fat	Sat. Fat	Chol.	Carb.	Fiber	Sug.	Prot.	Sod.
Banana Barge									
	970	46	24	95	128	7	95	19	290
Caramel									
	700	36	25	155	84	0	62	8	370
Hot Fudge									
	540	30	22	115	60	2	52	7	220
Strawberry									
	610	34	24	155	67	1	57	8	230

Food Serving size	Cal.	(g) Total Fat	(g) Sat. Fat	(mg) Chol.	(g) Carb.	(g) Fiber	(g) Sug.	(g) Prot.	(mg) Sod.
Cones (Small)									
Cake Cone with Chocolate	440	21	13	55	51	2	42	10	220
Cake Cone with Vanilla	470	26	17	130	50	0	40	6	220
Sugar Cone with Chocolate	460	21	13	55	59	2	46	11	250
Sugar Cone with Vanilla	490	26	17	130	57	0	43	6	230
Waffle Cone with Chocolate	490	23	13	60	63	2	49	10	220
Waffle Cone with Vanilla	510	24	14	90	61	1	47	11	260
Dashers (Small, 12 oz)									
Bananas Foster	660	23	15	90	105	2	67	6	420
Fudge Brownie	850	45	21	135	102	4	84	10	420
Mint Chocolate Chip	770	42	24	100	95	4	76	9	290
Peanut Butter Cup	1060	60	20	55	95	7	76	22	670
Strawberry Shortcake	580	29	19	145	74	2	60	7	240
Ice Cream - Small Cup (7.5 wt oz)									
Chocolate	410	21	13	55	48	2	42	10	220
No Sugar Added Vanilla	260	7	4.5	30	51	0	15	11	190
Sherbet	290	2.5	1.5	5	67	0	50	2	115
Vanilla	450	26	17	130	47	0	40	6	210
Low Fat									
Arctic Blender - Cookie Dough (Low Fat)	720	18	10	40	129	1	86	14	320

Food Serving size	Cal.	(g) Total Fat	(g) Sat. Fat	(mg) Chol.	(g) Carb.	(g) Fiber	(g) Sug.	(g) Prot.	(mg) Sod.
Arctic Blender - Fried Ice Cream (Low Fat)									
	500	10	6	25	95	1	61	12	210
Arctic Blender - Peanut Butter (Low Fat)									
	710	14	6	25	93	3	71	17	400
Cake Cone with Low Fat Chocolate									
	300	6	5	20	53	0	40	11	135
Cake Cone with Low Fat Vanilla									
	320	6	5	25	57	0	42	10	140
Carvelatte - Caramel Macchiato (Low Fat)									
	500	7	6	25	100	0	73	10	290
Carvelatte - Coffee (Low Fat)									
	450	8	6	30	89	0	72	12	180
Carvelatte - Mocha (Low Fat)									
	440	6	4.5	25	91	1	69	9	160
Flying Saucer (Low Fat Chocolate)									
	190	5	3	5	34	0	20	5	135
Flying Saucer (Low Fat Vanilla)									
	190	4.5	3	10	35	0	20	5	135
Small Cup (7.5 wt oz) Low Fat Chocolate									
	280	6	5	20	49	0	40	11	130
Small Cup (7.7 wt oz) Low Fat Vanilla									
	290	6	5	25	54	0	42	10	135
Sugar Cone with Low Fat Chocolate									
	320	6	5	20	59	0	43	11	140
Sugar Cone with Low Fat Vanilla									
	340	6	5	25	64	0	44	10	150
Waffle Cone with Low Fat Chocolate									
	360	8	6	25	64	0	47	12	130
Waffle Cone with Low Fat Vanilla									
	370	8	5	30	68	0	48	11	135

Menu Item

Slice of Carvel Ice Cream Cake									
	250	13	9	35	29	1	21	4	125

Food Serving size	Cal.	(g) Total Fat	(g) Sat. Fat	(mg) Chol.	(g) Carb.	(g) Fiber	(g) Sug.	(g) Prot.	(mg) Sod.
Smoothies (Small 16 oz)									
Raspberry - Strawberry	300	0	0	0	75	1	69	0	35
Strawberry	330	0	0	0	80	2	66	0	35
Strawberry - Banana	320	0	0	0	78	2	67	0	25
Take Home Treats									
Brown Bonnet	390	23	17	60	43	0	31	3	115
Carvel Sinful Love Bar	470	30	15	30	48	5	29	4	230
Chipster	350	17	9	45	45	4	27	4	230
Cupcake	270	12	8	45	36	0	28	3	180
Deluxe Flying Saucer - Sprinkles	350	16	10	45	49	0	20	3	160
Flying Saucer - Chocolate	230	10	5	20	33	1	20	4	160
Flying Saucer - Vanilla	250	11	7	45	33	0	20	3	160
Lil' Rounder - Chocolate Chip	180	9	5	20	23	1	15	2	125
Lil' Rounder - Double Chocolate Chip	180	9	5	20	23	1	16	2	135
Lil' Rounder - Oreo	160	7	2.5	15	25	1	12	3	200
Lil' Rounder - Sugar Cookie	190	9	5	25	22	0	13	2	140
Mini Sundae (Chocolate Syrup)	220	10	8	50	29	0	22	3	95
Olde Fashion Sundae	340	15	11	75	47	0	34	4	150
Sprinkle Cup	260	14	10	50	31	0	17	3	85

Food Serving size	Cal.	(g) Total Fat	(g) Sat. Fat	(mg) Chol.	(g) Carb.	(g) Fiber	(g) Sug.	(g) Prot.	(mg) Sod.

CiCi's PIZZA

12" Buffet Pizzas (Serving Size - 1 Slice)

Food	Cal.	Total Fat	Sat. Fat	Chol.	Carb.	Fiber	Sug.	Prot.	Sod.
Alfredo	120	3.5	1.5	5	19	<1	<1	4	270
Bacon Cheddar	110	4.5	1.5	5	19	<1	<1	5	350
BBQ	140	2.5	1	5	25	1	6	6	380
Beef	150	4	2	10	20	<1	1	6	380
Buffalo Chicken	140	4.5	1.5	10	19	<1	1	6	460
Cheese	150	3.5	2	10	20	<1	1	6	330
Classic Chicken	130	4	1.5	10	19	<1	<1	5	350
Ham	150	3.5	1.5	10	20	<1	1	6	370
Ham and Pineapple	150	3.5	1.5	10	21	<1	2	6	350
Macaroni and Cheese	170	2.5	1	5	29	1	2	6	250
Medium Pepperoni Deep Dish	180	6	3	15	19	<1	1.5	7	340
Ole'	70	2	1	<5	11	<1	1	4	240
Pepperoni	160	4.5	2	10	20	<1	1	6	370
Pepperoni and Jalapeno	150	4.5	2	10	20	<1	1	6	390
Pepperoni Flip	100	5	1.5	<5	9	0	<1	3	220
Pepperoni Sausage Italiano	90	5	2	10	8	0	<1	4	250

Food Serving size	Cal.	(g) Total Fat	(g) Sat. Fat	(mg) Chol.	(g) Carb.	(g) Fiber	(g) Sug.	(g) Prot.	(mg) Sod.
Philly Cheesesteak									
	130	4	1	<5	19	<1	1	4	300
Sausage									
	170	6	2.5	10	19	1	1	6	350
Spinach Alfredo									
	120	3.5	1.5	5	19	<1	<1	4	270
Tomato Alfredo									
	120	3	1.5	<5	19	<1	1	4	290
Vegetable Italiano									
	70	3.5	1	5	9	0	<1	3.5	210
Veggie									
	130	2	0.5	<5	20	<1	2	4	280
Zesty Ham and Cheddar									
	120	3	1	5	19	<1	<1	5	340
Zesty Pepperoni									
	130	4.5	1.5	5	19	<1	<1	5	340
Zesty Veggie									
	120	3	1	<5	20	<1	1	4	320

15" Buffet Pizzas (Serving Size - 1 Slice)

Food	Cal.	Total Fat	Sat. Fat	Chol.	Carb.	Fiber	Sug.	Prot.	Sod.
Alfredo									
	170	6	3	10	23	<1	1	6	400
Bacon Cheddar									
	150	8	2.5	15	25	<1	1	8	560
BBQ									
	240	6	3	20	36	2	12	11	710
Beef									
	210	7	3.5	20	24	1	2	9	560
Buffalo Chicken									
	190	7	2.5	20	23	<1	1	9	670
Cheese									
	190	5	2.5	15	24	<1	2	7	420
Classic Chicken									
	180	6	2	10	23	<1	1	8	490
Ham									
	190	6	2.5	20	24	<1	2	8	500

Food Serving size	Cal.	(g) Total Fat	(g) Sat. Fat	(mg) Chol.	(g) Carb.	(g) Fiber	(g) Sug.	(g) Prot.	(mg) Sod.
Ham and Pineapple	230	8	3.5	30	25	<1	3	12	740
Large Pepperoni Deepdish	200	7	3.5	20	22	<1	2	8	390
Macaroni and Cheese	230	3.5	1.5	10	39	1	2	8	310
Ole'	150	4.5	2	10	21	1	2	7	480
Pepperoni	210	8	3.5	20	24	<1	2	9	530
Pepperoni and Jalapeno	210	7	3.5	20	24	<1	2	8	590
Sausage	230	10	4.5	20	24	1	2	8	490
Spinach Alfredo	170	6	2.5	10	23	<1	1	6	380
Tomato Alfredo	160	5	2.5	10	24	<1	2	6	400
Veggie 15"	160	2.5	1	<5	25	1	2	5	340
Zesty Ham and Cheddar	180	6	2	15	23	<1	1	8	520
Zesty Pepperoni	190	7	2.5	15	23	<1	1	7	510
Zesty Veggie	160	4.5	1.5	5	24	<1	2	5	390

A La Carte

Food Serving size	Cal.	(g) Total Fat	(g) Sat. Fat	(mg) Chol.	(g) Carb.	(g) Fiber	(g) Sug.	(g) Prot.	(mg) Sod.
BBQ Wings (4 pieces)	270	18	5	115	6	<1	0	22	730
Hot Wings (4 pieces)	280	21	5	115	2	0	0	22	1130
Mild Wings (4 pieces)	320	26	6	115	1	0	0	22	980

Food Serving size	Cal.	(g) Total Fat	(g) Sat. Fat	(mg) Chol.	(g) Carb.	(g) Fiber	(g) Sug.	(g) Prot.	(mg) Sod.
Additional Menu Items									
Chicken Noodle Soup (4 oz)	60	1.5	0	<5	8	0	1	3	520
Garlic Bread Sticks (1 piece)	100	5	1.5	<5	10	0	0	4	120
Italian Signature Salad (1/2 cup)	35	1	0	0	2	<1	1	<1	280
Pasta (with sauce) (4 oz)	240	1	0	0	48	3	6	8	300
Dessert Items									
Bavarian Dessert (1 roll)	170	3	5	0	32	<1	11	3	210
Cinnamon Rolls (1 roll)	140	5	1	0	20	0	20	2	100
Fudge Brownies (1 slice)	140	6	1	0	23	<1	15	1	125
Iced Apple Crumb Pizza (1 slice)	240	6	1	0	43	<1	15	5	290

COLDSTONE CREAMERY

Ice Cream

Food Serving size	Cal.	(g) Total Fat	(g) Sat. Fat	(mg) Chol.	(g) Carb.	(g) Fiber	(g) Sug.	(g) Prot.	(mg) Sod.
Amaretto Ice Cream (142g)	330	20	12	80	33	0	29	5	80
Amaretto Ice Cream (227g)	530	31	20	125	53	0	46	8	130
Amaretto Ice Cream (340g)	790	47	30	185	80	0	69	12	190
Banana Ice Cream (142g)	310	18	12	70	33	0	28	5	70
Banana Ice Cream (227g)	500	29	18	115	53	0	46	8	115
Banana Ice Cream (340g)	750	44	28	175	80	<1	68	11	170

Food Serving size	Cal.	(g) Total Fat	(g) Sat. Fat	(mg) Chol.	(g) Carb.	(g) Fiber	(g) Sug.	(g) Prot.	(mg) Sod.
Black Cherry Ice Cream (142g)	330	19	12	75	36	0	32	5	75
Black Cherry Ice Cream (227g)	530	30	19	120	58	0	51	8	120
Black Cherry Ice Cream (340g)	790	44	28	175	86	0	76	11	180
Blueberry Ice Cream (142g)	320	20	13	75	33	0	31	5	55
Blueberry Ice Cream (227g)	510	31	21	120	53	0	49	9	90
Blueberry Ice Cream (340g)	760	47	31	185	79	0	74	13	130
Butter Pecan Ice Cream (142g)	320	19	12	75	32	0	28	5	105
Butter Pecan Ice Cream (227g)	520	31	20	125	53	0	45	8	170
Butter Pecan Ice Cream (340g)	780	47	30	185	79	0	68	12	260
Cake Batter Ice Cream (142g)	340	19	12	70	41	0	32	5	180
Cake Batter Ice Cream (227g)	550	30	19	115	66	0	51	8	280
Cake Batter Ice Cream (340g)	830	45	28	170	99	0	76	12	420
Cheesecake Ice Cream (142g)	320	19	13	50	36	0	32	4	85
Cheesecake Ice Cream (227g)	510	30	20	75	57	0	51	6	140
Cheesecake Ice Cream (340g)	760	45	30	115	86	1	76	10	210
Chocolate Cake Batter Ice Cream (142g)	340	19	11	70	42	1	33	5	210
Chocolate Cake Batter Ice Cream (227g)	550	30	18	110	68	2	53	9	340
Chocolate Cake Batter Ice Cream (340g)	820	45	27	160	101	3	79	13	510

Food Serving size	Cal.	(g) Total Fat	(g) Sat. Fat	(mg) Chol.	(g) Carb.	(g) Fiber	(g) Sug.	(g) Prot.	(mg) Sod.
Chocolate Dipped Strawberry (142g)									
	310	19	12	30	32	2	29	5	65
Chocolate Dipped Strawberry (227g)									
	490	30	20	45	51	3	46	8	100
Chocolate Dipped Strawberry (340g)									
	740	45	30	70	77	5	70	12	150
Chocolate Ice Cream (142g)									
	320	20	13	75	33	1	30	6	95
Chocolate Ice Cream (227g)									
	520	32	20	125	53	2	48	9	160
Chocolate Ice Cream (340g)									
	780	48	30	185	79	3	71	13	230
Chocolate Peanut Butter Ice Cream (142g)									
	410	28	13	25	36	3	31	10	200
Chocolate Peanut Butter Ice Cream (227g)									
	660	45	21	35	58	4	49	16	320
Chocolate Peanut Butter Ice Cream (340g)									
	990	67	31	55	86	6	74	24	480
Cinnamon Bun Ice Cream (142g)									
	350	18	12	45	47	1	37	4	190
Cinnamon Bun Ice Cream (227g)									
	560	28	18	70	75	2	59	7	310
Cinnamon Bun Ice Cream (340g)									
	840	42	28	105	112	2	89	10	460
Cinnamon Ice Cream (142g)									
	330	20	12	80	34	<1	29	5	80
Cinnamon Ice Cream (227g)									
	530	32	20	125	55	1	46	8	125
Cinnamon Ice Cream (340g)									
	790	47	30	185	82	2	69	12	190
Coconut Ice Cream (142g)									
	330	20	12	75	33	0	28	5	80
Coconut Ice Cream (227g)									
	520	31	20	125	52	0	45	8	125
Coconut Ice Cream (340g)									
	780	47	30	185	79	0	68	12	190

Food Serving size	Cal.	(g) Total Fat	(g) Sat. Fat	(mg) Chol.	(g) Carb.	(g) Fiber	(g) Sug.	(g) Prot.	(mg) Sod.
Coffee Ice Cream (142g)	330	20	12	80	34	0	29	5	80
Coffee Ice Cream (227g)	530	31	20	125	54	0	46	8	125
Coffee Ice Cream (340g)	790	47	30	185	81	0	69	12	190
Cookie Batter Ice Cream (142g)	360	20	12	40	43	0	37	4	270
Cookie Batter Ice Cream (227g)	580	33	19	65	68	1	59	7	430
Cookie Batter Ice Cream (340g)	860	49	28	100	102	1	89	10	650
Cotton Candy Ice Cream (142g)	330	19	12	75	34	0	28	5	75
Cotton Candy Ice Cream (227g)	530	31	20	125	55	0	45	8	120
Cotton Candy Ice Cream (340g)	790	47	29	185	82	0	68	12	180
Dark Chocolate Ice Cream (142g)	340	20	12	75	32	3	29	7	95
Dark Chocolate Ice Cream (227g)	540	32	20	115	51	5	46	11	150
Dark Chocolate Ice Cream (340g)	800	47	30	175	77	7	68	16	230
French Toast Ice Cream (142g)	330	19	12	75	35	0	30	5	150
French Toast Ice Cream (227g)	530	31	19	120	56	0	49	8	250
French Toast Ice Cream (340g)	790	46	29	180	84	0	73	12	370
French Vanilla Ice Cream (142g)	340	19	14	100	37	0	33	5	80
French Vanilla Ice Cream (227g)	540	30	22	60	60	0	52	8	125
French Vanilla Ice Cream (340g)	810	46	33	240	89	0	78	12	190

Food Serving size	Cal.	(g) Total Fat	(g) Sat. Fat	(mg) Chol.	(g) Carb.	(g) Fiber	(g) Sug.	(g) Prot.	(mg) Sod.
Fudge Brownie Batter Ice Cream (142g)									
	350	19	12	30	43	2	37	5	125
Fudge Brownie Batter Ice Cream (227g)									
	550	30	19	45	69	2	59	8	200
Fudge Brownie Batter Ice Cream (340g)									
	830	45	29	65	103	4	89	12	300
Ghirardelli Chocolate Ice Cream (142g)									
	330	20	12	75	37	4	27	7	75
Ghirardelli Chocolate Ice Cream (227g)									
	520	31	20	115	59	6	43	11	125
Ghirardelli Chocolate Ice Cream (340g)									
	780	47	30	175	88	8	64	16	180
Irish Cream Ice Cream (142g)									
	330	20	13	80	33	0	29	5	80
Irish Cream Ice Cream (227g)									
	530	32	20	125	54	0	46	8	125
Irish Cream Ice Cream (340g)									
	790	47	30	190	80	0	70	12	190
Key Lime Ice Cream (142g)									
	340	20	13	70	39	0	36	5	50
Key Lime Ice Cream (227g)									
	550	32	21	115	63	0	58	8	80
Key Lime Ice Cream (340g)									
	820	47	31	170	94	0	87	12	120
Macadamia Nut Ice Cream (142g)									
	330	20	12	80	34	0	29	5	75
Macadamia Nut Ice Cream (227g)									
	530	31	20	125	54	0	46	8	125
Macadamia Nut Ice Cream (340g)									
	790	47	30	185	81	0	70	12	190
Mango Ice Cream (142g)									
	310	18	12	70	33	0	28	5	70
Mango Ice Cream (227g)									
	490	29	18	115	53	0	45	7	115
Mango Ice Cream (340g)									
	740	44	28	175	80	0	68	11	170

Food Serving size	Cal.	(g) Total Fat	(g) Sat. Fat	(mg) Chol.	(g) Carb.	(g) Fiber	(g) Sug.	(g) Prot.	(mg) Sod.
Mint Ice Cream (142g)	330	19	12	75	36	0	31	5	75
Mint Ice Cream (227g)	530	30	19	120	57	0	50	8	120
Mint Ice Cream (340g)	790	45	29	180	86	0	75	12	180
Mocha Ice Cream (142g)	320	20	12	75	33	1	29	6	95
Mocha Ice Cream (227g)	520	31	20	120	53	2	47	9	150
Mocha Ice Cream (340g)	780	47	30	180	80	3	70	14	230
Oatmeal Cookie Batter Ice Cream (142g)	340	19	12	75	36	0	28	5	110
Oatmeal Cookie Batter Ice Cream (227g)	540	31	19	120	58	<1	45	9	170
Oatmeal Cookie Batter Ice Cream (340g)	810	46	29	180	87	<1	68	13	260
Orange Dreamsicle Ice Cream (142g)	320	19	12	75	35	0	28	5	75
Orange Dreamsicle Ice Cream (227g)	510	30	19	120	55	0	45	8	120
Orange Dreamsicle Ice Cream (340g)	760	45	28	180	83	0	68	11	180
Oreo Créme Ice Cream (142g)	440	31	14	60	41	0	38	4	80
Oreo Créme Ice Cream (227g)	710	49	23	95	65	0	61	7	125
Oreo Créme Ice Cream (340g)	1060	74	35	145	97	0	91	10	190
Peach Ice Cream (142g)	310	15	10	55	44	0	39	4	45
Peach Ice Cream (227g)	500	23	16	90	71	0	63	7	70
Peach Ice Cream (340g)	760	35	23	135	106	0	94	10	105

Food Serving size	Cal.	(g) Total Fat	(g) Sat. Fat	(mg) Chol.	(g) Carb.	(g) Fiber	(g) Sug.	(g) Prot.	(mg) Sod.
Peach Iced Tea Ice Cream (142g)	330	17	11	45	39	0	37	4	80
Peach Iced Tea Ice Cream (227g)	520	27	18	70	63	0	59	6	125
Peach Iced Tea Ice Cream (340g)	780	41	27	105	94	1	88	9	190
Peanut Butter Ice Cream (142g)	370	24	13	75	33	<1	28	7	130
Peanut Butter Ice Cream (227g)	590	39	20	115	53	1	44	12	210
Peanut Butter Ice Cream (340g)	890	58	30	175	79	2	66	18	310
Pecan Praline Ice Cream (142g)	330	19	12	75	37	0	31	5	90
Pecan Praline Ice Cream (227g)	530	30	19	115	58	0	49	8	150
Pecan Praline Ice Cream (340g)	800	45	28	175	88	0	73	11	220
Pistachio Ice Cream (142g)	330	20	12	80	34	0	29	5	85
Pistachio Ice Cream (227g)	520	31	20	125	54	0	46	8	135
Pistachio Ice Cream (340g)	780	47	30	185	80	0	70	12	200
Pistachio Jello Pudding Ice Cream (142g)	350	18	12	45	45	0	41	4	260
Pistachio Jello Pudding Ice Cream (227g)	560	29	19	70	73	1	66	6	410
Pistachio Jello Pudding Ice Cream (340g)	840	43	28	105	109	1	99	9	620
Pumpkin Ice Cream (142g)	290	15	10	60	33	1	28	4	105
Pumpkin Ice Cream (227g)	460	24	15	95	53	2	45	7	170
Pumpkin Ice Cream (340g)	680	37	23	145	80	3	67	10	260

Food Serving size	Cal.	(g) Total Fat	(g) Sat. Fat	(mg) Chol.	(g) Carb.	(g) Fiber	(g) Sug.	(g) Prot.	(mg) Sod.
Raspberry Ice Cream (142g)									
	330	19	12	75	36	0	31	5	75
Raspberry Ice Cream (227g)									
	520	30	19	120	57	0	50	8	125
Raspberry Ice Cream (340g)									
	780	44	28	175	85	0	75	12	180
Sinless Cake Batter Ice Cream (142g)									
	210	1	0.5	0	43	1	15	7	250
Sinless Cake Batter Ice Cream (227g)									
	340	1.5	1	0	68	1	25	12	400
Sinless Cake Batter Ice Cream (340g)									
	500	2.5	1	0	102	2	37	18	600
Sinless Sans Fat Sweet Cream (142g)									
	170	0	0	0	35	1	11	8	160
Sinless Sans Fat Sweet Cream (227g)									
	280	0	0	0	56	1	17	12	260
Sinless Sans Fat Sweet Cream (340g)									
	420	0.5	0	10	83	2	26	18	390
Strawberry Cheesecake Ice Cream (142g)									
	320	21	12	65	39	0	32	5	50
Strawberry Cheesecake Ice Cream (227g)									
	520	33	18	105	63	0	51	8	85
Strawberry Cheesecake Ice Cream (340g)									
	780	50	28	160	94	1	77	12	125
Strawberry Ice Cream (142g)									
	320	18	12	75	35	0	30	5	75
Strawberry Ice Cream (227g)									
	510	30	19	115	55	0	48	8	120
Strawberry Ice Cream (340g)									
	770	44	28	175	83	0	72	11	180
Sweet Cream Ice Cream (142g)									
	330	20	13	80	33	0	29	5	80
Sweet Cream Ice Cream (227g)									
	530	32	20	125	53	0	46	8	125
Sweet Cream Ice Cream (340g)									
	790	48	30	190	80	0	70	12	190

Food Serving size	Cal.	(g) Total Fat	(g) Sat. Fat	(mg) Chol.	(g) Carb.	(g) Fiber	(g) Sug.	(g) Prot.	(mg) Sod.
Vanilla Bean Ice Cream (142g)	330	19	12	75	32	0	28	5	75
Vanilla Bean Ice Cream (227g)	530	31	19	120	52	0	45	8	120
Vanilla Bean Ice Cream (340g)	790	46	29	180	77	0	67	12	180
White Chocolate Ice Cream (142g)	320	19	12	75	33	0	28	5	75
White Chocolate Ice Cream (227g)	520	31	20	125	53	0	45	8	125
White Chocolate Ice Cream (340g)	780	47	29	185	79	0	68	12	180

Sorbet and Yogurt

Food Serving size	Cal.	(g) Total Fat	(g) Sat. Fat	(mg) Chol.	(g) Carb.	(g) Fiber	(g) Sug.	(g) Prot.	(mg) Sod.
Countrytime Pink Lemonade Sorbet (142g)	240	0	0	0	59	0	59	0	25
Countrytime Pink Lemonade Sorbet (227g)	380	0	0	0	95	0	95	0	35
Countrytime Pink Lemonade Sorbet (340g)	570	0	0	0	142	0	142	0	55
Lemon Sorbet (142g)	150	0	0	0	40	0	34	0	15
Lemon Sorbet (227g)	250	0	0	0	64	0	54	0	25
Lemon Sorbet (340g)	370	0	0	0	96	<1	81	0	35
Raspberry Sorbet (142g)	160	0	0	0	42	0	36	0	15
Raspberry Sorbet (227g)	260	0	0	0	67	0	58	0	30
Raspberry Sorbet (340g)	390	0	0	0	101	<1	87	0	40
Strawberry Mango Banana Sorbet (142g)	220	0	0	0	55	0	52	0	15
Strawberry Mango Banana Sorbet (227g)	350	0	0	0	87	1	83	0	25

Food Serving size	Cal.	(g) Total Fat	(g) Sat. Fat	(mg) Chol.	(g) Carb.	(g) Fiber	(g) Sug.	(g) Prot.	(mg) Sod.
Strawberry Mango Banana Sorbet (340g)									
	520	0.5	0	0	131	1	125	0	35
Tart and Tangy Berry Yogurt (142g)									
	150	0	0	0	36	0	27	3	65
Tart and Tangy Berry Yogurt (227g)									
	240	0	0	0	58	0	44	5	105
Tart and Tangy Berry Yogurt (340g)									
	360	0	0	0	87	0	66	7	160
Tart and Tangy Yogurt (142g)									
	140	0	0	0	33	0	24	3	70
Tart and Tangy Yogurt (227g)									
	230	0	0	0	53	0	38	5	115
Tart and Tangy Yogurt (340g)									
	340	0	0	0	79	0	57	8	170
Watermelon Sorbet (142g)									
	160	0	0	0	41	0	35	0	15
Watermelon Sorbet (227g)									
	260	0	0	0	66	0	56	0	25
Watermelon Sorbet (340g)									
	380	0	0	90	99	<1	84	0	40

DUNKIN' DONUTS

AM Snacks

Hash Browns (9 pieces)									
	200	11	1.5	0	22	3	0	2	730
Sausage Pancake Bites (3 Pancake Bites)									
	300	20	7	20	23	1	7	7	550

Bagel Twist - Serving Size: 1 Bagel Twist

Cheddar Cheese Bagel Twist									
	400	9	4.5	20	63	5	5	17	800
Cinnamon Raisin Bagel Twist									
	350	3.5	0.5	0	72	5	19	11	460

Food Serving size	Cal.	(g) Total Fat	(g) Sat. Fat	(mg) Chol.	(g) Carb.	(g) Fiber	(g) Sug.	(g) Prot.	(mg) Sod.
Bagels - Serving Size: 1 Bagel									
Blueberry Bagel									
	330	3	1	0	65	5	10	11	620
Cinnamon Raisin Bagel									
	330	3.5	0.5	0	65	5	13	11	450
Everything Bagel									
	350	4.5	0.5	0	66	5	5	13	660
Garlic Bagel									
	340	2.5	0.5	0	68	6	5	12	660
Multigrain Bagel									
	390	8	0.5	0	65	9	7	14	560
Onion Bagel									
	310	2	0	0	63	3	3	11	380
Plain Bagel									
	320	2.5	0.5	0	63	5	5	11	660
Poppy Seed Bagel									
	350	6	0.5	0	64	5	5	13	660
Salt Bagel									
	320	2.5	0.5	0	63	5	5	11	3420
Sesame Bagel									
	360	6	0.5	0	63	5	5	13	660
Sour Cream and Onion Bagel									
	330	2.5	0.5	0	66	3	5	12	930
Wheat Bagel									
	320	3.5	0	0	61	5	4	12	550
Breakfast Sandwiches - Serving Size: 1 Sandwich									
Bacon, Egg and Cheese on Bagel									
	530	19	7	205	66	5	7	24	1340
Bacon, Egg and Cheese on Biscuit									
	490	30	14	205	35	1	4	18	1300
Bacon, Egg and Cheese on Croissant									
	530	33	13	205	38	2	6	20	1030
Bacon, Egg and Cheese on English Muffin									
	370	18	6	205	34	1	3	18	1030

Food Serving size	Cal.	(g) Total Fat	(g) Sat. Fat	(mg) Chol.	(g) Carb.	(g) Fiber	(g) Sug.	(g) Prot.	(mg) Sod.
Big n' Toasty	580	35	11	125	41	1	4	26	1370
Chicken Biscuit	500	25	10	35	48	2	5	20	1260
Egg and Cheese on Bagel	480	15	5	200	66	5	6	20	1130
Egg and Cheese on Biscuit	440	27	13	200	35	1	3	14	1090
Egg and Cheese on Croissant	480	29	12	200	38	2	6	16	820
Egg and Cheese on English Muffin	320	15	5	200	34	1	3	14	820
Ham, Egg and Cheese on Bagel	510	16	6	215	66	5	7	26	1390
Ham, Egg and Cheese on Biscuit	480	28	14	215	35	1	4	19	1350
Ham, Egg and Cheese on Croissant	510	31	12	215	38	2	6	21	1080
Ham, Egg and Cheese on English Muffin	360	16	6	215	34	1	3	20	1080
Sausage Biscuit	490	33	16	45	33	1	2	13	1140
Sausage, Egg and Cheese on Bagel	690	35	13	245	66	5	7	29	1650
Sausage, Egg and Cheese on Biscuit	650	46	20	245	36	1	4	22	1610
Sausage, Egg and Cheese on Croissant	690	48	19	245	39	2	6	24	1340
Sausage, Egg and Cheese on English Muffin	530	34	13	245	34	1	3	23	1340

Coffee

Blueberry Coffee - Small (10 fl oz)	15	0	0	0	2	0	0	0	5
Caramel Coffee - Small (10 fl oz)	10	0	0	0	2	0	0	0	5

Food Serving size	Cal.	(g) Total Fat	(g) Sat. Fat	(mg) Chol.	(g) Carb.	(g) Fiber	(g) Sug.	(g) Prot.	(mg) Sod.
Caramel Mocha Coffee - Large (20 fl oz)									
	230	0	0	0	53	1	48	3	40
Caramel Mocha Coffee - Medium (14 fl oz)									
	170	0	0	0	39	1	36	2	30
Caramel Mocha Coffee - Small (10 fl oz)									
	110	0	0	0	26	1	24	2	20
Caramel Mocha Coffee - XLarge (24 fl oz)									
	280	0	0	5	66	2	60	4	50
Caramel Mocha Coffee with Cream - Large (20 fl oz)									
	340	12	7	40	55	1	48	5	65
Caramel Mocha Coffee with Cream - Medium (14 fl oz)									
	260	9	6	30	41	1	36	3	50
Caramel Mocha Coffee with Cream - Small (10 fl oz)									
	170	6	3.5	20	27	1	24	2	30
Caramel Mocha Coffee with Cream - XLarge (24 fl oz)									
	430	15	9	55	68	2	60	6	80
Caramel Mocha Iced Coffee - Large (32 fl oz)									
	230	0	0	0	54	1	48	4	45
Caramel Mocha Iced Coffee - Medium (24 fl oz)									
	180	0	0	0	41	1	36	3	35
Caramel Mocha Iced Coffee - Small (16 fl oz)									
	120	0	0	0	27	1	24	2	25
Caramel Mocha Iced Coffee with Cream - Large (32 fl oz)									
	350	12	7	40	56	1	48	5	70
Caramel Mocha Iced Coffee with Cream - Medium (24 fl oz)									
	260	9	6	30	42	1	36	4	50
Caramel Mocha Iced Coffee with Cream - Small (16 fl oz)									
	180	6	3.5	20	28	1	24	3	35
Cinnamon Coffee - Small (10 fl oz)									
	15	0	0	0	2	0	0	0	5
Coconut Coffee - Small (10 fl oz)									
	10	0	0	0	1	0	0	0	5
Coffee - Extra Large (24 fl oz)									
	15	0	0	0	2	0	0	1	15
Coffee - Large (20 fl oz)									
	10	0	0	0	2	0	0	1	15

Food Serving size	Cal.	(g) Total Fat	(g) Sat. Fat	(mg) Chol.	(g) Carb.	(g) Fiber	(g) Sug.	(g) Prot.	(mg) Sod.
Coffee - Medium (14 fl oz)	10	0	0	0	1	0	0	1	10
Coffee - Small (10 fl oz)	5	0	0	0	1	0	0	0	5
Coffee with Cream - Small (10 fl oz)	60	6	4	20	2	0	0	1	20
Coffee with Cream and Sugar - Small (10 fl oz)	120	6	4	20	19	0	17	1	20
Coffee with Milk - Small (10 fl oz)	25	1	1	5	2	0	1	1	20
Coffee with Milk and Sugar - Small (10 fl oz)	80	1	1	5	20	0	19	1	20
Coffee with Skim Milk - Small (10 fl oz)	15	0	0	0	3	0	2	2	25
Coffee with Skim Milk and Splenda - Large (20 fl oz)	45	0	0	0	8	0	3	3	45
Coffee with Skim Milk and Splenda - Medium (14 fl oz)	30	0	0	0	6	0	2	2	35
Coffee with Skim Milk and Splenda - Small (10 fl oz)	25	0	0	0	5	0	2	2	25
Coffee with Skim Milk and Sugar - Small (10 fl oz)	70	0	0	0	20	0	19	2	25
Coffee with Splenda - Large (20 fl oz)	25	0	0	0	5	0	0	1	15
Coffee with Splenda - Medium (14 fl oz)	15	0	0	0	3	0	0	1	10
Coffee with Splenda - Small (10 fl oz)	15	0	0	0	3	0	0	0	5
Coffee with Sugar - Small (10 fl oz)	60	0	0	0	18	0	17	0	5
French Vanilla Coffee - Small (10 fl oz)	10	0	0	0	1	0	0	0	5
Hazelnut Coffee - Small (10 fl oz)	10	0	0	0	1	0	0	0	5
Iced Coffee - Large (32 fl oz)	20	0	0	0	3	0	0	1	15

Food Serving size	Cal.	(g) Total Fat	(g) Sat. Fat	(mg) Chol.	(g) Carb.	(g) Fiber	(g) Sug.	(g) Prot.	(mg) Sod.
Iced Coffee - Medium (24 fl oz)									
	15	0	0	0	2	0	0	1	10
Iced Coffee - Small (16 fl oz)									
	10	0	0	0	2	0	0	1	5
Iced Coffee with Cream - Small (16 fl oz)									
	70	6	4	20	3	0	0	1	20
Iced Coffee with Cream and Sugar - Small (16 fl oz)									
	120	6	4	20	20	0	17	1	20
Iced Coffee with Milk - Small (16 fl oz)									
	30	1	1	5	3	0	1	2	20
Iced Coffee with Milk and Sugar - Small (16 fl oz)									
	90	1	1	5	21	0	19	2	20
Iced Coffee with Skim Milk - Small (16 fl oz)									
	20	0	0	0	3	0	2	2	25
Iced Coffee with Skim Milk and Splenda - Large (32 fl oz)									
	60	0	0	0	10	0	3	3	45
Iced Coffee with Skim Milk and Splenda - Medium (24 fl oz)									
	40	0	0	0	8	0	2	3	35
Iced Coffee with Skim Milk and Splenda - Small (16 fl oz)									
	30	0	0	0	5	0	2	2	25
Iced Coffee with Skim Milk and Sugar - Small (16 fl oz)									
	80	0	0	0	21	0	19	2	25
Iced Coffee with Sugar - Small (16 fl oz)									
	70	0	0	0	19	0	17	1	5
Iced Dunkin' Dark Roast with Cream, Sugar - Large (32 fl oz)									
	250	12	7	40	40	0	35	3	40
Iced Dunkin' Dark Roast with Cream, Sugar - Medium (24 fl oz)									
	190	9	5	30	30	0	26	2	30
Iced Dunkin' Dark Roast with Cream, Sugar - Small (16 fl oz)									
	130	6	3.5	20	20	0	17	1	20
Iced Dunkin' Dark Roast with Skim Milk, Splenda - Large (32 fl oz)									
	60	0	0	0	10	0	3	3	50
Iced Dunkin' Dark Roast/Skim Milk, Splenda - Medium (24 fl oz)									
	40	0	0	0	8	0	2	3	35
Iced Dunkin' Dark Roast/Skim Milk, Splenda - Small (24 fl oz)									
	30	0	0	0	5	0	1	2	25

Food Serving size	Cal.	(g) Total Fat	(g) Sat. Fat	(mg) Chol.	(g) Carb.	(g) Fiber	(g) Sug.	(g) Prot.	(mg) Sod.
Mocha Coffee - Large (20 fl oz)									
	230	1	0	0	52	2	46	3	40
Mocha Coffee - Medium (14 fl oz)									
	170	0.5	0	0	39	2	34	2	30
Mocha Coffee - Small (10 fl oz)									
	110	0	0	0	26	1	23	1	20
Mocha Coffee Extra - Large (24 fl oz)									
	280	1	0.5	0	65	3	57	3	50
Mocha Coffee with Cream - Large (20 fl oz)									
	340	12	8	40	54	2	46	4	60
Mocha Coffee with Cream - Medium (14 fl oz)									
	260	9	6	30	41	2	34	3	45
Mocha Coffee with Cream - Small (10 fl oz)									
	170	6	4	20	27	1	23	2	30
Mocha Coffee with Cream Extra - Large (24 fl oz)									
	430	16	10	50	68	3	57	5	75
Mocha Iced Coffee with Cream - Large (32 fl oz)									
	350	12	8	40	56	2	46	5	70
Mocha Iced Coffee with Cream - Medium (24 fl oz)									
	260	9	6	30	42	2	34	3	50
Mocha Iced Coffee with Cream - Small (16 fl oz)									
	180	6	4	20	28	1	23	2	35
Raspberry Coffee - Small (10 fl oz)									
	15	0	0	0	2	0	0	0	5
Toasted Almond Coffee - Small (10 fl oz)									
	10	0	0	0	1	0	0	0	5

Cookies - Serving Size (1 Cookie)

Food	Cal.	Total Fat	Sat. Fat	Chol.	Carb.	Fiber	Sug.	Prot.	Sod.
Oatmeal Raisin Cookie									
	320	9	4.5	30	54	3	33	5	210
Reverse Chocolate Chunk Cookie									
	380	18	10	40	50	2	34	5	320
Triple Chocolate Chunk Cookie									
	360	15	8	35	53	2	31	5	380

Coolatta

Food	Cal.	Total Fat	Sat. Fat	Chol.	Carb.	Fiber	Sug.	Prot.	Sod.
Blue Raspberry Coolatta - Large (32 fl oz)									
	480	0	0	0	122	0	121	0	45

Food Serving size	Cal.	(g) Total Fat	(g) Sat. Fat	(mg) Chol.	(g) Carb.	(g) Fiber	(g) Sug.	(g) Prot.	(mg) Sod.
Blue Raspberry Coolatta - Medium (24 fl oz)									
	360	0	0	0	92	0	91	0	35
Blue Raspberry Coolatta - Small (16 fl oz)									
	240	0	0	0	61	0	60	0	25
Cherry Strawberry Coolatta - Large (32 fl oz)									
	530	0	0	0	131	0	130	0	60
Cherry Strawberry Coolatta - Medium (24 fl oz)									
	400	0	0	0	98	0	97	0	45
Cherry Strawberry Coolatta - Small (16 fl oz)									
	270	0	0	0	65	0	65	0	30
Coffee Coolatta with Cream - Large (32 fl oz)									
	800	46	29	160	98	0	87	7	150
Coffee Coolatta with Cream - Medium (24 fl oz)									
	600	35	22	120	73	0	65	5	110
Coffee Coolatta with Cream - Small (16 fl oz)									
	400	23	14	80	49	0	43	3	75
Coffee Coolatta with Milk - Large (32 fl oz)									
	480	8	5	35	100	0	98	8	180
Coffee Coolatta with Milk - Medium (32 fl oz)									
	360	6	3.5	25	75	0	73	6	130
Coffee Coolatta with Milk - Small (16 fl oz)									
	240	4	2.5	15	50	0	49	4	90
Coffee Coolatta with Skim Milk - Large (32 fl oz)									
	420	0	0	5	102	0	98	9	180
Coffee Coolatta with Skim Milk - Medium (24 fl oz)									
	310	0	0	0	76	0	73	7	135
Coffee Coolatta with Skim Milk - Small (16 fl oz)									
	210	0	0	0	51	0	49	4	90
Coffee-Mocha Coolatta with Cream - Large (32 fl oz)									
	990	47	29	160	141	2	125	8	170
Coffee-Mocha Coolatta with Cream - Medium (24 fl oz)									
	740	35	22	120	106	2	94	6	130
Coffee-Mocha Coolatta with Cream - Small (16 fl oz)									
	490	24	15	80	70	1	63	4	85
Coffee-Mocha Coolatta with Milk - Large (32 fl oz)									
	670	9	5	35	144	2	137	10	200

Food Serving size	Cal.	(g) Total Fat	(g) Sat. Fat	(mg) Chol.	(g) Carb.	(g) Fiber	(g) Sug.	(g) Prot.	(mg) Sod.
Coffee-Mocha Coolatta with Milk - Medium (24 fl oz)									
	500	6	4	25	108	2	102	7	150
Coffee-Mocha Coolatta with Milk - Small (16 fl oz)									
	330	4.5	2.5	15	72	1	68	5	100
Coffee-Mocha Coolatta with Skim Milk - Large (32 fl oz)									
	610	1	0	5	145	2	137	11	200
Coffee-Mocha Coolatta with Skim Milk - Medium (24 fl oz)									
	460	0.5	0	0	109	2	103	8	150
Coffee-Mocha Coolatta with Skim Milk - Small (16 fl oz)									
	300	0	0	0	72	1	68	5	100
Mountain Dew Coolatta - Large (32 fl oz)									
	390	0	0	0	104	0	101	0	135
Mountain Dew Coolatta - Medium (24 fl oz)									
	290	0	0	0	78	0	76	0	100
Moutain Dew Coolatta - Small (16 fl oz)									
	200	0	0	0	52	0	50	0	65
Strawberry Fruit Coolatta - Large (32 fl oz)									
	610	0	0	0	150	0	135	1	85
Strawberry Fruit Coolatta - Medium (24 fl oz)									
	460	0	0	0	112	0	102	1	65
Strawberry Fruit Coolatta - Small (16 fl oz)									
	310	0	0	0	75	0	68	0	45
Strawberry Lemonade Coolatta - Large (32 fl oz)									
	490	0	0	0	123	0	119	0	210
Strawberry Lemonade Coolatta - Medium (24 fl oz)									
	360	0	0	0	92	0	89	0	160
Strawberry Lemonade Coolatta - Small (16 fl oz)									
	240	0	0	0	61	0	60	0	105
Strawberry Tropicana Coolatta - Large (32 fl oz)									
	440	0	0	0	11	0	108	1	50
Strawberry Tropicana Coolatta - Medium (24 fl oz)									
	330	0	0	0	83	0	81	1	40
Strawberry Tropicana Coolatta - Small (16 fl oz)									
	220	0	0	0	56	0	54	1	25
Strawberry Vanilla Bean Coolatta - Large (32 fl oz)									
	800	0	0	5	196	0	188	4	290

Food Serving size	Cal.	(g) Total Fat	(g) Sat. Fat	(mg) Chol.	(g) Carb.	(g) Fiber	(g) Sug.	(g) Prot.	(mg) Sod.
Strawberry Vanilla Bean Coolatta - Medium (24 fl oz)									
	600	0	0	0	147	0	141	3	220
Strawberry Vanilla Bean Coolatta - Small (16 fl oz)									
	400	0	0	0	98	0	94	2	140
Tropicana Blue Raspberry Coolatta - Large (32 fl oz)									
	510	0	0	0	127	0	124	1	40
Tropicana Blue Raspberry Coolatta - Medium (24 fl oz)									
	380	0	0	0	95	0	93	1	30
Tropicana Blue Raspberry Coolatta - Small (16 fl oz)									
	250	0	0	0	64	0	62	1	20
Tropicana Orange Coolatta - Large (32 fl oz)									
	470	0	0	0	113	0	109	2	80
Tropicana Orange Coolatta - Medium (24 fl oz)									
	350	0	0	0	85	0	82	2	60
Tropicana Orange Coolatta - Small (16 fl oz)									
	230	0	0	0	57	0	54	1	40
Tropicana Vanilla Bean Coolatta - Large (32 fl oz)									
	770	0	0	5	193	0	183	5	270
Tropicana Vanilla Bean Coolatta - Medium (24 fl oz)									
	580	0	0	0	145	0	137	4	200
Tropicana Vanilla Bean Coolatta - Small (16 fl oz)									
	390	0	0	0	96	0	91	3	135
Vanilla Bean Coolatta - Large (32 fl oz)									
	860	12	7	45	181	0	172	6	350
Vanilla Bean Coolatta - Medium (24 fl oz)									
	650	9	5	30	136	0	129	4	260
Vanilla Bean Coolatta - Small (16 fl oz)									
	430	6	3.5	20	91	0	86	3	170

Cream Cheese - Serving: 1 Unit (50g)

Food Serving size	Cal.	Total Fat	Sat. Fat	Chol.	Carb.	Fiber	Sug.	Prot.	Sod.
Plain Cream Cheese									
	150	15	9	40	3	0	3	3	250
Reduced Fat Blueberry Cream Cheese Spread - 25% Less Fat than Cream Cheese Spread									
	150	9	6	25	15	0	11	2	210
Reduced Fat Onion and Chive Cream Cheese Spread - 25% Less Fat than Cream Cheese Spread									
	130	11	7	35	6	0	3	3	250

Food Serving size	Cal.	(g) Total Fat	(g) Sat. Fat	(mg) Chol.	(g) Carb.	(g) Fiber	(g) Sug.	(g) Prot.	(mg) Sod.
Reduced Fat Plain Cream Cheese - 50% Less Fat than Regular Cream Cheese									
	100	8	5	25	5	0	2	4	250
Reduced Fat Smoked Salmon Cream Cheese Spread - 25% Less Fat than Cream Cheese Spread									
	140	11	7	35	6	0	3	4	260
Reduced Fat Strawberry Cream Cheese Spread - 25% Less Fat than Cream Cheese Spread									
	150	10	6	30	15	0	11	2	200
Reduced Fat Veggie Cream Cheese Spread - 25% Less Fat than Cream Cheese Spread									
	120	10	6	30	6	0	2	2	240

Danish - Serving Size: 1 Danish

Food Serving size	Cal.	(g) Total Fat	(g) Sat. Fat	(mg) Chol.	(g) Carb.	(g) Fiber	(g) Sug.	(g) Prot.	(mg) Sod.
Apple Cheese Danish									
	330	16	7	0	41	1	18	4	270
Cheese Danish									
	330	17	8	5	39	1	17	5	270
Strawberry Cheese Danish									
	320	16	7	0	40	1	18	4	260

Donuts Serving Size: 1

Food Serving size	Cal.	(g) Total Fat	(g) Sat. Fat	(mg) Chol.	(g) Carb.	(g) Fiber	(g) Sug.	(g) Prot.	(mg) Sod.
Apple Crumb Donut									
	490	18	9	0	80	2	49	4	350
Apple 'n Spice Donut									
	270	14	6	0	32	1	8	3	350
Apple Pie Donut									
	320	15	7	0	42	1	19	3	360
Bavarian Kreme Donut									
	270	15	7	0	31	1	9	4	350
Blueberry Crumb Donut									
	500	18	9	0	84	2	52	4	350
Blueberry Cake Donut									
	340	17	8	30	44	1	21	4	570
Boston Kreme Donut									
	310	16	7	0	39	1	16	3	370
Bow Tie Donut									
	310	15	7	0	39	1	15	4	400

Food Serving size	Cal.	(g) Total Fat	(g) Sat. Fat	(mg) Chol.	(g) Carb.	(g) Fiber	(g) Sug.	(g) Prot.	(mg) Sod.
Chocolate Coconut Cake Donut	550	39	25	0	47	2	22	5	390
Chocolate Dipped Banana Donut	290	12	5	0	41	2	20	5	260
Chocolate Frosted Cake Donut	370	23	10	25	45	1	20	4	320
Chocolate Frosted Cocoa Donut	250	11	4.5	0	32	2	13	4	260
Chocolate Frosted Coffee Roll	410	19	8	0	53	3	19	7	420
Chocolate Frosted Donut	270	15	7	0	31	1	13	3	340
Chocolate Glazed Cake Donut	370	24	11	0	35	1	17	3	390
Chocolate Iced Bismark	390	19	8	0	52	2	21	5	360
Chocolate Kreme Filled Donut	370	21	10	0	42	1	21	4	370
Cinnamon Cake Donut	340	22	10	25	38	1	13	3	300
Cinnamon Cake Stick	350	18	8	35	44	2	19	4	420
Cocoa Boston Kreme Donut	280	13	5	0	39	2	16	5	270
Cocoa Butternut Donut	260	11	5	0	36	2	17	4	250
Cocoa Coconut Donut	260	13	6	0	33	2	13	5	260
Cocoa Coffee Roll	310	14	6	0	44	3	16	5	300
Cocoa Confetti Donut	270	12	5	0	35	2	15	4	260
Cocoa Glazed Donut	240	11	4.5	0	32	2	12	4	240
Cocoa Jelly Donut	300	12	5	0	45	2	15	5	260

Food Serving size	Cal.	(g) Total Fat	(g) Sat. Fat	(mg) Chol.	(g) Carb.	(g) Fiber	(g) Sug.	(g) Prot.	(mg) Sod.
Cocoa Kreme Puff Donut									
	300	16	7	0	34	2	16	4	260
Coffee Roll									
	400	18	7	0	53	3	19	7	400
Double Chocolate Cake Donut									
	380	25	11	0	36	2	17	4	410
Double Cocoa Coffee Roll									
	320	15	6	0	44	3	16	5	320
Double Cocoa Kreme Donut									
	300	16	7	0	36	2	14	5	260
Double Cocoa Kreme Puff Donut									
	290	16	6	0	34	2	13	5	260
Dulce de Chocolate Donut									
	350	17	7	5	45	1	21	4	360
Dulce de Leche Donut									
	290	16	7	0	31	1	10	4	340
Éclair									
	390	19	8	0	52	2	21	5	360
French Cruller									
	250	20	9	35	18	0	10	2	105
Glazed Cake Donut									
	360	22	10	25	44	1	19	3	300
Glazed Cake Stick									
	370	18	8	35	48	1	23	4	420
Glazed Chocolate Cake Stick									
	390	25	11	0	40	2	17	3	540
Glazed Cocoa Jelly Donut									
	290	11	4.5	0	44	2	14	4	250
Glazed Donut									
	260	14	6	0	31	1	12	3	330
Guayaba Burst Donut									
	300	15	7	0	38	1	15	4	330
Jelly Filled Donut									
	290	14	7	0	36	1	6	3	340
Jelly Stick									
	420	18	8	35	60	1	20	4	440

Food Serving size	Cal.	Total Fat (g)	Sat. Fat (g)	Chol. (mg)	Carb. (g)	Fiber (g)	Sug. (g)	Prot. (g)	Sod. (mg)
Lemon Filled Donut	270	15	7	0	31	1	9	4	350
Lemon Meringue Pie	320	16	7	0	42	1	19	3	360
Maple Frosted Cocoa Donut	250	11	4.5	0	33	2	14	4	250
Maple Frosted Coffee Roll	410	19	8	0	54	3	20	7	410
Maple Frosted Donut	270	15	7	0	32	1	14	3	340
Marble Frosted Cocoa Donut	260	11	4.5	0	36	2	17	4	250
Marble Frosted Donut	270	15	7	0	32	1	13	3	340
Old Fashioned Cake Donut	320	22	10	25	33	1	9	3	300
Pina Boom Donut	270	15	7	0	32	1	12	4	350
Pina Colada Donut	330	17	9	0	42	1	20	4	380
Plain Cake Stick	330	18	8	35	36	1	12	4	420
Powdered Cake Donut	340	22	10	25	38	1	13	4	300
Powdered Cake Stick	360	18	8	35	43	2	18	5	420
Powdered Cocoa Donut	220	11	4.5	0	25	2	6	5	240
Reverse Boston Kreme Donut	290	12	5	0	42	2	20	4	260
Sprinkle the Love Donut	310	14	6	0	43	1	19	4	270
Strawberry Frosted Cocoa Donut	250	11	4.5	0	33	2	14	4	250
Strawberry Frosted Donut	280	15	7	0	32	1	14	3	340

Food Serving size	Cal.	(g) Total Fat	(g) Sat. Fat	(mg) Chol.	(g) Carb.	(g) Fiber	(g) Sug.	(g) Prot.	(mg) Sod.
Strawberry Shortcake									
	330	15	7	0	47	1	23	3	360
Sugar Cocoa Donut									
	200	11	4.5	0	23	2	4	4	240
Sugar Raised Donut									
	230	14	6	0	22	1	4	3	330
Triple Cocoa Donut									
	260	12	5	0	35	2	14	5	260
Vanilla Cocoa Kreme Donut									
	310	17	7	0	36	2	17	5	260
Vanilla Frosted Cocoa Donut									
	250	11	4.5	0	33	2	14	4	250
Vanilla Frosted Coffee Roll									
	410	19	8	0	54	3	20	7	410
Vanilla Kreme Filled Donut									
	380	23	10	0	42	1	22	4	370

Dunkin' Deli

Food Serving size	Cal.	(g) Total Fat	(g) Sat. Fat	(mg) Chol.	(g) Carb.	(g) Fiber	(g) Sug.	(g) Prot.	(mg) Sod.
Broccoli Cheddar Soup (8 oz)									
	190	11	6	35	14	2	5	10	990
Caesar Salad (7.3 oz)									
	320	29	6	30	11	3	2	6	790
Cheeseburger Stuffed Breadstick (1 Breadstick)									
	200	6	2.5	10	28	1	2	9	400
Chicken Bruschetta Sandwich (1 Sandwich)									
	580	26	7	80	49	2	4	37	1200
Chicken Caesar Salad (10.4 oz)									
	440	33	7	75	11	3	2	25	1020
Chicken Noodle Soup (8 oz)									
	130	3	1	45	19	1	1	7	970
Chicken Salad on a Croissant (1 Sandwich)									
	560	37	10	45	38	2	6	17	890
Chicken Salad on an English Muffin (1 Sandwich)									
	400	23	4	45	33	1	3	15	890
Chipotle Chicken Sandwich (1 Sandwich)									
	600	25	8	85	50	3	5	43	1380

Food Serving size	Cal.	(g) Total Fat	(g) Sat. Fat	(mg) Chol.	(g) Carb.	(g) Fiber	(g) Sug.	(g) Prot.	(mg) Sod.
Garden Salad (12.3 oz)									
	180	6	3	15	21	4	6	8	500
Pastrami Supreme Sandwich (1 Sandwich)									
	750	39	16	125	51	3	4	48	2060
Pepperoni and Cheese Stuffed Breadstick (1 Breadstick)									
	210	7	3	15	27	1	2	11	380
Pressed Cuban Sandwich (1 Sandwich)									
	680	33	13	120	50	2	6	46	2000
Steak and Cheese Sandwich (1 Sandwich)									
	470	16	6	75	50	2	3	31	2040
Toasted Italian Sandwich (1 Sandwich)									
	560	25	9	75	52	3	5	33	2630
Tuna Melt on a Croissant (1 Sandwich)									
	630	40	14	50	42	2	5	19	900
Tuna Melt Sandwich (1 Sandwich)									
	770	30	7	70	57	3	8	36	1560
Tuna Salad Sandwich on a Plain Bagel (1 Sandwich)									
	540	20	3	30	69	5	6	18	1070
Tuna Salad Sandwich on an English Muffin (1 Sandwich)									
	380	19	3	30	37	1	2	12	750
Turkey and Bacon Club Sandwich (1 Sandwich)									
	440	13	3	45	51	3	5	35	1800
Turkey and Cheese Sandwich (1 Sandwich)									
	450	13	4.5	60	52	3	4	35	1500

Espresso Beverages

Food Serving size	Cal.	(g) Total Fat	(g) Sat. Fat	(mg) Chol.	(g) Carb.	(g) Fiber	(g) Sug.	(g) Prot.	(mg) Sod.
Cappuccino Small (10 fl oz)									
	80	4	2.5	15	7	0	7	4	70
Cappuccino with Sugar - Small (10 fl oz)									
	140	4	2.5	15	24	0	24	4	70
Caramel Mocha Latte with Milk - Large (20 fl oz)									
	450	12	8	55	70	1	67	14	230
Caramel Mocha Latte with Milk - Medium (16 fl oz)									
	330	9	6	40	52	1	50	11	170
Caramel Mocha Latte with Milk - Small (10 fl oz)									
	220	6	4	25	35	1	33	7	115

Food Serving size	Cal.	(g) Total Fat	(g) Sat. Fat	(mg) Chol.	(g) Carb.	(g) Fiber	(g) Sug.	(g) Prot.	(mg) Sod.
Caramel Mocha Latte with Skim Milk - Large (20 fl oz)									
	350	1	0.5	10	70	1	68	15	200
Caramel Mocha Latte with Skim Milk - Medium (16 fl oz)									
	260	0.5	0	5	53	1	51	11	150
Caramel Mocha Latte with Skim Milk - Small (10 fl oz)									
	170	0	0	5	35	1	34	7	100
Caramel Swirl Latte - Small (10 fl oz)									
	220	6	3.5	25	35	0	34	8	150
Espresso (1.75 fl oz)									
	5	0	0	0	1	0	1	0	5
Espresso with Sugar (1.75 fl oz)									
	30	0	0	0	7	0	7	0	5
Iced Caramel Mocha Latte with Milk - Large (32 fl oz)									
	450	12	8	55	70	1	67	14	240
Iced Caramel Mocha Latte with Milk - Medium (24 fl oz)									
	330	9	6	40	52	1	50	11	180
Iced Caramel Mocha Latte with Milk - Small (16 fl oz)									
	220	6	4	25	35	1	33	7	120
Iced Caramel Mocha Latte with Skim Milk - Large (32 fl oz)									
	350	1	0.5	10	70	1	68	15	210
Iced Caramel Mocha Latte with Skim Milk - Medium (24 fl oz)									
	260	0.5	0	5	53	1	51	11	150
Iced Caramel Mocha Latte with Skim Milk - Small (16 fl oz)									
	170	0	0	5	35	1	34	7	105
Iced Caramel Swirl Latte - Small (16 fl oz)									
	220	6	3.5	25	35	0	34	8	150
Iced Caramel Swirl Latte with Skim Milk - Small (16 fl oz)									
	180	0	0	5	36	0	35	9	150
Iced Latte - Small (16 fl oz)									
	120	6	3.5	25	10	0	10	6	105
Iced Latte Lite - Large (32 fl oz)									
	160	0	0	5	25	0	20	14	220
Iced Latte Lite - Medium (24 fl oz)									
	120	0	0	5	19	0	15	10	170
Iced Latte Lite - Small (16 fl oz)									
	80	0	0	0	13	0	10	7	110

Food Serving size	Cal.	(g) Total Fat	(g) Sat. Fat	(mg) Chol.	(g) Carb.	(g) Fiber	(g) Sug.	(g) Prot.	(mg) Sod.
Iced Latte with Skim Milk - Small (16 fl oz)									
	70	0	0	0	11	0	10	7	110
Iced Latte with Skim Milk and Sugar - Small (16 fl oz)									
	130	0	0	0	28	0	27	7	110
Iced Latte with Sugar - Small (16 fl oz)									
	170	6	3.5	25	27	0	27	6	100
Iced Mocha Raspberry Latte - Large (32 fl oz)									
	450	12	8	50	73	2	64	13	220
Iced Mocha Raspberry Latte - Medium (24 fl oz)									
	340	9	6	35	54	2	48	10	160
Iced Mocha Raspberry Latte - Small (16 fl oz)									
	230	6	4	25	36	1	32	7	110
Iced Mocha Spice Latte - Large (32 fl oz)									
	450	12	8	50	70	2	64	13	190
Iced Mocha Spice Latte - Medium (24 fl oz)									
	330	9	6	35	53	2	48	10	140
Iced Mocha Spice Latte - Small (16 fl oz)									
	220	6	4	25	35	1	32	7	95
Iced Mocha Swirl Latte - Small (16 fl oz)									
	220	6	4	25	35	1	32	7	115
Iced Mocha Swirl Latte with Skim Milk - Small (16 fl oz)									
	180	0	0	0	36	1	32	8	125
Iced Vanilla Latte Lite - Small (16 fl oz)									
	90	0	0	0	14	0	10	7	110
Latte - Small (10 fl oz)									
	120	6	3.5	25	10	0	10	6	105
Latte Lite - Large (20 fl oz)									
	160	0	0	5	25	0	20	14	220
Latte Lite - Medium (16 fl oz)									
	120	0	0	5	19	0	15	10	170
Latte Lite - Small (10 fl oz)									
	80	0	0	0	13	0	10	7	110
Latte with Sugar - Small (10 fl oz)									
	170	6	3.5	25	27	0	27	6	100
Mocha Raspberry Latte - Large (20 fl oz)									
	450	12	8	50	73	2	64	13	220

Food Serving size	Cal.	(g) Total Fat	(g) Sat. Fat	(mg) Chol.	(g) Carb.	(g) Fiber	(g) Sug.	(g) Prot.	(mg) Sod.
Mocha Raspberry Latte - Medium (16 fl oz)									
	340	9	6	35	54	2	48	10	160
Mocha Raspberry Latte - Small (10 fl oz)									
	230	6	4	25	36	1	32	7	110
Mocha Spice Latte - Large (20 fl oz)									
	450	12	8	50	70	2	64	13	190
Mocha Spice Latte - Medium (16 fl oz)									
	330	9	6	35	53	2	48	10	140
Mocha Spice Latte - Small (10 fl oz)									
	220	6	4	25	35	1	32	7	95
Mocha Swirl Latte - Small (10 fl oz)									
	220	6	4	25	35	1	32	7	115
Turbo Shot - Extra Large (4 fl oz)									
	10	0	0	0	2	0	2	0	15
Turbo Shot - Large (3.5 fl oz)									
	10	0	0	0	2	0	2	0	15
Turbo Shot - Medium (2.5 fl oz)									
	5	0	0	0	1	0	1	0	10
Turbo Shot - Small (1.75 fl oz)									
	5	0	0	0	1	0	1	0	5
Vanilla Latte Lite - Large (20 fl oz)									
	170	0	0	5	28	0	20	14	220
Vanilla Latte Lite - Medium (16 fl oz)									
	130	0	0	5	20	0	15	10	170
Vanilla Latte Lite - Small (10 fl oz)									
	90	0	0	0	14	0	10	7	110

Frozen Beverages

Food Serving size	Cal.	Total Fat	Sat. Fat	Chol.	Carb.	Fiber	Sug.	Prot.	Sod.
Frozen Hot Chocolate - Large (32 fl oz)									
	820	10	6	35	180	4	144	14	430
Frozen Hot Chocolate - Medium (24 fl oz)									
	610	7	4.5	25	135	3	108	10	320
Frozen Hot Chocolate - Small (16 fl oz)									
	410	5	3	20	90	2	72	7	220
Frozen Hot Chocolate Coconut - Large (32 fl oz)									
	870	10	6	35	190	4	154	14	440

Food Serving size	Cal.	(g) Total Fat	(g) Sat. Fat	(mg) Chol.	(g) Carb.	(g) Fiber	(g) Sug.	(g) Prot.	(mg) Sod.
Frozen Hot Chocolate Coconut - Medium (24 fl oz)									
	650	7	4.5	25	143	3	116	10	330
Frozen Hot Chocolate Coconut - Small (16 fl oz)									
	430	5	3	20	95	2	77	7	220
Frozen Iced Tea - Large (32 fl oz)									
	470	0	0	0	118	3	115	5	70
Frozen Iced Tea - Medium (24 fl oz)									
	350	0	0	0	88	2	86	4	50
Frozen Iced Tea - Small (16 fl oz)									
	240	0	0	0	59	1	58	2	35
Frozen Iced Tea Lemonade - Large (32 fl oz)									
	490	0	0	0	124	2	120	2	210
Frozen Iced Tea Lemonade - Medium (24 fl oz)									
	370	0	0	0	93	1	90	2	160
Frozen Iced Tea Lemonade - Small (16 fl oz)									
	240	0	0	0	62	1	60	1	105
Frozen Lemonade - Large (32 fl oz)									
	510	0	0	0	131	1	125	0	350
Frozen Lemonade - Medium (24 fl oz)									
	380	0	0	0	98	1	94	0	260
Frozen Lemonade - Small (16 fl oz)									
	250	0	0	0	65	0	62	0	180

Muffins - Serving Size (1 Muffin)

Food Serving size	Cal.	(g) Total Fat	(g) Sat. Fat	(mg) Chol.	(g) Carb.	(g) Fiber	(g) Sug.	(g) Prot.	(mg) Sod.
Blueberry Muffin									
	500	16	3	65	83	2	48	7	500
Chocolate Chip Muffin									
	610	23	7	70	92	3	55	8	520
Coffee Cake Muffin									
	650	27	9	70	95	1	56	8	530
Corn Muffin									
	510	18	3.5	75	80	1	35	7	840
Honey Bran Raisin Muffin									
	490	15	3	60	82	5	44	7	450
Reduced Fat Blueberry Muffin - 25% Less than Regular Blueberry Muffin									
	450	11	2	65	81	2	42	7	700

Food Serving size	Cal.	(g) Total Fat	(g) Sat. Fat	(mg) Chol.	(g) Carb.	(g) Fiber	(g) Sug.	(g) Prot.	(mg) Sod.
Munchkins - Serving Size (1 Munchkin)									
Cinnamon Cake Munchkin	60	3.5	1.5	5	6	0	3	1	65
Cocoa Glazed Munchkin	35	1	0	0	6	0	3	1	35
Cocoa Kreme Puff Munchkin	50	2.5	1	0	7	0	4	1	40
Double Cocoa Kreme Puff Munchkin	50	2.5	1	0	7	0	3	1	45
Glazed Cake Munchkin	70	3.5	1.5	5	8	0	4	1	65
Glazed Chocolate Cake Munchkin	70	3.5	1.5	0	8	0	4	1	85
Glazed Munchkin	70	4	2	0	7	0	3	1	80
Jelly Filled Munchkin	80	4	2	0	9	0	2	1	85
Plain Cake Munchkin	60	3.5	1.5	5	6	0	2	1	65
Powdered Cake Munchkin	60	3.5	1.5	5	7	0	3	1	65
Sugared Munchkin	60	3.5	1.5	5	6	0	2	1	65
Other Bakery - Serving Size (1 Item)									
Apple Fritter	410	17	7	0	60	2	27	6	380
Apple Pie	270	13	6	0	34	1	12	3	180
Biscuit	280	14	8	0	32	1	2	5	620
Brownie	440	23	5	55	58	1	49	3	250
Double Cocoa Fritter	430	19	8	0	63	2	30	5	370
English Muffin	160	2	0	0	31	1	1	5	350

Food Serving size	Cal.	(g) Total Fat	(g) Sat. Fat	(mg) Chol.	(g) Carb.	(g) Fiber	(g) Sug.	(g) Prot.	(mg) Sod.
Glazed Fritter									
	410	17	7	0	60	2	27	6	380
Plain Croissant									
	310	16	7	0	35	1	4	7	350
Vanilla Cocoa Fritter									
	440	20	8	0	63	2	34	5	360

Other Hot Beverages

Food Serving size	Cal.	(g) Total Fat	(g) Sat. Fat	(mg) Chol.	(g) Carb.	(g) Fiber	(g) Sug.	(g) Prot.	(mg) Sod.
Caramel Hot Chocolate - Extra Large (24 fl oz)									
	560	18	16	0	99	4	74	5	670
Caramel Hot Chocolate - Large (20 fl oz)									
	460	15	14	0	82	3	62	4	560
Caramel Hot Chocolate - Medium (14 fl oz)									
	330	11	10	0	59	2	44	3	400
Caramel Hot Chocolate - Small (10 fl oz)									
	230	7	7	0	40	2	30	2	270
Dunkaccino - Small									
	240	11	9	10	35	1	26	2	220
Hot Chocolate - Small (10 fl oz)									
	220	7	7	0	39	2	30	2	270
Vanilla Chai (14 fl oz)									
	330	8	8	10	53	1	45	11	180
White Hot Chocolate - Large (20 fl oz)									
	470	17	16	5	79	1	65	4	650
White Hot Chocolate - Medium (14 fl oz)									
	340	12	11	5	56	1	47	3	460
White Hot Chocolate - Small (10 fl oz)									
	230	8	8	5	38	1	32	2	310

PM Snacks - Serving Size (1 Sandwich)

Food Serving size	Cal.	(g) Total Fat	(g) Sat. Fat	(mg) Chol.	(g) Carb.	(g) Fiber	(g) Sug.	(g) Prot.	(mg) Sod.
Egg White Turkey Sausage Flatbread									
	280	8	3	15	32	3	4	19	770
Egg White Veggie Flatbread									
	280	10	4	20	32	3	3	16	690
Ham and Cheese Flatbread									
	310	11	4.5	40	35	1	2	19	880
Turkey, Cheddar and Bacon Flatbread									
	410	20	7	50	36	1	2	22	1140

Food Serving size	Cal.	(g) Total Fat	(g) Sat. Fat	(mg) Chol.	(g) Carb.	(g) Fiber	(g) Sug.	(g) Prot.	(mg) Sod.
Tea									
Decaffeinated Tea (10 fl oz)									
	0	0	0	0	0	0	0	0	5
Decaffeinated Tea with Milk (10 fl oz)									
	20	1	0.5	5	1	0	1	1	20
Decaffeinated Tea with Milk and Sugar (10 fl oz)									
	80	1	0.5	5	19	0	19	1	20
Decaffeinated Tea with Skim Milk (10 fl oz)									
	10	0	0	0	2	0	2	1	20
Decaffeinated Tea with Skim Milk and Sugar (10 fl oz)									
	70	0	0	0	19	0	19	1	20
Decaffeinated Tea with Sugar (10 fl oz)									
	60	0	0	0	17	0	17	0	5
Earl Grey Tea (10 fl oz)									
	0	0	0	0	0	0	0	0	5
Earl Grey Tea with Milk (10 fl oz)									
	20	1	0.5	5	1	0	1	1	20
Earl Grey Tea with Milk and Sugar (10 fl oz)									
	80	1	0.5	5	19	0	19	1	20
Earl Grey Tea with Skim Milk (10 fl oz)									
	10	0	0	0	2	0	2	1	20
Earl Grey Tea with Skim Milk and Sugar (10 fl oz)									
	70	0	0	0	19	0	19	1	20
Earl Grey Tea with Sugar (10 fl oz)									
	60	0	0	0	17	0	17	0	5
English Breakfast Tea (10 fl oz)									
	0	0	0	0	0	0	0	0	5
English Breakfast Tea with Milk (10 fl oz)									
	20	1	0.5	5	1	0	1	1	20
English Breakfast Tea with Milk and Sugar (10 fl oz)									
	80	1	0.5	5	19	0	19	1	20
English Breakfast Tea with Skim Milk (10 fl oz)									
	10	0	0	0	2	0	2	1	20
English Breakfast Tea with Skim Milk and Sugar (10 fl oz)									
	70	0	0	0	19	0	19	1	20
English Breakfast Tea with Sugar (10 fl oz)									
	60	0	0	0	17	0	17	0	5

Food Serving size	Cal.	(g) Total Fat	(g) Sat. Fat	(mg) Chol.	(g) Carb.	(g) Fiber	(g) Sug.	(g) Prot.	(mg) Sod.
Freshly Brewed Sweetened Iced Tea (16 fl oz)									
	80	0	0	0	20	0	19	0	0
Freshly Brewed Tea with Milk (10 fl oz)									
	20	1	0.5	5	1	0	1	1	20
Freshly Brewed Tea with Milk and Sugar (10 fl oz)									
	80	1	0.5	5	19	0	19	1	20
Freshly Brewed Tea with Skim Milk (10 fl oz)									
	10	0	0	0	2	0	2	1	20
Freshly Brewed Tea with Skim Milk and Sugar (10 fl oz)									
	70	0	0	0	19	0	19	1	20
Freshly Brewed Tea with Sugar (10 fl oz)									
	60	0	0	0	17	0	17	0	5
Freshly Brewed Unsweetened Iced Tea - Large (32 fl oz)									
	10	0	0	0	5	2	0	0	5
Freshly Brewed Unsweetened Iced Tea - Medium (24 fl oz)									
	5	0	0	0	2	0	0	0	0
Freshly Brewed Unsweetened Iced Tea (16 fl oz)									
	5	0	0	0	1	0	0	0	0
Freshly Brewed Unsweetened Tea (10 fl oz)									
	0	0	0	0	0	0	0	0	5
Green Tea (10 fl oz)									
	0	0	0	0	0	0	0	0	5
Green Tea with Milk (10 fl oz)									
	20	1	0.5	5	1	0	1	1	20
Green Tea with Milk and Sugar (10 fl oz)									
	80	1	0.5	5	19	0	19	1	20
Green Tea with Skim Milk (10 fl oz)									
	10	0	0	0	2	0	2	1	20
Green Tea with Skim Milk and Sugar (10 fl oz)									
	70	0	0	0	19	0	19	1	20
Green Tea with Sugar (10 fl oz)									
	60	0	0	0	17	0	17	0	5
Peach Flavored Iced Tea (16 fl oz)									
	15	0	0	0	2	0	0	0	0
Peach Flavored Sweetened Iced Tea (16 fl oz)									
	90	0	0	0	21	0	19	0	0

Food Serving size	Cal.	(g) Total Fat	(g) Sat. Fat	(mg) Chol.	(g) Carb.	(g) Fiber	(g) Sug.	(g) Prot.	(mg) Sod.
Raspberry Flavored Iced Tea (16 fl oz)									
	15	0	0	0	2	0	0	0	0
Raspberry Flavored Sweetened Iced Tea (16 fl oz)									
	90	0	0	0	21	0	19	0	0
Sweet Tea (16 fl oz)									
	120	0	0	0	29	0	28	0	0

Wake-Up Wraps

Food Serving size	Cal.	(g) Total Fat	(g) Sat. Fat	(mg) Chol.	(g) Carb.	(g) Fiber	(g) Sug.	(g) Prot.	(mg) Sod.
Bacon, Egg and Cheese Wake-Up Wrap									
	210	12	5	105	14	1	1	10	580
Egg and Cheese Wake-Up Wrap									
	180	11	4	105	14	1	1	8	470
Egg White Turkey Sausage Wake-Up Wrap									
	150	5	2.5	15	14	1	2	11	400
Egg White Veggie Wake-Up Wrap									
	150	6	3	15	14	1	1	10	340
Ham, Egg and Cheese Wake-Up Wrap									
	200	11	4.5	115	14	1	1	11	600
Sausage, Egg and Cheese Wake-Up Wrap									
	290	20	8	125	14	1	1	12	730

KFC

Food Serving size	Cal.	(g) Total Fat	(g) Sat. Fat	(mg) Chol.	(g) Carb.	(g) Fiber	(g) Sug.	(g) Prot.	(mg) Sod.
Fiery Buffalo Hot Wings (1) (29g)									
	70	4	0.5	20	5	0	0	4	270
HBBQ Hot Wings (1) (31g)									
	80	4	0.5	20	8	0	2	4	240

Beverages

Food Serving size	Cal.	(g) Total Fat	(g) Sat. Fat	(mg) Chol.	(g) Carb.	(g) Fiber	(g) Sug.	(g) Prot.	(mg) Sod.
7UP (16 fl oz)									
	180	0	0	0	46	0	45	0	55
7UP (20 fl oz)									
	230	0	0	0	59	0	55	0	70
7UP (30 fl oz)									
	350	0	0	0	91	0	90	0	110
7UP (64 fl oz)									
	780	0	0	0	202	0	195	0	235

Food Serving size	Cal.	(g) Total Fat	(g) Sat. Fat	(mg) Chol.	(g) Carb.	(g) Fiber	(g) Sug.	(g) Prot.	(mg) Sod.
Capri Sun Roarin' Waters Tropical Fruit (6 fl oz)									
	30	0	0	0	8	0	8	0	15
Code Red Mountain Dew (16 fl oz)									
	190	0	0	0	54	0	54	0	60
Code Red Mountain Dew (20 fl oz)									
	250	0	0	0	70	0	70	0	80
Code Red Mountain Dew (30 fl oz)									
	390	0	0	0	109	0	109	0	125
Code Red Mountain Dew (64 fl oz)									
	850	0	0	0	240	0	240	0	270
Diet Dr Pepper (16 fl oz)									
	0	0	0	0	0	0	0	0	60
Diet Dr Pepper (20 fl oz)									
	0	0	0	0	0	0	0	0	80
Diet Dr Pepper (30 fl oz)									
	0	0	0	0	0	0	0	0	125
Diet Dr Pepper (64 fl oz)									
	0	0	0	0	0	0	0	0	270
Diet Mountain Dew (16 fl oz)									
	0	0	0	0	0	0	0	0	70
Diet Mountain Dew (20 fl oz)									
	0	0	0	0	0	0	0	0	90
Diet Mountain Dew (30 fl oz)									
	0	0	0	0	0	0	0	0	140
Diet Mountain Dew (64 fl oz)									
	0	0	0	0	0	0	0	0	310
Diet Pepsi (16 fl oz)									
	0	0	0	0	0	0	0	0	45
Diet Pepsi (20 fl oz)									
	0	0	0	0	0	0	0	0	55
Diet Pepsi (30 fl oz)									
	0	0	0	0	0	0	0	0	90
Diet Pepsi (64 fl oz)									
	0	0	0	0	0	0	0	0	195
Diet Sierra Mist (16 fl oz)									
	0	0	0	0	0	0	0	0	45

Food Serving size	Cal.	(g) Total Fat	(g) Sat. Fat	(mg) Chol.	(g) Carb.	(g) Fiber	(g) Sug.	(g) Prot.	(mg) Sod.
Diet Sierra Mist (20 fl oz)	0	0	0	0	0	0	0	0	55
Diet Sierra Mist (30 fl oz)	0	0	0	0	0	0	0	0	90
Diet Sierra Mist (64 fl oz)	0	0	0	0	0	0	0	0	195
Dr Pepper (16 fl oz)	180	0	0	0	47	0	47	0	60
Dr Pepper (20 fl oz)	230	0	0	0	61	0	61	0	80
Dr Pepper (30 fl oz)	350	0	0	0	95	0	95	0	125
Dr Pepper (64 fl oz)	780	0	0	0	209	0	209	0	270
Lipton Brisk Green with Peach Tea (16 fl oz)	0	0	0	0	0	0	0	0	125
Lipton Brisk Green with Peach Tea (20 fl oz)	0	0	0	0	0	0	0	0	160
Lipton Brisk Green with Peach Tea (30 fl oz)	0	0	0	0	0	0	0	0	245
Lipton Brisk Green with Peach Tea (64 fl oz)	0	0	0	0	0	0	0	0	545
Lipton Brisk Lemon Tea (16 fl oz)	120	0	0	0	35	0	35	0	25
Lipton Brisk Lemon Tea (20 fl oz)	160	0	0	0	45	0	45	0	35
Lipton Brisk Lemon Tea (30 fl oz)	250	0	0	0	70	0	70	0	55
Lipton Brisk Lemon Tea (64 fl oz)	540	0	0	0	155	0	155	0	115
Lipton Brisk Peach Tea (16 fl oz)	140	0	0	0	37	0	37	0	45
Lipton Brisk Peach Tea (20 fl oz)	180	0	0	0	47	0	47	0	55
Lipton Brisk Peach Tea (30 fl oz)	280	0	0	0	74	0	74	0	90

Food Serving size	Cal.	(g) Total Fat	(g) Sat. Fat	(mg) Chol.	(g) Carb.	(g) Fiber	(g) Sug.	(g) Prot.	(mg) Sod.
Lipton Brisk Peach Tea (64 fl oz)									
	620	0	0	0	163	0	163	0	195
Lipton Brisk Raspberry Tea (16 fl oz)									
	140	0	0	0	37	0	37	0	45
Lipton Brisk Raspberry Tea (20 fl oz)									
	180	0	0	0	47	0	47	0	55
Lipton Brisk Raspberry Tea (30 fl oz)									
	280	0	0	0	74	0	74	0	90
Lipton Brisk Raspberry Tea (64 fl oz)									
	620	0	0	0	163	0	163	0	195
Lipton Brisk Tea (16 fl oz)									
	0	0	0	0	0	0	0	0	55
Lipton Brisk Tea (20 fl oz)									
	0	0	0	0	0	0	0	0	70
Lipton Brisk Tea (30 fl oz)									
	0	0	0	0	0	0	0	0	105
Lipton Brisk Tea (64 fl oz)									
	0	0	0	0	0	0	0	0	235
Manzanita Sol (16 fl oz)									
	190	0	0	0	51	0	49	0	45
Manzanita Sol (20 fl oz)									
	250	0	0	0	65	0	63	0	55
Manzanita Sol (30 fl oz)									
	390	0	0	0	102	0	98	0	90
Manzanita Sol (64 fl oz)									
	850	0	0	0	225	0	217	0	195
Milk 2% (10 fl oz)									
	170	6	4	25	17	0	16	12	180
Miranda Strawberry (16 fl oz)									
	190	0	0	0	51	0	51	0	90
Miranda Strawberry (20 fl oz)									
	250	0	0	0	65	0	65	0	115
Miranda Strawberry (30 fl oz)									
	390	0	0	0	102	0	102	0	175
Miranda Strawberry (64 fl oz)									
	850	0	0	0	225	0	225	0	390

Food Serving size	Cal.	(g) Total Fat	(g) Sat. Fat	(mg) Chol.	(g) Carb.	(g) Fiber	(g) Sug.	(g) Prot.	(mg) Sod.
Mountain Dew (16 fl oz)	190	0	0	0	51	0	51	0	60
Mountain Dew (20 fl oz)	250	0	0	0	65	0	65	0	80
Mountain Dew (30 fl oz)	390	0	0	0	102	0	102	0	125
Mountain Dew (64 fl oz)	850	0	0	0	225	0	225	0	270
Mug Root Beer (16 fl oz)	180	0	0	0	46	0	46	0	25
Mug Root Beer (20 fl oz)	230	0	0	0	59	0	59	0	35
Mug Root Beer (30 fl oz)	350	0	0	0	91	0	91	0	55
Mug Root Beer (64 fl oz)	780	0	0	0	202	0	202	0	115
Pepsi (16 fl oz)	180	0	0	0	49	0	49	0	35
Pepsi (20 fl oz)	230	0	0	0	63	0	63	0	45
Pepsi (30 fl oz)	350	0	0	0	98	0	98	0	70
Pepsi (64 fl oz)	780	0	0	0	217	0	217	0	155
Pepsi Max (16 fl oz)	0	0	0	0	0	0	0	0	45
Pepsi Max (20 fl oz)	0	0	0	0	0	0	0	0	55
Pepsi Max (30 fl oz)	0	0	0	0	0	0	0	0	90
Pepsi Max (64 fl oz)	0	0	0	0	0	0	0	0	195
Sierra Mist (16 fl oz)	180	0	0	0	47	0	47	0	35
Sierra Mist (20 fl oz)	230	0	0	0	61	0	61	0	45

Food Serving size	Cal.	(g) Total Fat	(g) Sat. Fat	(mg) Chol.	(g) Carb.	(g) Fiber	(g) Sug.	(g) Prot.	(mg) Sod.
Sierra Mist (30 fl oz)	350	0	0	0	95	0	95	0	70
Sierra Mist (64 fl oz)	780	0	0	0	209	0	209	0	155
Tropicana Fruit Punch (16 fl oz)	190	0	0	0	53	0	53	0	45
Tropicana Fruit Punch (20 fl oz)	250	0	0	0	68	0	68	0	55
Tropicana Fruit Punch (30 fl oz)	390	0	0	0	105	0	105	0	90
Tropicana Fruit Punch (64 fl oz)	850	0	0	0	233	0	233	0	195
Tropicana Lemonade (16 fl oz)	180	0	0	0	47	0	47	0	185
Tropicana Lemonade (20 fl oz)	230	0	0	0	61	0	61	0	235
Tropicana Lemonade (30 fl oz)	350	0	0	0	95	0	95	0	370
Tropicana Lemonade (64 fl oz)	780	0	0	0	209	0	209	0	815
Tropicana Pink Lemonade (16 fl oz)	180	0	0	0	47	0	47	0	185
Tropicana Pink Lemonade (20 fl oz)	230	0	0	0	61	0	61	0	235
Tropicana Pink Lemonade (30 fl oz)	350	0	0	0	95	0	95	0	370
Tropicana Pink Lemonade (64 fl oz)	780	0	0	0	209	0	209	0	815
Tropicana Sugar Free Lemonade (16 fl oz)	10	0	0	0	0	0	0	0	165
Tropicana Sugar Free Lemonade (20 fl oz)	10	0	0	0	0	0	0	0	215
Tropicana Sugar Free Lemonade (30 fl oz)	20	0	0	0	0	0	0	0	335
Tropicana Sugar Free Lemonade (64 fl oz)	40	0	0	0	0	0	0	0	735

Food Serving size	Cal.	(g) Total Fat	(g) Sat. Fat	(mg) Chol.	(g) Carb.	(g) Fiber	(g) Sug.	(g) Prot.	(mg) Sod.
Tropicana Twister Orange (16 fl oz)									
	190	0	0	0	54	0	53	0	45
Tropicana Twister Orange (20 fl oz)									
	250	0	0	0	70	0	68	0	55
Tropicana Twister Orange (30 fl oz)									
	390	0	0	0	109	0	109	0	90
Tropicana Twister Orange (64 fl oz)									
	850	0	0	0	240	0	233	0	195
Wild Cherry Pepsi (16 fl oz)									
	180	0	0	0	49	0	49	0	35
Wild Cherry Pepsi (20 fl oz)									
	230	0	0	0	63	0	63	0	45
Wild Cherry Pepsi (30 fl oz)									
	350	0	0	0	98	0	98	0	70
Wild Cherry Pepsi (64 fl oz)									
	780	0	0	0	217	0	217	0	155

Chicken

Food Serving size	Cal.	Total Fat	Sat. Fat	Chol.	Carb.	Fiber	Sug.	Prot.	Sod.
Extra Crispy, Breast (176g)									
	510	33	7	110	16	0	1	39	1010
Extra Crispy, Drumstick (59g)									
	150	10	2	55	5	0	0	12	360
Extra Crispy, Thigh (110g)									
	340	24	5	80	10	0	0	20	780
Extra Crispy, Whole Wing (56g)									
	190	13	2.5	55	6	0	0	12	410
Grilled, Breast (152g)									
	220	7	2	135	0	0	0	40	730
Grilled, Drumstick (50g)									
	90	4	1	60	0	0	0	13	290
Grilled, Thigh (88g)									
	170	10	3	90	0	0	0	19	530
Grilled, Whole Wing (37g)									
	80	4.5	1.5	50	1	0	0	10	250
Original Recipe, Breast (163g)									
	360	21	5	110	11	0	0	34	1080

Food Serving size	Cal.	(g) Total Fat	(g) Sat. Fat	(mg) Chol.	(g) Carb.	(g) Fiber	(g) Sug.	(g) Prot.	(mg) Sod.
Original Recipe, Breast Without Skin or Breading (116g)									
	160	3.5	1	85	2	0	0	31	580
Original Recipe, Drumstick (51g)									
	120	7	1.5	45	3	0	0	11	310
Original Recipe, Thigh (96g)									
	250	17	4.5	80	7	0	0	17	730
Original Recipe, Whole Wing (49g)									
	120	7	1.5	50	3	0	0	11	380
Spicy Crispy, Breast (178g)									
	420	25	5	110	12	1	0	38	1250
Spicy Crispy, Drumstick (55g)									
	160	10	2	50	5	0	0	11	440
Spicy Crispy, Thigh (111g)									
	360	27	6	85	13	1	0	17	1010
Spicy Crispy, Whole Wing (51g)									
	170	12	2.5	45	6	0	0	11	470

Desserts

Food Serving size	Cal.	(g) Total Fat	(g) Sat. Fat	(mg) Chol.	(g) Carb.	(g) Fiber	(g) Sug.	(g) Prot.	(mg) Sod.
Apple Turnover (1) (85g)									
	250	12	3	0	33	2	12	2	160
Caf Valley Bakery Chocolate Chip Cake (6 Slices per Cake)									
	300	15	3	50	39	1	27	4	260
Lil' Bucket Chocolate Céme Parfait Cup (113g)									
	280	13	8	0	37	1	23	2	240
Lil' Bucket Lemon Créme Parfait Cup (127g)									
	400	13	7	5	65	2	50	7	220
Lil' Bucket Strawberry Shortcake Parfait Cup (99g)									
	200	7	3.5	20	35	2	23	2	140
Oreo Cookies and Créme Pie Slice (74g)									
	290	16	10	5	34	1	23	3	210
Reese's Peanut Butter Pie Slice (71g)									
	310	19	10	5	31	1	22	5	200
Sweet Life Chocolate Chip Cookie (32g)									
	160	8	4	10	21	1	14	2	85
Sweet Life Oatmeal Raisin Cookie (32g)									
	150	6	2.5	10	22	1	12	2	90

Food Serving size	Cal.	(g) Total Fat	(g) Sat. Fat	(mg) Chol.	(g) Carb.	(g) Fiber	(g) Sug.	(g) Prot.	(mg) Sod.
Other									
Colonel's Buttery Spread (6g)									
	30	3.5	0.5	0	0	0	0	0	30
Country Fried Steak with Peppered White Gravy (162g)									
	420	29	9	40	25	2	0	16	1130
Country Fried Steak Without Peppered White Gravy (117g)									
	390	27	9	40	21	2	0	15	960
Creamy Ranch Dipping Sauce Cup (25g)									
	140	15	2.5	10	1	0	1	0	230
HBBQ Dipping Sauce Cup (25g)									
	40	0	0	0	9	0	8	0	310
Honey Mustard Dipping Sauce Cup (25g)									
	120	10	1.5	5	6	0	5	0	110
Honey Sauce Packet (9g)									
	30	0	0	0	8	0	5	0	0
Jalapeno Peppers (32g)									
	20	1.5	0	0	1	1	0	0	480
KFC Gizzards (55g)									
	200	11	2	100	15	1	0	11	800
KFC Livers (55g)									
	180	10	2	200	11	0	0	11	620
KFC Signature Sauce Dipping Cup (25g)									
	70	5	1	10	5	0	4	0	135
Sargento Light String Cheese (21g)									
	50	2.5	1.5	10	1	0	0	6	160
Spicy Chipotle Dipping Sauce Cup (25g)									
	70	3.5	1	10	8	1	3	0	220
Sweet and Sour Dipping Sauce Cup (25g)									
	45	0	0	0	12	0	10	0	95
Popcorn Chicken									
Individual (122g)									
	400	26	6	45	18	1	0	22	1040
Kids (81g)									
	260	17	3.5	30	12	1	0	15	690

Food Serving size	Cal.	(g) Total Fat	(g) Sat. Fat	(mg) Chol.	(g) Carb.	(g) Fiber	(g) Sug.	(g) Prot.	(mg) Sod.
Large (174g)	560	37	8	65	26	2	0	32	1480

Pot Pies, Bowls, and Value Boxes

Chicken Pot Pie (400g)	790	45	37	75	66	3	7	29	1970
Extra Crispy Drumstick Value Box (166g)	440	25	4.5	55	39	2	0	16	1160
Extra Crispy Thigh Value Box (217g)	630	39	8	80	45	2	0	24	1580
Fiery Buffalo Hot Wings Value Box (194g)	510	28	4.5	55	51	4	0	15	1610
Grilled Drumstick Value Box (158g)	380	19	3.5	60	34	2	0	17	1090
Grilled Thigh Value Box (196g)	460	25	5	90	34	2	0	23	1330
HBBQ Hot Wings Value Box (199g)	540	28	4.5	55	58	3	6	15	1530
Hot Wings Value Box (173g)	490	27	4.5	55	45	3	0	15	1220
KFC Famous Bowls - Mashed Potato with Gravy (525g)	680	31	8	45	74	6	3	26	2130
Original Recipe Drumstick Value Box (159g)	400	22	4	45	37	2	0	15	1110
Original Recipe Value Box (204g)	540	32	7	80	42	2	0	20	1540
Popcorn Chicken Value Box (230g)	680	41	8	45	53	4	0	26	1850
Snack-size Bowl (183g)	260	13	4	25	26	1	1	12	760

Salads and More

Caesar Side Salad Without Dressing and Croutons (91g)	40	2	1	5	2	1	1	3	90
Crispy Chicken BLT Salad Without Dressing (374g)	360	19	3.5	75	18	4	5	30	1120

Food Serving size	Cal.	(g) Total Fat	(g) Sat. Fat	(mg) Chol.	(g) Carb.	(g) Fiber	(g) Sug.	(g) Prot.	(mg) Sod.
Crispy Chicken Caesar Salad Without Dressing/Croutons (313g)									
	340	18	4.5	70	16	3	3	28	930
Heinz Buttermilk Ranch Dressing (1) (28g)									
	160	17	2	10	1	0	1	0	220
Hidden Valley - The Original Ranch Fat Free Dressing (1) (43g)									
	35	0	0	0	8	0	2	1	410
House Side Salad Without Dressing (105g)									
	15	0	0	0	3	1	2	1	10
KFC Creamy Parmesan Caesar Dressing (1) (57g)									
	260	26	5	15	4	0	2	2	540
Marzetti Light Italian Dressing (1) (28g)									
	15	0.5	0	0	2	0	1	0	510
Parmesan Garlic Croutons Pouch (1) (14g)									
	70	3	0	0	8	0	0	1	160

Sandwiches

Food Serving size	Cal.	(g) Total Fat	(g) Sat. Fat	(mg) Chol.	(g) Carb.	(g) Fiber	(g) Sug.	(g) Prot.	(mg) Sod.
Crispy Twister (247g)									
	610	33	6	75	52	3	4	28	1380
Crispy Twister Without Sauce (225g)									
	490	20	3.5	60	51	3	3	28	1260
Double Down with Original Recipe Filet (248g)									
	610	37	11	150	18	1	1	52	1880
Doublicious with Original Recipe Filet (188g)									
	520	25	7	85	40	2	6	32	1180
Honey BBQ Sandwich (161g)									
	320	3.5	1	70	47	3	21	24	770
KFC Snacker with Crispy Strip (120g)									
	310	15	2.5	35	30	2	4	15	600
KFC Snacker with Crispy Strip Without Sauce (110g)									
	260	9	1.5	30	29	2	4	15	550
KFC Snacker with Crispy Strip, Buffalo (120g)									
	270	9	1.5	30	31	2	4	15	720
KFC Snacker with Crispy Strip, Ultimate Cheese (119g)									
	280	11	2	30	31	2	4	15	700
KFC Snacker, Honey BBQ (98g)									
	210	3	1	35	32	2	12	13	470

Food Serving size	Cal.	(g) Total Fat	(g) Sat. Fat	(mg) Chol.	(g) Carb.	(g) Fiber	(g) Sug.	(g) Prot.	(mg) Sod.
Sides (Individual)									
BBQ Baked Beans (138g)	210	1.5	0	0	41	8	18	8	780
Biscuit (54g)	180	8	6	0	23	1	2	4	530
Cole Slaw (114g)	150	6	1	0	21	2	16	1	135
Corn on the Cob (3") (71g)	70	0.5	0	0	16	2	3	2	0
Corn on the Cob (5.5") (146g)	140	1	0	0	33	4	5	5	5
Green Beans (86g)	25	0	0	0	4	2	1	1	260
KFC Cornbread Muffin (52g)	210	9	1.5	35	28	0	11	3	240
Macaroni and Cheese (135g)	160	7	2.5	5	19	1	2	5	720
Macaroni Salad (117g)	190	10	2	5	22	1	6	4	430
Mashed Potatoes with Gravy (145g)	120	4	1	0	19	1	0	2	530
Mashed Potatoes Without Gravy (102g)	90	3	0.5	0	15	1	0	2	320
Potato Salad (135g)	210	11	2.5	10	26	3	6	2	560
Potato Wedges (108g)	290	15	2.5	0	35	2	0	4	810
Sweet Kernel Corn (95g)	100	0.5	0	0	21	2	3	3	0
Strips & Filets									
Crispy Strips (2) (110g)	260	14	2	60	11	0	0	21	750
Crispy Strips (3) (165g)	390	21	3	85	17	0	0	32	1130
KFC Original Recipe Filet (100g)	200	9	1.5	55	8	1	0	22	670

Food Serving size	Cal.	(g) Total Fat	(g) Sat. Fat	(mg) Chol.	(g) Carb.	(g) Fiber	(g) Sug.	(g) Prot.	(mg) Sod.
Wings									
Hot Wings (1) (22g)	70	4	0.5	20	4	0	0	4	140

LONG JOHN SILVER'S

Alaskan Pollock and Seafood

Food Serving size	Cal.	(g) Total Fat	(g) Sat. Fat	(mg) Chol.	(g) Carb.	(g) Fiber	(g) Sug.	(g) Prot.	(mg) Sod.
Battered Alaskan Pollock (1 Piece)	260	16	4	35	17	0	0	12	790
Battered Shrimp (3 Pieces)	130	9	2.5	45	8	0	0	5	480
Breaded Clam Strips (1 Snack Box)	320	19	4.5	35	29	2	1	9	1190
Buttered Langostino Lobster Bites (1 Snack Box)	230	9	3	60	24	2	0	13	520
Grilled Pacific Salmon (2 Filets)	150	5	1	50	2	0	1	24	440
Grilled Tilapia (1 Filet)	110	2.5	1	55	1	0	1	22	250
Langostino Lobster Stuffed Crab Cake (1 Cake)	170	9	2	30	16	1	0	6	390
Popcorn Shrimp (1 Snack Box)	270	16	4	75	23	1	1	9	570
Shrimp Scampi (8 Pieces)	200	13	2.5	135	3	0	1	17	650

Beverages

Food Serving size	Cal.	(g) Total Fat	(g) Sat. Fat	(mg) Chol.	(g) Carb.	(g) Fiber	(g) Sug.	(g) Prot.	(mg) Sod.
Diet Mountain Dew (Kids) (12 fl oz)	0	0	0	0	0	0	0	0	60
Diet Mountain Dew (Large) (40 fl oz)	0	0	0	0	0	0	0	0	200
Diet Mountain Dew (Medium) (32 fl oz)	0	0	0	0	0	0	0	0	160
Diet Mountain Dew (Small) (20 fl oz)	0	0	0	0	0	0	0	0	100

Food Serving size	Cal.	(g) Total Fat	(g) Sat. Fat	(mg) Chol.	(g) Carb.	(g) Fiber	(g) Sug.	(g) Prot.	(mg) Sod.
Diet Pepsi (Kids) (12 fl oz)									
	0	0	0	0	0	0	0	0	35
Diet Pepsi (Large) (40 fl oz)									
	0	0	0	0	0	0	0	0	125
Diet Pepsi (Medium) (32 fl oz)									
	0	0	0	0	0	0	0	0	100
Diet Pepsi (Small) (20 fl oz)									
	0	0	0	0	0	0	0	0	60
Dr Pepper (Kids) (12 fl oz)									
	150	0	0	0	40	0	40	0	50
Dr Pepper (Large) (40 fl oz)									
	500	0	0	0	135	0	135	0	175
Dr Pepper (Medium) (32 fl oz)									
	400	0	0	0	108	0	108	0	140
Dr Pepper (Small) (20 fl oz)									
	250	0	0	0	67	0	67	0	85
Iced Tea (Unsweetened) (Kids) (12 fl oz)									
	0	0	0	0	0	0	0	0	0
Iced Tea (Unsweetened) (Large) (40 fl oz)									
	0	0	0	0	0	0	0	0	0
Iced Tea (Unsweetened) (Medium) (32 fl oz)									
	0	0	0	0	0	0	0	0	0
Iced Tea (Unsweetened) (Small) (20 fl oz)									
	0	0	0	0	0	0	0	0	0
Lipton Raspberry Tea (Kids) (12 fl oz)									
	120	0	0	0	31	0	31	0	35
Lipton Raspberry Tea (Large) (40 fl oz)									
	400	0	0	0	105	0	105	0	125
Lipton Raspberry Tea (Medium) (32 fl oz)									
	320	0	0	0	84	0	84	0	100
Lipton Raspberry Tea (Small) (20 fl oz)									
	200	0	0	0	52	0	52	0	60
Mounatain Dew (Kids) (12 fl oz)									
	160	0	0	0	43	0	43	0	50
Mountain Dew (Large) (40 fl oz)									
	550	0	0	0	145	0	145	0	170

Food Serving size	Cal.	(g) Total Fat	(g) Sat. Fat	(mg) Chol.	(g) Carb.	(g) Fiber	(g) Sug.	(g) Prot.	(mg) Sod.
Mountain Dew (Medium) (32 fl oz)									
	440	0	0	0	116	0	116	0	140
Mountain Dew (Small) (20 fl oz)									
	270	0	0	0	72	0	72	0	85
Pepsi (Kids) (12 fl oz)									
	150	0	0	0	42	0	40	0	35
Pepsi (Large) (40 fl oz)									
	500	0	0	0	140	0	135	0	125
Pepsi (Medium) (32 fl oz)									
	400	0	0	0	112	0	108	0	100
Pepsi (Small) (20 fl oz)									
	250	0	0	0	70	0	67	0	60
Sierra Mist (Kids) (12 fl oz)									
	150	0	0	0	40	0	40	0	30
Sierra Mist (Large) (40 fl oz)									
	500	0	0	0	135	0	135	0	100
Sierra Mist (Medium) (32 fl oz)									
	400	0	0	0	108	0	108	0	80
Sierra Mist (Small) (20 fl oz)									
	250	0	0	0	67	0	67	0	50
Tropicana Fruit Punch (Kids)									
	160	0	0	0	45	0	45	0	35
Tropicana Fruit Punch (Large) (40 fl oz)									
	550	0	0	0	150	0	150	0	125
Tropicana Fruit Punch (Medium) (32 fl oz)									
	440	0	0	0	120	0	120	0	100
Tropicana Fruit Punch (Small) (20 fl oz)									
	270	0	0	0	75	0	75	0	60
Tropicana Lemonade (Kids) (12 fl oz)									
	150	0	0	0	41	0	41	0	160
Tropicana Lemonade (Large) (40 fl oz)									
	500	0	0	0	135	0	135	0	525
Tropicana Lemonade (Medium) (32 fl oz)									
	400	0	0	0	108	0	108	0	420
Tropicana Lemonade (Small) (20 fl oz)									
	250	0	0	0	68	0	68	0	265

Food Serving size	Cal.	(g) Total Fat	(g) Sat. Fat	(mg) Chol.	(g) Carb.	(g) Fiber	(g) Sug.	(g) Prot.	(mg) Sod.
Tropicana Twister Orange (Kids) (12 fl oz)									
	170	0	0	0	47	0	45	0	40
Tropicana Twister Orange (Large) (40 fl oz)									
	550	0	0	0	155	0	150	0	125
Tropicana Twister Orange (Medium) (32 fl oz)									
	440	0	0	0	124	0	120	0	100
Tropicana Twister Orange (Small) (20 fl oz)									
	280	0	0	0	78	0	75	0	65
Wild Cherry Pepsi (Kids) (12 fl oz)									
	150	0	0	0	42	0	42	0	30
Wild Cherry Pepsi (Large) (40 fl oz)									
	500	0	0	0	140	0	140	0	100
Wild Cherry Pepsi (Medium) (32 fl oz)									
	400	0	0	0	112	0	112	0	80
Wild Cherry Pepsi (Small) (20 fl oz)									
	250	0	0	0	70	0	70	0	50

Chicken Strips

Chicken Strips (1 Piece)									
	140	8	2	20	9	0	0	8	480

Desserts

Chocolate Cream Pie (1 Slice)									
	280	17	10	10	28	1	19	3	230
Pineapple Cream Pie (1 Slice)									
	300	17	11	10	35	0	25	3	250

Iceflow Lemonade

Iceflow Lemonade (16 oz Cup)									
	190	0	0	0	47	0	40	0	15
Iceflow Lemonade (20 oz Cup)									
	240	0	0	0	60	0	50	0	15
Strawberry Iceflow Lemonade (16 oz Cup)									
	240	0	0	0	60	0	48	0	15
Strawberry Iceflow Lemonade (20 oz Cup)									
	310	0	0	0	79	0	62	0	20

Food Serving size	Cal.	(g) Total Fat	(g) Sat. Fat	(mg) Chol.	(g) Carb.	(g) Fiber	(g) Sug.	(g) Prot.	(mg) Sod.
Sandwiches and More									
Alaskan Pollock Sandwich (1 Sandwich)									
	470	23	5	40	49	3	4	18	1180
Baja Chicken Strip Taco (1 Taco)									
	370	23	5	25	31	3	2	11	890
Baja Fish Taco (1 Taco)									
	360	23	4.5	25	30	3	2	9	810
Chicken Strip Sandwich (1 Sandwich)									
	440	30	6	50	47	4	2	22	1350
Freshside Grille Salmon Entrée (1 Plate)									
	280	7	2	50	27	3	5	27	1010
Freshside Grille Shrimp Scampi (1 Plate)									
	330	15	3.5	135	29	3	5	20	1230
Freshside Grille Tilapia Entrée (1 Plate)									
	250	4.5	2	60	27	3	4	25	820
Ultimate Alaskan Pollock Sandwich (1 Sandwich)									
	530	27	8	55	50	3	4	21	1500
Zesty Chicken Strip Sandwich (1 Sandwich)									
	380	19	4	25	39	3	2	14	880
Sauces/Condiments									
BBQ (1 Dipping Cup)									
	40	0	0	0	10	0	6	0	230
Cocktail Sauce (1 oz)									
	25	0	0	0	6	0	5	0	250
Honey Mustard (1 Dipping Cup)									
	100	6	1.5	0	12	0	6	0	170
Ketchup (1 Packet)									
	10	0	0	0	2	0	2	0	100
Lemon Juice (1 Packet)									
	0	0	0	0	0	0	0	0	0
Louisiana Hot Sauce (1 Teaspoon)									
	0	0	0	0	0	0	0	0	140
Malt Vinegar (0.5 oz)									
	0	0	0	0	0	0	0	0	35

Food Serving size	Cal.	(g) Total Fat	(g) Sat. Fat	(mg) Chol.	(g) Carb.	(g) Fiber	(g) Sug.	(g) Prot.	(mg) Sod.
Marina (1 Dipping Cup)									
	15	0	0	0	4	1	2	1	125
Ranch (1 Dipping Cup)									
	160	17	2.5	15	2	0	1	0	240
Sweet and Sour (1 Dipping Cup)									
	45	0	0	0	12	0	7	0	120
Tartar Sauce (1 oz)									
	100	9	1.5	15	4	0	3	0	250

Sides

Food Serving size	Cal.	(g) Total Fat	(g) Sat. Fat	(mg) Chol.	(g) Carb.	(g) Fiber	(g) Sug.	(g) Prot.	(mg) Sod.
Breaded Mozzarella Sticks (3 Pieces)									
	150	9	3.5	10	13	1	0	5	350
Breadstick (1 Breadstick)									
	170	3.5	1	0	29	1	2	6	290
Broccoli Cheese Bites (5 Pieces)									
	230	12	4.5	15	25	2	2	5	550
Broccoli Cheese Soup (1 Bowl)									
	220	18	8	30	8	1	2	5	650
Cole Slaw (4 oz)									
	200	15	2.5	20	15	3	10	1	340
Corn Cobbette with Butter Oil									
	150	10	2	0	14	3	6	3	30
Corn Cobbette Without Butter Oil									
	90	3	0.5	0	4	3	6	3	0
Crumblies (1 oz)									
	170	12	2.5	0	14	1	0	1	410
Fries - Basket Combo Portion (4 oz)									
	310	14	3.5	0	45	4	0	3	460
Fries - Platter Portion (3 oz)									
	230	10	2.5	0	34	3	0	3	350
Hushpuppy (1 Pup)									
	60	2.5	0.5	0	9	1	1	1	200
Jalapeno Cheddar Bites (5 Pieces)									
	240	14	5	15	23	2	2	6	730
Jalapeno Peppers (1 Whole Pepper)									
	15	0	0	0	2	0	1	1	190

Food Serving size	Cal.	(g) Total Fat	(g) Sat. Fat	(mg) Chol.	(g) Carb.	(g) Fiber	(g) Sug.	(g) Prot.	(mg) Sod.
Rice (5 oz)	180	1	0.5	0	37	2	1	4	470
Vegetable Medley (4 oz)	50	2	0.5	0	8	3	3	1	360

McDONALD's

Beverages

1% Low Fat Chocolate Milk (1 carton)	170	3	1.5	5	26	1	25	9	150
1% Low Fat Milk Jug (1 carton)	100	2.5	1.5	10	12	0	12	8	125
Coca-Cola Classic (Child) (12 fl oz)	110	0	0	0	29	0	29	0	5
Coca-Cola Classic (Large) (32 fl oz)	310	0	0	0	86	0	86	0	20
Coca-Cola Classic (Medium) (21 fl oz)	210	0	0	0	58	0	58	0	15
Coca-Cola Classic (Small) (16 fl oz)	150	0	0	0	40	0	40	0	10
Coffee (Large) (16 fl oz)	0	0	0	0	0	0	0	0	0
Coffee (Small) (12 fl oz)	0	0	0	0	0	0	0	0	0
Coffee Cream (0.4 fl oz)	20	2	1.5	10	0	0	0	0	15
Dasani Water (16.9 fl oz)	0	0	0	0	0	0	0	0	0
Diet Coke (Child) (12 fl oz)	0	0	0	0	0	0	0	0	15
Diet Coke (Large) (32 fl oz)	0	0	0	0	0	0	0	0	45
Diet Coke (Medium) (21 fl oz)	0	0	0	0	0	0	0	0	30
Diet Coke (Small) (16 fl oz)	0	0	0	0	0	0	0	0	20

Food Serving size	Cal.	(g) Total Fat	(g) Sat. Fat	(mg) Chol.	(g) Carb.	(g) Fiber	(g) Sug.	(g) Prot.	(mg) Sod.
Equal 0 Calorie Sweetener (1 Package)									
	0	0	0	0	1	0	1	0	0
Hi-C Orange Lavaburst (Child) (12 fl oz)									
	120	0	0	0	32	0	32	0	0
Hi-C Orange Lavaburst (Large) (32 fl oz)									
	350	0	0	0	94	0	94	0	10
Hi-C Orange Lavaburst (Medium) (21 fl oz)									
	240	0	0	0	64	0	64	0	10
Hi-C Orange Lavaburst (Small) (16 fl oz)									
	160	0	0	0	44	0	44	0	5
Iced Coffee - Caramel (Large) (17 fl oz)									
	270	11	7	40	41	0	41	2	160
Iced Coffee - Caramel (Medium) (11.5 fl oz)									
	190	8	5	30	27	0	27	2	115
Iced Coffee - Caramel (Small) (8 fl oz)									
	130	5	3.5	20	21	0	21	1	80
Iced Coffee - Hazelnut (Large) (17 fl oz)									
	270	11	7	40	43	0	43	2	85
Iced Coffee - Hazelnut (Medium) (11.5 fl oz)									
	190	8	5	30	29	0	29	2	60
Iced Coffee - Hazelnut (Small) (8 fl oz)									
	130	5	3.5	20	21	0	21	1	40
Iced Coffee - Regular (Large) (17 fl oz)									
	280	11	7	40	45	0	45	2	85
Iced Coffee - Regular (Medium) (11.5 fl oz)									
	200	8	5	30	30	0	30	2	60
Iced Coffee - Regular (Small) (8 fl oz)									
	140	5	3.5	20	22	0	22	1	40
Iced Coffee - Vanilla (Large) (32 fl oz)									
	270	11	7	40	43	0	43	2	80
Iced Coffee - Vanilla (Medium) (11.5 fl oz)									
	190	8	5	30	29	0	28	2	60
Iced Coffee - Vanilla (Small) (8 fl oz)									
	130	5	3.5	20	21	0	21	1	40
Iced Coffee with Sugar Free Vanilla Syrup (Large) (17 fl oz)									
	120	11	7	40	16	0	2	2	140

Food Serving size	Cal.	(g) Total Fat	(g) Sat. Fat	(mg) Chol.	(g) Carb.	(g) Fiber	(g) Sug.	(g) Prot.	(mg) Sod.
Iced Coffee with Sugar Free Vanilla Syrup (Medium) (11.5 fl oz)									
	90	8	5	30	11	0	2	2	100
Iced Coffee with Sugar Free Vanilla Syrup (Small) (8 fl oz)									
	60	5	3.5	20	8	0	1	1	70
Iced Tea (Child) (12 fl oz)									
	0	0	0	0	0	0	0	0	5
Iced Tea (Large) (32 fl oz)									
	0	0	0	0	1	0	0	0	20
Iced Tea (Medium) (21 fl oz)									
	0	0	0	0	0	0	0	0	15
Iced Tea (Small) (16 fl oz)									
	0	0	0	0	0	0	0	0	10
Minute Maid 100% Apple Juice Box (6.8 fl oz)									
	100	0	0	0	23	0	22	0	15
Minute Maid Orange Juice (Large) (22 fl oz)									
	280	0	0	0	58	0	58	4	5
Minute Maid Orange Juice (Medium) (16 fl oz)									
	190	0	0	0	39	0	39	3	0
Minute Maid Orange Juice (Small) (12 fl oz)									
	150	0	0	0	30	0	30	2	0
Powerade Mountain Blast (Child) (12 fl oz)									
	70	0	0	0	20	0	16	0	65
Powerade Mountain Blast (Large) (32 fl oz)									
	220	0	0	0	58	0	46	0	190
Powerade Mountain Blast (Medium) (21 fl oz)									
	150	0	0	0	39	0	31	0	130
Powerade Mountain Blast (Small) (16 fl oz)									
	100	0	0	0	27	0	21	0	85
Splenda No Calorie Sweetener (1 Package)									
	0	0	0	0	1	0	1	0	0
Sprite (Child) (12 fl oz)									
	110	0	0	0	28	0	28	0	30
Sprite (Large) (32 fl oz)									
	310	0	0	0	83	0	83	0	80
Sprite (Medium) (21 fl oz)									
	210	0	0	0	56	0	56	0	55

Food Serving size	Cal.	(g) Total Fat	(g) Sat. Fat	(mg) Chol.	(g) Carb.	(g) Fiber	(g) Sug.	(g) Prot.	(mg) Sod.
Sprite (Small) (16 fl oz)									
	150	0	0	0	39	0	39	0	40
Sugar Packet (1 package)									
	15	0	0	0	4	0	4	0	0
Sweet Tea (Child) (12 fl oz)									
	110	0	0	0	27	0	27	0	5
Sweet Tea (Large) (32 fl oz)									
	280	0	0	0	69	0	69	1	15
Sweet Tea (Medium) (21 fl oz)									
	180	0	0	0	45	0	45	1	10
Sweet Tea (Small) (16 fl oz)									
	150	0	0	0	36	0	36	1	10

Breakfast

Food Serving size	Cal.	Total Fat	Sat. Fat	Chol.	Carb.	Fiber	Sug.	Prot.	Sod.
Bacon, Egg and Cheese Bagel (6.5 oz)									
	560	27	9	260	56	3	7	24	1300
Bacon, Egg and Cheese Biscuit (Large Size Biscuit) (5.4 oz)									
	480	27	12	235	43	3	4	15	1270
Bacon, Egg and Cheese Biscuit (Regular Size Biscuit) (4.9 oz)									
	420	23	12	235	37	2	3	15	1160
Bacon, Egg and Cheese McGriddles (6.3 oz)									
	420	18	8	240	48	2	15	15	1110
Big Breakfast (Large Size Biscuit) (10 oz)									
	800	52	18	555	56	4	3	28	1680
Big Breakfast (Regular Size Biscuit) (9.5 oz)									
	740	48	17	555	51	3	3	28	1560
Big Breakfast with Hotcakes (Large Size Biscuit) (15.3 oz)									
	1150	60	20	575	116	7	17	36	2260
Big Breakfast with Hotcakes (Regular Size Biscuit) (14.8 oz)									
	1090	56	19	575	111	6	17	36	2150
Egg McMuffin (7.1 oz)									
	300	12	5	260	30	2	3	18	820
English Muffin (4.3 oz)									
	160	3	0.5	0	27	2	2	5	280
Fruit and Maple Oatmeal (9.2 oz)									
	290	4.5	2	10	57	5	32	5	160

Food Serving size	Cal.	(g) Total Fat	(g) Sat. Fat	(mg) Chol.	(g) Carb.	(g) Fiber	(g) Sug.	(g) Prot.	(mg) Sod.
Fruit and Maple Oatmeal Without Brown Sugar (9.2 oz)									
	260	4.5	2	10	48	5	18	5	115
Grape Jam (0.5 oz)									
	35	0	0	0	9	0	9	0	0
Hash Brown (2 oz)									
	150	9	1.5	0	15	2	0	1	310
Hotcake Syrup (1 Package)									
	180	0	0	0	45	0	32	0	20
Hotcakes (5.3 oz)									
	350	9	2	20	60	3	14	8	590
Hotcakes and Sausages (6.8 oz)									
	520	24	7	50	61	3	14	15	930
McSkillet Burrito with Sausage (8.4 oz)									
	610	36	14	410	44	3	4	27	1390
Sausage Biscuit (Large Size Biscuit) (4.6 oz)									
	480	31	13	30	39	3	3	11	1190
Sausage Biscuit (Regular Size Biscuit) (4.1 oz)									
	430	27	12	30	34	2	2	11	1080
Sausage Biscuit with Egg (Large Size Biscuit) (6.2 oz)									
	570	37	15	250	42	3	3	18	1280
Sausage Biscuit with Egg (Regular Size Biscuit) (5.7 oz)									
	510	33	14	250	36	2	2	18	1170
Sausage Burrito (3.9 oz)									
	300	16	7	115	26	1	2	12	830
Sausage McGriddles (5 oz)									
	420	22	8	35	44	2	15	11	1030
Sausage McMuffin (6.2 oz)									
	370	22	8	45	29	2	2	14	850
Sausage McMuffin with Egg (8 oz)									
	450	27	10	285	30	2	2	21	920
Sausage, Egg and Cheese McGriddles (7.6 oz)									
	560	32	12	265	48	2	15	20	1360
Southern Style Chicken Biscuit (Large Size Biscuit) (5.5 oz)									
	470	24	9	30	46	3	4	17	1290
Southern Style Chicken Biscuit (Regular Size Biscuit) (5 oz)									
	410	20	8	30	41	2	3	17	1180

Food Serving size	Cal.	(g) Total Fat	(g) Sat. Fat	(mg) Chol.	(g) Carb.	(g) Fiber	(g) Sug.	(g) Prot.	(mg) Sod.
Steak, Egg and Cheese Bagel (9.2 oz)									
	660	33	12	300	56	3	7	33	1580
Strawberry Preserves (0.5 oz)									
	35	0	0	0	9	0	9	0	0
Whipped Margarine (1 Pat)									
	40	4.5	1.5	0	0	0	0	0	55

Chicken McNuggets/Chicken Selects Premium Breast Strips/Sauces

Food Serving size	Cal.	(g) Total Fat	(g) Sat. Fat	(mg) Chol.	(g) Carb.	(g) Fiber	(g) Sug.	(g) Prot.	(mg) Sod.
Barbecue Sauce (1 Package)									
	50	0	0	0	12	0	10	0	260
Chicken McNuggets (10 Piece)									
	470	30	5	65	30	2	0	22	900
Chicken McNuggets (4 Piece)									
	190	12	2	25	12	1	0	9	360
Chicken McNuggets (6 Piece)									
	280	18	3	40	18	1	0	13	540
Chicken Select Premium Breast Strips (3 Pieces)									
	400	24	3.5	50	23	0	0	23	1010
Chicken Select Premium Breast Strips (5 Pieces)									
	660	40	6	85	39	0	0	38	1680
Creamy Ranch Sauce (1.3 oz)									
	170	18	3	10	2	0	1	0	270
Honey (1 Package)									
	50	0	0	0	12	0	11	0	0
Hot Mustard Sauce (1 Package)									
	60	2.5	0	5	9	2	6	1	250
Southwestern Chipotle Barbecue Sauce (1.3 oz)									
	60	0	0	0	15	1	11	0	210
Spicy Buffalo Sauce (1.3 oz)									
	60	6	1	0	1	1	0	0	800
Sweet 'N Sour Sauce (1 Package)									
	50	0	0	0	12	0	10	0	150
Tangy Honey Mustard Sauce (1.3 oz)									
	60	2	0	5	10	0	8	0	140

Food Serving size	Cal.	(g) Total Fat	(g) Sat. Fat	(mg) Chol.	(g) Carb.	(g) Fiber	(g) Sug.	(g) Prot.	(mg) Sod.
Desserts/Shakes									
Apple Dippers with Low Fat Caramel Dip (3.1 oz)									
	100	0.5	0	5	23	0	15	0	35
Baked Hot Apple Pie (2.7 oz)									
	250	13	7	0	32	4	13	2	170
Chocolate Chip Cookie (1 Cookie)									
	160	8	3.5	10	21	1	15	2	90
Chocolate McCafe Shake (10.2 oz Serving Size)									
	580	17	10	50	94	1	77	11	240
Chocolate McCafe Shake (12.9 oz Serving Size)									
	720	20	12	60	119	1	98	15	300
Chocolate McCafe Shake (15.8 oz Serving Size)									
	880	24	15	75	147	1	121	18	370
Chocolate Triple Thick Shake (12 fl oz Cup)									
	440	10	6	40	76	1	63	10	190
Chocolate Triple Thick Shake (16 fl oz Cup)									
	580	14	8	50	102	1	84	13	250
Chocolate Triple Thick Shake (21 fl oz Cup)									
	770	18	11	70	134	1	111	18	330
Chocolate Triple Thick Shake (32 fl oz Cup)									
	1160	27	16	100	203	2	168	27	510
Cinnamon Melts (4 oz)									
	460	19	9	15	66	3	32	6	370
Fruit 'n Yogurt Parfait (5.3 oz)									
	160	2	1	5	31	1	21	4	85
Hot Caramel Sundae (6.4 oz)									
	340	8	5	30	60	1	44	7	160
Hot Fudge Sundae (6.3 oz)									
	330	10	7	25	54	2	48	8	180
Kiddie Cone (1 oz)									
	45	1	0.5	5	8	0	6	1	20
Low Fat Caramel Dip (0.8 oz)									
	70	0.5	0	5	15	0	9	0	35
McDonaldland Cookies (2 oz)									
	260	8	2.5	0	43	1	13	4	300

Food Serving size	Cal.	(g) Total Fat	(g) Sat. Fat	(mg) Chol.	(g) Carb.	(g) Fiber	(g) Sug.	(g) Prot.	(mg) Sod.
McFlurry with M&M'S Candies (12.5 fl oz Serving Size)									
	710	25	16	60	105	4	97	15	220
McFlurry with Oreo Cookies (12 fl oz Cup)									
	580	19	10	50	89	3	73	13	320
Oatmeal Raisin Cookie (1 Cookie)									
	150	6	2.5	10	22	1	13	2	135
Peanuts (for Sundaes) (0.3 oz)									
	45	3.5	0.5	0	2	1	0	2	0
Snack Size McFlurry with M&M'S Candies (7.3 oz)									
	430	16	10	35	64	2	59	9	130
Snack Size McFlurry with Oreo Cookies (6.7 oz)									
	340	12	6	30	53	2	43	8	200
Strawberry McCafe Shake (10.5 oz Serving Size)									
	570	17	10	50	92	0	79	11	170
Strawberry McCafe Shake (13.4 oz Serving Size)									
	710	20	12	65	116	0	100	14	210
Strawberry McCafe Shake (16.5 oz Serving Size)									
	860	24	15	75	144	0	124	18	260
Strawberry Sundae (6.3 oz)									
	280	6	4	25	49	1	45	6	95
Strawberry Triple Thick Shake (12 fl oz Cup)									
	420	10	6	40	73	0	63	10	130
Strawberry Triple Thick Shake (16 fl oz Cup)									
	560	13	8	50	97	0	84	13	170
Strawberry Triple Thick Shake (21 fl oz Cup)									
	740	18	11	70	128	0	111	17	230
Strawberry Triple Thick Shake (32 fl oz Cup)									
	1110	26	16	100	194	0	168	25	350
Sugar Cookie (1 Cookie)									
	160	7	3	5	21	0	11	2	120
Vanilla McCafe Shake (12.8 oz Serving Size)									
	680	20	12	60	111	0	82	14	220
Vanilla McCafe Shake (16 oz Serving Size)									
	830	24	14	75	138	0	103	17	270
Vanilla McCafe Shake (9.9 oz Serving Size)									
	540	16	10	45	88	0	64	10	170

Food Serving size	Cal.	(g) Total Fat	(g) Sat. Fat	(mg) Chol.	(g) Carb.	(g) Fiber	(g) Sug.	(g) Prot.	(mg) Sod.
Vanilla Reduced Fat Ice Cream Cone (3.2 oz)									
	150	3.5	2	15	24	0	18	4	60
Vanilla Triple Thick Shake (12 fl oz Cup)									
	420	10	6	40	72	0	54	9	140
Vanilla Triple Thick Shake (16 fl oz Cup)									
	550	13	8	50	96	0	72	13	190
Vanilla Triple Thick Shake (21 fl oz Cup)									
	740	18	11	70	128	0	96	17	250
Vanilla Triple Thick Shake (32 fl oz Cup)									
	1110	26	16	100	193	0	145	25	370

French Fries

Food	Cal.	Total Fat	Sat. Fat	Chol.	Carb.	Fiber	Sug.	Prot.	Sod.
Ketchup Packet (1 Packet)									
	15	0	0	0	3	0	2	0	110
Large French Fries (5.4 oz)									
	500	25	3.5	0	63	6	0	6	350
Medium French Fries (4.1 oz)									
	380	19	2.5	0	48	5	0	4	270
Salt Packet (1 Package)									
	0	0	0	0	0	0	0	0	270
Small French Fries (2.5 oz)									
	230	11	1.5	0	29	3	0	3	160

McCafe Coffees - Non-fat Milk

Food	Cal.	Total Fat	Sat. Fat	Chol.	Carb.	Fiber	Sug.	Prot.	Sod.
Hot Chocolate with Non-fat Milk (Large) (20 fl oz)									
	390	6	3.5	10	68	0	59	16	250
Hot Chocolate with Non-fat Milk (Medium) (16 fl oz)									
	310	6	3.5	10	55	0	47	11	190
Hot Chocolate with Non-fat Milk (Small) (12 fl oz)									
	250	5	3	10	43	0	37	8	140
Iced Mocha with Non-fat Milk (Medium) (16 fl oz)									
	270	8	4.5	10	43	0	35	7	140
Iced Non-fat Caramel Latte (Large) (22 fl oz)									
	190	0	0	5	40	0	40	6	150
Iced Non-fat Caramel Latte (Medium) (16 fl oz)									
	150	0	0	5	32	0	32	5	120

Food Serving size	Cal.	(g) Total Fat	(g) Sat. Fat	(mg) Chol.	(g) Carb.	(g) Fiber	(g) Sug.	(g) Prot.	(mg) Sod.
Iced Non-fat Caramel Latte (Small) (12 fl oz)									
	140	0	0	0	30	0	30	3	105
Iced Non-fat Caramel Mocha (Large) (22 fl oz)									
	300	6	4	10	49	0	45	11	230
Iced Non-fat Caramel Mocha (Medium) (16 fl oz)									
	240	6	4	10	37	0	34	9	190
Iced Non-fat Caramel Mocha (Small) (12 fl oz)									
	200	6	4	10	29	0	26	6	140
Iced Non-fat Hazelnut Latte (Large) (22 fl oz)									
	190	0	0	5	42	0	42	6	80
Iced Non-fat Hazelnut Latte (Medium) (16 fl oz)									
	150	0	0	5	33	0	33	5	70
Iced Non-fat Hazelnut Latte (Small) (12 fl oz)									
	140	0	0	0	32	0	32	3	50
Iced Non-fat Latte (Large) (22 fl oz)									
	70	0	0	5	11	0	11	7	105
Iced Non-fat Latte (Medium) (16 fl oz)									
	60	0	0	5	9	0	9	6	90
Iced Non-fat Latte (Small) (12 fl oz)									
	50	0	0	5	7	0	7	5	70
Iced Non-fat Latte with Sugar Free Vanilla Syrup (Large) (22 fl oz)									
	60	0	0	5	19	0	8	6	130
Iced Non-fat Latte with Sugar Free Vanilla Syrup (Medium) (16 fl oz)									
	50	0	0	5	14	0	6	5	100
Iced Non-fat Latte with Sugar Free Vanilla Syrup (Small) (12 fl oz)									
	40	0	0	0	13	0	5	4	85
Iced Non-fat Vanilla Latte (Large) (22 fl oz)									
	190	0	0	5	41	0	41	6	85
Iced Non-fat Vanilla Latte (Medium) (16 fl oz)									
	150	0	0	5	33	0	33	5	70
Iced Non-fat Vanilla Latte (Small) (12 fl oz)									
	140	0	0	0	31	0	31	3	50
Mocha with Non-fat Milk (Large) (20 fl oz)									
	330	6	3.5	10	58	0	50	10	190
Mocha with Non-fat Milk (Medium) (16 fl oz)									
	280	6	3.5	10	50	0	42	8	160

Food Serving size	Cal.	(g) Total Fat	(g) Sat. Fat	(mg) Chol.	(g) Carb.	(g) Fiber	(g) Sug.	(g) Prot.	(mg) Sod.
Mocha with Non-fat Milk (Small) (12 fl oz)									
	240	5	3	5	41	0	34	7	130
Non-fat Cappuccino (Large) (20 fl oz)									
	90	0	0	5	13	0	13	9	130
Non-fat Cappuccino (Medium) (16 fl oz)									
	80	0	0	5	12	0	12	8	110
Non-fat Cappuccino (Small) (12 fl oz)									
	60	0	0	5	9	0	9	6	85
Non-fat Cappuccino with Sugar Free Vanilla Syrup (Large) (20 fl oz)									
	80	0	0	5	22	0	11	8	150
Non-fat Cappuccino with Sugar Free Vanilla Syrup (Medium) (16 fl oz)									
	70	0	0	5	19	0	10	7	130
Non-fat Cappuccino with Sugar Free Vanilla Syrup (Small) (12 fl oz)									
	50	0	0	5	15	0	8	5	100
Non-fat Caramel Cappuccino (Large) (20 fl oz)									
	230	0	0	5	49	0	49	7	180
Non-fat Caramel Cappuccino (Medium) (16 fl oz)									
	190	0	0	5	41	0	41	6	150
Non-fat Caramel Cappuccino (Small) (12 fl oz)									
	150	0	0	5	33	0	32	5	120
Non-fat Caramel Latte (Large) (20 fl oz)									
	260	0	0	5	53	0	53	10	220
Non-fat Caramel Latte (Medium) (16 fl oz)									
	220	0	0	5	45	0	45	9	180
Non-fat Caramel Latte (Small) (12 fl oz)									
	170	0	0	5	36	0	36	7	150
Non-fat Caramel Mocha (Large) (20 fl oz)									
	280	4	2.5	10	49	0	46	12	260
Non-fat Caramel Mocha (Medium) (16 fl oz)									
	240	4	2.5	5	41	0	38	9	200
Non-fat Caramel Mocha (Small) (12 fl oz)									
	200	4	2.5	5	34	0	31	8	170
Non-fat Hazelnut Cappuccino (Large) (20 fl oz)									
	230	0	0	5	51	0	51	7	100
Non-fat Hazelnut Cappuccino (Medium) (16 fl oz)									
	190	0	0	5	43	0	43	6	90

Food Serving size	Cal.	(g) Total Fat	(g) Sat. Fat	(mg) Chol.	(g) Carb.	(g) Fiber	(g) Sug.	(g) Prot.	(mg) Sod.
Non-fat Hazelnut Cappuccino (Small) (12 fl oz)									
	150	0	0	5	34	0	34	5	70
Non-fat Hazelnut Latte (Large) (20 fl oz)									
	260	0	0	5	55	0	55	10	135
Non-fat Hazelnut Latte (Medium) (16 fl oz)									
	220	0	0	5	46	0	46	9	115
Non-fat Hazelnut Latte (Small) (12 fl oz)									
	180	0	0	5	37	0	37	7	95
Non-fat Latte (Large) (20 fl oz)									
	120	0	0	5	18	0	18	12	160
Non-fat Latte (Medium) (16 fl oz)									
	110	0	0	5	15	0	15	10	140
Non-fat Latte (Small) (12 fl oz)									
	90	0	0	5	13	0	13	9	115
Non-fat Latte with Sugar Free Vanilla Syrup (Large) (20 fl oz)									
	110	0	0	5	27	0	15	11	190
Non-fat Latte with Sugar Free Vanilla Syrup (Medium) (16 fl oz)									
	90	0	0	5	22	0	13	9	160
Non-fat Latte with Sugar Free Vanilla Syrup (Small) (12 fl oz)									
	80	0	0	5	18	0	11	7	130
Non-fat Vanilla Cappuccino (Large) (20 fl oz)									
	230	0	0	5	51	0	51	7	100
Non-fat Vanilla Cappuccino (Medium) (16 fl oz)									
	190	0	0	5	42	0	42	6	90
Non-fat Vanilla Cappuccino (Small) (12 fl oz)									
	150	0	0	5	34	0	34	5	70
Non-fat Vanilla Latte (Large) (20 fl oz)									
	260	0	0	5	55	0	55	10	135
Non-fat Vanilla Latte (Medium) (16 fl oz)									
	220	0	0	5	46	0	46	9	115
Non-fat Vanilla Latte (Small) (12 fl oz)									
	180	0	0	5	37	0	37	7	95

McCafe Coffees - Whole Milk

Food Serving size	Cal.	(g) Total Fat	(g) Sat. Fat	(mg) Chol.	(g) Carb.	(g) Fiber	(g) Sug.	(g) Prot.	(mg) Sod.
Cappuccino (Large) (20 fl oz)									
	180	10	6	30	13	0	13	9	130

Food Serving size	Cal.	(g) Total Fat	(g) Sat. Fat	(mg) Chol.	(g) Carb.	(g) Fiber	(g) Sug.	(g) Prot.	(mg) Sod.
Cappuccino (Medium) (16 fl oz)									
	140	8	4.5	25	11	0	11	8	105
Cappuccino (Small) (12 fl oz)									
	120	7	4	20	9	0	9	6	85
Cappuccino with Sugar Free Vanilla Syrup (Large) (20 fl oz)									
	150	8	4.5	25	22	0	11	8	160
Cappuccino with Sugar Free Vanilla Syrup (Medium) (16 fl oz)									
	120	6	3.5	20	18	0	9	6	130
Cappuccino with Sugar Free Vanilla Syrup (Small) (12 fl oz)									
	100	5	3	15	15	0	7	5	105
Caramel Cappuccino (Large) (20 fl oz)									
	290	8	4.5	25	49	0	49	8	190
Caramel Cappuccino (Medium) (16 fl oz)									
	240	6	3.5	20	41	0	40	6	150
Caramel Cappuccino (Small) (12 fl oz)									
	200	5	3	15	32	0	32	5	125
Caramel Latte (Large) (20 fl oz)									
	330	9	5	30	52	0	51	9	210
Caramel Latte (Medium) (16 fl oz)									
	280	8	4.5	25	43	0	43	8	170
Caramel Latte (Small) (12 fl oz)									
	230	7	4	20	35	0	35	7	140
Caramel Mocha (Large) (20 fl oz)									
	360	14	8	35	47	0	46	10	220
Caramel Mocha (Medium) (16 fl oz)									
	290	12	7	25	39	0	38	8	180
Caramel Mocha (Small) (12 fl oz)									
	250	11	6	25	33	0	31	7	150
Hazelnut Cappuccino (Large) (20 fl oz)									
	290	8	4.5	25	51	0	51	7	105
Hazelnut Cappuccino (Medium) (16 fl oz)									
	240	6	3.5	20	42	0	42	6	85
Hazelnut Cappuccino (Small) (12 fl oz)									
	200	5	3	15	34	0	34	5	70
Hazelnut Latte (Large) (20 fl oz)									
	330	9	5	30	53	0	53	9	130

Food Serving size	Cal.	(g) Total Fat	(g) Sat. Fat	(mg) Chol.	(g) Carb.	(g) Fiber	(g) Sug.	(g) Prot.	(mg) Sod.
Hazelnut Latte (Medium) (16 fl oz)									
	280	8	4.5	25	45	0	45	8	110
Hazelnut Latte (Small) (12 fl oz)									
	230	7	4	20	36	0	36	7	90
Hot Chocolate (Large) (20 fl oz)									
	460	18	10	40	63	0	54	13	220
Hot Chocolate (Medium) (16 fl oz)									
	380	15	9	30	53	0	45	10	170
Hot Chocolate (Small) (12 fl oz)									
	300	12	7	25	41	0	35	8	135
Iced Caramel Latte (Large) (22 fl oz)									
	230	6	3.5	15	40	0	40	6	150
Iced Caramel Latte (Medium) (16 fl oz)									
	180	4.5	2.5	15	31	0	31	4	120
Iced Caramel Latte (Small) (12 fl oz)									
	160	3	1.5	10	29	0	29	3	100
Iced Caramel Mocha (Large) (22 fl oz)									
	380	16	9	35	48	0	46	10	210
Iced Caramel Mocha (Medium) (16 fl oz)									
	300	14	8	30	36	0	33	8	160
Iced Caramel Mocha (Small) (12 fl oz)									
	240	12	7	25	29	0	26	6	130
Iced Hazelnut Latte (Large) (22 fl oz)									
	230	6	3.5	15	41	0	41	6	85
Iced Hazelnut Latte (Medium) (16 fl oz)									
	180	4.5	2.5	15	33	0	33	4	65
Iced Hazelnut Latte (Small) (12 fl oz)									
	160	3	1.5	10	31	0	31	3	45
Iced Latte (Large) (22 fl oz)									
	140	8	4.5	25	10	0	10	7	105
Iced Latte (Medium) (16 fl oz)									
	100	6	3.5	15	8	0	8	6	80
Iced Latte (Small) (12 fl oz)									
	80	4.5	2.5	15	6	0	6	4	65
Iced Latte with Sugar Free Vanilla Syrup (Large) (22 fl oz)									
	110	6	3.5	15	19	0	8	6	130

Food Serving size	Cal.	(g) Total Fat	(g) Sat. Fat	(mg) Chol.	(g) Carb.	(g) Fiber	(g) Sug.	(g) Prot.	(mg) Sod.
Iced Latte with Sugar Free Vanilla Syrup (Medium) (16 fl oz)									
	90	5	3	15	14	0	6	5	105
Iced Latte with Sugar Free Vanilla Syrup (Small) (12 fl oz)									
	60	3	2	10	12	0	4	3	80
Iced Mocha (Medium) (16 fl oz)									
	310	13	8	25	42	0	35	7	140
Iced Vanilla Latte (Large) (22 fl oz)									
	230	6	3.5	15	41	0	41	6	85
Iced Vanilla Latte (Medium) (16 fl oz)									
	190	4.5	2.5	15	33	0	33	5	70
Iced Vanilla Latte (Small) (12 fl oz)									
	160	3	1.5	10	31	0	31	3	45
Latte (Large) (20 fl oz)									
	210	11	7	35	16	0	16	11	150
Latte (Medium) (16 fl oz)									
	180	10	6	30	13	0	13	10	130
Latte (Small) (12 fl oz)									
	150	8	4.5	25	11	0	11	8	105
Latte with Sugar Free Vanilla Syrup (Large) (20 fl oz)									
	180	10	6	30	25	0	13	10	180
Latte with Sugar Free Vanilla Syrup (Medium) (16 fl oz)									
	160	8	5	25	21	0	11	8	150
Latte with Sugar Free Vanilla Syrup (Small) (12 fl oz)									
	130	7	4	20	17	0	10	7	125
Mocha (Large) (20 fl oz)									
	400	14	8	30	58	0	49	10	190
Mocha (Medium) (16 fl oz)									
	330	12	7	25	48	0	41	7	150
Mocha (Small) (12 fl oz)									
	280	11	6	20	40	0	33	6	125
Vanilla Cappuccino (Large) (20 fl oz)									
	290	8	4.5	25	51	0	51	7	105
Vanilla Cappuccino (Medium) (16 fl oz)									
	240	6	3.5	20	42	0	42	6	85
Vanilla Cappuccino (Small) (12 fl oz)									
	200	5	3	15	34	0	34	5	70

Food Serving size	Cal.	(g) Total Fat	(g) Sat. Fat	(mg) Chol.	(g) Carb.	(g) Fiber	(g) Sug.	(g) Prot.	(mg) Sod.
Vanilla Latte (Large) (20 fl oz)									
	330	9	5	30	53	0	53	9	130
Vanilla Latte (Medium) (16 fl oz)									
	280	8	4.5	25	44	0	44	8	110
Vanilla Latte (Small) (12 fl oz)									
	230	7	4	20	36	0	36	7	90

McCafe Frappes

Food Serving size	Cal.	(g) Total Fat	(g) Sat. Fat	(mg) Chol.	(g) Carb.	(g) Fiber	(g) Sug.	(g) Prot.	(mg) Sod.
Frappe Caramel (Large) (22 fl oz)									
	680	29	18	85	94	0	88	10	200
Frappe Caramel (Medium) (16 fl oz)									
	550	24	15	70	76	0	71	8	160
Frappe Caramel (Small) (12 fl oz)									
	450	20	13	55	61	0	57	6	135
Frappe Mocha (Large) (22 fl oz)									
	680	28	18	80	96	1	87	10	200
Frappe Mocha (Medium) (16 fl oz)									
	560	24	15	65	78	1	70	8	160
Frappe Mocha (Small) (12 fl oz)									
	450	20	13	55	62	1	56	7	130

McCafe Smoothies

Food Serving size	Cal.	(g) Total Fat	(g) Sat. Fat	(mg) Chol.	(g) Carb.	(g) Fiber	(g) Sug.	(g) Prot.	(mg) Sod.
Mango Pineapple Smoothie (Large) (22 fl oz)									
	350	1.5	1	5	78	3	77	4	65
Mango Pineapple Smoothie (Medium) (16 fl oz)									
	270	1.5	1	5	61	2	60	3	50
Mango Pineapple Smoothie (Small) (12 fl oz)									
	220	1	1	5	49	2	49	3	40
Strawberry Banana Smoothie (Large) (22 fl oz)									
	330	1	0.5	5	77	4	70	3	55
Strawberry Banana Smoothie (Medium) (16 fl oz)									
	260	1	0	5	60	3	54	2	40
Strawberry Banana Smoothie (Small) (12 fl oz)									
	210	0.5	0	5	49	2	44	2	35
Wild Berry Smoothie (Large) (22 fl oz)									
	320	1	0.5	5	75	4	69	3	45

Food Serving size	Cal.	(g) Total Fat	(g) Sat. Fat	(mg) Chol.	(g) Carb.	(g) Fiber	(g) Sug.	(g) Prot.	(mg) Sod.
Wild Berry Smoothie (Medium) (16 fl oz)									
	260	1	0	5	60	4	55	3	35
Wild Berry Smoothie (Small) (12 fl oz)									
	210	0.5	0	5	48	3	44	2	30

Menu Item

Food Serving size	Cal.	Total Fat	Sat. Fat	Chol.	Carb.	Fiber	Sug.	Prot.	Sod.
Angus Bacon and Cheese (10.2 oz)									
	790	39	17	145	63	4	13	45	2070
Angus Bacon and Cheese Snack Wrap (5.1 oz)									
	390	21	9	75	28	1	4	21	1080
Angus Chipotle BBQ Bacon (10.3 oz)									
	800	39	18	145	66	4	16	45	2020
Angus Chipotle BBQ Bacon Snack Wrap (5.2 oz)									
	400	22	10	75	30	1	6	21	1060
Angus Deluxe (11.1 oz)									
	750	39	16	135	61	4	10	40	1700
Angus Deluxe Snack Wrap (6 oz)									
	410	25	10	75	27	2	3	20	990
Angus Mushroom and Swiss (10 oz)									
	770	40	17	135	59	4	8	44	1170
Angus Mushroom and Swiss Snack Wrap (5.7 oz)									
	430	26	10	75	27	2	2	22	730
Big Mac (7.5 oz)									
	540	29	10	75	45	3	9	25	1040
Big N' Tasty (7.2 oz)									
	460	24	8	70	37	3	8	24	720
Big N' Tasty with Cheese (7.7 oz)									
	510	28	11	85	38	3	8	27	960
Cheeseburger (4 oz)									
	300	12	6	40	33	2	6	15	750
Chipotle BBQ Snack Wrap (Crispy) (4.2 oz)									
	330	15	4.5	30	35	1	4	14	810
Chipotle BBQ Snack Wrap (Grilled) (4.4 oz)									
	260	9	3.5	45	28	1	5	18	830
Double Cheeseburger (5.8 oz)									
	440	23	11	80	34	2	7	25	1150

Food Serving size	Cal.	(g) Total Fat	(g) Sat. Fat	(mg) Chol.	(g) Carb.	(g) Fiber	(g) Sug.	(g) Prot.	(mg) Sod.
Double Quarter Pounder with Cheese (9.8 oz)									
	740	42	19	155	40	3	9	48	1380
Filet-O-Fish (5 oz)									
	380	18	3.5	40	38	2	5	15	640
Hamburger (3.5 oz)									
	250	9	3.5	25	31	2	6	12	520
Honey Mustard Snack Wrap (Crispy) (4.2 oz)									
	330	16	4.5	30	34	1	4	14	780
Honey Mustard Snack Wrap (Grilled) (4.4 oz)									
	260	9	3.5	45	27	1	4	18	800
Mac Snack Wrap (4.4 oz)									
	330	19	7	45	26	1	3	15	690
McChicken (5 oz)									
	360	16	3	35	40	2	5	14	830
McDouble (5.3 oz)									
	390	19	8	65	33	2	7	22	920
McRib (7.4 oz)									
	500	26	10	70	44	3	11	22	980
Premium Crispy Chicken Classic Sandwich (7.5 oz)									
	510	22	3.5	45	56	3	10	24	990
Premium Crispy Chicken Club Sandwich (8.4 oz)									
	620	29	7	70	57	3	11	31	1200
Premium Crispy Chicken Ranch BLT Sandwich (7.6 oz)									
	540	23	4.5	55	56	3	11	27	1160
Premium Grilled Chicken Classic Sandwich (7 oz)									
	350	9	2	65	42	3	8	28	820
Premium Grilled Chicken Club Sandwich (7.9 oz)									
	460	16	6	90	43	3	9	35	1030
Premium Grilled Chicken Ranch BLT Sandwich (7.1 oz)									
	380	10	3	75	42	3	9	31	1000
Quarter Pounder with Cheese (7 oz)									
	510	26	12	90	40	3	9	29	1190
Ranch Snack Wrap (Crispy) (4.1 oz)									
	340	17	4.5	30	33	1	2	14	810
Ranch Snack Wrap (Grilled) (4.3 oz)									
	270	10	4	45	26	1	2	18	830

Food Serving size	Cal.	(g) Total Fat	(g) Sat. Fat	(mg) Chol.	(g) Carb.	(g) Fiber	(g) Sug.	(g) Prot.	(mg) Sod.
Southern Style Crispy Chicken Sandwich (8.7 oz)									
	400	17	3	45	39	1	6	24	1030

Salad Dressings

Newman's Own Creamy Caesar Dressing (2 fl oz)									
	190	18	3.5	20	4	0	2	2	500
Newman's Own Creamy Southwest Dressing (1.5 fl oz)									
	100	6	1	20	11	0	3	1	340
Newman's Own Low Fat Balsamic Vinaigrette (1.5 fl oz)									
	40	3	0	0	4	0	3	0	730
Newman's Own Low Fat Family Recipe Italian Dressing (1.5 fl oz)									
	60	2.5	0	0	8	0	1	1	730
Newman's Own Ranch Dressing (2 fl oz)									
	170	15	2.5	20	9	0	4	1	530

Salads

Butter Garlic Croutons (0.5 oz)									
	60	1.5	0	0	10	1	0	2	140
Premium Bacon Ranch Salad (Without Chicken) (7.8 oz)									
	140	7	3.5	25	10	3	4	9	300
Premium Bacon Ranch Salad with Crispy Chicken (11.4 oz)									
	370	20	6	75	20	3	6	29	970
Premium Bacon Ranch Salad with Grilled Chicken (11.3 oz)									
	260	9	4	90	12	3	5	33	1010
Premium Caesar Salad (Without Chicken) (7.5 oz)									
	90	4	2.5	10	9	3	4	7	180
Premium Caesar Salad with Crispy Chicken (11.1 oz)									
	330	17	4.5	60	20	3	6	26	840
Premium Caesar Salad with Grilled Chicken (11 oz)									
	220	6	3	75	12	3	5	30	890
Premium Southwest Salad (Without Chicken) (8.1. oz)									
	140	4.5	2	10	20	6	6	6	150
Premium Southwest Salad with Crispy Chicken (12.5 oz)									
	430	20	4	55	38	6	12	26	920
Premium Southwest Salad with Grilled Chicken (12.3 oz)									
	320	9	3	70	30	6	11	30	960

Food Serving size	Cal.	(g) Total Fat	(g) Sat. Fat	(mg) Chol.	(g) Carb.	(g) Fiber	(g) Sug.	(g) Prot.	(mg) Sod.
Side Salad (3.1 oz)	20	0	0	0	4	1	2	1	10
Snack Size Fruit and Walnut Salad	210	8	1.5	5	31	2	25	4	60

MOE'S SOUTHWEST

Bowls

Chicken Bowl	854	42	11.8	110	77	12	4	46	1314
Pork Bowl	655	24	10.5	110	75	10	5	42	1659
Tofu Bowl	700	23	6	30	82	14	4	32	1583

Burritos

Art Vandalay	776	29	13.3	60	97	14	4	29	1446
Homewrecker	935	36	16.3	129	97	14	4	53	1686
Joey Bag of Donuts	784	24	10	99	91	11	2	50	1443
Joey Junior	407	13	5.5	50	48	5	2	25	714

Chili Soup

Baja Chicken Enchilada Soup Bowl	360	21	9	75	26	5	8	18	1730
Baja Chicken Enchilada Soup Cup	180	11	4.5	40	13	2	4	9	860
Chili Bowl	408	15	5.2	47	47	8	10	23	1716
Chili Cup	204	7	2.6	23	23	4	5	12	858

Chips, Add-Ons, and Sides

Black Beans 6 oz	240	2	0	0	40	18	0	16	636

Food Serving size	Cal.	(g) Total Fat	(g) Sat. Fat	(mg) Chol.	(g) Carb.	(g) Fiber	(g) Sug.	(g) Prot.	(mg) Sod.
Grilled Mushrooms 2 oz	40	0	0	0	3	0	0	0	0
Grilled Onions 2 oz	45	3	0	0	5	1	3	1	55
Grilled Peppers 2 oz	30	2	0	0	3	2	1	1	50
Pinto Beans 6 oz	110	0	0	0	38	16	0	14	258
Rice 6 oz	330	0	0	0	69	0	0	9	405
Side Guacamole	60	5	1	0	4	2	1	1	220
Side of Chips	660	26	4	0	96	6	0	10	210
Side Pico	15	0	0	0	3	1	1	1	220
Side Queso	150	13	8	40	5	0	1	6	590
Side Sour Cream	90	8	5.3	30	2	0	2	2	23

Desserts

Food Serving size	Cal.	(g) Total Fat	(g) Sat. Fat	(mg) Chol.	(g) Carb.	(g) Fiber	(g) Sug.	(g) Prot.	(mg) Sod.
Chocolate Chunk Cookie	170	8	4	10	23	1	14	2	125
Oatmeal Raisin	160	6	2.5	10	23	1	12	2	115
White Chocolate Macadamia	180	9	4	10	22	1	14	2	125

Dressings

Food Serving size	Cal.	(g) Total Fat	(g) Sat. Fat	(mg) Chol.	(g) Carb.	(g) Fiber	(g) Sug.	(g) Prot.	(mg) Sod.
Chipotle Ranch	225	23	3.8	11	3	0	2	1	225
Southwest Vinaigrette	195	20	3	0	4	0	0	0	533

Kids Menu

Food Serving size	Cal.	(g) Total Fat	(g) Sat. Fat	(mg) Chol.	(g) Carb.	(g) Fiber	(g) Sug.	(g) Prot.	(mg) Sod.
Mini Masterpiece	325	20	11.3	60	23	2	2	12	563

Food Serving size	Cal.	(g) Total Fat	(g) Sat. Fat	(mg) Chol.	(g) Carb.	(g) Fiber	(g) Sug.	(g) Prot.	(mg) Sod.
Moo Moo Mr. Cow	266	10	4.5	38	27	3	0	17	397
Power Wagon Hard Shell	625	31	7.5	50	65	5	0	23	215
Power Wagon Soft Shell	285	12	5	50	26	1	1	21	410

Nachos

Alfredo Garcia	961	45	19	198	66	7	5	73	1587
Billy Barou	1509	79	31	189	145	18	5	62	3656
Fat Sam	1108	57	25.3	228	71	9	7	75	1828
Ruprict	1300	70	28	120	137	17	4	36	3216

Quesadillas

Chicken Club	1115	79	27.3	200	31	1	3	62	1946
John Coctostan	774	38	19.8	159	52	11	3	53	1381
Super Kingpin	495	30	16.8	90	33	2	3	21	823

Salads

Closetalker	844	46	13	99	61	13	2	45	1438
Closetalker No Shell	454	20	8	99	27	12	1	40	1208
Personal Trainer	685	39	10	30	61	13	2	21	1198
Personal Trainer No Shell	295	13	5	30	27	12	1	16	968

Salsas

El Guapos Salsa	15	0	0	0	3	1	1	1	230

Food Serving size	Cal.	(g) Total Fat	(g) Sat. Fat	(mg) Chol.	(g) Carb.	(g) Fiber	(g) Sug.	(g) Prot.	(mg) Sod.
Kaiser Salsa	20	0	0	0	4	1	1	1	360
Tomatillo Salsa	15	0	0	0	3	2	1	0	250

Tacos

Food Serving size	Cal.	Total Fat	Sat. Fat	Chol.	Carb.	Fiber	Sug.	Prot.	Sod.
Funk Meister Hard Shell	693	31	7.5	50	77	10	1	27	484
Funk Meister Soft Shell	353	12	5	50	38	6	2	25	679
Overachiever Hard Shell	763	37	10.6	65	79	11	2	28	606
Overachiever Soft Shell	428	18	8.1	65	40	7	3	26	801
Unanimous Decision Hard Shell	673	33	8.3	25	79	11	1	16	482
Unanimous Decision Soft Shell	333	14	5.8	25	40	7	2	14	677

PIZZA HUT

12" Fit 'n Delicious Pizza (1 Slice = 1/8 Pizza)

Food Serving size	Cal.	Total Fat	Sat. Fat	Chol.	Carb.	Fiber	Sug.	Prot.	Sod.
Chicken, Mushrooms and Jalapeno	170	4.5	1.5	20	22	1	4	11	720
Chicken, Red Onion and Green Pepper	180	4.5	1.5	20	23	1	5	11	510
Diced Red Tomato, Mushroom and Jalapeno	150	4	1.5	10	23	2	4	6	610
Green Pepper, Red Onion and Diced Red Tomato	150	4	1.5	10	24	2	5	6	400
Ham, Pineapple and Diced Red Tomato	160	4.5	1.5	15	24	1	6	7	550
Ham, Red Onion and Mushroom	160	4.5	1.5	15	23	1	4	8	550

Food Serving size	Cal.	(g) Total Fat	(g) Sat. Fat	(mg) Chol.	(g) Carb.	(g) Fiber	(g) Sug.	(g) Prot.	(mg) Sod.
12" Medium Hand-Tossed Style Pizza (1 Slice = 1/8 Pizza)									
Cheese Only	220	8	4	25	26	1	4	10	550
Cheese Only Garlic Parmesan	220	8	4.5	25	26	1	4	10	580
Dan's Original	260	12	5	30	26	1	4	12	650
Dan's Original Garlic Parmesan	260	12	5	30	27	1	4	12	680
Ham and Pineapple	200	6	3	20	27	1	5	9	550
Ham and Pineapple Garlic Parmesan	210	6	3	20	28	1	5	9	570
Hawaiian Luau	240	9	4	25	27	1	5	11	640
Hawaiian Luau Garlic Parmesan	240	9	4	25	28	1	5	11	670
Italian Sausage and Red Onion	240	10	4.5	25	27	1	4	11	580
Italian Sausage and Red Onion Garlic Parmesan	250	10	4.5	25	28	1	4	11	610
Meat Lover's	300	16	7	40	26	1	4	14	860
Meat Lover's Garlic Parmesan	310	16	7	40	26	1	4	14	890
Pepperoni	230	9	4	25	25	1	3	10	610
Pepperoni and Mushroom	210	8	3.5	20	26	1	4	10	540
Pepperoni and Mushroom Garlic Parmesan	210	8	3.5	20	26	1	4	10	570
Pepperoni Garlic Parmesan	230	9	4.5	25	26	1	4	10	640
Pepperoni Lover's	270	13	6	35	26	1	4	13	770

Food Serving size	Cal.	(g) Total Fat	(g) Sat. Fat	(mg) Chol.	(g) Carb.	(g) Fiber	(g) Sug.	(g) Prot.	(mg) Sod.
Pepperoni Lover's Garlic Parmesan	280	13	6	35	27	1	4	13	790
Spicy Sicilian	240	11	4.5	25	26	1	4	11	730
Spicy Sicilian Garlic Parmesan	250	11	5	25	27	2	4	11	760
Supreme	260	12	5	30	26	1	4	12	680
Supreme Garlic Parmesan	260	12	5	30	27	1	4	12	700
Triple Meat Italiano	260	12	5	30	26	1	4	12	730
Triple Meat Italiano Garlic Parmesan	260	12	5	30	26	1	4	12	750
Ultimate Cheese Lover's	240	11	5	30	25	1	3	11	590
Ultimate Cheese Lover's Garlic Parmesan	250	11	5	30	26	1	3	11	620
Veggie Lover's	200	6	3	15	27	2	4	9	530
Veggie Lover's Garlic Parmesan	200	7	3	15	27	2	4	9	550

12" Medium Pan Pizza (1 Slice = 1/8 pizza)

Food Serving size	Cal.	(g) Total Fat	(g) Sat. Fat	(mg) Chol.	(g) Carb.	(g) Fiber	(g) Sug.	(g) Prot.	(mg) Sod.
Cheese Only	240	10	4.5	25	27	1	2	11	530
Dan's Original	280	14	5	30	27	1	2	12	630
Ham and Pineapple	230	9	3.5	20	28	1	3	10	520
Hawaiian Luau	260	12	4.5	25	28	1	3	11	610
Italian Sausage and Red Onion	270	13	4.5	25	28	1	3	11	560
Meat Lover's	330	18	7	40	27	1	2	14	830

Food Serving size	Cal.	(g) Total Fat	(g) Sat. Fat	(mg) Chol.	(g) Carb.	(g) Fiber	(g) Sug.	(g) Prot.	(mg) Sod.
Pepperoni									
	250	12	4.5	25	26	1	2	11	590
Pepperoni and Mushroom									
	240	10	4	20	27	1	2	10	520
Pepperoni Lover's									
	290	14	6	35	27	1	2	13	730
Spicy Sicilian									
	270	13	5	25	27	2	2	11	700
Supreme									
	290	14	5	30	27	2	2	12	650
Triple Meat Italiano									
	290	15	5	30	27	1	2	13	700
Ultimate Cheese Lover's									
	270	13	5	25	26	1	2	12	580
Veggie Lover's									
	230	9	3.5	15	28	2	3	9	500

12" Medium Thin 'N Crispy Pizza (1 Slice = 1/8 Pizza)

Food Serving size	Cal.	(g) Total Fat	(g) Sat. Fat	(mg) Chol.	(g) Carb.	(g) Fiber	(g) Sug.	(g) Prot.	(mg) Sod.
Cheese Only									
	190	8	4	25	22	1	4	9	550
Dan's Original									
	240	12	5	30	22	1	4	11	650
Ham and Pineapple									
	180	6	3	20	23	1	5	8	540
Hawaiian Luau									
	220	10	4	25	24	1	5	10	650
Italian Sausage and Red Onion									
	220	10	4	25	23	1	4	9	580
Meat Lover's									
	280	16	6	40	22	1	4	13	860
Pepperoni									
	200	9	4	25	21	1	4	9	610
Pepperoni and Mushroom									
	180	8	3.5	20	22	1	4	9	540
Pepperoni Lover's									
	250	13	6	35	22	1	4	12	760

Food Serving size	Cal.	(g) Total Fat	(g) Sat. Fat	(mg) Chol.	(g) Carb.	(g) Fiber	(g) Sug.	(g) Prot.	(mg) Sod.
Spicy Sicilian	220	10	4.5	25	22	1	4	9	750
Supreme	240	12	5	30	23	1	4	10	670
Triple Meat Italiano	240	12	5	30	22	1	4	11	720
Ultimate Cheese Lover's	220	11	5	25	21	1	4	10	600
Veggie Lover's	180	6	3	15	23	1	4	8	530

14" Large Hand-Tossed Style Pizza (1 Slice = 1/8 Pizza)

Food Serving size	Cal.	(g) Total Fat	(g) Sat. Fat	(mg) Chol.	(g) Carb.	(g) Fiber	(g) Sug.	(g) Prot.	(mg) Sod.
Cheese Only	320	12	6	35	38	2	5	15	800
Cheese Only Garlic Parmesan	320	12	6	35	39	2	5	15	840
Dan's Original	370	17	7	40	38	2	5	17	950
Dan's Original Garlic Parmesan	380	17	7	40	39	2	5	17	980
Ham and Pineapple	290	9	4.5	25	40	2	7	13	810
Ham and Pineapple Garlic Parmesan	300	9	4.5	25	41	2	7	14	840
Hawaiian Luau	340	13	6	35	40	2	7	15	930
Hawaiian Luau Garlic Parmesan	340	13	6	35	41	2	7	16	970
Italian Sausage and Red Onion	350	14	6	35	40	2	6	15	840
Italian Sausage and Red Onion Garlic Parmesan	350	15	6	35	40	2	6	15	870
Meat Lover's	440	23	9	60	38	2	5	20	1250
Meat Lover's Garlic Parmesan	440	23	10	60	39	2	5	20	1290

Food Serving size	Cal.	(g) Total Fat	(g) Sat. Fat	(mg) Chol.	(g) Carb.	(g) Fiber	(g) Sug.	(g) Prot.	(mg) Sod.
Pepperoni									
	330	14	6	35	38	2	5	15	910
Pepperoni and Mushroom									
	310	11	5	30	38	2	5	14	800
Pepperoni and Mushroom Garlic Parmesan									
	320	11	5	30	39	2	5	14	840
Pepperoni Garlic Parmesan									
	340	14	6	35	38	2	5	15	940
Pepperoni Lover's									
	400	19	9	55	39	2	5	19	1130
Pepperoni Lover's Garlic Parmesan									
	410	19	9	55	39	2	5	19	1170
Spicy Sicilian									
	350	15	7	40	39	2	6	15	1040
Spicy Sicilian Garlic Parmesan									
	360	15	7	40	40	2	6	16	1080
Supreme									
	380	17	7	45	39	2	6	17	990
Supreme Garlic Parmesan									
	380	17	8	45	40	2	6	17	1030
Triple Meat Italiano									
	380	17	7	45	38	2	5	18	1060
Triple Meat Italiano Garlic Parmesan									
	380	17	7	45	39	2	5	18	1100
Ultimate Cheese Lover's									
	350	15	7	40	37	1	5	16	840
Ultimate Cheese Lover's Garlic Parmesan									
	360	15	7	40	38	2	5	16	880
Veggie Lover's									
	290	9	4.5	25	39	2	6	13	760
Veggie Lover's Garlic Parmesan									
	300	10	4.5	25	40	2	6	13	790

14" Large Pan Pizza (1 Slice = 1/8 Pizza)

Food	Cal.	Total Fat	Sat. Fat	Chol.	Carb.	Fiber	Sug.	Prot.	Sod.
Cheese Only									
	360	17	7	35	37	2	3	15	740

Food Serving size	Cal.	(g) Total Fat	(g) Sat. Fat	(mg) Chol.	(g) Carb.	(g) Fiber	(g) Sug.	(g) Prot.	(mg) Sod.
Dan's Original	420	22	8	40	37	2	3	17	880
Ham and Pineapple	340	15	5	25	39	2	4	14	740
Hawaiian Luau	380	18	6	35	39	2	4	15	860
Italian Sausage and Red Onion	390	20	7	35	38	2	3	15	770
Meat Lover's	480	28	10	60	37	2	3	20	1180
Pepperoni	380	19	7	35	36	2	3	15	840
Pepperoni and Mushroom	350	17	6	30	37	2	3	14	730
Pepperoni Lover's	430	23	9	55	37	2	3	20	1070
Spicy Sicilian	400	21	7	35	38	2	3	16	960
Supreme	420	23	8	45	38	2	3	17	920
Triple Meat Italiano	420	23	8	45	37	2	3	18	1000
Ultimate Cheese Lover's	400	21	8	40	36	2	3	16	800
Veggie Lover's	330	15	5	20	38	2	4	13	690

14" Large Stuffed Crust Pizza (1 Slice = 1/8 Pizza)

Food Serving size	Cal.	(g) Total Fat	(g) Sat. Fat	(mg) Chol.	(g) Carb.	(g) Fiber	(g) Sug.	(g) Prot.	(mg) Sod.
Cheese Only	340	14	7	40	39	2	6	16	900
Dan's Original	410	20	9	50	40	2	6	19	1080
Ham and Pineapple	330	12	6	40	41	2	7	15	940
Hawaiian Luau	380	16	8	45	41	2	7	17	1050

Food Serving size	Cal.	(g) Total Fat	(g) Sat. Fat	(mg) Chol.	(g) Carb.	(g) Fiber	(g) Sug.	(g) Prot.	(mg) Sod.
Italian Sausage and Red Onion									
	390	17	8	45	41	2	6	17	970
Meat Lover's									
	480	26	11	70	39	2	6	22	1380
Pepperoni									
	370	17	8	45	39	2	5	17	1040
Pepperoni and Mushroom									
	350	14	7	40	39	2	6	16	930
Pepperoni Lover's									
	430	21	10	60	40	2	6	20	1230
Spicy Sicilian									
	390	18	9	50	40	2	6	17	1160
Supreme									
	420	20	9	55	40	2	6	19	1120
Triple Meat Italiano									
	420	20	9	55	39	2	6	20	1190
Ultimate Cheese Lover's									
	380	17	9	45	38	1	5	17	940
Veggie Lover's									
	330	12	6	35	41	2	6	15	880

14" Large Thin 'N Crispy Pizza (1 Slice = 1/8 Pizza)

Food Serving size	Cal.	(g) Total Fat	(g) Sat. Fat	(mg) Chol.	(g) Carb.	(g) Fiber	(g) Sug.	(g) Prot.	(mg) Sod.
Cheese Only									
	260	11	6	35	29	1	5	12	740
Dan's Original									
	320	16	7	40	29	1	5	15	890
Ham and Pineapple									
	240	9	4	25	31	1	7	11	750
Hawaiian Luau									
	300	14	6	35	31	1	7	13	900
Italian Sausage and Red Onion									
	300	14	6	35	30	1	6	13	780
Meat Lover's									
	390	23	9	60	28	1	5	18	1210
Pepperoni									
	280	13	6	35	28	1	5	13	850

Food Serving size	Cal.	(g) Total Fat	(g) Sat. Fat	(mg) Chol.	(g) Carb.	(g) Fiber	(g) Sug.	(g) Prot.	(mg) Sod.
Pepperoni and Mushroom	260	11	4.5	30	29	1	5	12	740
Pepperoni Lover's	350	18	8	55	29	1	5	17	1080
Spicy Sicilian	300	15	6	35	30	2	5	13	1020
Supreme	330	17	7	45	30	2	5	15	930
Triple Meat Italiano	320	17	7	45	28	1	5	15	1000
Ultimate Cheese Lover's	300	15	7	40	28	1	5	14	800
Veggie Lover's	240	9	4	20	30	2	6	10	710

6" Personal Pan Pizza (Whole Pizza)

Food Serving size	Cal.	(g) Total Fat	(g) Sat. Fat	(mg) Chol.	(g) Carb.	(g) Fiber	(g) Sug.	(g) Prot.	(mg) Sod.
Cheese Only	590	24	10	55	69	3	7	26	1290
Dan's Original	720	36	13	75	69	4	7	31	1600
Ham and Pineapple	550	20	8	45	71	3	9	23	1260
Hawaiian Luau	620	25	10	55	71	3	9	26	1440
Italian Sausage and Red Onion	690	32	12	65	71	4	8	28	1440
Meat Lover's	830	46	17	100	68	3	7	36	2110
Pepperoni	610	26	10	55	67	3	6	26	1410
Pepperoni and Mushroom	570	23	9	45	68	4	7	24	1250
Pepperoni Lover's	720	34	14	85	69	3	7	32	1760
Spicy Sicilian	680	32	12	70	69	4	7	29	1730

Food Serving size	Cal.	(g) Total Fat	(g) Sat. Fat	(mg) Chol.	(g) Carb.	(g) Fiber	(g) Sug.	(g) Prot.	(mg) Sod.
Supreme	720	36	14	80	69	4	7	30	1680
Triple Meat Italiano	730	36	13	80	68	3	6	32	1770
Ultimate Cheese Lover's	660	30	12	65	68	3	6	29	1400
Veggie Lover's	550	20	8	35	70	4	8	22	1190

Appetizers

Food Serving size	Cal.	(g) Total Fat	(g) Sat. Fat	(mg) Chol.	(g) Carb.	(g) Fiber	(g) Sug.	(g) Prot.	(mg) Sod.
Baked Hot Wings (2 Pieces)	100	6	2	55	1	0	0	10	430
Baked Mild Wings (2 Pieces)	110	7	2	55	1	0	0	10	430
Breadsticks (Each)	140	5	1	0	19	1	2	5	260
Cheese Breadsticks (Each)	170	6	2.5	15	20	1	2	8	390
Marinara Dipping Sauce (3 oz)	60	0	0	0	12	2	9	2	440
Wing Blue Cheese Dipping Sauce (1.5 oz)	230	24	4.5	20	2	0	2	1	420
Wing Ranch Dipping Sauce (1.5 oz)	220	23	3.5	10	2	0	1	0	420

Beverages

Food Serving size	Cal.	(g) Total Fat	(g) Sat. Fat	(mg) Chol.	(g) Carb.	(g) Fiber	(g) Sug.	(g) Prot.	(mg) Sod.
Diet Pepsi (16 oz)	0	0	0	0	0	0	0	0	50
Diet Pepsi (22 oz)	0	0	0	0	0	0	0	0	70
Diet Pepsi (32 oz)	0	0	0	0	0	0	0	0	100
Mountain Dew (16 oz)	220	0	0	0	58	0	58	0	70
Mountain Dew (22 oz)	300	0	0	0	80	0	80	0	100

Food Serving size	Cal.	(g) Total Fat	(g) Sat. Fat	(mg) Chol.	(g) Carb.	(g) Fiber	(g) Sug.	(g) Prot.	(mg) Sod.
Mountain Dew (32 oz)	440	0	0	0	116	0	116	0	140
Pepsi (16 oz)	200	0	0	0	56	0	54	0	50
Pepsi (22 oz)	280	0	0	0	77	0	74	0	70
Pepsi (32 oz)	400	0	0	0	112	0	108	0	100
Sierra Mist (16 oz)	200	0	0	0	54	0	54	0	40
Sierra Mist (22 oz)	275	0	0	0	74	0	74	0	60
Sierra Mist (32 oz)	400	0	0	0	108	0	108	0	80

Big Eat Tiny Price Menu: 9" Personal PANormous Pizza (Whole Pizza)

Food	Cal.	Total Fat	Sat. Fat	Chol.	Carb.	Fiber	Sug.	Prot.	Sod.
Cheese Only	1100	45	19	105	124	6	10	48	2400
Dan's Original	1270	62	23	125	124	7	10	55	2810
Ham and Pineapple	1020	37	14	80	128	6	14	43	2300
Hawaiian Luau	1150	49	18	105	129	6	14	49	2670
Italian Sausage and Red Onion	1210	56	21	110	128	7	12	50	2550
Meat Lover's	1470	80	30	175	123	6	10	64	3670
Pepperoni	1100	48	18	100	121	6	9	47	2540
Pepperoni and Mushroom	1050	42	16	85	123	7	10	45	2290
Pepperoni Lover's	1290	62	26	150	124	6	10	59	3160
Spicy Sicilian	1220	57	22	115	126	7	11	51	3150

Food Serving size	Cal.	(g) Total Fat	(g) Sat. Fat	(mg) Chol.	(g) Carb.	(g) Fiber	(g) Sug.	(g) Prot.	(mg) Sod.
Supreme	1270	62	24	130	125	7	11	54	2920
Triple Meat Italiano	1280	62	23	135	123	6	9	56	3070
Ultimate Cheese Lover's	1200	56	23	120	121	5	9	53	2560
Veggie Lover's	1010	38	14	70	127	8	12	42	2240

Bone Out Wings (2 Pieces)

Food Serving size	Cal.	(g) Total Fat	(g) Sat. Fat	(mg) Chol.	(g) Carb.	(g) Fiber	(g) Sug.	(g) Prot.	(mg) Sod.
All American	150	8	1.5	20	11	1	0	10	490
Buffalo Burnin' Hot	190	8	1.5	20	18	1	2	10	1000
Buffalo Medium	190	9	1.5	20	18	1	2	10	990
Buffalo Mild	190	9	1.5	20	18	1	2	10	1020
Garlic Parmesan	260	19	3.5	20	11	1	1	11	710
Honey BBQ	220	8	1.5	20	27	1	12	10	720
Lemon Pepper	220	12	2	20	18	1	7	10	620
Spicy Asian	210	8	1.5	20	24	1	13	10	690
Spicy BBQ	200	8	1.5	25	21	1	11	10	940

Crispy Bone in Wings (2 Pieces)

Food Serving size	Cal.	(g) Total Fat	(g) Sat. Fat	(mg) Chol.	(g) Carb.	(g) Fiber	(g) Sug.	(g) Prot.	(mg) Sod.
All American	200	14	2.5	45	8	1	0	9	500
Buffalo Burnin' Hot	230	15	3	45	16	1	2	9	1020
Buffalo Medium	230	15	3	45	16	2	2	9	1010

Food Serving size	Cal.	(g) Total Fat	(g) Sat. Fat	(mg) Chol.	(g) Carb.	(g) Fiber	(g) Sug.	(g) Prot.	(mg) Sod.
Buffalo Mild	230	15	3	45	16	1	2	9	1040
Garlic Parmesan	300	25	5	45	9	1	1	10	730
Honey BBQ	260	14	3	45	24	1	12	10	740
Lemon Pepper	270	19	3.5	45	16	1	7	9	640
Spicy Asian	250	14	2.5	45	21	1	13	10	710
Spicy BBQ	240	14	2.5	50	19	1	11	9	950

Desserts

Food Serving size	Cal.	Total Fat	Sat. Fat	Chol.	Carb.	Fiber	Sug.	Prot.	Sod.
Cinnamon Sticks (2 Pieces)	160	4.5	0.5	0	26	1	8	4	210
Hershey's Chocolate Dunkers	190	8	3	0	27	2	9	5	220
Hershey's Chocolate Sauce (1.5 oz)	120	2.5	1	0	24	1	18	1	75
White Icing Dipping Cup (2 oz)	170	0	0	0	44	0	38	0	5

P'Zone Pizza (1/2 Order)

Food Serving size	Cal.	Total Fat	Sat. Fat	Chol.	Carb.	Fiber	Sug.	Prot.	Sod.
Classic	470	16	7	40	61	2	3	20	1070
Marinara Dipping Sauce (3 oz)	60	0	0	0	12	2	9	2	440
Meaty	550	23	10	55	61	2	2	24	1370
Pepperoni	450	15	7	40	60	2	2	19	1120

Side Items

Food Serving size	Cal.	Total Fat	Sat. Fat	Chol.	Carb.	Fiber	Sug.	Prot.	Sod.
Apple Pie (2 Pies)	330	17	5	0	40	2	20	2	190

Food Serving size	Cal.	(g) Total Fat	(g) Sat. Fat	(mg) Chol.	(g) Carb.	(g) Fiber	(g) Sug.	(g) Prot.	(mg) Sod.
Fried Cheese Sticks (4 Pieces)									
	380	24	9	40	29	2	3	13	1020
Wedge Fries (Side Order)									
	320	18	3.5	0	35	3	0	4	530

Stuffed Pizza Rollers (Each)

Food Serving size	Cal.	(g) Total Fat	(g) Sat. Fat	(mg) Chol.	(g) Carb.	(g) Fiber	(g) Sug.	(g) Prot.	(mg) Sod.
Marinara Dipping Sauce (3 oz)									
	60	0	0	0	12	2	9	2	440
Ranch Dipping Sauce (1.5 oz)									
	220	23	3.5	10	2	0	1	0	420
Stuffed Pizza Rollers									
	220	10	4.5	25	24	1	3	10	580

Traditional Wings (2 Pieces)

Food Serving size	Cal.	(g) Total Fat	(g) Sat. Fat	(mg) Chol.	(g) Carb.	(g) Fiber	(g) Sug.	(g) Prot.	(mg) Sod.
All American									
	80	5	1.5	40	0	0	0	7	290
Buffalo Burnin' Hot									
	110	6	1.5	40	8	1	2	8	810
Buffalo Medium									
	110	6	1.5	40	8	1	2	8	800
Buffalo Mild									
	110	6	1.5	40	8	1	2	8	830
Garlic Parmesan									
	180	16	3.5	45	1	0	1	8	520
Honey BBQ									
	140	5	1.5	40	16	0	12	8	530
Lemon Pepper									
	150	10	2	40	8	0	7	8	430
Spicy Asian									
	130	5	1.5	40	13	0	13	8	500
Spicy BBQ									
	120	5	1.5	45	11	0	11	8	750

Tuscani Pastas (1/2 Pan)

Food Serving size	Cal.	(g) Total Fat	(g) Sat. Fat	(mg) Chol.	(g) Carb.	(g) Fiber	(g) Sug.	(g) Prot.	(mg) Sod.
Chicken Alfredo									
	580	32	9	50	49	4	4	23	1250

Food Serving size	Cal.	(g) Total Fat	(g) Sat. Fat	(mg) Chol.	(g) Carb.	(g) Fiber	(g) Sug.	(g) Prot.	(mg) Sod.
Meaty Marinara	450	20	8	70	44	5	8	22	1100

RED MANGO

Frozen Yogurt (Serving Size, 1/2 Cup) (93g)

Amaretto Non-fat Frozen Yogurt	110	0	0	0	24	0	24	2	95
Apricot Non-fat Frozen Yogurt	100	0	0	0	24	0	24	2	95
Banana Non-fat Frozen Yogurt	100	0	0	0	23	0	23	2	95
Black Cherry Non-fat Frozen Yogurt	80	0	0	0	18	0	18	2	105
Black Currant Non-fat Frozen Yogurt	100	0	0	0	24	0	24	2	95
Blackberry Non-fat Frozen Yogurt	100	0	0	0	24	0	24	2	90
Blueberry Non-fat Frozen Yogurt	100	0	0	0	23	0	23	2	90
Caribbean Coconut Non-fat Frozen Yogurt	100	0	0	0	24	0	24	2	90
Chai Non-fat Frozen Yogurt	90	0	0	0	21	0	21	2	95
Cinnamon Non-fat Frozen Yogurt	100	0	0	0	22	0	22	2	95
Cocoa Non-fat Frozen Yogurt	100	0	0	0	23	0	22	2	95
Dark Chocolate Frozen Yogurt	100	0.5	0	0	24	<1	23	2	110
Dulce de Leche Frozen Yogurt	80	0	0	0	18	0	18	2	110
Espresso Non-fat Frozen Yogurt	100	0	0	0	23	0	22	2	95
Ginger Non-fat Frozen Yogurt	90	0	0	0	21	0	21	2	95

Food Serving size	Cal.	(g) Total Fat	(g) Sat. Fat	(mg) Chol.	(g) Carb.	(g) Fiber	(g) Sug.	(g) Prot.	(mg) Sod.
Golden Peach Non-fat Frozen Yogurt									
	100	0	0	0	24	0	23	2	90
Green Tea (Sencha) Non-fat Frozen Yogurt									
	80	0	0	0	18	0	18	2	105
Hazelnut Non-fat Frozen Yogurt									
	100	0	0	0	23	0	23	2	95
Irish Cream Non-fat Frozen Yogurt									
	100	0	0	0	24	0	16	2	95
Key Lime Pie Non-fat Frozen Yogurt									
	80	0	0	0	18	0	18	2	105
Lemon Spritzer Non-fat Frozen Yogurt									
	80	0	0	0	18	0	18	2	105
Madagascar Vanilla Non-fat Frozen Yogurt									
	80	0	0	0	18	0	18	2	105
Mandarin Orange Non-fat Frozen Yogurt									
	100	0	0	0	23	0	23	2	95
Mojito Non-fat Frozen Yogurt									
	100	0	0	0	23	0	23	2	95
Original Non-fat Frozen Yogurt									
	80	0	0	0	19	0	19	2	110
Peppermint Dark Chocolate Frozen Yogurt									
	100	0.5	0	0	24	<1	23	2	110
Peppermint Non-fat Frozen Yogurt									
	100	0	0	0	23	0	22	2	95
Pineapple Non-fat Frozen Yogurt									
	80	0	0	0	18	0	18	2	105
Pomegranate by POM Wonderful Frozen Yogurt									
	90	0	0	0	21	0	20	2	100
Pumpkin Spice Non-fat Frozen Yogurt (Seasonal)									
	80	0	0	0	18	0	18	2	105
Raspberry Cheesecake Non-fat Frozen Yogurt									
	80	0	0	0	19	0	19	2	110
Raspberry Non-fat Frozen Yogurt									
	100	0	0	0	24	0	24	2	90
Sonoma Strawberry Non-fat Frozen Yogurt									
	100	0	0	0	24	0	23	3	95

Food Serving size	Cal.	(g) Total Fat	(g) Sat. Fat	(mg) Chol.	(g) Carb.	(g) Fiber	(g) Sug.	(g) Prot.	(mg) Sod.
Summer Melon Non-fat Frozen Yogurt									
	80	0	0	0	19	0	18	2	105
Tangomonium Non-fat Frozen Yogurt									
	80	0	0	0	18	0	18	2	105
White Peach Non-fat Frozen Yogurt									
	100	0	0	0	23	0	23	2	90
Wild Raspberry Non-fat Frozen Yogurt									
	100	0	0	0	24	0	24	2	90
Winter Caramel Non-fat Frozen Yogurt									
	100	0	0	0	24	0	24	2	90

Hot Chocolate Chiller

Food Serving size	Cal.	(g) Total Fat	(g) Sat. Fat	(mg) Chol.	(g) Carb.	(g) Fiber	(g) Sug.	(g) Prot.	(mg) Sod.
Dark Chocolate (Large)									
	410	2.5	1.5	<5	97	4	89	9	420
Dark Chocolate (Regular)									
	260	1.5	1	<5	60	3	55	6	260
Dark Chocolate + Banana (Large)									
	420	1.5	0.5	<5	99	4	87	7	340
Dark Chocolate + Banana (Regular)									
	270	1	0	<5	64	3	55	5	220
Dark Chocolate + Peppermint (Large)									
	430	2.5	1.5	<5	100	5	92	9	430
Dark Chocolate + Peppermint (Regular)									
	260	1.5	1	<5	62	3	57	6	260
Dark Chocolate + Strawberries (Large)									
	370	1.5	0.5	<5	86	4	80	7	340
Dark Chocolate + Strawberries (Regular)									
	230	1	0	<5	55	2	51	4	220
Dark Chocolate + Strawberries + Banana (Large)									
	420	2	0.5	<5	99	5	88	8	340
Dark Chocolate + Strawberries + Banana (Regular)									
	270	1	0	<5	64	3	56	5	220

Parfaits

Food Serving size	Cal.	(g) Total Fat	(g) Sat. Fat	(mg) Chol.	(g) Carb.	(g) Fiber	(g) Sug.	(g) Prot.	(mg) Sod.
Key Lime Pie Frozen Yogurt Parfait (Regular)									
	310	5	0	0	63	5	42	6	180

Food Serving size	Cal.	(g) Total Fat	(g) Sat. Fat	(mg) Chol.	(g) Carb.	(g) Fiber	(g) Sug.	(g) Prot.	(mg) Sod.
Mixed Berry Frozen Yogurt Parfait (Regular)									
	280	4.5	0	0	57	5	38	6	150
Tropical Frozen Yogurt Parfait (Regular)									
	320	4.5	0	0	67	5	47	6	150

Probiotic Lemonade

Food Serving size	Cal.	Total Fat	Sat. Fat	Chol.	Carb.	Fiber	Sug.	Prot.	Sod.
Lemonade with Real Honey (Large)									
	220	0	0	0	56	0	52	0	0
Lemonade with Real Honey (Regular)									
	150	0	0	0	37	0	35	0	0
Pomegranate Lemonade (Large)									
	260	0	0	0	66	0	60	0	0
Pomegranate Lemonade (Regular)									
	160	0	0	0	41	0	37	0	0

Probiotic Teas

Food Serving size	Cal.	Total Fat	Sat. Fat	Chol.	Carb.	Fiber	Sug.	Prot.	Sod.
Green Tea (Sweetened with Stevia) (Large)									
	20	0	0	0	8	0	2	0	5
Green Tea (Sweetened with Stevia) (Regular)									
	15	0	0	0	5	0	1	0	0
Green Tea (Unsweetened) (Large)									
	10	0	0	0	2	0	0	0	5
Green Tea (Unsweetened) (Regular)									
	5	0	0	0	1	0	0	0	0
Lemon Honey Iced Green Tea (Large)									
	240	0	0	0	59	0	48	0	0
Lemon Honey Iced Green Tea (Regular)									
	160	0	0	0	40	0	32	0	0
Mango Passion Iced Green Tea (Large)									
	240	0	0	0	55	0	51	0	0
Mango Passion Iced Green Tea (Regular)									
	160	0	0	0	37	0	34	0	0
Pomegranate Green Tea by POM Wonderful (Large)									
	250	0	0	0	63	0	51	0	0
Pomegranate Green Tea by POM Wonderful (Regular)									
	170	0	0	0	43	0	34	0	0

Food Serving size	Cal.	(g) Total Fat	(g) Sat. Fat	(mg) Chol.	(g) Carb.	(g) Fiber	(g) Sug.	(g) Prot.	(mg) Sod.
Smoothies									
4 Berry Blend Smoothie (Large)									
	280	1	0	<5	65	6	58	6	260
4 Berry Blend Smoothie (Regular)									
	200	0.5	0	<5	46	4	41	4	190
Acai Berry Smoothie (Large)									
	420	2.5	0.5	<5	95	2	92	5	230
Acai Berry Smoothie (Regular)									
	280	2	0	0	63	1	62	3	160
Antioxidants Smoothie (Large)									
	420	1	0	<5	98	<1	92	5	270
Antioxidants Smoothie (Regular)									
	290	0.5	0	<5	67	0	63	3	190
Berry Banana Smoothie (Large)									
	300	0.5	0	<5	69	3	61	6	260
Berry Banana Smoothie (Regular)									
	210	0.5	0	<5	49	2	43	4	190
Healthy Bones Smoothie (Large)									
	300	0	0	<5	70	3	64	5	260
Healthy Bones Smoothie (Regular)									
	210	0	0	<5	49	2	45	4	190
Mandarin Mango Smoothie (Large)									
	330	0.5	0	<5	78	3	72	6	270
Mandarin Mango Smoothie (Regular)									
	230	0	0	<5	55	2	51	4	190
Pomegranate by POM Wonderful Smoothie (Large)									
	380	0	0	<5	91	<1	83	5	270
Pomegranate by POM Wonderful Smoothie (Regular)									
	260	0	0	<5	62	0	57	3	190
Protein Power Smoothie (Large)									
	530	8	1	<5	95	8	65	21	360
Protein Power Smoothie (Regular)									
	380	5	0.5	<5	67	5	47	18	280
Revitalizing Energy Smoothie (Large)									
	290	0.5	0	<5	68	4	62	6	260

Food Serving size	Cal.	(g) Total Fat	(g) Sat. Fat	(mg) Chol.	(g) Carb.	(g) Fiber	(g) Sug.	(g) Prot.	(mg) Sod.
Revitalizing Energy Smoothie (Regular)									
	210	0.5	0	<5	48	3	44	4	190
Strawberry Banana Smoothie (Large)									
	300	0.5	0	<5	69	4	61	6	260
Strawberry Banana Smoothie (Regular)									
	210	0.5	0	<5	49	3	43	4	190
Tropical Mango Smoothie (Large)									
	330	0.5	0	<5	76	3	71	5	260
Tropical Mango Smoothie (Regular)									
	220	0	0	<5	53	2	49	4	190
Tropical Pineapple Smoothie (Large)									
	340	0.5	0	0	81	4	71	6	260
Tropical Pineapple Smoothie (Regular)									
	240	0	0	0	57	2	50	4	190

SUBWAY

6" Flatbread Sandwiches with 7 Grams of Fat or Less.

Values include 9-grain wheat bread, lettuce. tomatoes. onions, green peppers, and cucumbers. Double values for approximate footlong flatbread nutrition.

Food Serving size	Cal.	(g) Total Fat	(g) Sat. Fat	(mg) Chol.	(g) Carb.	(g) Fiber	(g) Sug.	(g) Prot.	(mg) Sod.
Black Forest Ham on Flatbread									
	300	7	1.5	25	44	3	5	17	980
Oven Roasted Chicken on Flatbread									
	330	7	1.5	25	45	3	6	22	790
Roast Beef on Flatbread									
	330	7	2	45	43	3	4	23	840
Subway Club on Flatbread									
	320	7	2	40	44	3	5	22	1030
Sweet Onion Chicken Teriyaki on Flatbread									
	390	7	1.5	50	57	3	16	25	1050
Turkey Breast and Black Forest Ham on Flatbread									
	290	6	1.5	25	44	3	5	17	970
Turkey Breast on Flatbread									
	290	6	1.5	20	44	3	4	17	950
Veggie Delite on Flatbread									
	240	4.5	1	0	42	3	4	8	450

Food Serving size	Cal.	(g) Total Fat	(g) Sat. Fat	(mg) Chol.	(g) Carb.	(g) Fiber	(g) Sug.	(g) Prot.	(mg) Sod.

6" Limited Time Offer/Regional Subs

Values include 9-grain wheat bread, lettuce. tomatoes. onions, green peppers, and cucumbers.

6" Barbecue Chicken									
	310	5	1.5	35	52	6	15	15	900
6" Barbecue Rib Patty									
	430	18	6	50	47	5	8	19	620
6" Chicken Pizziola (Includes Cheese)									
	450	15	6	75	50	6	10	31	1250
6" Orchard Chicken									
	370	4	1.5	50	51	5	9	25	560
6" Pastrami, Big (Includes Cheese)									
	580	28	9	65	49	5	7	31	1700
6" Pulled Pork									
	570	17	6	95	68	5	11	56	1340
6" Subway Seafood Sensation (Includes Cheese)									
	460	22	5	25	51	5	8	15	950
6" Turkey Bacon Avacado (Includes Cheese)									
	420	15	5	40	49	7	8	24	1200
6" Veggie Patty									
	390	7	1	10	56	8	8	23	830

6" Low Fat Sandwiches with 6 Grams of Fat or Less

Values include 9-grain wheat bread, lettuce. tomatoes. onions, green peppers, and cucumbers.

6" Black Forest Ham									
	290	4.5	1	25	46	5	8	18	830
6" Oven Roasted Chicken									
	320	5	1.5	25	47	5	8	23	640
6" Roast Beef									
	320	5	1.5	45	45	5	7	24	700
6" Subway Club									
	310	4.5	1.5	40	46	5	7	23	880
6" Sweet Onion Chicken Teriyaki									
	380	4.5	1	50	59	5	18	26	900
6" Turkey Breast									
	280	3.5	1	20	46	5	7	18	810

Food Serving size	Cal.	(g) Total Fat	(g) Sat. Fat	(mg) Chol.	(g) Carb.	(g) Fiber	(g) Sug.	(g) Prot.	(mg) Sod.
6" Turkey Breast and Black Forest Ham									
	280	4	1	20	46	5	8	18	820
6" Veggie Delite									
	230	2.5	0.5	0	44	5	6	8	310

6" Omelet Sandwich (with Egg White)

Values include 9-grain wheat bread, egg white and cheese.

Food Serving size	Cal.	(g) Total Fat	(g) Sat. Fat	(mg) Chol.	(g) Carb.	(g) Fiber	(g) Sug.	(g) Prot.	(mg) Sod.
6" Bacon, Egg White and Cheese									
	370	11	4.5	20	45	4	5	23	1120
6" Breakfast B.M.T.									
	460	17	7	45	48	5	7	29	1680
6" Egg White and Cheese									
	320	8	3	10	44	4	5	19	940
6" Egg White and Cheese (with Ham)									
	350	9	3.5	25	45	4	6	24	1200
6" Mega									
	610	35	14	55	45	4	5	30	1640
6" Sausage, Egg White and Cheese									
	570	31	12	45	45	4	5	26	1460
6" Steak, Egg White and Cheese									
	390	10	4	35	47	4	6	28	1300
6" Sunrise Melt									
	430	13	5	45	48	4	7	32	1640

6" Omelet Sandwiches (with Regular Egg)

Values include 9-grain wheat bread, regular egg and cheese.

Food Serving size	Cal.	(g) Total Fat	(g) Sat. Fat	(mg) Chol.	(g) Carb.	(g) Fiber	(g) Sug.	(g) Prot.	(mg) Sod.
6" Bacon, Egg and Cheese									
	410	16	6	240	45	5	6	23	1080
6" Breakfast B.M.T.									
	500	21.95	8	265	47	5	9	29	1640
6" Egg and Cheese									
	360	12	4.5	230	44	5	6	19	890
6" Egg and Cheese (with Ham)									
	390	13	5	240	45	5	7	24	1150
6" Mega									
	650	39	15	275	45	5	7	30	1600

Food Serving size	Cal.	(g) Total Fat	(g) Sat. Fat	(mg) Chol.	(g) Carb.	(g) Fiber	(g) Sug.	(g) Prot.	(mg) Sod.
6" Sausage, Egg and Cheese									
	610	36	14	265	45	5	6	26	1410
6" Steak, Egg and Cheese									
	430	15	5	255	47	5	7	28	1260
6" Sunrise Melt									
	470	17	7	260	48	5	8	32	1600

6" Sandwiches

Values include 9-grain wheat bread, lettuce, tomatoes, onions, green peppers, cucumbers, and cheese.

Food Serving size	Cal.	(g) Total Fat	(g) Sat. Fat	(mg) Chol.	(g) Carb.	(g) Fiber	(g) Sug.	(g) Prot.	(mg) Sod.
6" Big Philly Cheesesteak									
	520	18	9	90	52	6	8	39	1370
6" BLT									
	360	13	6	30	44	5	6	17	890
6" Buffalo Chicken (with Regular Ranch Dressing)									
	460	19	5	65	47	5	9	27	1390
6" Chicken and Bacon Ranch									
	570	28	10	95	47	5	8	35	1080
6" Cold Cut Combo									
	410	16	6	60	47	5	7	21	1340
6" Italian B.M.T.									
	450	20	8	55	47	5	8	22	1500
6" Meatball Marinara									
	580	23	9	45	69	9	18	24	1420
6" Spicy Italian									
	520	28	11	65	46	5	8	22	1720
6" Steak and Cheese									
	380	10	4.5	50	48	5	8	26	1060
6" Subway Melt									
	370	11	5	45	47	5	8	23	1210
6" Tuna									
	530	30	6	45	44	5	7	21	830

8" Pizza

Food Serving size	Cal.	(g) Total Fat	(g) Sat. Fat	(mg) Chol.	(g) Carb.	(g) Fiber	(g) Sug.	(g) Prot.	(mg) Sod.
Cheese									
	680	22	9	40	96	4	7	32	1070

Food Serving size	Cal.	(g) Total Fat	(g) Sat. Fat	(mg) Chol.	(g) Carb.	(g) Fiber	(g) Sug.	(g) Prot.	(mg) Sod.
Cheese and Veggies									
	740	25	11	50	100	5	9	36	1270
Pepperoni									
	790	32	13	60	96	4	8	38	1350
Sausage									
	820	34	14	70	97	4	8	39	1420

Beverages

Food Serving size	Cal.	(g) Total Fat	(g) Sat. Fat	(mg) Chol.	(g) Carb.	(g) Fiber	(g) Sug.	(g) Prot.	(mg) Sod.
Bottled Juice/Drink									
	0-300	0	0	0	54-68	0	48-64	0	40-160
Fountain Drink, Diet/Unsweetened Tea - 16 oz, No Ice									
	0-10	0	0	0	0	0	0	0	0-60
Fountain Drink, Diet/Unsweetened Tea - 21 oz, No Ice									
	0-15	0	0	0	0	0	0	0	0-80
Fountain Drink, Diet/Unsweetened Tea - 30 oz, No Ice									
	0-25	0	0	0	0	0	0	0	0-60
Fountain Drink, Diet/Unsweetened Tea - 40 oz, No Ice									
	0-30	0	0	0	0	0	0	0	0-100
Fountain Drink/Sweetened Tea, Regular - 16 oz, No Ice									
	120-240	0	0	0	34-66	0	34-66	0	0-110
Fountain Drink/Sweetened Tea, Regular - 21 oz, No Ice									
	160-320	0	0	0	45-87	0	45-87	0	0-140
Fountain Drink/Sweetened Tea, Regular - 30 oz, No Ice									
	230-460	0	0	0	65-120	0	65-120	0	0-200
Fountain Drink/Sweetened Tea, Regular - 40 oz, No Ice									
	310-620	0	0	0	90-160	0	90-160	0	0-260
Juice Box									
	100	0	0	0	24	0	21	0	15
Milk, Chocolate Flavored Reduced Fat									
	300	8	5	35	43	<1	43	15	300
Milk, Low Fat									
	160	3.5	2.5	20	19	0	17	12	180
Milk, Strawberry Flavored Reduced Fat									
	300	7	4.5	35	44	0	42	15	220

Food Serving size	Cal.	(g) Total Fat	(g) Sat. Fat	(mg) Chol.	(g) Carb.	(g) Fiber	(g) Sug.	(g) Prot.	(mg) Sod.
Breads									
6" 9-Grain Wheat Bread	210	2	0.5	0	40	4	5	8	310
6" Flatbread	220	4.5	1	0	38	2	2	7	450
6" Hearty Italian Bread	210	2.5	0.5	0	41	2	5	7	290
6" Honey Oat	260	3	0.5	0	48	5	9	9	330
6" Italian (White) Bread	200	2	0.5	0	38	1	5	7	290
6" Italian Herbs and Cheese	250	5	2.5	10	40	2	5	9	490
6" Monterey Cheddar	240	6	2.5	10	38	2	5	10	360
6" Parmesan Oregano Bread	220	2.5	1	0	40	2	5	8	440
6" Roasted Garlic	230	2.5	0.5	0	45	2	7	8	1260
6" Wheat Bread with Omega-3 ALA (CA Only)	230	3	0.5	0	44	4	3	9	310
Light Wheat English Muffin	100	0.5	0	0	22	5	1	6	170
Mini Italian Bread	130	1.5	0	0	25	1	3	5	190
Mini Wheat Bread	140	1.5	0	0	27	3	3	5	200
Wrap	310	8	2.5	0	51	1	0	8	610
Breakfast Sides									
Hash Browns (4 Pieces)	150	9	1	0	17	2	0	1	440
Cheese (Amount on 6-inch Sub, 6" Flatbread or Salad)									
American, Processed	40	3.5	2	10	1	0	0	2	200

Food Serving size	Cal.	(g) Total Fat	(g) Sat. Fat	(mg) Chol.	(g) Carb.	(g) Fiber	(g) Sug.	(g) Prot.	(mg) Sod.
Monterey Cheddar, Shredded									
	50	4.5	3	15	1	0	0	3	90
Mozzarella, Shredded									
	40	2	1	10	0	0	0	2	100
Natural Cheddar									
	60	5	3	15	0	0	0	4	100
Pepperjack									
	50	4	2.5	15	0	0	0	3	140
Provolone									
	50	4	2	10	0	0	0	4	125
Swiss									
	50	4.5	2.5	15	0	0	0	4	30

Chips

Food Serving size	Cal.	(g) Total Fat	(g) Sat. Fat	(mg) Chol.	(g) Carb.	(g) Fiber	(g) Sug.	(g) Prot.	(mg) Sod.
Baked Lay's									
	130	2	0	0	23	2	2	2	200
Baked Lay's Sour Cream and Onion									
	140	3.5	0.5	0	24	2	3	3	240
Chips, 1 Bag									
	75-340	0-22	0-4.5	0-35	13-36	0-3	0-9	0-7	150-940
Doritos Nacho									
	250	13	2.5	<5	30	2	2	4	310
Lay's Classic									
	230	15	1.5	0	23	2	0	3	270
Sunchips Harvest Cheddar									
	210	9	1.5	0	29	3	3	4	240

Cookies and Desserts

Food Serving size	Cal.	(g) Total Fat	(g) Sat. Fat	(mg) Chol.	(g) Carb.	(g) Fiber	(g) Sug.	(g) Prot.	(mg) Sod.
Apple Pie									
	250	10	2	0	37	1	25	0	290
Apple Slices - 1 Package									
	35	0	0	0	9	2	7	0	0
Chocolate Chip									
	210	10	6	15	30	1	18	2	150
Chocolate Chunk									
	220	10	5	10	30	<1	17	2	100
Double Chocolate Chip									
	210	10	6	15	30	1	20	2	170

Food Serving size	Cal.	(g) Total Fat	(g) Sat. Fat	(mg) Chol.	(g) Carb.	(g) Fiber	(g) Sug.	(g) Prot.	(mg) Sod.
M&M	210	10	5	10	32	<1	18	2	100
Oatmeal Raisin	200	8	4	15	30	1	17	3	170
Peanut Butter	220	12	5	15	26	1	16	4	190
Raspberry Cheesecake	210	9	4.5	13	29	0	16	2	180
Sugar	220	12	6	15	28	<1	14	2	140
White Chip Macadamia Nut	220	11	5	15	29	<1	18	2	160
Yogurt Dannon Light and Fit	80	0	0	<5	16	0	11	5	80
Yogurt Parfait	160	2	1.004	10	30	2	24	6	75

Egg Muffin Melts (with Egg White)

Values include light wheat English muffin, egg white, and cheese.

Food Serving size	Cal.	(g) Total Fat	(g) Sat. Fat	(mg) Chol.	(g) Carb.	(g) Fiber	(g) Sug.	(g) Prot.	(mg) Sod.
Bacon, Egg (White) and Cheese	180	5	2	10	24	5	1	13	580
Breakfast B.M.T.	220	8	3	20	25	5	2	16	860
Egg White and Cheese	150	3.5	1.5	5	24	5	1	12	480
Egg White and Cheese (with Ham)	170	4	1.5	10	24	5	1	14	610
Mega	300	17	7	30	24	5	1	17	840
Sausage, Egg (White) and Cheese	270	15	6	25	24	5	1	15	740
Steak, Egg (White) and Cheese	180	4	1.5	15	25	5	1	15	620
Sunrise Melt	210	6	2.5	20	26	5	2	18	830

Food Serving size	Cal.	(g) Total Fat	(g) Sat. Fat	(mg) Chol.	(g) Carb.	(g) Fiber	(g) Sug.	(g) Prot.	(mg) Sod.

Egg Muffin Melts (with Regular Egg)

Values include light wheat English muffin, regular egg, and cheese.

Food Serving size	Cal.	Total Fat	Sat. Fat	Chol.	Carb.	Fiber	Sug.	Prot.	Sod.
Bacon, Egg and Cheese	200	7	3	120	24	6	1	13	550
Breakfast B.M.T.	240	10	4	130	25	6	2	16	830
Egg and Cheese	170	6	2	115	24	6	1	12	460
Egg and Cheese (with Ham)	190	6	2	120	24	6	2	14	590
Mega	320	19	7	140	24	6	2	17	810
Sausage, Egg and Cheese	290	17	7	130	24	6	1	15	720
Steak, Egg and Cheese	200	6	2.5	125	25	6	2	15	610
Sunrise Melt	230	8	3	130	26	6	2	18	810

Egg Whites on Mornin' Flatbreads

Values include mornin' flatbread, egg white, and cheese.

Food Serving size	Cal.	Total Fat	Sat. Fat	Chol.	Carb.	Fiber	Sug.	Prot.	Sod.
Bacon, Egg White and Cheese	190	7	2.5	10	21	1	1	11	630
Breakfast B.M.T.	230	10	3.5	20	22	1	2	14	910
Egg White and Cheese	170	5	1.5	5	21	1	1	9	540
Egg White and Cheese (with Ham)	180	5	2	10	22	1	1	12	670
Mega	310	19	7	30	22	1	1	15	830
Sausage, Egg White and Cheese	290	17	6	25	21	1	1	13	800
Steak, Egg White and Cheese	190	6	2	15	22	1	1	13	670

Food Serving size	Cal.	(g) Total Fat	(g) Sat. Fat	(mg) Chol.	(g) Carb.	(g) Fiber	(g) Sug.	(g) Prot.	(mg) Sod.
Sunrise Melt	220	8	3	20	23	1	2	16	890

Individual Meats (Amount on 6" Sub or Salad)

Food Serving size	Cal.	(g) Total Fat	(g) Sat. Fat	(mg) Chol.	(g) Carb.	(g) Fiber	(g) Sug.	(g) Prot.	(mg) Sod.
Chicken Patty, Roasted	90	2.5	0.5	25	4	0	2	15	330
Chicken Strips	80	1.5	0.5	50	0	0	0	16	210
Cold Cut Combo Meals	140	11	3.5	50	2	0	1	10	830
Egg Patty (Regular)	110	7	2	220	3	1	1	9	380
Egg White Patty	70	2	0	0	3	0	0	9	430
Ham	60	2	0.5	25	2	0	2	9	520
Italian B.M.T. Meats	180	14	5	45	2	0	2	11	990
Meatballs	310	17	6	30	25	4	11	13	910
Roast Beef	90	2.5	1	45	1	0	1	16	390
Sausage, Breakfast	240	24	9	35	1	0	0	7	520
Seafood Sensation	190	16	2.5	15	7	0	1	5	430
Steak (No Cheese)	110	2	1.5	40	1	0	1	16	550
Subway Club Meats	90	2.5	1	39	2	0	1	15	570
Tuna	260	24	4	35	0	0	0	10	310
Turkey Breast	50	1	0	20	2	0	1	9	500
Veggie Patty	160	5	0.5	10	12	3	2	15	520

Food Serving size	Cal.	(g) Total Fat	(g) Sat. Fat	(mg) Chol.	(g) Carb.	(g) Fiber	(g) Sug.	(g) Prot.	(mg) Sod.
Kids Meal Sandwiches									
Values include 9-grain wheat bread, lettuce. tomatoes. onions, green peppers, and cucumbers.									
Black Forest Ham									
	180	2.5	0.5	10	30	3	5	10	470
Roast Beef									
	200	3	1	25	30	4	5	14	410
Turkey Breast									
	180	2	0.5	10	30	3	5	10	460
Veggie Delite									
	150	1.5	0	0	29	3	4	6	210
Low Fat Footlong Sandwiches									
Values include 9-grain wheat bread, lettuce. tomatoes. onions, green peppers, and cucumbers.									
Footlong Black Forest Ham									
	570	9	2.5	50	92	10	16	35	1670
Footlong Oven Roasted Chicken									
	640	10	2.5	45	95	11	17	46	1290
Footlong Roast Beef									
	630	10	3.5	90	90	11	14	48	1390
Footlong Subway Club									
	630	9	3	80	92	10	15	46	1770
Footlong Sweet Onion Chicken Teriyaki									
	750	9	2.5	100	117	10	37	51	1810
Footlong Turkey Breast									
	560	7	2	40	92	10	14	35	1620
Footlong Turkey Breast and Black Forest Ham									
	570	8	2	45	92	10	15	35	1650
Footlong Veggie Delite									
	460	4.5	1	0	87	10	13	17	620
Omelet on 6" Flatbread (with Egg White)									
Values include 6" flatbread, egg white, and cheese.									
Bacon, Egg White and Cheese on 6" Flatbread									
	380	13	5	20	43	2	2	22	1270
Breakfast B.M.T. on 6" Flatbread									
	470	20	7	45	45	2	4	28	1830

Food Serving size	Cal.	(g) Total Fat	(g) Sat. Fat	(mg) Chol.	(g) Carb.	(g) Fiber	(g) Sug.	(g) Prot.	(mg) Sod.
Egg White and Cheese (with Ham) on 6" Flatbread									
	360	11	3.5	25	43	2	3	23	1340
Egg White and Cheese on 6" Flatbread									
	330	10	3.5	10	42	2	2	19	1080
Mega on 6" Flatbread									
	620	37	14	60	43	2	2	29	1790
Sausage, Egg White and Cheese on 6" Flatbread									
	570	34	13	45	43	2	2	26	1600
Steak, Egg (White) and Cheese on 6" Flatbread									
	400	12	4.5	35	45	2	3	28	1450
Sunrise Melt on 6" Flatbread									
	440	15	6	45	46	2	4	31	1780

Omelet on 6" Flatbread (with Regular Egg)

Values include 6" flatbread, regular egg, and cheese.

Bacon, Egg and Cheese on 6" Flatbread									
	420	18	7	240	42	3	4	22	1220
Breakfast B.M.T. on 6" Flatbread									
	510	24	8	265	45	3	6	28	1780
Egg and Cheese (with Ham) on 6" Flatbread									
	400	15	5	240	43	3	4	23	1290
Egg and Cheese on 6" Flatbread									
	370	14	5	230	42	3	3	19	1030
Mega on 6" Flatbread									
	660	42	16	275	43	3	4	29	1740
Sausage, Egg and Cheese on 6" Flatbread									
	610	38	14	265	43	3	4	26	1550
Steak, Egg and Cheese on 6" Flatbread									
	440	17	6	255	44	3	4	28	1363
Sunrise Melt on 6" Flatbread									
	480	20	7	260	46	3	6	32	1730

Regular Egg on Mornin' Flatbreads

Values include Mornin' flatbread, regular egg and cheese

Bacon, Egg and Cheese									
	210	9	3.5	120	21	1	2	11	610

Food Serving size	Cal.	(g) Total Fat	(g) Sat. Fat	(mg) Chol.	(g) Carb.	(g) Fiber	(g) Sug.	(g) Prot.	(mg) Sod.
Breakfast B.M.T.	250	12	4	130	22	1	3	14	890
Egg and Cheese	190	7	2.5	115	21	1	2	9	520
Egg and Cheese (with Ham)	200	8	2.5	120	22	1	2	12	650
Mega	330	21	8	140	22	1	2	15	870
Sausage, Egg and Cheese	310	19	7	135	21	1	2	13	770
Steak, Egg and Cheese	210	8	3	125	22	1	2	13	650
Sunrise Melt	240	10	3.5	130	23	1	3	16	870

Salad Dressing

Food Serving size	Cal.	(g) Total Fat	(g) Sat. Fat	(mg) Chol.	(g) Carb.	(g) Fiber	(g) Sug.	(g) Prot.	(mg) Sod.
Fat-free Italian	35	0	0	0	7	0	4	1	720
Ranch	290	30	4.5	15	3	0	3	1	540

Salads with 6 Grams of Fat or Less

Values include lettuce, tomatoes, onions, green peppers, cucumbers, and olives. Values do not include dressing or croutons.

Food Serving size	Cal.	(g) Total Fat	(g) Sat. Fat	(mg) Chol.	(g) Carb.	(g) Fiber	(g) Sug.	(g) Prot.	(mg) Sod.
Black Forest Ham	110	3	1	25	11	4	6	12	590
Grilled Chicken and Baby Spinach	130	2.5	0.5	50	10	3	4	20	330
Oven Roasted Chicken Breast	130	2.5	0.5	50	9	4	4	19	270
Roast Beef	140	3.5	1	45	10	4	5	18	450
Subway Club	140	3.5	1	40	11	4	5	17	640
Sweet Onion Chicken Teriyaki	200	3	1	50	24	4	16	20	660
Turkey Breast	110	2	0.5	20	11	4	5	12	570

Food Serving size	Cal.	(g) Total Fat	(g) Sat. Fat	(mg) Chol.	(g) Carb.	(g) Fiber	(g) Sug.	(g) Prot.	(mg) Sod.
Turkey Breast and Ham	110	2.5	0.5	20	11	4	5	12	580
Veggie Delite	50	1	0	0	9	4	4	3	65

Sandwich Condiments (Amount on 6-inch Sub or Flatbread)

Food	Cal.	Total Fat	Sat. Fat	Chol.	Carb.	Fiber	Sug.	Prot.	Sod.
Bacon	45	3.5	1.5	10	0	0	0	3	190
Chipotle Southwest Sauce	100	10	1.5	10	1	0	0	0	220
Honey Mustard Sauce, Fat Free	30	0	0	0	7	0	6	0	120
Light Mayonnaise (1 Tablespoon)	50	5	1	5	<1	0	0	0	100
Mayonnaise (1 Tablespoon)	110	12	2	10	0	0	0	0	80
Mustard Yellow or Deli Brown	5	0	0	0	<1	0	0	0	115
Olive Oil Blend (1 Teaspoon)	45	5	0	0	0	0	0	0	0
Pepperoni, 3 Slices	80	7	2.5	15	1	0	1	4	400
Ranch Dressing	110	11	1.5	5	1	0	1	0	200
Red Wine Vinaigrette, Fat Free	30	0	0	0	6	0	3	0	340
Sweet Onion Sauce, Fat Free	40	0	0	0	9	0	8	0	85
Vinegar (1 Teaspoon)	0	0	0	0	0	0	0	0	0

Soup (10 oz Bowl)

Food	Cal.	Total Fat	Sat. Fat	Chol.	Carb.	Fiber	Sug.	Prot.	Sod.
Chicken and Dumpling	170	5	2	35	23	2	2	8	810
Chicken Tortilla	110	1.5	0.5	10	11	3	4	6	440

Food Serving size	Cal.	(g) Total Fat	(g) Sat. Fat	(mg) Chol.	(g) Carb.	(g) Fiber	(g) Sug.	(g) Prot.	(mg) Sod.
Chili Con Carne									
	340	11	5	60	35	10	7	20	950
Chipotle Chicken Corn Chowder									
	140	3	1.5	15	22	2	4	6	900
Cream of Potato with Bacon									
	240	13	5	15	26	3	3	5	870
Fire-Roasted Tomato Orzo									
	130	1	0.5	5	24	2	4	6	410
Golden Broccoli and Cheese									
	180	11	5	25	16	4	3	5	990
Minestrone									
	90	1	0	<5	17	3	4	4	910
New England Style Clam Chowder									
	150	5	1	10	20	4	2	6	990
Roasted Chicken Noodle									
	80	2	0.5	15	12	1	2	6	950
Rosemary Chicken and Dumpling									
	90	1.5	0.5	25	14	1	3	6	810
Spanish Style Chicken and Rice with Pork									
	110	2.5	1	5	16	1	1	6	980
Tomato Garden Vegetable with Rotini									
	90	0.5	0	0	20	3	8	3	820
Vegetable Beef									
	100	2	0.5	10	17	3	5	5	960
Wild Rice with Chicken									
	230	11	3.5	50	26	1	3	6	900

Vegetables (Amount on 6-inch Sub or Flatbread)

Food Serving size	Cal.	(g) Total Fat	(g) Sat. Fat	(mg) Chol.	(g) Carb.	(g) Fiber	(g) Sug.	(g) Prot.	(mg) Sod.
Avocado									
	70	7	1	0	3	2	0	1	0
Banana Peppers (3 Rings)									
	0	0	0	0	0	0	0	0	20
Cucumbers (3 Slices)									
	<5	0	0	0	<1	0	0	0	0
Green Peppers (3 Strips)									
	0	0	0	0	0	0	0	0	0

Food Serving size	Cal.	(g) Total Fat	(g) Sat. Fat	(mg) Chol.	(g) Carb.	(g) Fiber	(g) Sug.	(g) Prot.	(mg) Sod.
Jalapeno Peppers (3 Rings)									
	<5	0	0	0	0	0	0	0	70
Lettuce									
	<5	0	0	0	0	0	0	0	0
Olives (3 Rings)									
	<5	0	0	0	0	0	0	0	25
Onions									
	<5	0	0	0	1	0	0	0	0
Pickles (3 Chips)									
	0	0	0	0	0	0	0	0	115
Tomatoes (3 Wheels)									
	5	0	0	0	2	0	0	0	0

TACO BELL

Beverages

Food Serving size	Cal.	(g) Total Fat	(g) Sat. Fat	(mg) Chol.	(g) Carb.	(g) Fiber	(g) Sug.	(g) Prot.	(mg) Sod.
Cherry Limeade Sparkler (16 oz)									
	180	0	0	0	43	0	43	0	105
Cherry Limeade Sparkler (20 oz)									
	270	0	0	0	66	0	65	0	160
Classic Limeade Sparkler (16 oz)									
	150	0	0	0	39	0	38	0	80
Classic Limeade Sparkler (20 oz)									
	230	0	0	0	60	0	59	0	125
Diet Pepsi (16 oz)									
	0	0	0	0	0	0	0	0	50
Diet Pepsi (20 oz)									
	0	0	0	0	0	0	0	0	65
Diet Pepsi (30 oz)									
	0	0	0	0	0	0	0	0	95
Diet Pepsi (40 oz)									
	0	0	0	0	0	0	0	0	125
Dr Pepper (16 oz)									
	200	0	0	0	54	0	54	0	70
Dr Pepper (20 oz)									
	250	0	0	0	68	0	68	0	88

Food Serving size	Cal.	(g) Total Fat	(g) Sat. Fat	(mg) Chol.	(g) Carb.	(g) Fiber	(g) Sug.	(g) Prot.	(mg) Sod.
Dr Pepper (30 oz)	375	0	0	0	102	0	102	0	132
Dr Pepper (40 oz)	500	0	0	0	135	0	135	0	175
Lipton Raspberry Iced Tea (16 oz)	160	0	0	0	42	0	42	0	50
Lipton Raspberry Iced Tea (20 oz)	200	0	0	0	53	0	53	0	65
Lipton Raspberry Iced Tea (30 oz)	300	0	0	0	79	0	79	0	95
Lipton Raspberry Iced Tea (40 oz)	400	0	0	0	105	0	105	0	125
Mango Strawberry Frutista Freeze (16 oz)	250	0	0	0	62	0	59	0	10
Mango Strawberry Frutista Freeze (20 oz)	300	0	0	0	75	0	73	0	15
Mountain Dew (16 oz)	220	0	0	0	58	0	58	0	70
Mountain Dew (20 oz)	280	0	0	0	73	0	73	0	90
Mountain Dew (30 oz)	410	0	0	0	109	0	109	0	130
Mountain Dew (40 oz)	550	0	0	0	145	0	145	0	175
Mountain Dew Baja Blast (16 oz)	220	0	0	0	58	0	58	0	60
Mountain Dew Baja Blast (20 oz)	280	0	0	0	73	0	73	0	75
Mountain Dew Baja Blast (30 oz)	410	0	0	0	109	0	109	0	115
Mountain Dew Baja Blast (40 oz)	550	0	0	0	145	0	145	0	150
Mug Root Beer (16 oz)	200	0	0	0	52	0	52	0	30
Mug Root Beer (20 oz)	250	0	0	0	65	0	65	0	40

Food Serving size	Cal.	(g) Total Fat	(g) Sat. Fat	(mg) Chol.	(g) Carb.	(g) Fiber	(g) Sug.	(g) Prot.	(mg) Sod.
Mug Root Beer (30 oz)	380	0	0	0	98	0	98	0	55
Mug Root Beer (40 oz)	500	0	0	0	130	0	130	0	75
Pepsi (16 oz)	200	0	0	0	56	0	56	0	40
Pepsi (20 oz)	250	0	0	0	70	0	70	0	50
Pepsi (30 oz)	380	0	0	0	105	0	105	0	75
Pepsi (40 oz)	500	0	0	0	140	0	140	0	100
Sierra Mist (16 oz)	200	0	0	0	54	0	54	0	40
Sierra Mist (20 oz)	250	0	0	0	68	0	68	0	50
Sierra Mist (30 oz)	380	0	0	0	101	0	101	0	75
Sierra Mist (40 oz)	500	0	0	0	135	0	135	0	100
Strawberry Frutista Freeze (16 oz)	230	0	0	0	57	0	57	0	55
Strawberry Frutista Freeze (20 oz)	280	0	0	0	70	0	69	0	65
Tropical Fruit Lemonade (20 oz)	250	0	0	0	68	0	68	0	265
Tropical Fruit Lemonade (30 oz)	380	0	0	0	101	0	101	0	395
Tropical Fruit Lemonade (40 oz)	500	0	0	0	135	0	135	0	525
Tropical Fruit Punch (16 oz)	220	0	0	0	60	0	60	0	50
Tropical Fruit Punch (20 oz)	280	0	0	0	75	0	75	0	65
Tropical Fruit Punch (30 oz)	410	0	0	0	113	0	113	0	95

Food Serving size	Cal.	(g) Total Fat	(g) Sat. Fat	(mg) Chol.	(g) Carb.	(g) Fiber	(g) Sug.	(g) Prot.	(mg) Sod.
Tropical Fruit Punch (40 oz)	550	0	0	0	150	0	150	0	125
Tropical Pink Lemonade (16 oz)	200	0	0	0	54	0	54	0	210

Burritos

Food Serving size	Cal.	Total Fat	Sat. Fat	Chol.	Carb.	Fiber	Sug.	Prot.	Sod.
1/2 lb. Cheesy Potato Burrito	540	26	8	50	59	7	4	19	1430
1/2 lb. Combo Burrito	460	18	7	50	53	10	3	21	1400
7-Layer Burrito	500	18	6	20	69	12	5	17	1090
Burrito Supreme - Beef	420	15	7	35	53	9	5	17	1140
Burrito Supreme - Chicken	400	12	5	40	51	7	5	21	1060
Burrito Supreme - Steak	390	13	5	30	51	7	5	17	1100
Cheesy Bean and Rice Burrito	480	21	5	10	60	7	5	12	1020
Grilled Stuft Burrito - Beef	700	30	10	60	79	12	5	27	1740
Grilled Stuft Burrito - Chicken	650	24	7	65	76	9	5	34	1580
Grilled Stuft Burrito - Steak	640	25	8	50	76	9	5	28	1670

Chalupas

Food Serving size	Cal.	Total Fat	Sat. Fat	Chol.	Carb.	Fiber	Sug.	Prot.	Sod.
Chalupa Baja - Beef	430	29	6	35	30	4	3	13	570
Chalupa Baja - Chicken	410	26	4	35	28	2	3	17	490
Chalupa Baja - Steak	400	26	4.5	30	28	2	3	13	530
Chalupa Nacho Cheese - Beef	390	24	4	20	31	3	4	12	540

Food Serving size	Cal.	(g) Total Fat	(g) Sat. Fat	(mg) Chol.	(g) Carb.	(g) Fiber	(g) Sug.	(g) Prot.	(mg) Sod.
Chalupa Nacho Cheese - Chicken	360	21	2.5	25	30	1	3	15	460
Chalupa Nacho Cheese - Steak	360	21	2.5	20	30	1	4	12	500
Chalupa Supreme - Beef	390	24	6	35	31	3	4	13	480
Chalupa Supreme - Chicken	370	21	4	35	29	2	3	17	410
Chalupa Supreme - Steak	360	21	4.5	30	29	2	4	14	450

Fresco Menu

Food	Cal.	Total Fat	Sat. Fat	Chol.	Carb.	Fiber	Sug.	Prot.	Sod.
Fresco Bean Burrito	350	8	2.5	0	57	11	4	12	990
Fresco Burrito Supreme - Chicken	350	8	2.5	25	50	7	4	18	1060
Fresco Burrito Supreme - Steak	340	8	2.5	15	50	7	4	15	1100
Fresco Chicken Soft Taco	150	3.5	1	25	18	2	2	12	480
Fresco Crunchy Taco	150	7	2.5	20	13	3	1	7	350
Fresco Grilled Steak Soft Taco	150	4	1.5	15	19	2	2	9	520
Fresco Soft Taco - Beef	180	7	2.5	20	20	3	2	8	560

Fully Loaded Taco Salads

Food	Cal.	Total Fat	Sat. Fat	Chol.	Carb.	Fiber	Sug.	Prot.	Sod.
Chicken Ranch Taco Salad	910	55	10	70	69	8	5	34	1200
Chipotle Steak Taco Salad	900	57	11	65	69	8	6	27	1480
Fiesta Taco Salad	770	42	10	60	74	12	8	26	1420
Fiesta Taco Salad Without Shell	460	24	8	60	41	10	7	21	1260

Food Serving size	Cal.	(g) Total Fat	(g) Sat. Fat	(mg) Chol.	(g) Carb.	(g) Fiber	(g) Sug.	(g) Prot.	(mg) Sod.
Gorditas									
Gordita Baja - Beef	340	19	5	35	30	4	5	13	580
Gordita Baja - Chicken	320	15	3.5	35	28	2	5	17	500
Gordita Baja - Steak	310	16	3.5	30	28	2	5	13	540
Gordita Nacho Cheese - Beef	300	14	3.5	20	31	3	6	12	540
Gordita Nacho Cheese - Chicken	270	11	1.5	25	30	1	5	15	470
Gordita Nacho Cheese - Steak	260	11	2	20	30	1	6	12	510
Gordita Supreme - Beef	300	14	5	35	31	3	6	13	490
Gordita Supreme - Chicken	280	10	3.5	35	29	2	5	17	410
Gordita Supreme - Steak	270	11	4	30	29	2	6	14	450
Nachos and Sides									
Cheesy Fiesta Potatoes	290	17	2.5	10	32	3	2	4	620
Mexican Rice	120	3.5	0	0	20	1	0	2	200
Nachos	320	20	2	0	31	2	2	4	360
Nachos BellGrande	770	42	7	30	79	14	5	19	1050
Nachos Supreme	440	24	5	30	42	8	3	12	680
Pintos 'n Cheese	170	6	3	10	20	8	1	9	580
Regional Menu Items									
Cheese Quesadilla	480	27	11	50	40	4	3	19	1000

Food Serving size	Cal.	(g) Total Fat	(g) Sat. Fat	(mg) Chol.	(g) Carb.	(g) Fiber	(g) Sug.	(g) Prot.	(mg) Sod.
Chili Cheese Burrito	380	17	8	35	41	5	2	16	930
Tostada	250	10	3.5	15	30	9	2	10	550

Specialties

Food Serving size	Cal.	Total Fat	Sat. Fat	Chol.	Carb.	Fiber	Sug.	Prot.	Sod.
Chicken Quesadilla	530	28	12	75	41	4	3	28	1210
Chicken Taquitos	320	11	4.5	40	37	3	2	18	770
Crunchwrap Supreme	540	21	7	30	71	7	6	16	1150
Enchirto - Beef	360	17	8	45	34	8	2	18	1160
Enchirto - Chicken	340	14	7	50	32	6	2	22	1080
Enchirto - Steak	330	14	7	45	32	6	2	19	1120
Express Taco Salad	580	28	10	60	59	9	7	23	1350
Guacamole Side	35	3	0	0	2	1	0	0	85
Mexican Pizza	540	30	8	45	47	8	2	20	910
MexiMelt	270	14	7	45	21	4	2	15	800
Reduced Fat Sour Cream Side	30	2	1	5	2	0	1	1	20
Salsa Side	5	0	0	0	1	0	1	0	80
Steak Quesadilla	520	28	12	65	41	4	3	25	1250
Steak Taquitos	310	11	5	30	37	3	2	15	810

Food Serving size	Cal.	(g) Total Fat	(g) Sat. Fat	(mg) Chol.	(g) Carb.	(g) Fiber	(g) Sug.	(g) Prot.	(mg) Sod.
Tacos									
Chicken Soft Taco	180	6	2.5	30	18	1	1	14	460
Crunchy Taco Supreme	200	12	5	35	15	3	2	9	350
Double Decker Taco	320	13	4.5	30	37	8	2	13	690
Double Decker Taco Supreme	350	15	6	35	40	8	3	14	710
Grilled Steak Soft Taco	250	14	4	30	19	2	2	11	550
Soft Taco Supreme - Beef	230	11	5	35	22	3	3	11	560
Volcano Menu									
Volcano Burrito	780	41	12	70	80	9	6	24	1660
Volcano Nachos	980	60	9	45	89	15	6	20	1620
Volcano Taco	230	16	5	35	14	3	1	8	440
Why Pay More!									
Bean Burrito	370	10	3.5	5	56	10	3	13	980
Beefy 5-Layer Burrito	540	21	8	35	68	9	6	19	1320
Caramel Apple Empanada	310	15	2.5	0	39	2	13	3	310
Cheese Roll-Up	190	9	5	20	18	2	1	9	450
Cheesy Nachos	280	17	1.5	0	28	2	1	3	230
Chicken Burrito	430	18	5	35	48	3	3	18	870
Cinnamon Twists	170	7	0	0	26	1	10	1	200

Food Serving size	Cal.	(g) Total Fat	(g) Sat. Fat	(mg) Chol.	(g) Carb.	(g) Fiber	(g) Sug.	(g) Prot.	(mg) Sod.
Crispy Potato Soft Taco	270	13	3	10	31	3	1	6	520
Crunchy Taco	170	10	3.5	30	12	3	1	8	330
Soft Taco - Beef	200	9	4	30	19	3	1	10	540

TASTI D-LITE

Blended Coffee and Tea

	Cal.	Total Fat	Sat. Fat	Chol.	Carb.	Fiber	Sug.	Prot.	Sod.
Green Tea (16 fl oz)	210	1.5	1	5	38	0	34	6	115
Green Tea (24 fl oz)	310	2	1.5	10	57	0	51	9	170
Java D-Lite, with Whipped Cream and Caramel (16 fl oz)	330	1.5	1	5	66	0	39	7	230
Java D-Lite, with Whipped Cream and Caramel (24 fl oz)	460	2	1.5	10	92	0	58	11	320
Java D-Lite, Without Whipped Cream and Caramel (16 fl oz)	270	1.5	1	5	66	0	39	7	230
Java D-Lite, Without Whipped Cream and Caramel (24 fl oz)	410	2	1.5	10	92	0	58	11	320
Mocha D-Lite, with Whipped Cream and Caramel (16 fl oz)	380	1.5	1	5	78	0	51	8	240
Mocha D-Lite, with Whipped Cream and Caramel (24 fl oz)	540	2	1.5	10	109	1	75	11	340
Mocha D-Lite, Without Whipped Cream and Caramel (16 fl oz)	320	1.5	1	5	78	0	51	8	240
Mocha D-Lite, Without Whipped Cream and Caramel (24 fl oz)	480	2	1.5	10	109	1	75	11	340

Cakes

	Cal.	Total Fat	Sat. Fat	Chol.	Carb.	Fiber	Sug.	Prot.	Sod.
Apple Pie, 6" Round Cake (Serving Size, 102g)	150	4.5	2.5	5	25	1	19	3	65
Apple Pie, 8" Round Cake (Serving Size, 97g)	140	4	2.5	5	24	1	18	3	60

Food Serving size	Cal.	(g) Total Fat	(g) Sat. Fat	(mg) Chol.	(g) Carb.	(g) Fiber	(g) Sug.	(g) Prot.	(mg) Sod.
Cake Batter Up! 6" Round Cake (Serving Size, 103g)									
	130	4	3	5	20	0	17	2	65
Cake Batter Up! 8" Round Cake (Serving Size, 100g)									
	120	4	3	5	20	0	17	2	65
Caramel Apple Pie, 6" Round Cake (Serving Size, 120g)									
	180	4.5	3	5	31	1	22	3	85
Caramel Apple Pie, 8" Round Cake (Serving Size, 111g)									
	160	4	2.5	5	28	1	21	3	75
Chocolate Chip, 6" Round Cake (Serving Size, 115g)									
	170	6	4	0	28	1	21	4	100
Chocolate Chip, 8" Round Cake (Serving Size, 113g)									
	180	7	4.5	0	29	1	20	4	100
Chocolate Covered Strawberry Cake (Serving Size, 116g)									
	230	8	5	0	38	1	23	4	70
Classic Black and White, 6" Round Cake (Serving Size, 111g)									
	160	6	4	5	27	1	22	3	90
Classic Black and White, 8" Round Cake (Serving Size, 109g)									
	160	6	4	5	28	1	22	3	90
Neapolitan, 6" Round Cake (Serving Size, 110g)									
	130	3.5	2.5	5	21	1	19	3	70
Neapolitan, 8" Round Cake (Serving Size, 101g)									
	120	3.5	2.5	5	20	0	18	2	70
Oreo Cookie, 6" Round Cake (Serving Size, 97g)									
	160	6	3	5	25	0	19	3	115
Oreo Cookie, 8" Round Cake (Serving Size, 94g)									
	160	6	3	5	24	0	19	3	110
Peanut Buddy, 6" Round Cake (Serving Size, 112g)									
	220	10	5	5	27	1	18	5	120
Peanut Buddy, 8" Round Cake (Serving Size, 109g)									
	210	10	5	5	27	1	17	5	115
Pumpkin Cheesecake, 6" Round Cake (Serving Size, 102g)									
	150	4	3	5	25	0	19	3	95
Pumpkin Cheesecake, 8" Round Cake (Serving Size, 98g)									
	140	4.5	3	5	24	0	19	3	90
Pumpkin Pie, 6" Round Cake (Serving Size, 110g)									
	150	4.5	3	5	25	0	20	3	105

Food Serving size	Cal.	(g) Total Fat	(g) Sat. Fat	(mg) Chol.	(g) Carb.	(g) Fiber	(g) Sug.	(g) Prot.	(mg) Sod.
Pumpkin Pie, 8" Round Cake (Serving Size, 106g)									
	150	4.5	3	5	24	0	19	3	100
Raspberry Chocolate Truffle Cake (Serving Size, 120g)									
	240	8	5	0	39	2	23	4	75
Triple Berry D-Lite, 6" Round Cake (Serving Size, 127g)									
	150	3.5	2.5	5	26	0	23	2	65
Triple Berry D-Lite, 8" Round Cake (Serving Size, 123g)									
	140	4	2.5	5	25	1	22	2	60
Vanilla Chip, 6" Round Cake (Serving Size, 109g)									
	180	6	4.5	5	28	0	19	3	75
Vanilla Chip, 8" Round Cake (Serving Size, 108g)									
	190	7	4.5	5	29	0	19	3	75

Dry Toppings

Food Serving size	Cal.	(g) Total Fat	(g) Sat. Fat	(mg) Chol.	(g) Carb.	(g) Fiber	(g) Sug.	(g) Prot.	(mg) Sod.
Butterfinger Crumbles Topping (1 fl oz)									
	100	4	2	0	16	0	10	1	50
Chocolate Cookie Crunch Topping (1 fl oz)									
	50	1	0	NA	10	0	4	1	50
Chocolate Dipping Sauce Topping (0.5 fl oz)									
	110	9	5	0	8	1	7	0	10
Chocolate Sprinkles Topping (1 fl oz)									
	140	6	4	10	20	NA	NA	2	20
Chopped Peanuts Topping (1 fl oz)									
	100	8	1	0	3	1	1	4	0
Cinnamon Toast Granola Topping (1 fl oz)									
	60	2	0	0	10	2	3	2	5
Graham Cracker Crunch Topping (1 fl oz)									
	70	1.5	0	0	13	1	4	1	110
Heath Bar Chunk Topping (1 fl oz)									
	110	7	3.5	5	13	0	12	1	70
Honey Nut O's Topping (1 fl oz)									
	15	0	0	0	3	0	1	0	30
Mini Chocolate Chips Topping (1 fl oz)									
	160	8	5	0	20	NA	NA	2	0
Mini M&M's Topping (1 fl oz)									
	140	7	4	10	20	0	18	2	20

Food Serving size	Cal.	(g) Total Fat	(g) Sat. Fat	(mg) Chol.	(g) Carb.	(g) Fiber	(g) Sug.	(g) Prot.	(mg) Sod.
Oreo Cookie Pieces Topping (1 fl oz)	70	3	0	0	10	0	5	0	80
Peanut Butter Chips Topping (1 fl oz)	160	8	8	0	14	NA	12	6	70
Rainbow Sprinkles Topping (1 fl oz)	20	0	0	0	5	0	5	0	0
Vanilla Cookie Crunch Topping (1 fl oz)	60	2	1	NA	9	1	3	1	55

Fruit Toppings (Serving Size, 1 fl oz)

Food Serving size	Cal.	(g) Total Fat	(g) Sat. Fat	(mg) Chol.	(g) Carb.	(g) Fiber	(g) Sug.	(g) Prot.	(mg) Sod.
Banana Fruit Topping	15	0	0	0	4	0	2	0	0
Blackberry Fruit Topping	10	0	0	0	2	1	1	0	0
Blueberry Fruit Topping	10	0	0	0	3	0	2	0	0
Kiwi Fruit Topping	15	0	0	0	3	1	2	0	0
Mango Fruit Topping	15	0	0	0	4	0	3	0	0
Pineapple Fruit Topping	15	0	0	0	4	0	3	0	0
Raspberry Fruit Topping	10	0	0	0	2	1	1	0	0
Strawberry Fruit Topping	5	0	0	0	2	0	1	0	0

Parfaits (Serving Size, 140g)

Food Serving size	Cal.	(g) Total Fat	(g) Sat. Fat	(mg) Chol.	(g) Carb.	(g) Fiber	(g) Sug.	(g) Prot.	(mg) Sod.
Fruit Parfait - Regular	160	3	1.5	5	29	1	21	4	75

Pies

Food Serving size	Cal.	(g) Total Fat	(g) Sat. Fat	(mg) Chol.	(g) Carb.	(g) Fiber	(g) Sug.	(g) Prot.	(mg) Sod.
Apple Pie Square (Serving Size, 93g)	160	6	4	5	24	0	19	3	60
Caramel Apple Pie (Square) (Serving Size, 114g)	190	6	4	5	32	1	22	3	90
Caramel Toffee Square Pie (Serving Size, 104g)	190	7	5	5	30	0	22	3	105

Food Serving size	Cal.	Total Fat (g)	Sat. Fat (g)	Chol. (mg)	Carb. (g)	Fiber (g)	Sug. (g)	Prot. (g)	Sod. (mg)
Oreo Cookie Square Pie (Serving Size, 106g)									
	170	7	4	5	25	0	19	2	110
Peanut Buddy Square Pie (Serving Size, 118g)									
	230	7	4	0	38	1	16	5	125
Pumpkin Cheesecake Pie (Square) (Serving Size, 94g)									
	160	6	4	5	24	0	19	2	85
Pumpkin Pie Square									
	140	5	4	5	22	1	19	2	70
Triple Berry D-Lite Square Pie (Serving Size, 129g)									
	130	3.5	2.5	5	23	1	20	2	55

Smoothies

Food Serving size	Cal.	Total Fat (g)	Sat. Fat (g)	Chol. (mg)	Carb. (g)	Fiber (g)	Sug. (g)	Prot. (g)	Sod. (mg)
Acai Smoothie (16 fl oz)									
	270	4.5	2	5	53	4	41	4	70
Acai Smoothie (24 fl oz)									
	440	7	3	10	91	8	68	7	105
Blueberry Banana Classic Smoothie (16 fl oz)									
	190	1.5	1	5	43	3	34	3	70
Blueberry Banana Classic Smoothie (24 fl oz)									
	330	3	1.5	5	73	5	56	5	100
Goji Smoothie (16 fl oz)									
	260	2	1	5	59	3	34	3	65
Goji Smoothie (24 fl oz)									
	420	3	1.5	5	95	5	54	6	95
Mango Classic Smoothie (16 fl oz)									
	220	1.5	1	5	49	2	45	3	95
Mango Classic Smoothie (24 fl oz)									
	330	2	1	5	74	4	68	4	140
Mangosteen Smoothie (16 fl oz)									
	230	2	1	5	53	5	40	4	75
Mangosteen Smoothie (24 fl oz)									
	380	3	1.5	10	86	8	64	6	115
Mixed Berry Classic Smoothie (16 fl oz)									
	170	1.5	1	5	37	2	31	3	100
Mixed Berry Classic Smoothie (24 fl oz)									
	270	2.5	1	5	58	3	49	4	150

Food Serving size	Cal.	(g) Total Fat	(g) Sat. Fat	(mg) Chol.	(g) Carb.	(g) Fiber	(g) Sug.	(g) Prot.	(mg) Sod.
Peanut Butter Banana Smoothie (16 fl oz)	370	7	3	10	67	2	54	12	230
Peanut Butter Banana Smoothie (24 fl oz)	580	11	4.5	20	107	4	85	18	340
Pineapple Mango Classic Smoothie (16 fl oz)	260	1.5	1	5	59	3	48	3	115
Pineapple Mango Classic Smoothie (24 fl oz)	440	2.5	1.5	5	102	7	82	6	170
Pineapple Strawberry Classic Smoothie (16 fl oz)	250	1.5	1	5	56	3	45	3	105
Pineapple Strawberry Classic Smoothie (24 fl oz)	420	2.5	1.5	5	95	5	74	5	160
Pomegranate Smoothie (16 fl oz)	250	1.5	1	5	56	4	42	3	65
Pomegranate Smoothie (24 fl oz)	400	2.5	1.5	5	91	6	66	5	95
Strawberry Banana Smoothie (16 fl oz)	290	1.5	1	5	64	3	51	3	125
Strawberry Banana Smoothie (24 fl oz)	470	2.5	1.5	5	107	5	85	5	190

Sundaes

Food Serving size	Cal.	(g) Total Fat	(g) Sat. Fat	(mg) Chol.	(g) Carb.	(g) Fiber	(g) Sug.	(g) Prot.	(mg) Sod.
Large Caramel Sundae (8 fl oz)	170	2	1	5	44	0	20	4	170
Large Hot Fudge Sundae (8 fl oz)	200	2	1.5	5	42	1	35	4	90
Large Strawberry Sundae (8 fl oz)	200	2	1	5	43	0	37	3	70
Regular Caramel Sundae (6 fl oz)	140	1.5	1	5	37	0	15	3	150
Regular Hot Fudge Sundae (6 fl oz)	170	1.5	1	5	35	1	29	3	70
Regular Strawberry Sundae (6 fl oz)	170	1.5	1	5	36	0	32	2	45

Food Serving size	Cal.	(g) Total Fat	(g) Sat. Fat	(mg) Chol.	(g) Carb.	(g) Fiber	(g) Sug.	(g) Prot.	(mg) Sod.
Tasti Rounds and Bars									
Chocolate Tasti Bar (7 fl oz)									
	320	19	11	0	36	2	33	4	120
Tasti D-Lite Chocolate Round (74g)									
	180	2.5	1.5	0	36	1	17	3	230
Tasti D-Lite Chocolate Round with Rainbow Sprinkles (97g)									
	200	2.5	1.5	0	41	1	22	3	230
Tasti D-Lite Vanilla Round (71g)									
	180	2.5	1.5	0	36	1	16	3	220
Tasti D-Lite Vanilla Round with Rainbow Sprinkles (94g)									
	200	2.5	1.5	0	41	1	21	3	220
Vanilla Tasti Bar (7 fl oz)									
	310	19	11	5	35	1	31	4	85

TCBY

Soft Serve Frozen Yogurt, Based on 4 fl oz (1/2 Cup) Serving

Food Serving size	Cal.	(g) Total Fat	(g) Sat. Fat	(mg) Chol.	(g) Carb.	(g) Fiber	(g) Sug.	(g) Prot.	(mg) Sod.
Cake Batter									
	120	2	1	5	23	3	17	4	65
Cheesecake									
	110	2	1	5	23	3	17	4	65
Chocolate									
	110	1.5	1	5	23	3	18	4	90
Coffee									
	120	2	1	5	23	3	17	4	80
Golden Vanilla									
	120	2	1	5	23	3	17	4	65
Mango Sorbet									
	110	0	0	0	26	0	21	0	10
Non-fat Classic Tart									
	90	0	0	0	21	2	17	3	60
Non-fat Dutch Chocolate									
	100	0	0	0	24	4	16	4	65
Non-fat Old Fashioned Vanilla									
	110	0	0	0	23	3	17	4	65

Food Serving size	Cal.	(g) Total Fat	(g) Sat. Fat	(mg) Chol.	(g) Carb.	(g) Fiber	(g) Sug.	(g) Prot.	(mg) Sod.
NSA Non-fat Chocolate	70	0	0	0	21	6	6	4	70
NSA Non-fat Mountain Blackberry	80	0	0	0	22	4	6	4	70
NSA Non-fat Strawberry	80	0	0	0	22	4	6	4	70
NSA Non-fat Vanilla	80	0	0	0	21	4	6	4	65
NSA Non-fat White Chocolate Macadamia	80	0	0	0	21	4	6	4	65
Orange Sorbet	100	0	0	0	25	0	19	0	15
Peach Mango	120	2	1	5	23	3	17	4	65
Peanut Butter	130	2	1	0	26	3	20	4	95
Raspberry	120	2	1	5	24	3	17	4	65
Ruby Red Grapefruit Sorbet	100	0	0	0	24	0	19	0	10
Strawberry	110	2	1	5	23	3	17	4	70
Strawberry Kiwi Sorbet	100	0	0	0	24	0	19	0	15
White Chocolate Mousse	120	2	1	5	23	3	17	4	65

WENDY's
Additional Salad Dressings

Food Serving size	Cal.	(g) Total Fat	(g) Sat. Fat	(mg) Chol.	(g) Carb.	(g) Fiber	(g) Sug.	(g) Prot.	(mg) Sod.
Classic Ranch	100	10	1.5	10	2	0	1	1	150
Fat-free French	40	0	0	0	9	0	8	0	95
Italian Vinaigrette	70	6	1	0	4	0	3	0	180
Light Classic Ranch	50	4.5	1	10	2	0	1	1	150

Food Serving size	Cal.	(g) Total Fat	(g) Sat. Fat	(mg) Chol.	(g) Carb.	(g) Fiber	(g) Sug.	(g) Prot.	(mg) Sod.
Thousand Island	160	15	2.5	15	5	0	4	0	290

Beverages

Food Serving size	Cal.	(g) Total Fat	(g) Sat. Fat	(mg) Chol.	(g) Carb.	(g) Fiber	(g) Sug.	(g) Prot.	(mg) Sod.
Barq's Root Beer (Small Cup)	180	0	0	0	50	0	50	0	40
Coca-Cola (Small Cup)	160	0	0	0	44	0	44	0	0
Coke Zero (Small Cup)	0	0	0	0	0	0	0	0	5
Diet Coke (Small Cup)	0	0	0	0	0	0	0	0	15
Dr Pepper (Small Cup)	160	0	0	0	43	0	43	0	40
Fanta Orange (Small Cup)	180	0	0	0	49	0	49	0	25
Hi-C Flashin' Fruit Punch (Small Cup)	170	0	0	0	46	0	46	0	15
Juicy Juice Apple Juice	90	0	0	0	22	0	20	0	5
Minute Maid Light Lemonade (Small Cup)	5	0	0	0	1	0	0	0	5
Nestea Sweetened Iced Tea	100	0	0	0	28	0	27	0	10
Nestea Unsweetened Iced Tea	0	0	0	0	0	0	0	0	10
Nestle Pure Life Bottled Water	0	0	0	0	0	0	0	0	0
Pibb Xtra (Small Cup)	160	0	0	0	43	0	43	0	25
Sprite (Small Cup)	160	0	0	0	43	0	43	0	35
TruMoo Low-fat Chocolate Milk	140	2.5	1.5	10	22	0	20	7	170

Food Serving size	Cal.	(g) Total Fat	(g) Sat. Fat	(mg) Chol.	(g) Carb.	(g) Fiber	(g) Sug.	(g) Prot.	(mg) Sod.
TruMoo Low-fat White Milk	100	2.5	1.5	10	12	0	11	8	125

Crispy Chicken Nuggets

Food Serving size	Cal.	Total Fat	Sat. Fat	Chol.	Carb.	Fiber	Sug.	Prot.	Sod.
10 Piece Chicken Nuggets	450	29	6	65	26	2	1	21	930
4 Piece Kids' Meal Chicken Nuggets	180	11	2.5	25	11	1	1	8	370
5 Piece Chicken Nuggets	220	14	3	35	13	1	1	10	460
Babecue Nugget Sauce	45	0	0	0	11	0	4	0	120
Heartland Ranch Dipping Sauce	120	12	1.5	10	3	0	2	0	240
Honey Mustard Nugget Sauce	80	6	1	10	7	0	3	0	220
Sweet and Sour Nugget Sauce	50	0	0	0	12	0	11	0	120

Frosty Treats

Food Serving size	Cal.	Total Fat	Sat. Fat	Chol.	Carb.	Fiber	Sug.	Prot.	Sod.
Caramel Apple Parfait	400	9	5	30	71	1	57	8	180
Caramel Frosty Shake (Large)	1020	19	12	65	198	0	157	14	510
Caramel Frosty Shake (Small)	680	15	9	50	126	0	102	11	330
Chocolate Frosty (Small)	250	6	4	25	41	0	35	6	115
Chocolate Frosty Shake (Large)	890	18	11	55	168	4	151	16	380
Chocolate Frosty Shake (Small)	610	14	9	45	109	2	98	12	260
Oreo Frosty Parfait	400	10	6	30	68	1	56	8	220
Strawberry Frosty Shake (Large)	820	16	10	55	156	1	142	13	240

Food Serving size	Cal.	Total Fat (g)	Sat. Fat (g)	Chol. (mg)	Carb. (g)	Fiber (g)	Sug. (g)	Prot. (g)	Sod. (mg)
Strawberry Frosty Shake (Small)	580	14	8	45	104	1	94	10	190
Vanilla Bean Frosty Shake (Large)	890	16	10	55	172	0	119	13	710
Vanilla Bean Frosty Shake (Small)	620	14	8	45	115	0	83	10	450
Vanilla Frosty (Small)	260	7	4.5	25	43	0	37	7	125
Vanilla Frosty Float with Coca-Cola	380	7	4.5	30	75	0	69	7	135
Wild Berry Frosty Shake (Large)	750	16	10	55	137	2	120	13	250
Wild Berry Frosty Shake (Small)	550	14	8	45	96	1	84	11	190

Garden Sensations Salads

Food Serving size	Cal.	Total Fat (g)	Sat. Fat (g)	Chol. (mg)	Carb. (g)	Fiber (g)	Sug. (g)	Prot. (g)	Sod. (mg)
Apple Pecan Chicken Salad	340	11	7	105	28	5	20	35	1150
Apple Pecan Chicken Salad (Half-size)	170	6	3.5	50	15	3	11	18	580
Avocado Ranch Dressing	100	10	2	10	2	0	1	1	210
Baja Salad	550	33	14	90	34	12	12	32	1650
Baja Salad (Half-size)	280	17	7	45	18	6	6	16	840
BLT Cobb Salad	450	25	11	275	9	3	5	46	1610
BLT Cobb Salad (Half-size)	230	13	6	140	5	1	3	23	810
Creamy Red Jalapeno Dressing	100	10	2	10	2	0	1	1	270
Gourmet Croutons	80	3	0	0	12	0	0	2	220
Lemon Garlic Caesar Dressing	110	11	2	10	2	0	1	2	180

Food Serving size	Cal.	(g) Total Fat	(g) Sat. Fat	(mg) Chol.	(g) Carb.	(g) Fiber	(g) Sug.	(g) Prot.	(mg) Sod.
Pomegranate Vinaigrette Dressing	60	3	0	0	8	0	7	0	160
Roasted Pecans	110	9	1	0	5	1	4	1	60
Seasoned Tortilla Strips	80	4.5	1.5	0	11	1	0	1	105
Spicy Chicken Caesar Salad	460	25	12	85	27	6	3	33	1410
Spicy Chicken Caesar Salad (Half-size)	240	13	6	40	15	4	3	17	710

Sandwich Components

Food Serving size	Cal.	(g) Total Fat	(g) Sat. Fat	(mg) Chol.	(g) Carb.	(g) Fiber	(g) Sug.	(g) Prot.	(mg) Sod.
1/4 lb. Hamburger Patty	220	15	7	70	0	0	0	19	170
American Cheese	40	3.5	2	10	0	0	0	2	200
Applewood Smoked Bacon - 1 Strip	30	2.5	1	5	0	0	0	2	100
Crispy Chicken Patty	200	12	2.5	30	13	1	0	11	460
Dill Pickles - 4 Each	0	0	0	0	0	0	0	0	150
Homestyle Chicken Fillet	240	11	2	50	16	1	0	19	770
Honey Mustard Sauce	40	3.5	0	5	3	0	2	0	75
Iceberg Lettuce Leaf	0	0	0	0	0	0	0	0	0
Junior Hamburger Patty	90	7	3	30	0	0	0	8	70
Ketchup	10	0	0	0	2	0	2	0	80
Mayonnaise	40	3.5	0.5	5	1	0	0	0	55
Mustard	5	0	0	0	0	0	0	0	50

Food Serving size	Cal.	(g) Total Fat	(g) Sat. Fat	(mg) Chol.	(g) Carb.	(g) Fiber	(g) Sug.	(g) Prot.	(mg) Sod.
Natural Asiago Cheese									
	50	4	2.5	15	1	0	0	3	100
Premium Bun									
	190	2	0	0	36	1	6	6	360
Ranch Sauce									
	40	4	0.5	5	1	0	0	0	55
Red Onion - 2 Rings									
	0	0	0	0	0	0	0	0	0
Sandwich Bun									
	120	1	0	0	24	1	4	4	240
Spicy Chicken Fillet									
	250	11	2.5	50	17	1	0	19	950
Tomato - 1 Slice									
	5	0	0	0	1	0	1	0	0
Tortilla									
	130	3.5	1	0	21	0	0	3	280
Ultimate Chicken Grill Fillet									
	120	1.5	0	80	1	0	0	26	670

Sandwiches

Food Serving size	Cal.	(g) Total Fat	(g) Sat. Fat	(mg) Chol.	(g) Carb.	(g) Fiber	(g) Sug.	(g) Prot.	(mg) Sod.
1/2 lb Double									
	770	43	19	160	43	2	10	50	1430
1/4 lb Single									
	550	28	12	95	43	2	10	30	1270
3/4 lb Triple									
	1030	62	28	240	44	2	10	71	1800
Asiago Ranch Club with Homestyle Chicken									
	660	33	9	90	56	3	8	34	1650
Asiago Ranch Club with Spicy Chicken									
	670	34	10	90	57	3	8	35	1830
Asiago Ranch Club with Ultimate Chicken Grill									
	540	24	8	120	41	2	8	41	1550
Bacon Deluxe Double									
	850	51	22	180	43	2	11	54	1690
Bacon Deluxe Single									
	640	36	15	110	43	2	11	35	1520

Food Serving size	Cal.	(g) Total Fat	(g) Sat. Fat	(mg) Chol.	(g) Carb.	(g) Fiber	(g) Sug.	(g) Prot.	(mg) Sod.
Baconator Double	930	58	25	195	41	1	10	59	1840
Baconator Single	620	35	15	110	41	1	9	35	1370
Cheeseburger, Kids' Meal	260	11	5	40	26	1	6	14	570
Crispy Chicken Caesar Wrap	430	25	7	45	35	2	1	17	950
Crispy Chicken Sandwich	350	16	3.5	35	38	2	4	15	740
Crispy Chicken Sandwich, Kids' Meal	330	13	3	30	36	2	4	15	700
Double Junior Bacon Cheeseburger	440	25	11	85	26	1	5	26	820
Double Stack	360	18	8	70	27	1	6	23	740
Grilled Chicken Go Wrap	260	10	3.5	50	25	1	3	19	730
Hamburger, Kids' Meal	220	8	3	30	26	1	5	12	370
Homestyle Chicken Fillet Sandwich	470	16	3	55	55	3	7	26	1190
Homestyle Chicken Go Wrap	320	16	4.5	35	30	1	1	15	770
Junior Bacon Cheeseburger	350	19	8	55	26	1	5	18	750
Junior Cheeseburger	270	11	5	40	27	1	6	15	670
Junior Cheeseburger Deluxe	300	14	6	45	29	2	7	15	710
Junior Hamburger	230	8	3	30	26	1	6	12	470
Spicy Chicken Fillet Sandwich	480	17	3.5	55	56	3	7	26	1370
Spicy Chicken Go Wrap	330	16	4.5	40	31	1	1	16	860

Food Serving size	Cal.	(g) Total Fat	(g) Sat. Fat	(mg) Chol.	(g) Carb.	(g) Fiber	(g) Sug.	(g) Prot.	(mg) Sod.
Ultimate Chicken Grill Sandwich									
	360	7	1.5	80	42	2	9	33	1110

Side Selections

Food Serving size	Cal.	(g) Total Fat	(g) Sat. Fat	(mg) Chol.	(g) Carb.	(g) Fiber	(g) Sug.	(g) Prot.	(mg) Sod.
Apple Slices									
	40	0	0	0	9	2	7	0	0
Buttery Best Spread									
	50	5	1	0	0	0	0	0	95
Caesar Side Salad									
	60	3.5	2.5	10	5	2	2	4	115
Cheddar Cheese, Shredded									
	70	6	3.5	15	1	0	0	4	110
Garden Side Salad									
	25	0	0	0	5	2	3	1	30
Gourmet Croutons									
	80	3	0	0	12	0	0	2	220
Gourmet Croutons									
	80	3	0	0	12	0	0	2	220
Hot Chili Seasoning Packet									
	5	0	0	0	1	0	1	0	270
Ketchup (1 Packet)									
	10	0	0	0	3	0	2	0	95
Large Chili									
	310	9	3.5	60	31	10	10	26	1330
Large Natural-cut Fries									
	530	25	5	0	68	7	0	6	570
Lemon Garlic Caesar Dressing									
	110	11	2	10	2	0	1	2	180
Medium Natural-cut Fries									
	420	21	4	0	55	6	0	5	460
Plain Baked Potato (Average Weight 10 oz)									
	270	0	0	0	61	7	3	7	25
Saltine Crackers									
	25	0.5	0	0	5	0	0	1	80
Small Chili									
	210	6	2.5	40	21	6	6	17	880

Food Serving size	Cal.	(g) Total Fat	(g) Sat. Fat	(mg) Chol.	(g) Carb.	(g) Fiber	(g) Sug.	(g) Prot.	(mg) Sod.
Small Natural-cut Fries	320	16	3	0	42	4	0	4	350
Sour Cream and Chives Baked Potato	320	3.5	2	10	63	7	4	8	50
Value Natural-cut Fries	230	11	2.5	0	30	3	0	3	250

WHITE CASTLE

Breakfast Condiments

Food	Cal.	Total Fat	Sat. Fat	Chol.	Carb.	Fiber	Sug.	Prot.	Sod.
Butter	30	3.5	2.5	10	0	0	0	0	30
Cream Cheese	100	10	6	30	0	0	0	2	110
Grape Jelly - New York, Indianapolis, Minneapolis, Louisville and Chicago regions (1 container)	35	0	0	0	9	0	7	0	0
Maple Syrup - 1 Container	120	0	0	0	31	0	21	0	25
Strawberry Jam - Chicago, New York, Indianapolis and Louisville regions (1 container)	40	0	0	0	10	0	7	0	0

Breakfast Sides. Hash Rounds/Hash Bites/Hash Round/Potato Snackers (Select Regions)

Food	Cal.	Total Fat	Sat. Fat	Chol.	Carb.	Fiber	Sug.	Prot.	Sod.
Awrey Apple Danish (Select Regions)	450	24	6	30	52	1	22	6	390
Awrey Cheese Danish (Select Regions)	450	24	6	30	52	1	22	6	390
Awrey Cinnamon Roll (Select Regions)	420	20	8	5	56	2	22	6	460
Awrey Strawberry Danish (Select Regions)	480	21	8	5	67	2	34	6	400
French Toast Sticks	460	31	4.5	0	39	2	10	5	410

Food Serving size	Cal.	(g) Total Fat	(g) Sat. Fat	(mg) Chol.	(g) Carb.	(g) Fiber	(g) Sug.	(g) Prot.	(mg) Sod.
Haas Apple Danish (Select Regions)									
	470	22	10	5	62	1	29	6	520
Haas Cheese Danish (Select Regions)									
	490	25	11	10	62	1	28	6	550
Haas Chocolate Frosted Donuts (Twin Pack) (Select Regions)									
	460	24	12	40	120	4	52	12	760
Haas Cinnamon Danish (Select Regions)									
	490	25	6	20	60	2	26	6	380
Haas French Twist Donuts (Twin Pack) (Select Regions)									
	460	24	10	20	58	2	34	6	580
Haas Plain Old Fashion Donut (Single) (Select Regions)									
	385	21	9	18	51	2	23	5	403
Medium									
	600	46	6	0	42	4	0	4	760
Sack									
	1440	110	14	0	101	10	0	10	1830
Saver									
	360	28	3.5	0	25	2	0	2	460

Breakfast Slider Alterations

Food Serving size	Cal.	Total Fat	Sat. Fat	Chol.	Carb.	Fiber	Sug.	Prot.	Sod.
Bologna - Louisville and Nashville Regions									
	150	12	4	30	2	0	1	6	500
Egg									
	70	5	1.5	210	0	0	0	6	70
Hamburger Meat (100 % Beef)									
	70	6	2.5	10	0	0	0	4	15
Hashbrown (Varies by Region)									
	310	28	5	0	14	3	0	1	250
Sausage									
	150	14	5	25	0	0	0	5	310
Strip of Bacon									
	30	3	1	5	0	0	0	2	100
Wheat Toast (Select Regions)									
	130	2	0.5	0	24	2	3	6	260
White Toast (Select Regions)									
	130	2	0.5	0	25	1	2	4	250

Food Serving size	Cal.	(g) Total Fat	(g) Sat. Fat	(mg) Chol.	(g) Carb.	(g) Fiber	(g) Sug.	(g) Prot.	(mg) Sod.
Breakfast Sliders on a Bun									
Bacon	130	6	2	10	12	1	1	5	330
Bacon, Cheese	150	9	3.5	15	12	1	2	7	460
Bacon, Egg	200	11	3.5	220	12	1	2	12	400
Bacon, Egg, Cheese	190	11	4	225	13	1	2	12	430
Bologna, Cheese - Louisville and Nashville Regions	240	15	6	35	14	1	3	10	760
Bologna, Egg - Louisville and Nashville Regions	290	18	6	240	14	1	3	15	690
Bologna, Egg, Cheese - Louisville and Nashville Regions	310	20	7	250	15	1	3	16	830
Egg	140	6	2	210	12	1	2	9	190
Egg, Cheese	160	8	3	220	13	1	2	10	330
Hamburger, Egg	200	11	4	220	12	1	2	13	210
Hamburger, Egg, Cheese	230	14	6	225	13	1	2	14	350
Huevos Rancheros with Bacon Slider (Cincinnati Region)	190	11	4.5	225	14	1	2	12	500
Huevos Rancheros with Sausage Slider (Cincinnati Region)	310	23	9	245	14	1	2	15	710
Sausage	220	15	6	25	12	1	1	8	430
Sausage, Cheese	250	17	7	30	13	1	2	9	570
Sausage, Egg	290	20	7	240	13	1	2	14	500
Sausage, Egg, Cheese	320	22	9	245	13	1	2	15	640

Food Serving size	Cal.	(g) Total Fat	(g) Sat. Fat	(mg) Chol.	(g) Carb.	(g) Fiber	(g) Sug.	(g) Prot.	(mg) Sod.
Buffalo Chicken Rings									
20 Rings	1790	158	27	355	47	2	2	59	2940
6 Rings	540	48	8	105	14	1	1	18	870
9 Rings	810	71	12	160	22	1	1	26	1390
Buffalo Chicken Rings - New Jersey Region									
20 Rings	1790	158	31	355	47	2	2	59	2940
6 Rings	540	48	9	110	14	1	1	18	870
9 Rings	810	71	14	160	22	1	1	26	1390
Cheese Fries									
Cheese Fries (Medium)	410	28	4.5	0	35	3	2	4	350
Cheese Fries (New Jersey Region) (Medium)	410	28	5	0	35	3	2	4	350
Loaded Fries (Bacon, Ranch) - New Jersey Region (Medium)	560	49	9	25	20	2	4	3	810
Loaded Fries (Bacon, Ranch) (Medium)	560	49	9	25	20	2	4	3	810
Loaded Fries (Cheddar, Bacon) - New Jersey Region (Medium)	330	24	5	20	18	2	2	4	690
Loaded Fries (Cheddar, Bacon) (Medium)	330	24	4	20	20	2	1	4	780
Loaded Fries (Cheddar, Bacon, Ranch) - New Jersey Region (Medium)	460	38	8	20	20	2	3	4	900
Loaded Fries (Cheddar, Bacon, Ranch) (Medium)	470	38	6	20	21	2	3	4	990
Chicken Rings									
20 Rings	1760	158	27	355	41	2	1	58	2020

Food Serving size	Cal.	(g) Total Fat	(g) Sat. Fat	(mg) Chol.	(g) Carb.	(g) Fiber	(g) Sug.	(g) Prot.	(mg) Sod.
6 Rings	530	47	10	105	12	0	0	18	610
9 Rings	790	71	12	160	18	1	0	26	910

Chicken Rings - New Jersey Region

20 Rings	1760	158	31	355	41	2	1	58	2020
6 Rings	530	47	9	105	12	0	0	18	610
9 Rings	790	71	14	160	18	1	0	26	910

Clam Strips

Regular	210	17	2	15	5	0	1	8	620
Sack	410	34	4	35	9	0	2	16	1250

Clam Strips - New Jersey Region

Medium	210	17	2.5	15	5	0	1	8	620
Sack	410	34	5.5	35	9	0	2	16	1250

Coffee

Large	5	0	0	0	0	0	0	1	10
Medium	5	0	0	0	0	0	0	1	10
Small	5	0	0	0	0	0	0	0	5

Coffee (Decaffeinated)

Large	0	0	0	0	0	0	0	1	10
Medium	0	0	0	0	0	0	0	0	10

Food Serving size	Cal.	(g) Total Fat	(g) Sat. Fat	(mg) Chol.	(g) Carb.	(g) Fiber	(g) Sug.	(g) Prot.	(mg) Sod.
Small	0	0	0	0	0	0	0	0	5

Condiments

Food Serving size	Cal.	Total Fat	Sat. Fat	Chol.	Carb.	Fiber	Sug.	Prot.	Sod.
BBQ Sauce - 1 Packet	10	0	0	0	3	0	2	0	130
Fat-free Honey Mustard Sauce - 1 Packet	20	0	0	0	5	0	3	0	50
Hot Sauce - 1 Packet	5	0	0	0	1	1	0	0	170
Ketchup - 1 Packet	10	0	0	0	2	0	2	0	100
Lemon Juice - 1 Packet	5	0	0	0	1	0	0	0	0
Mayonnaise - 1 Packet	60	7	1	5	0	0	0	0	55
Mustard - Columbus, Detroit, Minneapolis, Nashville, NE Ohio, New Jersey and New York Regions - 1 Packet	5	0	0	0	<1	0	0	0	85
Mustard - Dusseldorf - Chicago, Cincinnati, Louisville and Nashville Regions - 1 Packet	5	0	0	0	0	0	0	0	65
Mustard - Horseradish - Indianapolis and St. Louis Regions - 1 Packet	5	0	0	0	0	0	0	0	65
Tartar Sauce - 1 Packet	25	1.5	0	0	1	0	1	0	85

Condiments Delivered on Sliders

Food Serving size	Cal.	Total Fat	Sat. Fat	Chol.	Carb.	Fiber	Sug.	Prot.	Sod.
Mustard (1 tsp) - Minneapolis, Columbus, Detroit & NE Ohio Regions	0	0	0	0	0	0	0	0	60
Golden BBQ Sauce	15	0	0	0	3	0	3	0	80
Hamburger Sauce (1 1/2 tsp) Detroit Region	0	0	0	0	0	0	0	0	75
Ketchup - Chicago, Cincinnati, Columbus, Detroit, Louisville, Minneapolis, Nashville, New York, New Jersey and NE Ohio Regions	5	0	0	0	1	0	1	0	50

Food Serving size	Cal.	(g) Total Fat	(g) Sat. Fat	(mg) Chol.	(g) Carb.	(g) Fiber	(g) Sug.	(g) Prot.	(mg) Sod.
Marinara Sauce	5	0	0	0	2	0	1	0	105
Mustard (1 tsp) - Indianapolis Region	0	0	0	0	0	0	0	0	85
Ranch Dressing	90	9	1.5	0	1	0	1	0	140
Spicy Hamburger Sauce (1 1/2 tsp) - Chicago Region	0	0	0	0	1	0	0	0	45

Crave Coolers

Food Serving size	Cal.	(g) Total Fat	(g) Sat. Fat	(mg) Chol.	(g) Carb.	(g) Fiber	(g) Sug.	(g) Prot.	(mg) Sod.
Crave Cooler Coke - Kids	40	0	0	0	12	0	12	0	0
Crave Cooler Coke - Large	200	0	0	0	56	0	56	0	20
Crave Cooler Coke - Medium	140	0	0	0	39	0	39	0	15
Crave Cooler Coke - Saver	90	0	0	0	24	0	24	0	10
Crave Cooler Coke - Small	110	0	0	0	29	0	29	0	10
Crave Cooler Fanta Wild Cherry - Kids	40	0	0	0	12	0	12	0	0
Crave Cooler Fanta Wild Cherry - Large	210	0	0	0	56	0	56	0	15
Crave Cooler Fanta Wild Cherry - Medium	140	0	0	0	39	0	39	0	10
Crave Cooler Fanta Wild Cherry - Saver	90	0	0	0	24	0	24	0	5
Crave Cooler Fanta Wild Cherry - Small	110	0	0	0	29	0	29	0	10

Desserts

Food Serving size	Cal.	(g) Total Fat	(g) Sat. Fat	(mg) Chol.	(g) Carb.	(g) Fiber	(g) Sug.	(g) Prot.	(mg) Sod.
Chocolate Chunk Cookie (Select Regions)	170	8	4	10	23	1	13	2	130
Oatmeal Raisin Cookie (Select Regions)	160	6	2.5	10	23	1	12	2	115

Food Serving size	Cal.	(g) Total Fat	(g) Sat. Fat	(mg) Chol.	(g) Carb.	(g) Fiber	(g) Sug.	(g) Prot.	(mg) Sod.
White Chocolate Macadamia Cookie (Select Regions)									
	180	9	4	10	22	1	14	2	125

Doubles

Double Bacon Cheddar									
	370	23	10	50	21	1	2	17	1240
Double Bacon Cheeseburger									
	350	22	10	40	21	1	2	18	1050
Double Cheeseburger									
	300	17	8	30	20	1	3	15	940
Double Fish Slider with Cheese									
	610	48	9	45	25	23	2	19	700
Double Fish Slider Without Cheese									
	550	43	6	30	24	23	1	17	420
Double Jalapeno Cheeseburger									
	280	17	8	30	21	1	2	15	860
Double Original Slider									
	240	12	5	20	21	1	2	12	660
Double Smokey Bacon Ranch									
	420	29	8	40	22	1	4	13	1100

Fish Nibblers

Medium									
	320	16	2.5	10	28	1	1	16	700
Sack									
	1100	53	8	35	95	3	3	55	2390

Fish Nibblers - New Jersey Region

Medium									
	320	16	3	10	28	1	1	16	700
Sack									
	1100	53	10	35	95	3	3	55	2390

French Fries

Medium									
	370	25	4	0	33	3	2	3	50
Sack									
	850	57	9	0	76	8	4	8	115

Food Serving size	Cal.	(g) Total Fat	(g) Sat. Fat	(mg) Chol.	(g) Carb.	(g) Fiber	(g) Sug.	(g) Prot.	(mg) Sod.
Saver	350	24	4	0	32	3	2	3	50

French Fries - New Jersey Region

Medium	360	22	5	0	36	3	2	5	40
Sack	810	49	11	0	81	8	4	12	95
Saver	350	21	5	0	34	3	1	5	40

Gold Peak Iced Tea, Black (Sweetened) (Select Regions)

Gallon	1230	0	0	0	336	0	336	0	130
Kids	70	0	0	0	20	0	20	0	10
Large	320	0	0	0	88	0	88	0	35
Medium	220	0	0	0	59	0	59	0	25
Saver	120	0	0	0	32	0	32	0	10
Small	160	0	0	0	45	0	45	0	20

Gold Peak Iced Tea, Black (Unsweetened) (Select Regions)

Gallon	0	0	0	0	1	0	0	1	130
Kids	0	0	0	0	0	0	0	0	10
Large	0	0	0	0	0	0	0	0	35
Medium	0	0	0	0	0	0	0	0	25
Saver	0	0	0	0	0	0	0	0	10
Small	0	0	0	0	0	0	0	0	15

Food Serving size	Cal.	(g) Total Fat	(g) Sat. Fat	(mg) Chol.	(g) Carb.	(g) Fiber	(g) Sug.	(g) Prot.	(mg) Sod.

Gold Peak Iced Tea, Southern Style (Select Regions)

Food Serving size	Cal.	Total Fat	Sat. Fat	Chol.	Carb.	Fiber	Sug.	Prot.	Sod.
Gallon	1550	0	0	0	432	0	416	0	130
Kids	90	0	0	0	25	0	25	0	10
Large	410	0	0	0	113	0	109	0	35
Medium	270	0	0	0	76	0	73	0	25
Saver	150	0	0	0	41	0	39	0	10
Small	210	0	0	0	57	0	55	0	15

Gold Peak Iced Tea, White Citrus (Select Regions)

Food Serving size	Cal.	Total Fat	Sat. Fat	Chol.	Carb.	Fiber	Sug.	Prot.	Sod.
Gallon	1340	0	0	0	350	0	350	0	110
Half and Half	15	1.5	0	0	0	0	0	0	15
Kids	80	0	0	0	21	0	21	0	5
Large	350	0	0	0	92	0	92	0	30
Medium	240	0	0	0	62	0	62	0	20
Saver	130	0	0	0	33	0	33	0	10
Small	180	0	0	0	47	0	47	0	15

Home-style Onion Rings - Chicago, Louisville and St. Louis Regions

Food Serving size	Cal.	Total Fat	Sat. Fat	Chol.	Carb.	Fiber	Sug.	Prot.	Sod.
Medium	480	33	4.5	0	40	2	7	6	580
Sack	890	61	8.5	0	74	3	14	11	1070

Food Serving size	Cal.	(g) Total Fat	(g) Sat. Fat	(mg) Chol.	(g) Carb.	(g) Fiber	(g) Sug.	(g) Prot.	(mg) Sod.
Saver	290	19	2.5	0	25	1	5	4	360

Hot Chocolate

Large	300	7	2	0	52	2	43	2	370
Medium	240	6	1.5	0	41	2	34	2	300
Small	170	4	1	0	31	1	25	1	220

Hot Tea

Large	0	0	0	0	0	0	0	0	0
Medium	0	0	0	0	0	0	0	0	0
Small	0	0	0	0	0	0	0	0	0

Hot Tea (Orange Pekoe) - Select Regions

Large	5	0	0	0	0	0	0	0	0
Medium	5	0.	0	0	0	0	0	0	0
Small	5	0	0	0	0	0	0	0	0

Iced Tea Sweetened

Gallon	1100	0	0	0	286	0	274	0	115
Kids'	80	0	0	0	22	0	22	0	10
Large	180	0	0	0	46	0	44	0	20
Medium	130	0	0	0	33	0	31	0	15

Food Serving size	Cal.	(g) Total Fat	(g) Sat. Fat	(mg) Chol.	(g) Carb.	(g) Fiber	(g) Sug.	(g) Prot.	(mg) Sod.
Saver	130	0	0	0	35	0	35	0	15
Small	80	0	0	0	20	0	19	0	10

Iced Tea Unsweetened

Food	Cal.	Total Fat	Sat. Fat	Chol.	Carb.	Fiber	Sug.	Prot.	Sod.
Gallon	40	0	0	0	11	0	0	0	115
Kids'	0	0	0	0	0	0	0	0	0
Large	5	0	0	0	2	0	0	0	20
Medium	5	0	0	0	1	0	0	0	15
Saver	0	0	0	0	1	0	0	0	5
Small	5	0	0	0	1	0	0	0	10

Juices

Food	Cal.	Total Fat	Sat. Fat	Chol.	Carb.	Fiber	Sug.	Prot.	Sod.
Large	290	0	0	0	70	0	70	5	5
Minute Maid Orange Juice NTC	140	0	0	0	33	0	33	2	0
Small	220	0	0	0	54	0	48	0	0
Vita Fresh Orange Juice Box	140	0.5	0	0	34	1	30	2	15

Minute Maid Raspberry Lemonade

Food	Cal.	Total Fat	Sat. Fat	Chol.	Carb.	Fiber	Sug.	Prot.	Sod.
Kids'	100	0	0	0	28	0	26	0	0
Large	460	0	0	0	126	0	117	0	10
Medium	310	0	0	0	85	0	79	0	0
Minute Maid Apple Juice Box	100	0	0	0	23	0	21	0	15

Food Serving size	Cal.	(g) Total Fat	(g) Sat. Fat	(mg) Chol.	(g) Carb.	(g) Fiber	(g) Sug.	(g) Prot.	(mg) Sod.
Saver	170	0	0	0	45	0	42	0	0
Small	230	0	0	0	64	0	60	0	5

Mozzarella Cheese Sticks

10 Sticks	1470	111	28	100	73	4	4	41	2850
3 Sticks	440	33	8	30	22	1	1	12	850
5 Sticks	740	55	14	50	36	2	2	21	1420

Mozzarella Cheese Sticks - New Jersey Region

10 Sticks	1470	111	31	100	73	4	4	41	2850
3 Sticks	440	33	9	30	22	1	1	12	850
5 Sticks	740	55	15	50	36	2	2	21	1420

Onion Chips

Medium	670	50	8	0	46	8	5	5	970
Sack	1350	101	15	0	92	16	11	11	1950
Saver	510	38	6	0	35	6	4	4	730

Onion Rings - New Jersey Region

Medium	340	22	4	0	33	3	5	2	310
Sack	640	41	7	0	62	6	9	4	580
Saver	220	14	2.5	0	21	2	3	1	190

Food Serving size	Cal.	(g) Total Fat	(g) Sat. Fat	(mg) Chol.	(g) Carb.	(g) Fiber	(g) Sug.	(g) Prot.	(mg) Sod.
Ranch Chicken Rings									
20 Rings	1790	159	28	360	46	2	2	60	2760
6 Rings	540	48	8	107	14	1	1	18	820
9 Rings	810	71	12	160	21	1	1	27	1300
Ranch Chicken Rings - New Jersey Region									
20 Rings	1790	159	31	360	46	2	2	60	2760
6 Rings	540	48	9	110	14	1	1	18	820
9 Rings	810	71	14	160	21	1	1	27	1300
Shakes									
Chocolate Shake - Chicago Region - Kids	260	4.5	2.5	15	51	1	43	6	160
Chocolate Shake - Chicago Region - Large	1150	21	12	70	220	5	189	24	700
Chocolate Shake - Chicago Region - Medium	780	14	8	50	152	3	129	16	480
Chocolate Shake - Chicago Region - Saver	420	8	4	25	81	2	69	9	250
Chocolate Shake - Chicago Region - Small	550	10	5.5	35	106	2	90	12	330
Chocolate Shake - Cincinnati Region - Kids	310	8	5	15	53	0	42	7	170
Chocolate Shake - Cincinnati Region - Large	1350	35	22	70	234	0	185	29	730
Chocolate Shake - Cincinnati Region - Medium	930	24	15	50	160	0	126	20	500
Chocolate Shake - Cincinnati Region - Saver	490	13	8	25	85	0	67	11	270
Chocolate Shake - Cincinnati Region - Small	650	17	11	35	111	0	88	14	350

Food Serving size	Cal.	(g) Total Fat	(g) Sat. Fat	(mg) Chol.	(g) Carb.	(g) Fiber	(g) Sug.	(g) Prot.	(mg) Sod.
Chocolate Shake - Columbus Region - Kids									
	240	6	3.5	20	42	0	39	6	220
Chocolate Shake - Columbus Region - Large									
	1040	26	16	100	183	0	171	27	980
Chocolate Shake - Columbus Region - Medium									
	710	18	11	65	126	0	117	19	670
Chocolate Shake - Columbus Region - Saver									
	380	9	6	35	67	0	62	10	360
Chocolate Shake - Columbus Region - Small									
	500	12	8	45	88	0	82	13	470
Chocolate Shake - Detroit Region - Kids									
	210	6	3	20	32	0	32	6	190
Chocolate Shake - Detroit Region - Large									
	920	25	13	85	141	0	141	25	830
Chocolate Shake - Detroit Region - Medium									
	620	17	9	55	96	0	96	17	570
Chocolate Shake - Detroit Region - Saver									
	330	9	4.5	30	52	0	52	9	300
Chocolate Shake - Detroit Region - Small									
	440	12	6	40	68	0	68	12	400
Chocolate Shake - Indianapolis Region - Kids									
	230	7	4.5	35	42	1	32	6	170
Chocolate Shake - Indianapolis Region - Large									
	1020	32	19	160	184	6	140	25	730
Chocolate Shake - Indianapolis Region - Medium									
	690	22	13	110	126	4	95	17	500
Chocolate Shake - Indianapolis Region - Saver									
	370	12	7	60	67	2	51	9	270
Chocolate Shake - Indianapolis Region - Small									
	490	15	9	75	88	3	67	12	350
Chocolate Shake - Louisville Region - Kids									
	230	7	4.5	35	42	1	32	6	170
Chocolate Shake - Louisville Region - Large									
	1020	32	19	160	184	6	140	25	730
Chocolate Shake - Louisville Region - Medium									
	690	22	13	110	126	4	95	17	500

Food Serving size	Cal.	(g) Total Fat	(g) Sat. Fat	(mg) Chol.	(g) Carb.	(g) Fiber	(g) Sug.	(g) Prot.	(mg) Sod.
Chocolate Shake - Louisville Region - Saver									
	370	12	7	60	67	2	51	9	270
Chocolate Shake - Louisville Region - Small									
	490	15	9	75	88	3	67	12	350
Chocolate Shake - Minneapolis Region - Kids									
	200	4	2	20	37	0	30	4	200
Chocolate Shake - Minneapolis Region - Large									
	860	19	10	95	163	0	134	19	860
Chocolate Shake - Minneapolis Region - Medium									
	590	13	7	65	111	0	91	13	590
Chocolate Shake - Minneapolis Region - Saver									
	310	7	3.5	35	59	0	49	7	310
Chocolate Shake - Minneapolis Region - Small									
	410	9	4.5	45	78	0	64	9	410
Chocolate Shake - Nashville Region - Kids									
	270	6	4	20	48	0	37	6	110
Chocolate Shake - Nashville Region - Large									
	1190	27	18	90	210	0	165	27	500
Chocolate Shake - Nashville Region - Medium									
	810	19	13	60	143	0	112	19	340
Chocolate Shake - Nashville Region - Saver									
	430	10	7	35	77	0	60	10	180
Chocolate Shake - Nashville Region - Small									
	570	13	9	45	100	0	79	13	240
Chocolate Shake - New Jersey Region - Kids									
	210	6	3	20	35	1	27	6	170
Chocolate Shake - New Jersey Region - Large									
	910	26	14	85	153	6	119	28	760
Chocolate Shake - New Jersey Region - Medium									
	620	17	10	60	104	4	81	19	520
Chocolate Shake - New Jersey Region - Saver									
	330	9	5	30	56	2	43	10	280
Chocolate Shake - New Jersey Region - Small									
	430	12	7	40	73	3	57	14	370
Chocolate Shake - St. Louis Region - Kids									
	240	5	3.5	20	42	2	31	5	75

Food Serving size	Cal.	(g) Total Fat	(g) Sat. Fat	(mg) Chol.	(g) Carb.	(g) Fiber	(g) Sug.	(g) Prot.	(mg) Sod.
Chocolate Shake - St. Louis Region - Large									
	1030	24	16	80	182	8	134	24	320
Chocolate Shake - St. Louis Region - Medium									
	700	16	11	55	124	5	92	16	220
Chocolate Shake - St. Louis Region - Saver									
	370	9	6	30	66	3	49	9	120
Chocolate Shake - St. Louis Region - Small									
	490	11	8	40	87	4	64	11	150
Strawberry Shake - Chicago Region - Kids									
	260	4	2.5	15	49	1	43	6	170
Strawberry Shake - Chicago Region - Large									
	1140	18	11	70	217	5	189	25	750
Strawberry Shake - Chicago Region - Medium									
	780	12	7	50	148	3	129	17	510
Strawberry Shake - Chicago Region - Saver									
	410	6	4	25	79	2	69	9	270
Strawberry Shake - Chicago Region - Small									
	540	8	5	35	103	2	90	12	360
Strawberry Shake - Cincinnati Region - Kids									
	300	8	5	15	52	0	42	7	170
Strawberry Shake - Cincinnati Region - Large									
	1330	33	22	75	229	0	185	29	730
Strawberry Shake - Cincinnati Region - Medium									
	910	23	15	50	156	0	126	20	500
Strawberry Shake - Cincinnati Region - Saver									
	480	12	8	25	83	0	67	11	270
Strawberry Shake - Cincinnati Region - Small									
	630	16	11	35	109	0	88	14	350
Strawberry Shake - Columbus Region - Kids									
	230	5	3.5	20	41	0	39	6	220
Strawberry Shake - Columbus Region - Large									
	1010	23	16	100	180	0	171	27	980
Strawberry Shake - Columbus Region - Medium									
	690	16	11	65	122	0	117	19	670
Strawberry Shake - Columbus Region - Saver									
	370	9	6	35	65	0	62	10	360

Food Serving size	Cal.	(g) Total Fat	(g) Sat. Fat	(mg) Chol.	(g) Carb.	(g) Fiber	(g) Sug.	(g) Prot.	(mg) Sod.
Strawberry Shake - Columbus Region - Small									
	480	11	8	45	85	0	81	13	470
Vanilla Shake - Chicago Region - Kids									
	220	4	2.5	15	41	1	34	6	170
Vanilla Shake - Chicago Region - Large									
	980	18	11	70	179	5	151	25	750
Vanilla Shake - Chicago Region - Medium									
	670	12	7	50	122	3	103	17	510
Vanilla Shake - Chicago Region - Saver									
	360	6.5	4	25	65	2	55	9	270
Vanilla Shake - Chicago Region - Small									
	470	8	5	35	85	2	72	12	360
Vanilla Shake - Cincinnati Region - Kids									
	300	8	5	15	52	0	42	7	170
Vanilla Shake - Cincinnati Region - Large									
	1330	33	22	75	229	0	185	29	730
Vanilla Shake - Cincinnati Region - Medium									
	910	23	15	50	156	0	126	20	500
Vanilla Shake - Cincinnati Region - Saver									
	480	12	8	25	83	0	67	11	270
Vanilla Shake - Cincinnati Region - Small									
	630	16	11	35	109	0	88	14	350
Vanilla Shake - Columbus Region - Kids									
	200	5	3.5	20	32	0	30	6	220
Vanilla Shake - Columbus Region - Large									
	860	23	16	100	141	0	133	27	980
Vanilla Shake - Columbus Region - Medium									
	590	16	11	65	96	0	91	19	670
Vanilla Shake - Columbus Region - Saver									
	310	9	6	35	51	0	48	10	360
Vanilla Shake - Columbus Region - Small									
	410	11	8	45	67	0	63	13	470
Vanilla Shake - New Jersey Region - Kids									
	210	6	4	25	31	0	26	8	220
Vanilla Shake - New Jersey Region - Large									
	910	26	17	115	137	0	114	34	970

Food Serving size	Cal.	(g) Total Fat	(g) Sat. Fat	(mg) Chol.	(g) Carb.	(g) Fiber	(g) Sug.	(g) Prot.	(mg) Sod.
Vanilla Shake - New Jersey Region - Medium									
	620	18	12	80	94	0	78	23	660
Vanilla Shake - New Jersey Region - Saver									
	330	9	6	40	50	0	42	12	350
Vanilla Shake - New Jersey Region - Small									
	440	12	8	55	65	0	54	16	460

Side Sauces

Food Serving size	Cal.	(g) Total Fat	(g) Sat. Fat	(mg) Chol.	(g) Carb.	(g) Fiber	(g) Sug.	(g) Prot.	(mg) Sod.
Apple Sauce (Select Regions) - 1 Container									
	100	0	0	0	24	2	19	0	10
BBQ Sauce - 1 Container									
	35	0.5	0	0	8	0	8	0	390
Cheese Sauce - Nashville and Louisville Regions									
	130	10	3.5	10	6	0	3	3	560
Cheese Sauce (Nacho) - Cincinnati, Chicago, Indianapolis, Minneapolis, New Jersey and St. Louis Regions									
	50	4	1	0	3	0	0	0	400
Cinnamon Sauce - 1 Container									
	110	4	0.5	0	20	0	17	0	85
Fat-free Honey Mustard Sauce - 1 Container									
	50	0	0	0	13	0	7	0	120
Marinara Sauce - 1 Container									
	15	0	0	0	4	0	2	0	260
Ranch Dressing - 1 Container									
	150	17	2.5	10	1	0	1	0	210
Seafood Sauce - 1 Container									
	30	0	0	0	7	0	3	0	340
Tartar Sauce - Chicago, Minneapolis and New Jersey Regions - 1 Container									
	90	8	1	10	4	0	2	0	220
White Castle Zesty Zing Sauce - 1 Container									
	120	11	1.5	15	4	0	3	0	190

Slider Alterations

Food Serving size	Cal.	(g) Total Fat	(g) Sat. Fat	(mg) Chol.	(g) Carb.	(g) Fiber	(g) Sug.	(g) Prot.	(mg) Sod.
American Cheese Slice									
	30	2	2	5	0	0	0	2	140
Bacon									
	30	3	1	4	0	0	0	2	105

Food Serving size	Cal.	(g) Total Fat	(g) Sat. Fat	(mg) Chol.	(g) Carb.	(g) Fiber	(g) Sug.	(g) Prot.	(mg) Sod.
Bacon Topping	40	2.5	1	10	0	0	0	1	180
Cheddar Cheese Slice	30	2.5	1.5	10	0	0	0	2	160
Jalapeno Cheese Slice	20	3	2	5	1	0	0	1	140
Traditional Bun	70	1	0	0	12	1	1	2	120

Sliders

Food Serving size	Cal.	(g) Total Fat	(g) Sat. Fat	(mg) Chol.	(g) Carb.	(g) Fiber	(g) Sug.	(g) Prot.	(mg) Sod.
Bacon Cheddar	200	12	5	25	13	1	2	9	650
Bacon Cheddar Chicken with BBQ	440	31	6	30	23	1	5	14	850
Bacon Cheeseburger	190	11	5	20	13	1	2	9	550
Bacon Jalapeno Cheeseburger	190	12	5	20	14	1	2	9	560
Bacon Ranch	260	18	5	20	14	1	3	7	640
Cheese Supreme Slider - Detroit and Cincinnati Regions	420	31	6	30	20	1	2	14	750
Cheeseburger	170	9	4	15	15	1	3	8	550
Chicken Breast Slider	360	26	3.5	20	20	1	1	11	510
Chicken Breast Slider with Cheese	390	28	5	25	20	1	2	13	650
Chicken Ring Slider	350	28	4.5	35	16	1	1	8	320
Chicken Ring Slider with Cheese	380	30	6	40	16	1	2	10	460
Fish Slider	310	22	3	15	18	12	1	9	270
Fish Slider with Cheese	340	24	4.5	20	18	12	2	11	410

Food Serving size	Cal.	(g) Total Fat	(g) Sat. Fat	(mg) Chol.	(g) Carb.	(g) Fiber	(g) Sug.	(g) Prot.	(mg) Sod.
Jalapeno Cheeseburger	160	9	4	15	14	1	2	8	460
Mushroom Cheddar (Select Regions)	170	9	4.5	20	14	1	1	8	600
Original Slider	140	6	2.5	10	13	1	1	7	360
Pulled Pork BBQ Slider	170	4.5	1	25	25	1	12	9	460
Surf and Turf	480	33	8	35	26	13	2	19	720
Surf and Turf with Cheese	540	38	11	45	27	13	2	22	990
Traditional Bun with Cheese	90	3	1.5	5	12	1	2	4	260

Soft Drinks (Carbonated)

Food Serving size	Cal.	(g) Total Fat	(g) Sat. Fat	(mg) Chol.	(g) Carb.	(g) Fiber	(g) Sug.	(g) Prot.	(mg) Sod.
Barq's Red Cream Soda - Kids	110	0	0	0	29	0	29	0	20
Barq's Red Cream Soda - Large	480	0	0	0	130	0	130	0	80
Barq's Red Cream Soda - Medium	320	0	0	0	87	0	87	0	50
Barq's Red Cream Soda - Saver	170	0	0	0	47	0	47	0	30
Barq's Red Cream Soda - Small	240	0	0	0	66	0	66	0	40
Barq's Root Beer - Kids	100	0	0	0	28	0	28	0	25
Barq's Root Beer - Large	470	0	0	0	126	0	126	0	100
Barq's Root Beer - Medium	310	0	0	0	85	0	85	0	70
Barq's Root Beer - Saver	170	0	0	0	45	0	45	0	35
Barq's Root Beer - Small	240	0	0	0	64	0	64	0	50

Food Serving size	Cal.	(g) Total Fat	(g) Sat. Fat	(mg) Chol.	(g) Carb.	(g) Fiber	(g) Sug.	(g) Prot.	(mg) Sod.
Big Red - Kids	100	0	0	0	24	0	24	0	0
Big Red - Large	440	0	0	0	105	0	103	0	10
Big Red - Medium	290	0	0	0	71	0	70	0	5
Big Red - Saver	160	0	0	0	38	0	37	0	5
Big Red - Small	220	0	0	0	53	0	53	0	5
Cherry Coca-Cola - Kids	100	0	0	0	26	0	26	0	5
Cherry Coca-Cola - Large	440	0	0	0	117	0	117	0	15
Cherry Coca-Cola - Medium	290	0	0	0	79	0	79	0	10
Cherry Coca-Cola - Saver	160	0	0	0	42	0	42	0	5
Cherry Coca-Cola - Small	220	0	0	0	60	0	60	0	10
Coca-Cola Classic - Kids	90	0	0	0	25	0	25	0	6
Coca-Cola Classic - Large	420	0	0	0	113	0	113	0	25
Coca-Cola Classic - Medium	280	0	0	0	76	0	76	0	15
Coca-Cola Classic - Saver	150	0	0	0	41	0	41	0	10
Coca-Cola Classic - Small	210	0	0	0	57	0	57	0	15
Coke Zero - Kids	0	0	0	0	0	0	0	0	25
Coke Zero - Large	5	0	0	0	0	0	0	0	115
Coke Zero - Medium	0	0	0	0	0	0	0	0	80

Food Serving size	Cal.	(g) Total Fat	(g) Sat. Fat	(mg) Chol.	(g) Carb.	(g) Fiber	(g) Sug.	(g) Prot.	(mg) Sod.
Coke Zero - Saver	0	0	0	0	0	0	0	0	40
Coke Zero - Small	0	0	0	0	0	0	0	0	60
Diet Coke - Kids	0	0	0	0	0	0	0	0	10
Diet Coke - Large	0	0	0	0	0	0	0	0	40
Diet Coke - Medium	0	0	0	0	0	0	0	0	25
Diet Coke - Saver	0	0	0	0	0	0	0	0	15
Diet Coke - Small	0	0	0	0	0	0	0	0	20
Diet Coke, Caffeine Free - Kids	0	0	0	0	0	0	0	0	10
Diet Coke, Caffeine Free - Large	0	0	0	0	0	0	0	0	40
Diet Coke, Caffeine Free - Medium	0	0	0	0	0	0	0	0	30
Diet Coke, Caffeine Free - Saver	0	0	0	0	0	0	0	0	15
Diet Coke, Caffeine Free - Small	0	0	0	0	0	0	0	0	20
Fanta Grape Soda - Kids	110	0	0	0	31	0	31	0	30
Fanta Grape Soda - Large	510	0	0	0	138	0	138	0	125
Fanta Grape Soda - Medium	340	0	0	0	93	0	93	0	85
Fanta Grape Soda - Saver	180	0	0	0	50	0	50	0	45
Fanta Grape Soda - Small	260	0	0	0	70	0	70	0	65
Fanta Orange Soda - Kids	100	0	0	0	33	0	33	0	35

Food Serving size	Cal.	(g) Total Fat	(g) Sat. Fat	(mg) Chol.	(g) Carb.	(g) Fiber	(g) Sug.	(g) Prot.	(mg) Sod.
Fanta Orange Soda - Large	470	0	0	0	147	0	147	0	150
Fanta Orange Soda - Medium	310	0	0	0	99	0	99	0	100
Fanta Orange Soda - Saver	170	0	0	0	53	0	53	0	55
Fanta Orange Soda - Small	240	0	0	0	74	0	74	0	75
Fanta Strawberry Soda - Kids	110	0	0	0	31	0	31	0	30
Fanta Strawberry Soda - Large	500	0	0	0	138	0	138	0	125
Fanta Strawberry Soda - Medium	340	0	0	0	93	0	93	0	85
Fanta Strawberry Soda - Saver	180	0	0	0	50	0	50	0	45
Fanta Strawberry Soda - Small	260	0	0	0	70	0	70	0	65
Pibb Xtra - Kids	90	0	0	0	24	0	24	0	25
Pibb Xtra - Large	410	0	0	0	109	0	109	0	115
Pibb Xtra - Medium	270	0	0	0	73	0	73	0	80
Pibb Xtra - Saver	150	0	0	0	39	0	39	0	40
Pibb Xtra - Small	210	0	0	0	55	0	55	0	60
Powerade Mountain Blast - Kids	60	0	0	0	16	0	16	0	50
Powerade Mountain Blast - Large	270	0	0	0	71	0	71	0	220
Powerade Mountain Blast - Medium	180	0	0	0	48	0	48	0	150
Powerade Mountain Blast - Saver	100	0	0	0	26	0	26	0	80

Food Serving size	Cal.	(g) Total Fat	(g) Sat. Fat	(mg) Chol.	(g) Carb.	(g) Fiber	(g) Sug.	(g) Prot.	(mg) Sod.
Powerade Mountain Blast - Small									
	140	0	0	0	36	0	36	0	115
Sprite - Kids									
	90	0	0	0	24	0	24	0	20
Sprite - Large									
	410	0	0	0	109	0	109	0	90
Sprite - Medium									
	270	0	0	0	73	0	73	0	60
Sprite - Saver									
	150	0	0	0	39	0	39	0	30
Sprite - Small									
	210	0	0	0	55	0	55	0	45
Vault - Kids									
	100	0	0	0	26	0	26	0	10
Vault - Large									
	450	0	0	0	117	0	117	0	40
Vault - Medium									
	300	0	0	0	79	0	79	0	25
Vault - Saver									
	160	0	0	0	42	0	42	0	15
Vault - Small									
	230	0	0	0	60	0	60	0	20

Soft Drinks (Non-carbonated)

Food Serving size	Cal.	(g) Total Fat	(g) Sat. Fat	(mg) Chol.	(g) Carb.	(g) Fiber	(g) Sug.	(g) Prot.	(mg) Sod.
Hi-C Flashing Fruit Punch - Kids									
	100	0	0	0	26	0	26	0	10
Hi-C Flashing Fruit Punch - Large									
	440	0	0	0	117	0	117	0	40
Hi-C Flashing Fruit Punch - Medium									
	290	0	0	0	79	0	79	0	25
Hi-C Flashing Fruit Punch - Saver									
	160	0	0	0	42	0	42	0	15
Hi-C Flashing Fruit Punch - Small									
	220	0	0	0	60	0	60	0	20
Hi-C Orange Lavaburst - Kids									
	100	0	0	0	28	0	28	0	0

Food Serving size	Cal.	(g) Total Fat	(g) Sat. Fat	(mg) Chol.	(g) Carb.	(g) Fiber	(g) Sug.	(g) Prot.	(mg) Sod.
Hi-C Orange Lavaburst - Large									
	470	0	0	0	126	0	126	0	0
Hi-C Orange Lavaburst - Medium									
	310	0	0	0	85	0	85	0	0
Hi-C Orange Lavaburst - Saver									
	170	0	0	0	45	0	45	0	0
Hi-C Orange Lavaburst - Small									
	240	0	0	0	64	0	64	0	0
Hi-C Poppin' Pink Lemonade Pink - Kids									
	90	0	0	0	23	0	23	0	38
Hi-C Poppin' Pink Lemonade Pink - Large									
	400	0	0	0	101	0	101	0	170
Hi-C Poppin' Pink Lemonade Pink - Medium									
	270	0	0	0	68	0	68	0	115
Hi-C Poppin' Pink Lemonade Pink - Saver									
	140	0	0	0	36	0	36	0	60
Hi-C Poppin' Pink Lemonade Pink - Small									
	200	0	0	0	51	0	51	0	85

Sweet Potato Fries

Medium									
	480	30	3	0	47	6	13	4	380
Sack									
	900	56	6	0	89	11	25	7	710
Saver									
	420	26	3	0	41	5	12	3	330

Sweet Potato Fries (New Jersey Region)

Medium									
	480	30	4	0	47	6	13	4	380
Sack									
	900	56	7	0	89	11	25	7	710
Saver									
	420	26	3	0	41	5	12	3	330

Food Serving size	Cal.	(g) Total Fat	(g) Sat. Fat	(mg) Chol.	(g) Carb.	(g) Fiber	(g) Sug.	(g) Prot.	(mg) Sod.
MISC. RESTAURANT ITEMS									
Biscuit with Egg and Sausage 1 item (162g)	505	34	10	261	34	0.3	2	18	1089
Burrito, Bean and Cheese, Frozen 1 oz (28.35g)	60	2	0	--	9	2.9	3	2	117
Burrito, Bean and Cheese, Microwaved 1 oz (28g)	73	2	1	1	11	2.9	0	2	178
Burrito, Beef and Bean, Frozen 1 oz (28.35g)	68	3	1	2	9	1.2	2	2	166
Burrito, Beef and Bean, Microwaved 1 oz (28.35g)	84	3	1	3	11	2.0	0	2	187
Crispy Chicken, Bacon and Tomato Club Sandwich, with Cheese, Lettuce and Mayonnaise 1 sandwich (271g)	696	32	9	103	61	3.3	7	42	1640
Fast Food, Pizza Chain, 14" Pizza, Cheese Topping, Regular Crust 1 pie (905g)	2389	86	38	190	295	15.4	8	108	4842
Fast Food, Pizza Chain, 14" Pizza, Cheese Topping, Thick Crust 1 pie (976g)	2655	107	46	234	306	14.6	--	117	5202
Fast Food, Pizza Chain, 14" Pizza, Cheese Topping, Thin Crust 1 pie (627g)	1906	98	43	219	166	12.5	17	89	3643
Fast Food, Pizza Chain, 14" Pizza, Meat and Vegetable Topping, Regular Crust 1 pie (1168g)	2850	127	51	315	296	25.7	57	129	6880
Fast Food, Pizza Chain, 14" Pizza, Pepperoni Topping, Regular Crust 1 pie (959g)	2647	108	47	259	302	14.4	60	118	6061
Fast Food, Pizza Chain, 14" Pizza, Pepperoni Topping, Thick Crust 1 pie (995g)	2826	124	50	279	302	17.9	51	124	6139
Fast Food, Bagel with Breakfast Steak, Eggs, Cheese and Condiment 1 item (217g)	612	31	12	282	50	0.4	8	35	1150
Fast Food, Bagel with Egg, Sausage Patty, Cheese and Condiment 1 item (219g)	646	37	14	291	50	0.4	9	28	1205
Fast Food, Bagel with Ham, Egg and Cheese 1 item (191g)	483	18	8	243	52	0.4	8	27	1259
Fast Food, Biscuit with Egg 1 biscuit (136g)	373	22	5	245	32	0.8	--	12	891

Food Serving size	Cal.	(g) Total Fat	(g) Sat. Fat	(mg) Chol.	(g) Carb.	(g) Fiber	(g) Sug.	(g) Prot.	(mg) Sod.
Fast Food, Biscuit with Egg and Bacon 1 biscuit (150g)	458	31	8	353	29	0.8	3	17	999
Fast Food, Biscuit with Egg and Ham 1 biscuit (192g)	442	27	6	300	31	0.8	4	20	1382
Fast Food, Biscuit with Egg and Steak 1 biscuit (148g)	410	28	9	272	21	--	--	18	888
Fast Food, Biscuit with Egg, Cheese and Bacon 1 item (145g)	436	25	9	241	35	0.3	3	17	1183
Fast Food, Biscuit with Ham 1 biscuit (113g)	386	18	11	25	44	0.8	2	13	1433
Fast Food, Biscuit with Sausage 1 item (111g)	412	27	8	31	33	0.4	2	11	904
Fast Food, Brownie 1 brownie, (2" square) (60g)	243	10	3	10	39	--	--	3	153
Fast Food, Burrito, with Beans 2 pieces (217g)	447	13	7	4	71	--	--	14	985
Fast Food, Burrito, with Beans and Cheese 2 pieces (186g)	378	12	7	28	55	--	--	15	1166
Fast Food, Burrito, with Beans and Chili Peppers 2 pieces (204g)	412	15	8	33	58	--	--	16	1044
Fast Food, Burrito, with Beans and Meat 2 pieces (231g)	508	18	8	49	66	--	--	22	1335
Fast Food, Burrito, with Beans, Cheese and Beef 2 pieces (203g)	331	13	7	124	40	--	--	15	991
Fast Food, Burrito, with Beans, Cheese and Chili Peppers 2 pieces (336g)	662	23	11	158	85	--	--	33	2060
Fast Food, Burrito, with Beef 2 pieces (220g)	524	21	10	64	59	--	--	27	1492
Fast Food, Burrito, with Beef and Chili Peppers 2 pieces (201g)	426	17	8	54	49	--	--	22	1116
Fast Food, Burrito, with Beef, Cheese and Chili Peppers 2 pieces (304g)	632	25	10	170	64	--	--	41	2092
Fast Food, Burrito, with Fruit (Apple or Cherry) 1 burrito, small (74g)	231	10	5	4	35	--	--	3	212

Food Serving size	Cal.	(g) Total Fat	(g) Sat. Fat	(mg) Chol.	(g) Carb.	(g) Fiber	(g) Sug.	(g) Prot.	(mg) Sod.
Fast Food, Cheeseburger, Double Regular Patty, Double Bun with Condiment and Special Sauce									
1 item (219g)	572	31	11	79	47	3.1	11	26	1062
Fast Food, Cheeseburger, Double, Large Patty with Condiment									
1 item (280g)	762	45	18	160	40	2.8	--	47	1344
Fast Food, Cheeseburger, Double, Large Patty, with Condiment and Vegetable									
1 sandwich (258g)	704	44	18	142	40	--	--	38	1148
Fast Food, Cheeseburger, Double, Large Patty, with Condiment, Vegetable and Mayonnaise									
1 item (355g)	898	55	23	174	45	4.6	2	55	1438
Fast Food, Cheeseburger, Double, Regular Patty and Bun, with Condiment and Vegetable									
1 sandwich (228g)	650	35	13	93	53	--	--	30	921
Fast Food, Cheeseburger, Double, Regular Patty, Plain									
1 item (149g)	459	26	11	82	31	1.0	6	26	925
Fast Food, Cheeseburger, Double, Regular Patty, with Condiment									
1 item (173g)	474	26	11	83	34	1.4	--	26	1137
Fast Food, Cheeseburger, Double, Regular Patty, with Condiment and Vegetable									
1 sandwich (166g)	417	21	9	60	35	--	--	21	1051
Fast Food, Cheeseburger, Regular, Double Patty, Bun, Plain									
1 sandwich (201g)	613	28	11	82	60	2.0	11	30	1184
Fast Food, Cheeseburger, Single, Large Patty, Plain									
1 item (166g)	506	28	11	93	35	2.3	6	29	885
Fast Food, Cheeseburger, Single, Large Patty, with Condiment									
1 item (199g)	535	29	14	96	39	2.4	--	30	1176
Fast Food, Cheeseburger, Single, Large Patty, with Condiment and Bacon									
1 item (211g)	595	33	13	106	40	2.7	10	33	1422
Fast Food, Cheeseburger, Single, Large Patty, with Condiment and Vegetable									
1 sandwich (233g)	480	24	9	79	39	3.3	9	27	897
Fast Food, Cheeseburger, Single, Large Patty, with Condiment, Vegetable and Ham									
1 sandwich (254g)	726	48	21	122	33	--	--	39	1712
Fast Food, Cheeseburger, Single, Large Patty, with Condiment, Vegetable and Mayonnaise									
1 item (266g)	625	36	15	98	41	3.2	--	35	1237
Fast Food, Cheeseburger, Single, Regular Patty, Plain									
1 item (100g)	303	14	5	41	30	1.0	5	15	589

Food Serving size	Cal.	(g) Total Fat	(g) Sat. Fat	(mg) Chol.	(g) Carb.	(g) Fiber	(g) Sug.	(g) Prot.	(mg) Sod.
Fast Food, Cheeseburger, Single, Regular Patty, with Condiment									
1 item (127g)	343	16	7	50	32	2.4	7	17	798
Fast Food, Cheeseburger, Single, Regular Patty, with Condiment and Vegetable									
1 sandwich (154g)	359	20	9	52	28	--	--	18	976
Fast Food, Cheeseburger, Triple, Regular Patty, Plain									
1 item (249g)	772	48	20	157	40	1.2	8	45	1586
Fast Food, Chicken Fillet Sandwich, Plain									
1 sandwich (182g)	515	29	9	60	39	--	--	24	957
Fast Food, Chicken Fillet Sandwich, with Cheese									
1 sandwich (228g)	632	39	12	78	42	--	--	29	1238
Fast Food, Chicken Tenders									
5 pieces (77g)	223	13	2	35	12	0.6	3	14	660
Fast Food, Chicken, Breaded and Fried, Boneless Pieces, Plain									
4 pieces (64g)	190	12	3	35	10	0.6	5	10	367
Fast Food, Chicken, Breaded and Fried, Dark Meat (Drumstick or Thigh)									
2 pieces (148g)	431	27	7	166	16	--	--	30	755
Fast Food, Chicken, Breaded and Fried, Light Meat (Breast or Wing)									
2 pieces (163g)	494	30	8	148	20	--	--	36	975
Fast Food, Chili Con Carne									
1 cup, (8 fl oz) (253g)	256	8	3	134	22	--	--	25	1007
Fast Food, Chimichanga, with Beef									
1 chimichanga (174g)	425	20	9	9	43	--	--	20	910
Fast Food, Chimichanga, with Beef and Cheese									
1 chimichanga (183g)	443	23	11	51	39	--	--	20	957
Fast Food, Chimichanga, with Beef and Red Chili Peppers									
1 chimichanga (190g)	424	19	8	10	46	--	--	18	1169
Fast Food, Chimichanga, with Beef, Cheese and Red Chili Peppers									
1 chimichanga (180g)	364	18	8	50	38	--	--	15	895
Fast Food, Clams, Breaded and Fried									
.75 cup (115g)	451	26	7	87	39	--	--	13	834
Fast Food, Cole Slaw									
1 package (116g)	177	11	2	5	17	2.2	14	1	235
Fast Food, Cookie, Chocolate Chip									
1 box (55g)	233	12	5	12	36	--	--	3	188

Food Serving size	Cal.	(g) Total Fat	(g) Sat. Fat	(mg) Chol.	(g) Carb.	(g) Fiber	(g) Sug.	(g) Prot.	(mg) Sod.
Fast Food, Cookies, Animal Crackers									
1 box (67g)	299	9	4	11	50	--	--	4	273
Fast Food, Corn on the Cob, with Butter									
1 ear (146g)	155	3	2	6	32	--	--	4	29
Fast Food, Crispy Chicken Filet Sandwich, with Lettuce, Tomato and Mayonnaise									
1 item (219g)	537	26	5	64	49	3.1	14	27	1424
Fast Food, Croissant, with Egg and Cheese									
1 croissant (127g)	368	25	14	216	24	--	--	13	551
Fast Food, Croissant, with Egg, Cheese and Bacon									
1 croissant (129g)	413	28	15	215	24	--	--	16	889
Fast Food, Croissant, with Egg, Cheese and Ham									
1 croissant (152g)	474	34	17	213	24	--	--	19	1081
Fast Food, Croissant, with Egg, Cheese and Sausage									
1 croissant (160g)	523	38	18	216	25	--	--	20	1115
Fast Food, Danish Pastry, Cheese									
1 pastry (91g)	353	25	5	20	29	--	--	6	319
Fast Food, Danish Pastry, Cinnamon									
1 pastry (88g)	349	17	3	27	47	--	--	5	326
Fast Food, Danish Pastry, Fruit									
1 pastry (94g)	335	16	3	19	45	--	--	5	333
Fast Food, Egg and Cheese Sandwich									
1 sandwich (146g)	340	19	7	291	26	--	--	16	804
Fast Food, Egg, Scrambled									
2 eggs (94g)	199	15	6	400	2	0.0	2	13	211
Fast Food, Enchilada, with Cheese									
1 enchilada (163g)	319	19	11	44	29	--	--	10	784
Fast Food, Enchilada, with Cheese and Beef									
1 enchilada (192g)	323	18	9	40	30	--	--	12	1319
Fast Food, Enchirito, with Cheese, Beef and Beans									
1 enchirito (193g)	344	16	8	50	34	--	--	18	1251
Fast Food, English Muffin, with Butter									
1 muffin (63g)	189	6	2	13	30	--	--	5	386
Fast Food, English Muffin, with Cheese and Sausage									
1 item (108g)	365	22	9	46	27	0.5	2	14	721

Food Serving size	Cal.	(g) Total Fat	(g) Sat. Fat	(mg) Chol.	(g) Carb.	(g) Fiber	(g) Sug.	(g) Prot.	(mg) Sod.
Fast Food, English Muffin, with Egg, Cheese and Canadian Bacon									
1 sandwich (139g)	307	13	5	234	30	0.6	3	19	773
Fast Food, English Muffin, with Egg, Cheese and Sausage									
1 item (165g)	472	30	11	269	29	0.3	2	22	776
Fast Food, Fish Sandwich, with Tartar Sauce									
1 sandwich (158g)	431	23	5	55	41	--	--	17	615
Fast Food, Fish Sandwich, with Tartar Sauce and Cheese									
1 sandwich (183g)	523	29	8	68	48	--	--	21	939
Fast Food, French Toast Sticks									
5 pieces (109g)	371	19	4	0	45	1.5	11	7	467
Fast Food, French Toast with Butter									
2 slices (135g)	356	19	8	116	36	--	--	10	513
Fast Food, Fried Chicken, Breast, Meat and Skin with Breading									
1 breast, without skin (136g)	343	20	5	120	11	0.7	--	30	749
Fast Food, Fried Chicken, Breast, Meat Only, Skin and Breast, Breading Removed									
1 breast, bone and skin removed (118g)	179	5	1	113	1	0.0	--	32	512
Fast Food, Fried Chicken, Drumstick, Meat and Skin with Breading									
1 drumstick, without skin (56g)	150	9	2	62	4	0.3	--	12	331
Fast Food, Fried Chicken, Drumstick, Meat Only, Skin and Breading Removed									
1 drumstick, without skin (56g)	96	4	1	74	0	0.0	--	15	276
Fast Food, Fried Chicken, Thigh, Meat and Skin and Breading									
1 thigh, without skin (84g)	246	17	5	85	8	0.5	--	15	519
Fast Food, Fried Chicken, Thigh, Meat Only, Skin and Breading Removed									
1 thigh, bone and skin removed (66g)	120	7	2	82	0	0.0	--	15	333
Fast Food, Fried Chicken, Wing, Meat and Skin and Breading									
1 wing, without skin (39g)	124	8	2	42	4	0.2	--	8	273
Fast Food, Fried Chicken, Wing, Meat Only, Skin and Breading Removed									
1 wing, bone and skin removed (27g)	62	3	1	36	1	0.0	--	8	176
Fast Food, Frijoles with Cheese									
1 cup (167g)	225	8	4	37	29	--	--	11	882

Food Serving size	Cal.	(g) Total Fat	(g) Sat. Fat	(mg) Chol.	(g) Carb.	(g) Fiber	(g) Sug.	(g) Prot.	(mg) Sod.
Fast Food, Griddle Cake Sandwich, Egg, Cheese and Sausage 1 item, 7.017 oz (199g)	579	35	11	263	44	1.2	8	21	1297
Fast Food, Griddle Cake Sandwich, Sausage 1 item, 4.744 oz (135g)	429	24	7	32	42	1.4	0	11	995
Fast Food, Griddle Food, Griddle Cake Sandwich, Egg, Cheese and Bacon 1 item, 5.923 oz (168g)	457	22	7	247	44	1.3	--	20	1263
Fast Food, Ham and Cheese Sandwich 1 sandwich (146g)	352	15	6	58	33	--	--	21	771
Fast Food, Ham, Egg and Cheese Sandwich 1 sandwich (143g)	347	16	7	246	31	--	--	19	1005
Fast Food, Hamburger, Double, Large Patty, with Condiment and Vegetable 1 sandwich (226g)	540	27	11	122	40	--	--	34	791
Fast Food, Hamburger, Double, Large patty, with Condiment, Vegetable and Mayonnaise 1 item (374g)	942	59	22	172	51	5.2	--	52	1081
Fast Food, Hamburger, Double, Regular Patty, Plain 1 item (120g)	354	17	6	56	29	1.1	5	20	497
Fast Food, Hamburger, Double, Regular Patty, with Condiment 1 item (215g)	576	32	12	103	39	--	--	32	742
Fast Food, Hamburger, Large, Single Patty, with Condiment 1 item (171g)	438	20	8	68	38	1.9	20	27	640
Fast Food, Hamburger, Large, Triple Patty, with Condiment 1 sandwich (259g)	692	41	16	142	29	--	--	50	712
Fast Food, Hamburger, Single, Large Patty, Plain 1 sandwich (137g)	426	23	8	71	32	--	--	23	474
Fast Food, Hamburger, Single, Large Patty, with Condiment 1 item (171g)	438	20	9	68	38	1.9	--	27	640
Fast Food, Hamburger, Single, Large Patty, with Condiment and Vegetable 1 sandwich (218g)	512	27	10	87	40	--	--	26	824
Fast Food, Hamburger, Single, Large Patty, with Condiments, Vegetable and Mayonnaise 1 item (247g)	558	31	10	82	43	3.7	--	28	845
Fast Food, Hamburger, Single, Regular Patty, Double Bun with Condiment and Special Sauce 1 item (205g)	531	27	9	66	47	2.9	--	25	791

Food Serving size	Cal.	(g) Total Fat	(g) Sat. Fat	(mg) Chol.	(g) Carb.	(g) Fiber	(g) Sug.	(g) Prot.	(mg) Sod.
Fast Food, Hamburger, Single, Regular Patty, Plain									
1 item (86g)	254	10	3	28	29	1.0	5	13	378
Fast Food, Hamburger, Single, Regular Patty, with Condiment									
1 item (114g)	294	11	5	33	33	2.1	6	15	560
Fast Food, Hamburger, Single, Regular Patty, with Condiment and Vegetable									
1 item (110g)	279	13	4	26	27	--	--	13	504
Fast Food, Hot Dog (with Chili)									
1 sandwich (114g)	296	13	5	51	31	--	--	14	480
Fast Food, Hot Dog, Plain									
1 sandwich (98g)	242	15	5	44	18	--	--	10	670
Fast Food, Hot Dog, with Corn Flour Coating (Corn Dog)									
1 sandwich (175g)	460	19	5	79	56	--	--	17	973
Fast Food, Hush Puppies									
5 pieces (78g)	257	12	3	135	35	--	--	5	965
Fast Food, Miniature Cinnamon Rolls									
1 each (25g)	101	4	1	5	13	0.6	--	2	139
Fast Food, Nachos, with Cheese									
1 portion, (6-8 nachos) (113g)	346	19	8	18	36	--	--	9	816
Fast Food, Nachos, with Cheese and Jalapeno Peppers									
1 portion, (6-8 nachos) (204g)	608	34	14	84	60	--	--	17	1736
Fast Food, Nachos, with Cheese, Beans, Ground Beef and Peppers									
1 portion, (6-8 nachos) (255g)	569	31	12	20	56	--	--	20	1800
Fast Food, Nachos, with Cinnamon and Sugar									
1 portion, (6-8 nachos) (109g)	592	36	18	39	63	--	--	7	439
Fast Food, Onion Rings, Breaded and Fried									
1 portion, (8-9 onion rings) (83g)	276	16	7	14	31	--	--	4	430
Fast Food, Oysters, Battered or Breaded and Fried									
6 pieces (139g)	368	18	5	108	40	--	--	13	677
Fast Food, Pancakes, with Butter and Syrup									
2 cakes (232g)	520	14	6	58	91	--	--	8	1104

Food Serving size	Cal.	(g) Total Fat	(g) Sat. Fat	(mg) Chol.	(g) Carb.	(g) Fiber	(g) Sug.	(g) Prot.	(mg) Sod.
Fast Food, Potato, Baked and Topped with Sour Cream and Chives									
1 piece (302g)	393	22	10	24	50	--	--	7	181
Fast Food, Potato, Baked and Topped with Cheese Sauce									
1 piece (296g)	474	29	11	18	47	--	--	15	382
Fast Food, Potato, Baked and Topped with Cheese Sauce and Bacon									
1 piece (299g)	451	26	10	30	44	--	--	18	972
Fast Food, Potato, Baked and Topped with Cheese Sauce and Broccoli									
1 piece (339g)	403	21	9	20	47	--	--	14	485
Fast Food, Potato, Baked and Topped with Cheese Sauce and Chili									
1 piece (395g)	482	22	13	32	56	--	--	23	699
Fast Food, Potato, French Fried in Vegetable Oil									
1 medium (134g)	421	22	3	0	52	4.7	1	5	389
Fast Food, Potato, Mashed									
.333 cup (80g)	66	1	0	2	13	--	--	2	182
Fast Food, Potatoes, Hashed Brown									
1 cup (144g)	471	31	7	0	46	3.9	0	4	746
Fast Food, Roast Beef Sandwich, Plain									
1 sandwich (139g)	346	14	4	51	33	--	--	22	792
Fast Food, Salad, Vegetable, Tossed, Without Dressing									
.75 cup (104g)	17	0	0	0	3	--	--	1	27
Fast Food, Salad, Vegetable, Tossed, Without Dressing, with Cheese and Egg									
1.5 cup (217g)	102	6	3	98	5	--	--	9	119
Fast Food, Salad, Vegetable, Tossed, Without Dressing, with Chicken									
1.5 cup (218g)	105	2	1	72	4	--	--	17	209
Fast Food, Salad, Vegetable, Tossed, Without Dressing, with Pasta and Seafood									
1.5 cup (417g)	379	21	3	50	32	--	--	16	1572
Fast Food, Salad, Vegetable, Tossed, Without Dressing, with Shrimp									
1.5 cup (236g)	106	2	1	179	7	--	--	15	489
Fast Food, Salad, Vegetable, Tossed, Without Dressing, with Turkey, Ham and Cheese									
1.5 cup (326g)	267	16	8	140	5	--	--	26	743
Fast Food, Scallops, Breaded and Fried									
6 pieces (144g)	386	19	5	108	38	--	--	16	919
Fast Food, Shrimp, Breaded and Fried									
6-8 shrimp (164g)	454	25	5	200	40	--	--	19	1446

Food Serving size	Cal.	(g) Total Fat	(g) Sat. Fat	(mg) Chol.	(g) Carb.	(g) Fiber	(g) Sug.	(g) Prot.	(mg) Sod.
Fast Food, Submarine Sandwich, with Cold Cuts									
1 submarine (228g)	456	19	7	36	51	--	--	22	1651
Fast Food, Submarine Sandwich, with Roast Beef									
1 submarine (216g)	410	13	7	73	44	--	--	29	845
Fast Food, Submarine Sandwich, with Tuna Salad									
1 submarine (256g)	584	28	5	49	55	--	--	30	1293
Fast Food, Sundae, Caramel									
1 sundae (155g)	304	9	5	25	49	0.0	--	7	195
Fast Food, Sundae, Hot Fudge									
1 sundae (158g)	284	9	5	21	48	0.0	--	6	182
Fast Food, Sundae, Strawberry									
1 sundae (153g)	268	8	4	21	45	0.0	--	6	92
Fast Food, Taco									
1 small (171g)	371	21	11	56	27	--	--	21	802
Fast Food, Taco Salad									
1.5 cup (198g)	279	15	7	44	24	--	--	13	762
Fast Food, Taco Salad with Chili Con Carne									
1.5 cup (261g)	290	13	6	5	27	--	--	17	885
Fast Food, Tostada, with Beans and Cheese									
1 piece (144g)	223	10	5	30	27	--	--	10	543
Fast Food, Tostada, with Beans, Beef and Cheese									
1 piece (225g)	333	17	11	74	30	--	--	16	871
Fast Food, Tostada, with Beef and Cheese									
1 piece (163g)	315	16	10	41	23	--	--	19	897
Fast Food, Vanilla, Light, Soft Serve Ice Cream, with Cone									
1 item (90g)	149	4	2	14	24	0.1	18	4	60
Grilled Chicken, Bacon and Tomato Club Sandwich, with Cheese, Lettuce and Mayonnaise									
1 sandwich (268g)	590	22	8	123	53	3.2	9	46	1688
Restaurant, Chinese, Beef and Vegetables									
1 order (574g)	603	30	6	80	42	8.6	--	41	2348
Restaurant, Chinese, Egg Roll, Assorted									
1 piece (89g)	223	11	2	14	24	2.3	--	7	417
Restaurant, Chinese, Fried Rice									
1 cup (140g)	228	3	1	32	43	1.5	--	7	554

Food Serving size	Cal.	(g) Total Fat	(g) Sat. Fat	(mg) Chol.	(g) Carb.	(g) Fiber	(g) Sug.	(g) Prot.	(mg) Sod.
Restaurant, Chinese, General Tso's Chicken									
3 pieces (53g)	156	9	1	28	13	0.5	--	7	231
Restaurant, Chinese, Kung Pao Chicken									
1 order (604g)	779	42	8	157	41	9.1	0	59	2428
Restaurant, Chinese, Lemon Chicken									
3 pieces (73g)	165	9	1	23	14	0.8	--	8	177
Restaurant, Family Style, Chicken Fingers (from Kid's Menu)									
1 serving (113g)	305	16	3	51	17	1.1	9	23	664
Restaurant, Family Style, French Fries									
1 serving (208g)	607	30	6	2	76	7.3	3	8	653
Restaurant, Family Style, Fried Mozzarella Sticks									
1 serving (233g)	767	44	16	77	58	4.2	15	35	1850
Restaurant, Family Style, Macaroni and Cheese (from Kid's Menu)									
1 serving (226g)	346	14	5	25	41	2.7	2	15	832
Restaurant, Family Style, Shrimp, Breaded and Fried									
1 piece (12.2g)	36	2	0	11	2	0.1	0	2	104
Restaurant, Family Style, Sirloin Steak									
1 steak (144g)	268	11	4	114	0	--	9	41	442
Restaurant, Latino, Arepa (Unleavened Cornmeal Bread)									
1 piece (98g)	215	5	3	5	36	2.5	3	5	265
Restaurant, Latino, Arroz Con Abichuelas Colorados (Rice and Red Beans)									
1 cup (157g)	223	5	1	--	37	4.1	6	6	581
Restaurant, Latino, Arroz Con Frijoles Negros (Rice and Black Beans)									
1 cup (146g)	220	6	1	--	36	5.0	4	7	613
Restaurant, Latino, Arroz Con Grandules (Rice and Pigeon Peas)									
1 cup (115g)	209	6	1	--	35	1.6	4	4	670
Restaurant, Latino, Arroz Con Leche (Rice Pudding)									
1 cup (253g)	369	9	5	20	63	1.3	8	8	268
Restaurant, Latino, Black Bean Soup									
1 cup (246g)	253	6	1	2	36	12.1	8	13	765
Restaurant, Latino, Bunuelos (Fried Yeast Bread)									
1 piece (70g)	323	18	5	--	34	1.1	2	6	293
Restaurant, Latino, Chicken and Rice, Entrée, Prepared									
1 cup (141g)	245	7	2	51	28	1.7	4	17	730
Restaurant, Latino, Empanadas, Beef, Prepared									
1 piece (89g)	298	16	5	23	28	1.8	3	10	392

Food Serving size	Cal.	(g) Total Fat	(g) Sat. Fat	(mg) Chol.	(g) Carb.	(g) Fiber	(g) Sug.	(g) Prot.	(mg) Sod.
Restaurant, Latino, Pupusas Con Frijoles (Pupusas, Bean)									
1 piece (126g)	289	11	3	--	40	7.3	4	7	384
Restaurant, Latino, Pupusas Con Queso (Pupusas, Cheese)									
1 piece (117g)	300	16	8	37	26	3.4	4	14	468
Restaurant, Latino, Pupusas Del Cerdo (Pupusas, Pork)									
1 piece (122g)	283	13	4	35	28	3.2	4	14	520
Restaurant, Latino, Tamale, Corn									
1 piece (166g)	309	12	4		44	5.3	5	6	460
Restaurant, Latino, Tamale, Pork									
1 piece (142g)	247	13	4	28	22	3.4	5	10	672
Restaurant, Latino, Tripe Soup									
1 cup (200g)	148	5	2	118	8	--	4	17	822
Rice, White, Steamed, Chinese Restaurant									
1 cup, loosely packed (132g)	199	0	--	--	45	1.2	--	4	7
Soup, Wonton, Chinese Restaurant									
1 cup (223g)	71	1	0	9	12	0.4	0	5	905